MATERNITY NURSING

MATERNITY NURSING

Eleventh Edition

ELISE FITZPATRICK, R.N., M.A.

*Associate Professor of Maternity Nursing, Frances Payne
Bolton School of Nursing, Western Reserve University*

NICHOLSON J. EASTMAN, M.D.

*Professor Emeritus of Obstetrics, Johns Hopkins University;
Formerly Obstetrician-in-Chief, Johns Hopkins Hospital*

SHARON R. REEDER, R.N., M.S.

*Assistant Professor of Maternity Nursing, School of Nursing,
University of California, Los Angeles*

J. B. LIPPINCOTT COMPANY

Philadelphia   ·   Toronto

Preface

In this revision of *Zabriskie's Obstetrics for Nurses* the authors have changed the title to *Maternity Nursing*. The various changes which recently have evolved in the total care of child-bearing women have brought to maternity nursing a broader meaning of care of the mother and her offspring throughout the child-bearing experience. The new title reflects the greatly increased emphasis on the family and the maternal-child continuum, psychosocial as well as physical and emotional considerations, and the role of the nurse in nursing management.

Comprehensive maternity care is a quality of patient care that is goal-directed toward the total health and the well-being of the mother and the infant. The therapy of all patients should be individualized but considered in the context of the family as a basic unit of society.

Maternity care involves the combined efforts of the expectant parents, the obstetrician, the professional nurse and other members of the health team. To meet the central objective of maternity care, the combined efforts of several disciplines, in addition to those of medicine and nursing, may be required in the cooperative plan to achieve the ultimate goals. A positive effort on the part of the health team becomes possible if each member has a clear understanding of his own role, appreciates and understands the contribution of other professions represented on the team, understands the processes involved in the differing approaches, recognizes the commonality of interest and skills, and has the intellectual and

emotional capacity to enter into a team relationship. Thus, skilled nursing management can make a significant contribution in the quality and quantity of maternity care available to expanding families everywhere.

Adequate maternity care provides the best of medical science to protect the life and the health of the childbearing mother and her infant. It considers the physical, emotional and psychosocial needs of the woman and her new baby, and it relates these needs to those of her husband and their other children so that the mother may pass through pregnancy and childbirth with maximum mental and physical fitness.

Almost every chapter of this edition has been revised, some of the content has been reorganized, and many chapters have been rewritten extensively. Dimensions of effective nursing care have been explored, particularly in the areas of antepartal care, conduct of normal labor, nursing care during the puerperium and care of the newborn infant. However, the general sequence of subject matter introduced in the 10th edition has been retained.

Every effort has been made to include new developments and expanded approaches in maternity care. A beginning orientation to maternity nursing is found in the first chapter, together with an introduction to some of the current concepts and current problems in the broad area of maternity care.

An overview of the various programs and methods of antepartal education is presented, though the major focus is on psychophysical preparation for childbearing. "The Mental Hygiene of Pregnancy and Childbirth," a chapter by Dr. Leo Kanner which has been well received in previous editions, has been retained. In addition, mental health concepts have been introduced in appropriate sections throughout the text to reinforce this important facet of patient care. Passages on parental guidance and instruction have been enlarged and used to explore new possibilities for nursing to further mother-infant adaptation, and for the first time there is a major section on family planning. New information has been added to the material on nurse-midwifery.

In this revision the authors have attempted to introduce some of the vast new knowledge on the complications associated with the childbearing cycle. Some of the subject matter included concerns uterine dysfunction, Down's syndrome, phocomelia, inborn errors of metabolism, amniotic fluid evaluation and intrauterine fetal transfusion, hyperbilirubinemia of the newborn, drug addiction in the neonate and care of the newborn of a diabetic mother.

Many new illustrations, both photographs and original drawings, have been added to this edition. The suggested reading lists that accompany each chapter have been enlarged and brought up to date with references from current professional literature. The conference material and study questions at the end of the various units, as well as the glossary, have been found useful by our readers and therefore have been retained.

The authors, the illustrators and the publishers have made a coordinated effort to present a textbook for students of maternity nursing which hopefully will stimulate them to achieve their maximum potential for professional development and to find the challenge and personal satisfaction which can be realized in the practice of truly professional maternity nursing.

ELISE FITZPATRICK, R.N.
NICHOLSON J. EASTMAN, M.D.
SHARON R. REEDER, R.N.

Acknowledgments

We acknowledge with sincere gratitude the help and encouragement of many colleagues and friends in the revision of this text. We are indebted to Miss Hazel Corbin, now retired, and to Miss Vera R. Keane, General Director of Maternity Center Association of New York, for permission to publish the exercises taught by Maternity Center Association in its program "Psychophysical Preparation for Childbirth." We are deeply grateful to Mrs. Jayne deClue Wiggins, Counselor, Maternity Center Association, for her assistance in preparation of this section of the manuscript.

We are also grateful to Dr. Arthur J. Lesser, Deputy Chief of the United States Children's Bureau, for reviewing the section "Current Problems in Maternity Care" and granting us permission to quote generously from his own writings on the subject. Our sincere appreciation goes to Dr. Margaret Foley, Executive Secretary, Conference of Catholic Schools of Nursing, and Consultant in Nursing Education, Catholic Hospital Association, who reviewed pertinent sections of this manuscript.

We are deeply grateful to Miss Olive Rich, Assistant Professor of Maternity Nursing, Western Reserve University, for sharing her observations in the study of nurse-patient interaction and nursing intervention. Her writings have particular significance in the application of psychosocial concepts in the nursing care of the maternity patient and her newborn infant.

To Dr. Eleanor P. Hunt, Consultant on Biostatistical Research, Division of Research, United States Children's Bureau, we are again indebted for generous assistance in compiling data on vital statistics. We are grateful also to Dr. Robert A. Hingson, Professor of Anesthesia, and to Dr. William A. Cull, Associate Professor of Anesthesia, both of Western Reserve University School of Medicine, for their editorial assistance in this edition. The authors would like to thank particularly Mrs. Colette Kerlin, Mrs. Margo McCafferey and Mrs. Marjorie Byrne of the UCLA School of Nursing faculty, whose constructive criticism and suggestions made a valuable contribution to this revision. To Miss Esther Leihgeber, Professor Emeritus of Public Health Nursing, Western Reserve University, the authors wish to express gratitude for untiring assistance in proofreading. To Mrs. Geraldine Mink, Librarian, School of Nursing, Western Reserve University; to Mr. Robert T. Lentz, Librarian, and Mr. Samuel A. Davis, Assistant Librarian, Jefferson Medical College Library, Philadelphia, Pa.; and many librarians at Freiberger Library, Western Reserve University, we wish also to express our thanks.

This book and its authors owe much to those who contributed illustrative material. Miss Ellen Cole of Philadelphia, Medical Illustrator, has contributed some superb original art work to this edition. We are indebted also to Mr. Wesley Kaswell, Department of Photography, University Hospitals of Cleveland, for his outstanding photography and, moreover, for his generous cooperation in giving his personal time and energy to secure certain special photographs. We are grateful to Mr. Frederick C. Schlein, Associate Curator of Education, Cleveland Health Museum, for his guidance and cooperation in photographing the Dickinson-Belskie Birth Models displayed in the MacDonald House classroom, University Hospitals of Cleveland. We wish to express our gratitude also to Dr. John J. Beeston, Director, Cleveland Health Museum, and to Dr. Neil Macintyre, Department of Anatomy, Western Reserve University School of Medicine, for their contributions.

The authors express their appreciation to colleagues, publishers and organizations who have granted permission to use their illustrations in this text. We wish to express our gratitude to our students of nursing and the many parents who granted permission for photographs to appear in this book. It is particularly appropriate that we mention Mr. and Mrs. Harrison P. Crowell and their family for making it possible to have the series of photographs of the "expanding family" which appear throughout this text. Kathy, Flip and Jeff are charming youngsters and entered into the spirit of many long sessions of picture snapping like real "pros," never realizing at the time that they were helping to teach students who will perhaps become our nursing leaders in the future.

Finally, we take this opportunity to thank the J. B. Lippincott Company, particularly Mr. David T. Miller, Dr. Walter Kahoe and Mr. Stanley A. Gillet, for their unwavering interest, cooperation and assistance.

THE AUTHORS

Contents

UNIT ONE   Human Reproduction

1. ORIENTATION TO MATERNITY NURSING 3

    Introduction 3
    Obstetrics 3
    Maternity Nursing 3
    Maternal and Child Health . . 4
    Expanding Families in America 5
    Vital Statistics 8
    Natality 9
    Population 11
    Maternal Mortality 12
    Infant Mortality 15
    Current Problems in Maternity
    Care 17

2. ANATOMY RELATED TO THE RE-
PRODUCTIVE SYSTEM 21

    Pelvis 21
    Female Organs of Reproduction 39
    Mammary Glands 50
    Male Organs of Reproduction . 51

3. PHYSIOLOGY IN RELATION TO
HUMAN REPRODUCTION . . . 53

    Sexual Maturity 53
    Menstrual Cycle 55
    The Use of the Basal Tempera-
    ture Graphs 61
    Infertility 62
    Menopause 62

4. DEVELOPMENT AND PHYSIOLOGY
OF THE FETUS 64

    Maturation of Ovum and Sperm
    Cells 64
    Determination of Sex 69
    Fertilization and Changes Fol-
    lowing Fertilization 73
    Implantation of the Ovum . . 75
    Decidua 75
    The Three Germ Layers . . . 77
    Amnion, Chorion and Placenta 78
    Size and Development of the
    Fetus 81
    Duration of Pregnancy . . . 85
    Calculation of the Expected
    Date of Confinement . . . 86
    Physiology of the Fetus . . . 86
    Periods of Development . . . 90
    Maternal Impressions 91

5. PRESENTATIONS AND POSITIONS . 92

    Fetal Habitus 92
    Fetal Head 92
    Presentation 93
    Positions 94
    Diagnosis of Fetal Position . . 97
    Conference Material 101
    Self-Examination Questions for the
    Student 101
    Study Questions 103

ix

x   *Contents*

UNIT TWO   Nursing in Pregnancy

6. NORMAL PREGNANCY 109

    Introduction 109
    Physiologic Changes of Pregnancy 109
    Local Changes 109
    Metabolic Changes 116
    Changes in the Various Systems 116
    Effects on the Nervous System . 118
    Endocrine Changes 118

7. SIGNS AND SYMPTOMS OF PREGNANCY 121

    Classification of Signs and Symptoms 121
    Presumptive Signs 121
    Probable Signs 123
    Positive Signs 127

8. ANTEPARTAL CARE 131

    Introduction 131
    The Importance of Preventive Care 131
    Medical Care 132
    Nursing Care 137
    Nutrition in Pregnancy . . . 145
    General Hygiene 153
    Minor Discomforts 163
    Preparation for Parenthood . . 170
    Psychophysical Preparation for Childbearing 174
    Preparations for the Baby . . 185
    Plans for After-Care of Mother and Baby 188

9. THE MENTAL HYGIENE OF PREGNANCY AND CHILDBIRTH—Leo Kanner, M.D. 191

    Introduction 191
    The Mother's Attitude Toward Her Pregnancy 192
    The Mother's Attitude Toward Labor 197
    The Mother's Attitude Toward the Newborn 198

    The Psychoses of Pregnancy . 200
    The Nurse's Contribution to the Mental Hygiene of Pregnancy 200
    Summary 203
    Conference Material 204
    Study Questions 205

UNIT THREE   Nursing During Labor and Delivery

10. PHENOMENA OF LABOR 211

    Premonitory Signs of Labor . . 211
    Cause of Onset of Labor . . . 214
    Uterine Contractions 215
    Duration of Labor 216
    The Three Stages of Labor . . 216

11. ANALGESIA AND ANESTHESIA FOR LABOR 226

    Types of Pain Relief 226
    General Principles 226
    Obstetric Analgesia 228
    Obstetric Anesthesia 230

12. CONDUCT OF NORMAL LABOR . 241

    Dimensions of Effective Nursing Care 241
    Prelude to Labor 242
    The Onset of Labor 243
    Admission to the Hospital . . 246
    Establishment of the Nurse-Patient Relationship . . . 246
    Continuing Care 247
    Examinations in Labor . . . 249
    Conduct of the First Stage . . 251
    Conduct of the Second Stage . 261
    Conduct of the Third Stage . . 269
    Immediate Care of the Infant . 277
    Emergency Delivery by the Nurse 284
    Lacerations of the Birth Canal 286
    Episiotomy and Repair . . . 286
    Conference Material 289
    Study Questions 291

UNIT FOUR   Nursing in the Normal Puerperium

13. THE PHYSIOLOGY OF THE PUER-
    PERIUM   297

    Introduction   297
    Anatomic Changes   297
    Clinical Aspects   300
    Postpartal Examinations . . .   302

14. NURSING CARE DURING THE
    PUERPERIUM   304

    Introduction   304
    Changes and Reactions During
       the Puerperium   304
    Immediate Care   312
    General Physical Care . . .   312
    Special Physical Care Aspects .   317
    The Mother Who Is Nursing .   322
    Parental Guidance and Instruc-
       tion   335
    Conference Material   344
    Study Questions   346

UNIT FIVE   Nursing the Normal Newborn

15. CARE OF THE NEWBORN INFANT   352

    Introduction   352
    Physiology of the Newborn . .   352
    Characteristics of the Newborn .   359
    The Environment of the New-
       born   365
    Nursing Care of the Newborn .   373
    Infant Feeding   385
    The Primigravida and Her New-
       born   394

16. CARE OF THE PREMATURE INFANT   406

    Introduction   406
    Causes of Prematurity . . .   407
    Causes of Premature Deaths .   407
    Description at Birth   407
    Nursing Management   409
    Parental Reactions   414
    Growth and Development . .   417
    Conference Material   418
    Study Questions   419

UNIT SIX   Operative Procedures in Obstetrics

17. OPERATIVE OSTETRICS   425

    Episiotomy and Repair of Lac-
       erations   425
    Forceps   425
    Version   428
    Cesarean Section   429
    Destructive Operations . . .   434
    Induction of Labor   434
    Conference Material   437
    Study Questions   438

UNIT SEVEN   Maternal Disorders Associated With the Childbearing Cycle

18. COMPLICATIONS OF PREGNANCY   443

    Introduction   443
    Toxemias of Pregnancy . . .   444
    Hemorrhagic Complications . .   455
    Blood Groups and the RH Factor   466
    Hyperemesis Gravidarum . .   469
    Coincidental Diseases and Preg-
       nancy   472

19. COMPLICATIONS OF LABOR . . .   482

    Introduction   482
    Mechanical Dystocia   482
    Hemorrhagic Complications . .   493
    Amniotic Fluid Embolism . .   497
    Accidental Complications . .   497
    Multiple Pregnancy   500

20. COMPLICATIONS OF THE PUER-
    PERIUM   503

    Puerperial Infection   403
    Subinvolution of the Uterus .   508
    Hemorrhage   508
    Vulvar Hematomas   508
    Disorders of the Breasts . . .   509
    Bladder Complications . . .   513
    Puerperal Psychoses   514
    Pulmonary Embolism   514
    Conference Material   515
    Study Questions   516

UNIT EIGHT   Abnormalities of the Fetus and the Newborn

21. DISORDERS OF THE NEWBORN. .   523

     Introduction   523
     Parental and Staff Reactions to
        Defects and Disorders . . .   523
     Neonatal Respiratory Diseases .   527
     Injuries   532
     Infections   536
     Malformations   539
     Inborn Errors of Metabolism .   545
     Hemolytic Disease of the New-
        born   547
     Miscellaneous Disorders . . .   550
     Conference Material   554
     Study Questions   555

UNIT NINE   Related Information

22. HOME DELIVERY; NURSE-MID-
     WIFERY   561

     Preparations for Home Delivery   561
     Delivery in the Home   565
     Nurse-Midwifery   569
     Midwifery in the United States   571

23. OBSTETRICS DURING EMERGENCY   576

     Disaster Insurance for Mothers
        and Babies   576

24. HISTORY OF OBSTETRICS . . .   581

     Obstetrics Among Primitive
        Peoples   581
     Egyptian Obstetrics   581
     Oriental Obstetrics   582
     Grecian Obstetrics   582
     Byzantine, Mohammedan, Jew-
        ish and Medieval Periods . .   582
     The Renaissance Period . . .   583
     The Seventeenth Century . . .   583
     The Eighteenth Century . . .   584
     The Nineteenth and the Twen-
        tieth Centuries   585
     Background and Development
        of Antepartal Care in the
        United States   587

APPENDIX

     Answer Key for Study Questions .   597
     Glossary   599
     Conversion Table for Weights of
        Newborn   609
     Aid for Visualization of Cervical
        Dilatation   610

INDEX   613

UNIT ONE

Human Reproduction

Orientation to Maternity Nursing
Anatomy Related to the Reproductive System
Physiology in Relation to Human Reproduction
Development and Physiology of the Fetus
Presentations and Positions

Chapter 1

Orientation to Maternity Nursing

INTRODUCTION

The study of obstetrics and of the nursing care of women during the various phases of childbearing includes the study of anatomic and physiologic adaptations to human reproduction and, in the full meaning, the study of human growth and development and the many interdependent relationships concerned. The vast importance of professional maternity care to mothers, infants and families of our country must be fully understood by all who participate in their care.

This chapter is planned to begin the student's orientation to maternity nursing. Certain basic terminology will be defined. Basic concepts of maternity care will be introduced, as well as the childbearing mother and her infant—all as they form a part of the expanding family found in our society.

The subsequent chapters of this unit survey the anatomy and the physiology related to human reproduction. Knowledge of the anatomy and the physiology of the reproductive organs and of the development of the unborn child from conception to birth is basic to the understandings required of every maternity nurse. The physiologic mechanism by which conception takes place and a new human being develops is not only a fascinating story in itself but also one that has far-reaching implications for the mother, the child and the family. All that a human being comes to be depends on many factors: his heritage, his prenatal en-

vironment, his care at birth and his care thereafter throughout infancy and childhood. Thus, it is all the more important that the safety, the health and the well-being of each mother and infant be protected, and, simultaneously, that the highest level of health possible for every childbearing family be achieved in the broader sense of physical, emotional and social well-being.

Unit One concludes with a consideration of the various positions which the fetus in utero may occupy. A clear grasp of the material in this unit is essential to a basic understanding of maternity care. The illustrations should be studied in close correlation with the text.

OBSTETRICS

Obstetrics is defined as that branch of medicine which deals with parturition, its antecedents and its sequels. It is concerned principally, therefore, with the phenomena and the management of pregnancy, labor and the puerperium under both normal and abnormal circumstances.[1]

The etymology of "obstetrics" is mentioned here to serve as basic information. For many students it will undoubtedly arouse curiosity and interest for further study. Briefly, the word "obstetrics" is derived from the Latin *obstetricia* or *obstetrix*, meaning midwife. The

[1] Eastman, N. J., and Hellman, L. M.: Williams Obstetrics, ed. 12, p. 1, New York, Appleton, 1961.

3

verb form *obsto* (*ob*, before, plus *sto*, stand) means "to stand by." Thus, in ancient Rome a person who cared for women at childbirth was known as an *obstetrix*, or a person who "stood by" the woman in labor. In both the United States and Great Britain this branch of medicine was called "midwifery" for several centuries—in fact, until the latter part of the 19th century. The term "obstetrics" really came into usage little more than a century ago, although reference to a variety of words of common derivation can be found occasionally in earlier writings. With the use of new terminology that has developed down through the years it is not unusual to find that from the standpoint of semantics changes have developed also in the present era. Today, in light of the various changes which have evolved in the total care of childbearing women, the usage of the term "obstetric care" is open to question. In the current frame of reference it seems more appropriate to use the term "maternity care," since this term implies a broader meaning of the care of the mother and her offspring throughout the childbearing experience. Moreover, it focuses attention on the care of a *person*, on the importance of interpersonal relationships—particularly those relationships which are *significant to her*—and the kind of patient care which will assist in promoting the health and the well-being of the expanding family group.

The World Health Organization Expert Committee on Maternity Care has defined maternity care as follows:

The object of maternity care is to ensure that every expectant and nursing mother maintains good health, learns the art of child care, has a normal delivery, and bears healthy children. Maternity care in the narrower sense consists in the care of the pregnant woman, her safe delivery, her postnatal examination, the care of her newly born infant, and the maintenance of lactation. In the wider sense it begins much earlier in measures aimed to promote the health and well-being of the young people who are potential parents, and to help them develop the right approach to family life and to the place of the family in the community. It should also include guidance in parentcraft and in problems associated with infertility and family planning.[2]

[2] World Health Organization Technical Report Series, No. 51, Geneva, Switzerland, World Health Organization, 1952.

MATERNITY NURSING

Maternity nursing involves direct, personal ministrations to maternity patients and their newborn infants, or related activities on their behalf, during the various phases of the childbearing experience. Maternity nursing differs from the practice of nursing in any of the other areas only in that the clinical focus primarily involves the care of maternity patients (in contrast, for example, with the care of surgical patients or psychiatric patients). How the maternity nurse meets the nursing needs of mothers and their newborn infants cannot be spelled out in stereotyped activities any more than it can in any other situation in which individualized nursing care is the underlying objective. In fact, the nurse may be called on at times to perform what superficially appears to be rather elementary nursing tasks; for example, in relation to body cleanliness. It is *how* the nurse carries out her care of the patient, the depth of problem-solving ability she employs, that makes the difference between truly professional nursing and nursing on a technical level.

In the practice of nursing the nurse intervenes to relieve or to reduce the patient's problems due to physical, physiologic or psychologic stress. A significant aspect of maternity nursing on the professional level is that patient care involves purposeful, sustained interaction between the nurse and the patient, during which the nurse assesses the patient's problems, i.e., makes a nursing diagnosis as to the nature of the discomfort or the dysfunction, and takes action to relieve the problem if it can be alleviated properly with nursing measures.

Begetting children is a family affair; thus the nursing care of maternity patients is properly a family-centered activity. In most situations today the maternity patient is a healthy woman involved in the normal physiologic process of childbearing. However, like individuals facing any other new experience in the family life cycle, maternity patients may begin the experience at various stages of preparation for pregnancy and childbirth, with various kinds of stress and at various levels of contentment. It is safe to say that in almost no other normal physiologic process does one find such individual extremes of reactions within a normal context. These individual reactions may be based on events going back to childhood, to certain experiences shared in growing up, or to later happenings. Certainly, they are influenced by the home environment from which the mother comes and to which, a short time after the delivery, she will return with her newborn infant. The level of satisfaction with which the expectant mother leaves the clinic or the level of contentment with which the newly delivered mother leaves the hospital environment with her baby will be modified somewhat by the interpersonal relationships of those most significant to her in that environment. Thus, the nurse, who has more continuity in the time spent with patients than other professionals, by the very nature of her position has it within her ability to make a significant contribution to maternity care.

MATERNAL AND CHILD HEALTH

Despite the fact that today the use of the term "maternal and child health" seems to imply a relatively new concept of care, it actually was in usage more than 50 years ago. In 1912 the United States Children's Bureau was created by an act of Congress for the purpose of promoting maternal and child health "among all classes of people." It was said to be a public health nurse who first conceived the idea of a Federal bureau of this kind and originally suggested the plan to President Theodore Roosevelt in 1905. The Children's Bureau has continually stressed the importance of public health nursing in maternal and child welfare. Between the years 1921 and 1929 public health nursing consultants were employed by the Bureau, and their services were offered to the states for maternal and infant hygiene. In rural areas public health nursing services throughout the United States were greatly extended, and 2,978 centers for prenatal and child health work were established.

Since these early beginnings the Children's Bureau has continued to make significant contributions to the promotion of maternal and child health in this country (see Suggested Reading).

Maternal and child health nursing has been interpreted in many different ways, often de-

pending on the individual's frame of reference. To some it means a combination of the traditional courses in maternity and pediatric nursing. To others it is a concept of patient care which takes into consideration the relationship of the mother to the care of a child, or the relationship of the mother and her newborn infant in maternity care. To still others it refers to the care of healthy mothers and children, of families.

The authors of this textbook refer to maternal and child health nursing as a philosophy of patient care rather than a special area of nursing. Whether it concerns maternity nursing, pediatric nursing, the nursing of children or maternal-child health nursing, the patient care involves the nursing of mothers or children. Thus the crux lies in the care of families. There is a body of knowledge which specifically pertains to maternity nursing, and, likewise, there is a closely related but separate body of knowledge which pertains to the nursing of children or pediatric nursing. As one develops knowledge, understanding and skills in these areas, a philosophy of maternal and child health also evolves.

This is a philosophy of nursing that is shared by many colleagues. For example, Bruce and Hall have said:

When maternity and pediatric nurses study and work together in providing nursing care for parents and children, the whole family benefits. . . . The members of each field bring with them their own unique skills and understandings which, when put together, cannot help but enrich the total practice.[3]

EXPANDING FAMILIES IN AMERICA

An awareness of the many facets involved in a changing society, especially as they relate to young childbearing families, should help the maternity nurse to develop an understanding of the forces that these changes exert on family life and, in addition, to see wherein they have implications for maternity care.

In recent years it has been said repeatedly that family life in the United States is rapidly changing due to the impact of socioeconomic

---

[3] Bruce, S. J., and Hall, E. J.: Maternity and pediatric nurses study and work together, Am. J. Nurs. 63:105, March, 1963.

pressures. This is reflected in a change in American family structure, a change in traditional male and female roles, a change in family relationships, and even a change in concepts of maternity care.

The objective of this brief discussion is merely to introduce some observations that concern young childbearing families in our society and to stimulate the student's interest. It is in no way any attempt to pursue the broad and complex subject of trends in American family life.

Young couples today marry at a younger age than their elders did. The average age of the young bride is 20 years, and many brides are in their late teens. The average age of the groom is a little more than 2 years older than his bride. Nearly all young couples establish a household of their own when they marry. In many situations the young bride may still be completing her formal education; if she has been employed, she is likely to continue working outside the home. These couples not only spend more of their leisure time together, but they share in the homemaking responsibilities as well.

Young married couples today appear to be interested in having children, not only more children than their parents did, but having them spaced closer together. The average size family today has 3 or 4 children, and often the last child is born by the time that the wife is 26 years old. When the wife becomes pregnant, the husband and the wife are likely to attend some kind of expectant parents' classes together. He is likely also to accompany his wife on her visits to the obstetrician, if his job requirements and responsibilities make it at all possible. It has become customary for husbands to stay with their wives during labor if they wish to, since the majority of modern maternity hospitals no longer exclude them. And after the baby is born, husbands more often are helping at home with the care of their babies—something which was considered to be strictly the role of the mother in the Victorian era.

As a consequence of the mobility of our population, smaller living quarters and other social changes, the more typical family in an urban industrial community usually consists of the husband, the wife and their children—

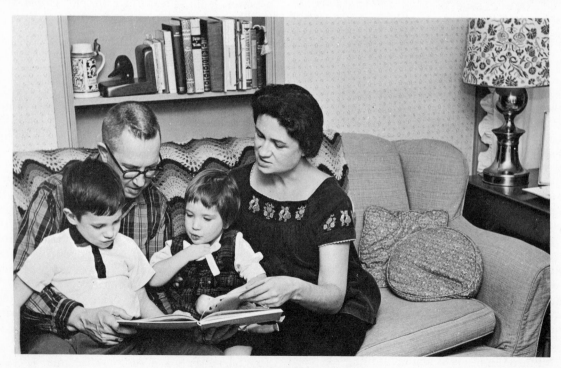

FIG. 1-1. An expectant family.

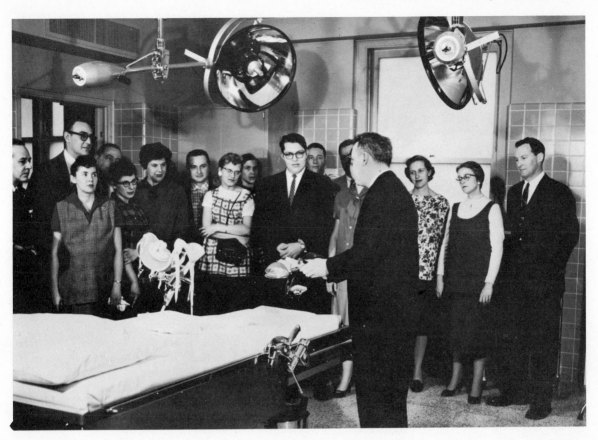

FIG. 1-2. Expectant couples on conducted tour of the maternity hospital. (Cleveland Clinic Hospital, Cleveland)

the so-called "nuclear family." Since they live apart from their original families, there are fewer close relatives near at hand to help out in time of need; for example, when the new baby arrives. Much has been said about the added stress which young couples must cope with because they live unto themselves and therefore lack the so-called advantages to be gained from living in the "family" home with the large 3-generation household. One cannot help wondering whether such thinking does not stem from those of the older generation who look at the young pregnant woman through the lens of their own past experiences, for many women of this older generation had to face childbirth with poor preparation for the experiences of childbearing.

From observations of mothers who enter the hospital to have their babies today, the average middle-class young woman in general is fairly well prepared for the experience. Most of them have done some reading from the current literature for expectant parents, many have attended some kind of parents' classes, and most of them have taken advantage of getting their questions answered by their doctors. And since most of the hospitals now have conducted tours of the maternity unit regularly scheduled for maternity patients, the husband and wife are likely to have taken advantage of this together sometime during the latter part of pregnancy. Granted, all of this preparation does not always hold true for the majority of women who come from the disadvantaged, low-income families, but it is in evidence as the quality of *total* maternity care in the clinics progresses.

One of the concerns about the 2-generation family found in most of the United States is the need for greater support for young couples who have married early and have children; i.e.,

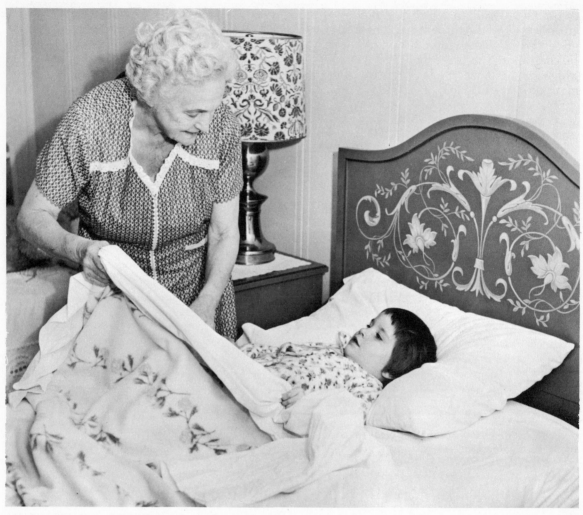

Fig. 1-3. Grandmother comes to visit and help. Putting 2-year-old Kathy to bed.

there is no one there to help them. From observations it can be said that most of the expectant parents have made some satisfactory arrangements for help upon returning home from the hospital with the new baby. It is not unusual to find that the patient's mother or mother-in-law or a close relative is coming to be with her and to manage the household for a short period of time. Often it is said, "She'll be with me as long as I need her." Even when parents live out of the state, the mobility of the population so prevalent today takes form in the ease with which relatives travel great distances when there is a need. Sussman

questions the notion that the nuclear family in modern society is the atomistic and isolated unit

it has often been reputed to be. Empirical evidence indicates that the nuclear family is functioning today within a network of other nuclear families, particularly with families of orientation and in-law families, and that this network offers services and help of all kinds—during emergencies, on ceremonial occasions, and in everyday situations.[4]

VITAL STATISTICS

With reference to frequency distribution, an examination of the vital statistics reports gives

[4] Sussman, M. B.: The isolated nuclear family: Fact or fiction? *in* Sussman, M. B. (ed.): Sourcebook in Marriage and the Family, ed. 2, p. 49, Boston, Houghton, 1963.

us quantitative data which has been systematically gathered and collated. These data are presented in this chapter because they relate to change in the large body of people with which we are concerned—statistics on births, marriages, population, morbidity and mortality.

In this country these data are published officially by the United States Public Health Service, National Center for Health Statistics, Vital Statistics Division. To understand the significance of the vital statistics quoted in the following discussion, the nurse should be familiar with the following terms, explained according to the definitions of the National Center for Health Statistics. Deaths are classified according to the World Health Organization Manual of International Classification of Diseases, Injuries and Causes of Death, based on recommendations of the Seventh Revision Conference, 1955, volume 1, Geneva, Switzerland, 1957.

Birth Rate. The number of births per 1,000 population

Marriage Rate. The number of marriages per 1,000 total population

Fertility Rate. The number of births per 1,000 women aged 15 to 44 years

Neonatal. Pertaining to the first 4 weeks after birth

Neonatal Death Rate. The number of neonatal deaths per 1,000 live births

Fetal Death or "Stillbirth." One in which the infant of 20 weeks or more gestational age dies in utero prior to birth

Perinatal Mortality. The sum of deaths of fetuses and infants weighing 1,000 Gm. or over which occur between 28 weeks of gestation and 4 weeks of age, i.e., to the end of the neonatal period

Infant Mortality Rate. The number of deaths before the first birthday per 1,000 live births

Maternal Mortality Rate. The number of maternal deaths per *100,000* live births

Race and Color.[5] Births in the United States are classified for vital statistics according to the race of the parents in the categories of white, Negro, American Indian, Chinese, Japa-

nese, Aleut and Eskimo combined, Hawaiian and part-Hawaiian combined, and "other nonwhite." In most tables a less detailed classification of "white" and "nonwhite" is used.

The category "white" includes births to parents classified as white, Mexican, Puerto Rican or "not stated." If one parent is Hawaiian and the other is not, the birth is classified as part-Hawaiian. If one parent is Negro, and the other is not Hawaiian, the birth is classified as Negro. In other cases of mixed parentage in which both parents are nonwhite, the child is assigned the father's race; if the father is white, the child is assigned the mother's race.

NATALITY

The number of registered births in the United States has remained relatively stable for the last 10 years, between 4.0 million and 4.3 million births per year. In the 1930's the average rate was 19 births per 1,000 population. There was a sharp rise during and immediately following World War II to a birth rate of 25.8 in 1947, but after this peak the birth rate for the total population declined slightly and maintained itself at about 25.0 during the next decade. The total number of live births in this country began to decline gradually in 1958; in 1963 the number of registered births totaled 4,098,020, which represented a birth rate of 21.7 (see Table 1). As in previous years, about 5 of every 6 births were white. In 1963 the birth rate ratios of white and of nonwhite population were 20.7 per 1,000 white population and 29.7 per 1,000 nonwhite population. The birth rates for both groups declined about 3 per cent between 1962 and 1963.

The frequency of twin births is always a subject of great interest and bears mention in this brief discussion of natality. Of the 4,098,-020 live births in the United States in 1963, some 81,158 (about 2%) were born in plural deliveries. One of every 54 white live births was a twin delivery, whereas the nonwhite twinning rate was 1 of every 39 live births.

An important consideration which influences the number of children being born annually is the size and the age composition of the female population of childbearing age. Although the *fertility rate* is computed on the basis of the

[5] U. S. Department of Health, Education, and Welfare, Public Health Service, National Center for Health Statistics: Vital Statistics of the United States 1963, vol. 1, Natality, Washington, D. C., U. S. Government Printing Office, 1965.

TABLE 1. LIVE BIRTHS AND POPULATION, UNITED STATES, 1930-1963*

YEAR	LIVE BIRTHS† TOTAL	WHITE	NONWHITE	BIRTH RATE	POPULATION OF UNITED STATES
1963‡	4,098,020	3,326,344	638,928	21.7	189,375,000§
1960‡	4,258,000	3,601,000	657,000	23.7	180,000,000‖
1957	4,308,000	3,621,400	633,300	25.3	171,300,000
1954	4,078,000	3,475,000	603,000	25.3	162,409,000
1950	3,632,000	3,108,000	524,000	24.1	151,700,000
1940	2,559,000	2,199,000	360,000	19.4	132,100,000
1930	2,618,000	2,274,000	344,000	21.3	123,100,000

* Beginning 1959, includes Alaska, and beginning 1960, includes Hawaii.

† Refers to births occurring within the United States. Adjusted for underregistration 1930-1957. Figures rounded to nearest thousand.

‡ Registered births. Figures by color exclude data for residents of New Jersey.

§ Revised estimate of total population.

‖ Census of April 1, 1960.

Sources:

Birth Statistics: Department of Health, Education, and Welfare, Welfare Administration, Children's Bureau; based on data from Public Health Service, National Center for Health Statistics, Vital Statistics Division.

Total Population: Department of Commerce, Bureau of the Census, Current Population Reports: Population Estimates, Series P-25, No. 286 (July, 1964) and No. 289 (August 31, 1964).

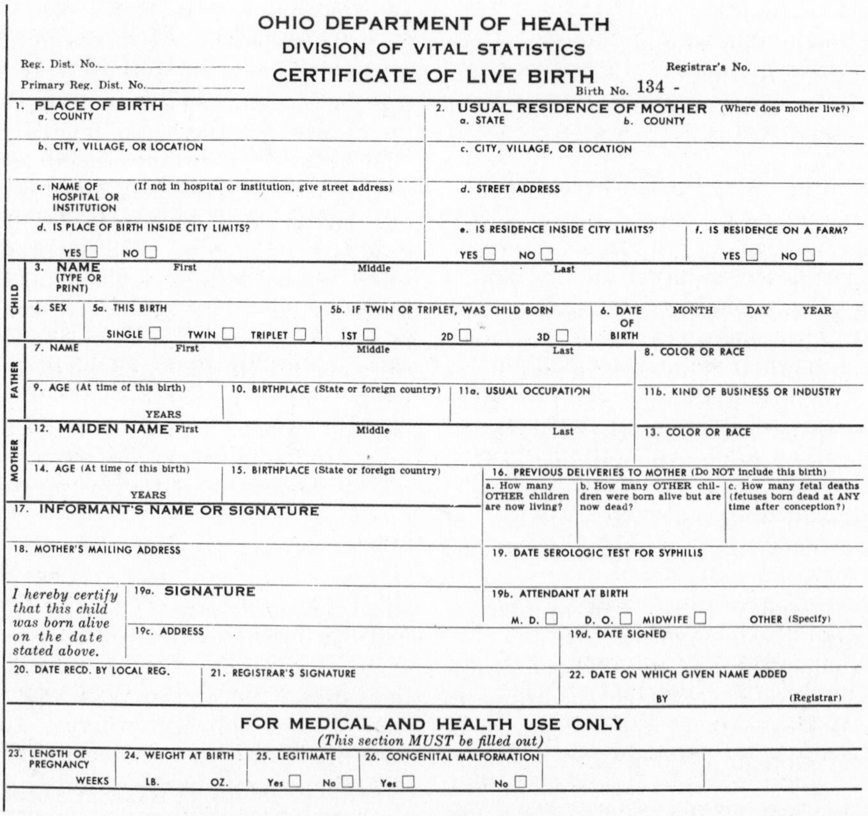
OHIO DEPARTMENT OF HEALTH
DIVISION OF VITAL STATISTICS
Reg. Dist. No.
Primary Reg. Dist. No.
CERTIFICATE OF LIVE BIRTH
Registrar's No.
Birth No. 134 -
1. PLACE OF BIRTH a. COUNTY
b. CITY, VILLAGE, OR LOCATION
c. NAME OF HOSPITAL OR INSTITUTION (If not in hospital or institution, give street address)
d. IS PLACE OF BIRTH INSIDE CITY LIMITS? YES ☐ NO ☐
2. USUAL RESIDENCE OF MOTHER (Where does mother live?) a. STATE b. COUNTY
c. CITY, VILLAGE, OR LOCATION
d. STREET ADDRESS
e. IS RESIDENCE INSIDE CITY LIMITS? YES ☐ NO ☐
f. IS RESIDENCE ON A FARM? YES ☐ NO ☐
CHILD
3. NAME (TYPE OR PRINT) First Middle Last
4. SEX
5a. THIS BIRTH SINGLE ☐ TWIN ☐ TRIPLET ☐
5b. IF TWIN OR TRIPLET, WAS CHILD BORN 1ST ☐ 2D ☐ 3D ☐
6. DATE OF BIRTH MONTH DAY YEAR
FATHER
7. NAME First Middle Last
8. COLOR OR RACE
9. AGE (At time of this birth) YEARS
10. BIRTHPLACE (State or foreign country)
11a. USUAL OCCUPATION
11b. KIND OF BUSINESS OR INDUSTRY
MOTHER
12. MAIDEN NAME First Middle Last
13. COLOR OR RACE
14. AGE (At time of this birth) YEARS
15. BIRTHPLACE (State or foreign country)
16. PREVIOUS DELIVERIES TO MOTHER (Do NOT include this birth)
a. How many OTHER children are now living?
b. How many OTHER children were born alive but are now dead?
c. How many fetal deaths (fetuses born dead at ANY time after conception?)
17. INFORMANT'S NAME OR SIGNATURE
18. MOTHER'S MAILING ADDRESS
19. DATE SEROLOGIC TEST FOR SYPHILIS
I hereby certify that this child was born alive on the date stated above.
19a. SIGNATURE
19b. ATTENDANT AT BIRTH M. D. ☐ D. O. ☐ MIDWIFE ☐ OTHER (Specify)
19c. ADDRESS
19d. DATE SIGNED
20. DATE RECD. BY LOCAL REG.
21. REGISTRAR'S SIGNATURE
22. DATE ON WHICH GIVEN NAME ADDED BY (Registrar)
FOR MEDICAL AND HEALTH USE ONLY
(This section MUST be filled out)
23. LENGTH OF PREGNANCY WEEKS
24. WEIGHT AT BIRTH LB. OZ.
25. LEGITIMATE Yes ☐ No ☐
26. CONGENITAL MALFORMATION Yes ☐ No ☐

FIG. 1-4. Certificate of live birth used by Ohio State Department of Health. Similar forms are used by other cities and states.

number of births per 1,000 women between the ages of 15 and 44, most of the childbearing is concentrated among women in their 20's. In 1963, for example, about 3 of every 5 births were to women who were 20 to 29 years of age. In that same year, when there were an estimated 37.8 million between the ages of 15 and 44, the fertility rate was 108.4.

Another factor which influences the number of infants being born annually is the number of marriages. According to the provisional vital statistics for the United States, in the 12 months ending with July, 1964, there were 1,720,000 marriages, or some 100,000 in excess of the previous year. This increase explains the reason that the marriage rate has reached 9.0 for the first time, having been approximately 8.5 for a number of years.

The Birth Certificate

In 1915 the Federal Government began to collect data on registered births and organized birth registration. At first only 10 states and the District of Columbia were included in this method of reporting births, but it gradually expanded so that by 1933 the entire country was included. The dependencies were admitted to the area: the Virgin Islands in 1924, the Territory of Hawaii in 1929, Puerto Rico in 1943 and Alaska in 1950. At the present time all 50 states and the District of Columbia demand that a birth certificate be filled out on every birth, and that it be submitted promptly to the local registrar. After the birth has been registered, the local registrar sends a notification to the parents of the child. Also, a complete report is forwarded from the local registrar to the state authorities, and then to the National Office of Vital Statistics in Washington.

Complete and accurate registration of births is a legal responsibility (see Fig. 1-4). The birth certificate gives evidence of age, citizenship and family relationships and as such often is required for military service, passports and even to collect benefits on retirement. On the basis of birth certificates, information which is essential to those agencies concerned with human reproduction is compiled by the National Office of Vital Statistics. The brief reports of statistics presented in this chapter are only a fraction of the volume of such studies compiled by that office.

POPULATION

The population of the United States has more than doubled in the last 50 years. In 1910 the population was 92.4 million; by mid-1962 the population had increased to 186.6 million, including those in the armed forces overseas. The United States Census Bureau projections have indicated that by 1970 the total population will be over 200 million, and by 1980 the population may reach 260 million.

Three vital factors determine the rate at which population grows: births, deaths and migration. The decline in the death rate that was so apparent in the first half of this century has fluctuated near the same relatively low level (9.6 deaths per 1,000 population) for the last decade. Control of immigration began in this country about a half century ago, and even with recent modifications it still continues to exert an influence on this factor in our population growth. The 1963 report from the National Vital Statistics Division states that "the dynamic factor in population growth in the United States is, and will continue to be, the number of births—births of Native parentage."[6]

One should not be deceived by the falling birth rate, which at first glance gives the impression that there is no need to have any concern about a "population problem" in the United States. The impression left by the tabulation of birth rates is that the number of live births has been relatively stable. However, it must be remembered that the birth rate relates to the number of births *per 1,000 population*. Table 1 shows the relationship of live births to population of the United States since 1930. The number of infants added to the population during the 1950's was greater than for any previous decade in the Nation's history. Although the birth rate declined 2 per cent from 1960 to 1963, in those same years, according to population estimates, the population increased by some 9,375,000 persons. The slight decline in births we have experienced in the 1960's is anticipated to continue for perhaps 2 or 3 years.

This decline in the annual number of births

[6] U. S. Department of Health, Education, and Welfare, National Vital Statistics Division, Public Health Service: Indicators, March, 1963, Washington, D. C., U. S. Government Printing Office, 1963.

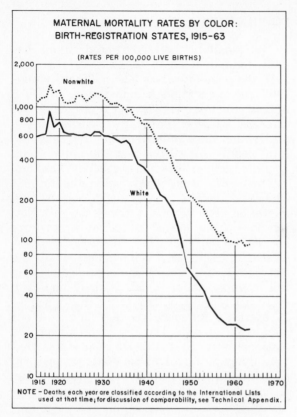

MATERNAL MORTALITY RATES BY COLOR:
BIRTH-REGISTRATION STATES, 1915-63

(RATES PER 100,000 LIVE BIRTHS)

Nonwhite

White

NOTE – Deaths each year are classified according to the International Lists
used at that time; for discussion of comparability, see Technical Appendix.

FIG. 1-5. Maternal mortality by color: birth-registration states, 1915-1963. Deaths from complications of pregnancy, childbirth and the puerperium per 100,000 live births in the specified groups. (Department of Health, Education, and Welfare, Welfare Administration, Children's Bureau; based on data from Public Health Service, National Center for Health Statistics, Vital Statistics Division)

is partly related to the age and the sex structure of the population. In 1960, for example, there were over one million fewer women in the most fertile age group (20-29 years) than in 1950. These women represented a 5 per cent smaller proportion of the total childbearing population than in 1950. Not until the sizeable groups of potential mothers now under the age of 20 move into the main childbearing years will there be an increase in the number of births. It was estimated that in 1963 there were 37.8 million women between the ages of 15 and 44 years, some 600,000 more than the

previous year. According to population projections made by the Bureau of the Census, during the next 10 years the number of women of childbearing age probably will rise to 44.7 million in this country.

MATERNAL MORTALITY

Maternal mortality refers to the deaths which occur as a direct result of childbearing; in other words, the underlying cause of the woman's death is the result of complications of pregnancy, childbirth or the puerperium.

During 1963 the 1,466 maternal deaths registered in the United States represented a maternal death rate of 35.8 per 100,000 live births. It must be noted that the maternal mortality rate was computed in 1960 for the first time on the larger base of 100,000 live births. Prior to this year the computation was made on the base of 10,000 live births. The Bureau of Vital Statistics explains that such a change was made, i.e., presenting the rates per 100,000 live births, to facilitate a comparison of the differences in rates from one year to another in the categories in which frequencies are small.

The reduction in maternal mortality rates has been rather consistent since 1915 (Fig. 1-5). The dramatic decline in these rates began about the mid-30's and continued until 1956. During the next succeeding 5 years the maternal mortality rate declined more slowly, reaching an all-time minimum in 1962. In 1963 the maternal death rate rose slightly to 35.8 per 100,000 live births, 1.7 per cent above the comparable figure for 1962 (35.2).

The risk of maternal death for all mothers is lowest in the group under 25 years of age. At age 25 and over the maternal death rate increases with age to such a degree that by 40 to 44 the figure is almost 7 times that at 20 to 24.

If the number of mothers who die in childbirth is to be reduced even further, it is necessary to know first why these women succumb. Three most common causes are responsible for about 70 per cent of all maternal deaths: hemorrhage, toxemias and puerperal infection (Fig. 1-6). Subsequently, these three conditions will be discussed in detail, but it would seem important to stress the fact that deaths from these causes are for the most part preventable. Substantial achievements in maternity care have caused the death rate from puerperal infection and toxemias of pregnancy to fall more dramatically than from hemorrhage. Consequently, hemorrhage has become the predominant cause of death in childbirth. According to the *official classification*, only the direct cause of death is considered, even though the predisposing cause may be an important factor. For example, in a case in which the mother has a massive hemorrhage and then (in her weakened condition) develops a puerperal infection that eventually causes her death, the death is classified as due to puerperal infection. Hemorrhage is often a predisposing factor, and in this manner its toll in maternal mortality probably exceeds all other causes combined.

Puerperal infection is a wound infection of the birth canal after childbirth, which sometimes extends to cause phlebitis or peritonitis. The nurse can play an important role in helping to prevent such infections, not only in terms of flawless technic in performing nursing procedures but also in protecting the mother from exposure to anyone with an infection.

The toxemias of pregnancy are certain disturbances peculiar to gravid women, characterized mainly by hypertension, edema, albuminuria and in some severe cases by convulsions and coma. Antepartal care plays an important role in prevention or early detection of symptoms, and with suitable treatment the disturbance often can be allayed.

Many factors are responsible for achieving the overall reduction in maternal mortality in this country during the past 25 years. Most important perhaps is the development of widespread training and educational programs in obstetrics which have provided more and better qualified specialists, professional nurses and other personnel in maternity programs. Better hospital facilities, multiple safeguards provided in the modern maternity hospitals and advances in therapy have all played major roles.

The distinct change in attitudes of doctors, nurses and parents also has contributed to this progressive saving of mothers. Childbirth is no longer an event to be awaited helplessly by the expectant mother with what fortitude she is

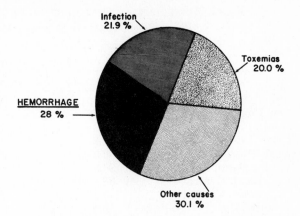

FIG. 1-6. Causes of maternal mortality, percentage distribution by cause, 1963. (Department of Health, Education, and Welfare, Welfare Administration, Children's Bureau; based on data from Division of Vital Statistics, National Center for Health Statistics, Public Health Service)

able to muster; instead, it is the climax of a period of preparation—a true state of preparedness attained through the cooperation of the physician, the nurse and the expectant mother or parents. As indicated before, this preparation for childbirth, based on careful medical and nursing supervision throughout pregnancy, is called antepartal (sometimes termed prenatal) care.

Antepartal care is one of the most important achievements in maternity care during the present century. It will be of interest to the nurse to know that this salutary contribution to the mother's welfare was initiated by the nursing profession. It had its beginning in 1901, when the Instructive Nursing Association in Boston began to pay antepartal visits to some of the expectant mothers who were to be delivered at the Boston Lying-In Hospital. This work gradually spread until, in 1906, all of these women prior to confinement were paid at least one visit by a nurse from the association. By 1912 this association was making about three antepartal visits to each patient. In 1907 another pioneer effort in prenatal work was instituted when George H. F. Schrader gave the Association for Improving the Condition of the Poor, New York City, funds to pay the salary of 2 nurses to do this work. In 1909 the Committee on Infant Social Service of the

TABLE 2. PERCENTAGE DISTRIBUTION OF LIVE BIRTHS BY ATTENDANT, BY COLOR:
UNITED STATES, EACH AREA, 1963*

	ATTENDED BY PHYSICIAN		ATTENDED BY MIDWIFE	ATTENDED BY OTHER OR NOT SPECIFIED ATTENDANT
	IN HOSPITAL†	NOT IN HOSPITAL		
United States	97.4	0.8	1.7	0.2
New England	99.7	0.3	0.0	0.0
Middle Atlantic	99.3	0.6	0.0	0.1
East North Central	99.2	0.7	0.0	0.1
West North Central	99.3	0.5	0.1	0.1
South Atlantic	94.3	1.3	4.1	0.2
East South Central	88.6	1.7	9.4	0.3
West South Central	95.3	0.8	3.5	0.3
Mountain	98.5	0.7	0.5	0.4
Pacific‡	99.2	0.6	0.1	0.2

* Source: Department of Health, Education, and Welfare, Welfare Administration, Children's Bureau; based on data from Public Health Service, National Center for Health Statistics, Vital Statistics Division: Advance Report, Final Natality Statistics 1963, September 11, 1964.
    † It is assumed that all births in hospitals or institutions are attended by physicians.
    ‡ Includes Alaska and Hawaii.

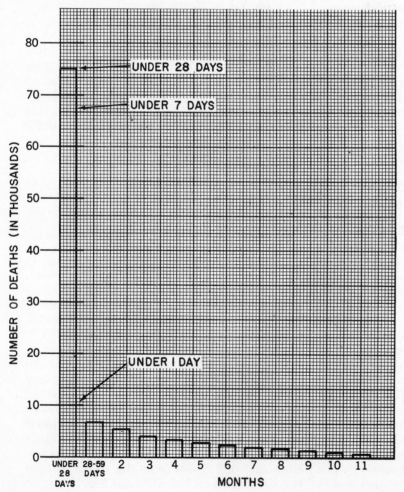

FIG. 1-7. Infant mortality by age, United States, 1963. Note the magnitude of neonatal deaths (under 28 days) as compared with mortality in later months.

In 1963 the total number of registered infant deaths under 1 year was 103,390. (Department of Health, Education, and Welfare, Welfare Administration, Children's Bureau; based on data from Public Health Service, National Center for Health Statistics, Vital Statistics Division)

Women's Municipal League, Boston, organized an experiment in antepartal work. The pregnant women were visited every 10 days—oftener if necessary. Blood pressure readings and urine tests were made at each visit. This important work was limited because of the effort to make it as nearly self-supporting as possible; therefore, only mothers under the care of physicians and hospitals were accepted. Thus began this movement for antepartal care which has done more than any other single effort to save mothers' lives in our time.

Another important factor in the reduction of maternal mortality has been the development of maternal and child health programs in State Departments of Public Health, particularly the work of public health nurses in maternal hygiene. These nurses visit a large number of the mothers who otherwise would receive little or no medical care, bringing them much-needed aid in pregnancy, labor and the puerperium. This service fills a great need not only in rural areas but also in metropolitan centers.

Still another factor responsible for the decline in maternal mortality is the trend toward hospitalization for childbirth—a trend that is gaining ground every year. In the early years of the century women rarely went to a hospital for such care. In 1935, 37 per cent of live births occurred in hospitals, and in 1963, 97.4 of the live births were attended by physicians in hospitals (see Table 2). This means that the percentage of hospital births has increased more than 2½ times during a 25-year period. In our larger cities the vast majority of babies are born in hospitals. This table also shows that in the United States the great majority of women are attended by physicians in childbirth, some 98.2 per cent in 1963.

INFANT MORTALITY

The two groups of problems in infant mortality which are of chief concern in maternity care are (1) those in which the fetus dies in the uterus prior to birth (so-called stillbirth) and (2) those in which it dies within a short period of time after birth (neonatal death). The phrase *perinatal mortality* often is used to designate all deaths in these two categories.

In May, 1950, in an effort to end confusion arising from usage of a variety of terms such

INFANT MORTALITY RATES BY COLOR: UNITED STATES, 1933-63

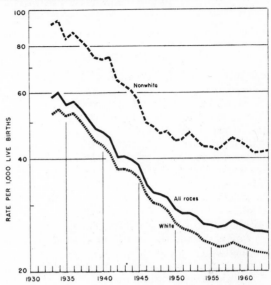

FIG. 1-8. (Department of Health, Education, and Welfare, Welfare Administration, Children's Bureau; based on data from Public Health Service, National Center for Health Statistics, Vital Statistics Division)

as stillbirth, abortion, miscarriage, etc., the World Health Organization recommended the adoption of the following definition of fetal death:

Fetal death is a death prior to complete expulsion or extraction from its mother of a product of conception, irrespective of duration of pregnancy; the death is indicated by the fact that after such separation, the fetus does not breathe or show any other evidence of life such as beating of the heart, pulsation of the umbilical cord, or definite movement of voluntary muscles.[7]

WHO further defined fetal death by indicating 4 subgroups, according to gestation age in weeks.

In the United States in 1963 there was reported a total of 103,390 infant deaths before the first birthday. Approximately 10 per cent of the infant deaths occurred on the first day after birth and 72 per cent under 28 days of age. The great toll taken in the first day of life in this country can be compared with the

[7] National Summaries: Fetal Deaths, U. S., 1954, National Office of Vital Statistics, vol. 44, No. 11, August 17, 1956.

TABLE 3. CAUSES OF NEONATAL MORTALITY, UNITED STATES, 1963*

CAUSE OF DEATH†	NUMBER OF DEATHS		
	TOTAL	WITH IMMATURITY	WITHOUT MENTION OF IMMATURITY
Certain diseases of early infancy:	61,373	....	....
Birth injuries	8,944	5,532	3,412
Postnatal asphyxia and atelectasis	17,692	12,964	4,728
Pneumonia of the newborn	3,181	877	2,304
Diarrhea of the newborn	384	66	318
Other infections of the newborn	835	334	501
Neonatal disorders arising from certain diseases of mother during pregnancy	721	466	225
Hemolytic disease of newborn (erythroblastosis)	1,821	401	1,420
Hemorrhagic disease of newborn	564	226	338
Ill-defined disease peculiar to early infancy, including nutritional maladjustment	9,683	7,510	2,173
Immaturity with mention of any other subsidiary condition	881	....	....
Immaturity, unqualified	16,667	....	....
Congenital malformations	9,454	....	....

* Department of Health, Education, and Welfare: Vital Statistics of the United States 1963, vol. II, Part A, Table 1-20, Washington, D. C., U. S. Government Printing Office, 1965.
† Classified according to the Seventh Revision of International Lists, 1955.

number of deaths occurring in the rest of the first year (Figs. 1-7, 8). The relatively favorable health conditions experienced by the general population of the United States in 1963 were reflected in a decline in the infant mortality rate to the lowest figure on record for this country. The neonatal mortality rate for 1963 was 18.2, the lowest it ever has been. Despite the fact that the reduction in infant mortality is indeed gratifying, it is not comparable with the fall in maternal mortality in the United States. Moreover, when it is compared with other infant mortality rates throughout the world, the United States ranks 11th.*

A consideration of the infant losses is incomplete unless the potential lives lost because of fetal death also is considered. In 1963 there were 64,640 fetal deaths (so-called stillbirths) reported. These deaths added to the 74,648 neonatal deaths in 1963 show the overwhelming sum of 139,288 infant losses associated with pregnancy, labor and the early weeks of life.

Many causes are responsible for this staggering infant mortality. The vast number of

* The United States dropped from 10th to 11th place among 15 modern industrial countries in 1962.

infant deaths is the result of several main causes: premature birth, asphyxia and atelectasis, congenital malformations and birth injuries.

During the first 4 weeks of life prematurity is the most important cause of death (Table 3). Birth injuries, another of the main causes of infant loss, accounted for almost 9,000 infant deaths in 1963. Almost one third of these deaths were due to intracranial and spinal injury at birth; for example, cerebral injury as a result of anoxia in utero or traumatic injury to the brain suffered in passing through the birth canal. In the vast majority of these cases death occurred under 7 days of life. Congenital malformations was another cause of some 9,454 neonatal deaths in 1963. Subsequently, these conditions will be discussed in detail. It suffices to say that one of the first and most important of them, prematurity, is largely a nursing problem. Indeed, in all the wide range of nursing care there is no area which offers such a challenge to the nurse or such lifesaving possibilities as that of caring for the premature infant.

The welfare of some 4,000,000 babies born annually in the United States is very much the concern of maternity nurses and obstetricians and one of the main objectives of the entire field of maternity care. To reduce the enormous loss of newborn lives, to protect the infant not only at birth but also in the prenatal period, and during the early days of the life of the infant to lay a solid foundation for his health throughout life—these are the problems and the challenge.

Abortion

The vast number of infants lost by abortion, the spontaneous or artificial termination of pregnancy prior to the period of viability, is a matter of grave importance (see Chap. 18). The abortion rate in this country exceeds stillbirths and neonatal deaths in fetal wastage. About 10 per cent of all pregnancies terminate in spontaneous abortion due to such factors as faulty germ plasm; unsatisfactory environmental conditions, hormonal and otherwise; many unknown etiologic causes; and an unknown number of criminal interruptions. The nurse should be aware of three major considerations in regard to criminal abortion: (1) that the mother is in immediate danger, (2) that the effects of such practices often impair the woman's childbearing potential, and (3) that there are legal implications for those involved.

CURRENT PROBLEMS IN MATERNITY CARE

An orientation to maternity nursing would be incomplete without calling attention to the broad problems in maternity care which reflect on the childbearing potential of families in the United States. In 1965 Dr. Arthur Lesser, the Deputy Chief of the United States Children's Bureau, made the analogy that some of the current problems in maternal and child care are like the old moving pictures shown on TV: "They are old and familiar. The problems which faced us 25 years ago are the same today."[8]

Today the problems for the United States as a whole reflect also a symptom of the far-reaching social changes since the last war. The

[8] Lesser, A. J.: Current problems in maternal and child care, paper presented at First Ohio Congress, Maternal and Child Health, Columbus, Ohio, March 3, 1965.

tremendous reduction in maternal and infant mortality rates presents concrete evidence of the noteworthy progress that has been achieved in maternity care in this country. Nevertheless, the problems of maternity care which are currently a major cause of concern relate to the kind of maternity care that a large segment of our population is receiving. Maternal and infant mortality rates are valuable in analyzing the current problems; moreover, they help to identify some of the areas in which difficulties exist.

Infant mortality has continued to decrease; in fact, the lowest figure on record for this country was recorded in 1961, when the infant mortality rate reached 25.3 (deaths under 1 year per 1,000 live births). Although the decline in infant mortality during the previous decade was substantial, 11 per cent, the greatest percentage of this decline was achieved between 1950 and 1955. In addition, 7 of the 10 largest cities had significant increases in infant mortality, increases ranging as high as 26.4 per cent, with infant mortality rates exceeding the national average of 26.0. Although the overall maternal mortality has been reduced dramatically in the last 35 years, in 1963 the maternal death rate rose slightly to 35.8 per 100,000 live births—1.7 per cent above the comparable figure for the previous year (Fig. 1-5).

The needs resulting from problems of maternal and child health in rural areas continues today, but what is new and alarming is that now there is a parallel situation in the larger cities.

Since the last war major shifts in population have occurred; urban middle-class families have migrated to suburban areas, whereas large numbers of families from rural areas have moved to the large urban industrial areas. Despite the increase in employment and in income generally, the population still includes a large segment of disadvantaged, low-income families which recently have concentrated in the major cities. With the increased cost of health services in general and the cost of hospital care in particular, these low-income families are straining the local resources of the communities in which they reside. Also, the number of maternity patients in these areas has greatly increased as a result of migration, producing overcrowding of clinics and hospital maternity in-service divisions. To accommodate such large numbers of maternity patients, many of the hospitals with large maternity services have had to resort to limiting the mother's hospital stay, some women being discharged 24 hours after delivery. The most serious problem by far is that many of these women are receiving poor or, often, no antepartal care, due in part to dissatisfaction with the kind of care provided. Inadequate care during pregnancy has been demonstrated to bear a direct relationship to the rate of prematurity (see Chap. 16).

It has been mentioned already that social factors play a role in morbidity and mortality and in fact influence the reproduction efficiency of childbearing women.

Much of the difficulty in providing adequate care is due to a shortage of professional personnel; i.e., there are not enough physicians, nurses and social workers to provide the necessary services for maternity patients. The rapid growth of the population has not been accompanied by a proportionate increase in physicians and nurses. This shortage is compounded by the fact that not enough physicians and nurses are being attracted into this area of specialization. Student nurses might well investigate the reason for this apathy and in good time provide some solution to this problem.

In a previous paper Dr. Arthur Lesser summarized some of the recommendations which were proposed on the national level to alleviate the current problems of maternity care. A part of the summary states:

The problems of maternity care led the President's Panel on Mental Retardation to make them the focus of one of its major recommendations. The Panel urged that a new program be established with Federal funds authorized on a project basis to assist state and local health departments in meeting the costs of administering programs of comprehensive maternity and infant care for women who have problems associated with pregnancy which increase the hazards of childbearing for themselves and for their infants and who are unlikely to receive the care they need because of low income or for other reasons. These programs would make it possible to:

1. increase the number of prenatal and postnatal clinics,

2. bring the prenatal and postpartum clinics close to the population served,

3. establish special clinics for some patients with complications of pregnancy (where more time by obstetricians, nurses, social workers, nutritionists and others can be provided),

4. pay for hospital care not only for the delivery but also during the prenatal period as needed,

5. relieve overcrowding in tax-supported hospitals by paying for care in voluntary hospitals,

6. pay for hospital care of premature infants and other infants needing special attention,

7. provide consultation services.

The Panel also recommended that the Children's Bureau support some comprehensive demonstration programs, including the provision of long-range child health supervision, especially among families which lack motivation, are apathetic and uncooperative.[9]

These and other recommendations related to the work of the Children's Bureau were enacted into legislation in 1963 with the maternal and the child health and the mental retardation amendments to the Social Security Act. The maternity care provisions of this statute authorize grants not only for new programs in preventive service, care, treatment and research but also provide for increased grants to the states for maternal and child health services, beginning in 1964. The funds are granted to the various state health departments or, with their agreement, directly to a local health department. These grants are for support of medical care programs—they are not demonstration projects—and upon request are granted to specific areas where they are most needed (see Suggested Reading).

SUGGESTED READING

Baird, Sir Dugold: The social aspect of obstetric practice, Obstet. Gynec. Survey 20, No. 3:410-430, June, 1965.

Bruce, S. J., and Hall, E.: Maternity and pediatric nurses study and work together, Am. J. Nurs. 63, No. 3:105-108, March, 1963.

Chambers, W.: Nursing diagnosis, Am. J. Nurs. 62, No. 11:102-104, November, 1962.

Children's Bureau: Five Decades of Action for Children (Pub. No. 3581), Washington, D. C., U. S. Government Printing Office, 1962.

Children and Youth at the Mid-Decade, Children 12, No. 2: entire issue, March-April, 1965.

9 Lesser, A. J.: Current Problems of Maternity Care, pp. 8-9, Washington, D. C., U. S. Department of Health, Education, and Welfare, Welfare Administration, Children's Bureau, 1963.

Close, Kathryn: Giving babies a healthy start in life, Children 12, No. 5:179-184, September-October, 1965.

Duvall, E. M.: Family Development, ed. 2, Philadelphia, Lippincott, 1962.

Gold, E. M.: A Broad View of Maternity Care, Children 9, No. 2:52-58, March-April, 1962.

Harpine, F.: Concepts in maternal and child health, Am. J. Nurs. 63, No. 3:84-87, March, 1963.

Herzog, E., and Bernstein, R.: Health Services for Unmarried Mothers, Children's Bureau Publication No. 425, Washington, D. C., U. S. Government Printing Office, 1964.

Johnson, D. E.: The nature of a science of nursing, Nurs. Outlook 7, No. 5:291-294, May, 1959.

————: A philosophy of nursing, Nurs. Outlook 7, No. 4:198-200, April, 1959.

Johnson, M. M., and Martin, H. W.: A sociological analysis of the nurse role, Am. J. Nurs. 58, No. 3:373-377, March, 1958.

Kreuter, F. R.: What is good nursing care?, Nurs. Outlook 5, No. 5:302-304, May, 1957.

Lemat, A.: The public health nurse in maternity service, Nurs. Outlook 12, No. 10:58-61, October, 1964.

Lesser, A. J.: Accent on prevention through improved service, Children 2, No. 1:13-18, January-February, 1964.

————: Current Problems of Maternity Care, Washington, D. C., U. S. Children's Bureau, 1963.

————: National needs and resources in newborn and maternity care, Bull. Am. Coll. Nurs. Midwifery 5, No. 3:49-58, September, 1960.

Lesser, M. S., and Keane, V. R.: Nurse-Patient Relationships in a Hospital Maternity Service, St. Louis, Mosby, 1956.

Malinowski, B.: Parenthood—the basis of social structure, *in* Sussman, M. B. (ed.): Sourcebook in Marriage and the Family, pp. 40-48, Boston, Houghton, 1963.

Maternity Center Association: Twenty Years of Nurse-Midwifery, New York, Maternity Center Association, 1955.

————: Meeting the Childbearing Needs of Families in a Changing World, New York, [Maternity Center] The Association, 1960.

————: The Forty-Fifth Annual Report, New York, [Maternity Center] The Association, 1965.

Monahan, H. B., and Spencer, E. C.: Deterrants to prenatal care, Children 9, No. 3:114-119, May-June, 1962.

Murray, B. L., McConnell, N., and Claypool, J. M.: Implications for learning: Persistent aspects of maternal-child nursing situations, J. Nurs. Ed. 2:5-9, 22-24, February-March, 1963.

Oettinger, K. B.: This Most Profound Challenge, U. S. Department of Health, Education, and Welfare, Welfare Administration, Children's Bureau, 1965.

Peplau, H. E.: Interpersonal techniques: The crux of psychiatric nursing, Am. J. Nurs. 62, No. 6:50-54, June, 1962.

Pollak, O.: Some Challenges to the American Family, Children 2, No. 1:19-20, January-February, 1964.

Rubin, R.: Maternity care in our society, Nurs. Outlook 11, No. 7:519-522, July, 1963.

Shyne, A. W., *et al.*: Evaluating public health nursing service to the maternity patient, Nurs. Outlook 11:56-58, January, 1963.

Sussman, M. B.: The isolated nuclear family: Fact or fiction? *in* Sussman, M. B. (ed.): Sourcebook in Marriage and the Family, pp. 48-53, Boston, Houghton, 1963.

Taylor, H. C., Jr.: Once again retrospect and prospect, Am. J. Obstet. Gynec. 87:839-847, December 1, 1963.

Taylor, R. G.: Some significant developments in maternal and child health nursing, Nurs. Outlook 8, No. 8:442-447, August, 1960.

U. S. Children's Bureau: It's Your Children's Bureau, Publication No. 357, Washington, D. C., U. S. Department of Health, Education, and Welfare, 1964.

————: Trends in Infant and Childhood Mortality, 1961, Statistical Series, No. 76, Washington, D. C., U. S. Government Printing Office, 1964.

U. S. Department of Commerce, Bureau of the Census: Current Population Reports: Population Estimates, Series P-25, Washington, D. C., U. S. Government Printing Office, 1965.

U. S. Department of Health, Education, and Welfare: The President's Panel on Mental Retardation: A Proposed Program for National Action to Combat Mental Retardation; Report to the President, October 1962, Washington, D. C., U. S. Government Printing Office, 1963.

————: Vital Statistics of The United States 1963, vols. I and II, Washington, D. C., U. S. Government Printing Office, 1965.

————: Health, Education, and Welfare Trends, 1964 ed., Washington, D. C., U. S. Government Printing Office, 1964.

Wallace, H. M.: Health Services for Mothers and Children, Philadelphia, Saunders, 1962.

Wessel, M. A.: A Physician Looks at Maternity Nursing, Bull. Am. Coll. Nurs. Midwifery 9, No. 3:44-55, Fall, 1964.

Wooden, H. E.: Impact of the industrial revolution on hospital maternity care, Nurs. Forum 1:90, Winter, 1961-1962.

————: The family-centered approach to maternity care, Nurs. Forum 1, No. 2:61-77, Spring, 1962.

World Health Organization: Manual of the International Statistical Classification of Diseases, Injuries and Causes of Death, 7th rev. of the Lists of Diseases, Injuries and Causes of Death, Geneva, Switzerland, World Health Organization, 1957.

————: First Report of Expert Committee on Maternity Care, WHO Technical Report Series, No. 51, Geneva, Switzerland, World Health Organization, 1952.

————: Social Aspects in the Teaching of Obstetrics and Gynecology, WHO Technical Report Series, No. 266, Geneva, Switzerland, World Health Organization, 1963.

Chapter 2

Anatomy Related to the Reproductive System

PELVIS

The pelvis, so called from its resemblance to a basin (*pelvis*, a basin), is a bony ring interposed between the trunk and the thighs. The vertebral column, or backbone, passes into it from above, transmitting to it the weight of the upper part of the body, which the pelvis in turn transmits to the lower limbs. From an obstetric point of view, however, we have to consider it as the cavity which contains the generative organs, and particularly as the canal through which the baby must pass during birth.

Structure

The pelvis is made up of 4 united bones: the 2 hip bones (*os coxae* or innominate) situated laterally and in front, and the sacrum and the coccyx behind (Figs. 2-1 to 3). Anatomically, the hip bones are divided into 3 parts: the ilium, the ischium and the pubis. These bones become firmly joined into one by the time the growth of the body is completed, i.e., at about the age of 20 to 25, so that on examining them in the prepared pelvis no trace of the original edges or divisions of these 3 bones can be discovered. Each of these bones may be roughly described as follows.

The ilium, which is the largest portion of the bones, forms the upper and back part of the pelvis. Its upper flaring border forms the prominence of the hip or crest of the ilium (hip bone). The ischium is the lower part below the hip joint; from it projects the tuberosity of the ischium on which the body rests when in a sitting posture. The pubis is the front part of the hip bone; it extends from the hip joint to the joint in front between the 2 hip bones, the symphysis pubis, and then turns down toward the ischial tuberosity, thus forming with the bone of the opposite side the arch below the symphysis, the pubic or subpubic arch. This articulation closes anteriorly the cavity of the pelvis.

The sacrum and the coccyx form the lowest portions of the spinal column. The former is a triangular wedge-shaped bone, consisting of 5 vertebrae fused together; it serves as the back part of the pelvis. The coccyx forms a tail end to the spine. In the child the coccyx consists of 4 or 5 very small, separate vertebrae; in the adult these bones are fused into one. The coccyx is usually movable at its attachment to the sacrum (the sacrococcygeal joint) and may become pressed back during labor to give more room for the passage of the fetal head.

Of special importance is the marked projection which is formed by the junction of the last lumbar vertebra with the sacrum; this is known as the sacral promontory and is one of the most important landmarks in obstetric anatomy.

21

Articulation and Surfaces

The articulations (joints) of the pelvis, which possess obstetric importance, are 4 in number. Two are behind, between the sacrum and the ilia on either side, and are termed the sacro-iliac articulations (Fig. 2-1 A); one is in front between the two pubic bones and is called the symphysis pubis (Fig. 2-1 B), and the fourth, of little consequence, is between the sacrum and coccyx, the sacrococcygeal articulation (Fig. 2-1 C).

All of these articular surfaces are lined with fibrocartilage, which becomes thickened and softened during pregnancy; likewise, the ligaments which bind the pelvic joints together become softened, and as a result greater mobility of the pelvic bones develops. A certain definite though very limited motion in the joints is desirable for a normal labor; however, there is no change in the actual size of the pelvis. From a practical standpoint, one of the most important facts for the nurse to know about these joints is that the increased mobility which they develop in pregnancy produces a slight "wobbliness" in the pelvis and throws greater strain on the surrounding muscles and ligaments. This accounts in large part for the frequency of backache and legache in the latter months of pregnancy.

The pelvis is lined with muscular tissue which provides a smooth, somewhat cushioned surface over which the fetus has to pass during labor; these muscles also help to support the abdominal contents.

Divisions

Regarded as a whole, the pelvis may be described as a two-storied, bony basin that is divided by a natural line of division (the inlet or brim) into 2 parts. These parts are called the false pelvis (above) and the true pelvis (below) (Fig. 2-4).

The false pelvis, or upper flaring part, is much less concerned with the problems of labor than is the true pelvis, but it is considered in obstetrics because it offers certain landmarks for the practice of pelvimetry or

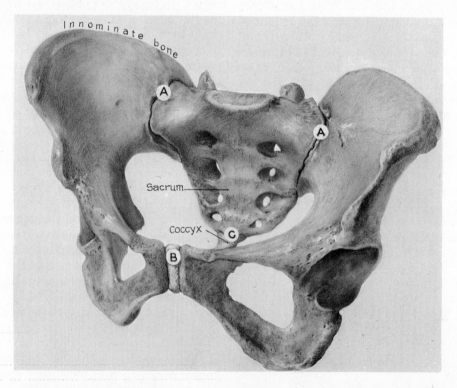

Fig. 2-1. Pelvis. (A) Sacro-iliac articulations. (B) Symphysis pubis. (C) Sacrococcygeal articulation.

FIG. 2-2. Lateral view of left innominate bone showing its 3 constituent parts (erect position).

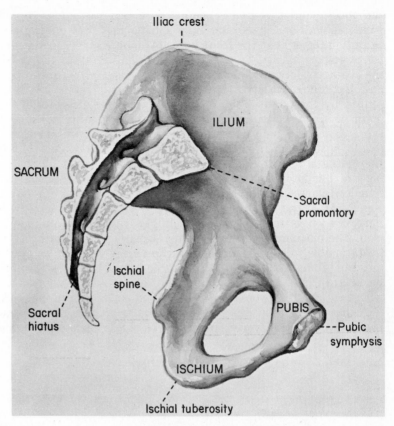

Iliac crest

ILIUM

SACRUM

Sacral promontory

Ischial spine

Sacral hiatus

PUBIS

Pubic symphysis

ISCHIUM

Ischial tuberosity

pelvic measurements, and because its shape and inclination aid in estimating the nature of the true pelvis. It also supports the uterus during late pregnancy and directs the fetus into the true pelvis at the proper time.

The true pelvis, or lower part, forms the bony canal through which the baby must pass during parturition; for convenience in description it is divided into 3 parts: an inlet or brim, a cavity and an outlet.

Pelvic Inlet. Continuous with the sacral promontory and extending along the ilium on each side in circular fashion is a ridge called the linea terminalis (brim). This bounds an area or plane called the inlet, so named because it is the entryway or inlet through which the baby's head must pass in order to enter the true pelvis. The pelvic inlet, sometimes also referred to as the pelvic brim or superior strait, divides the false from the true pelvis. It is roughly heart-shaped, the promontory of the sacrum forming a slight projection into it from behind (Fig. 2-5); it is widest from side to side, and narrowest from back to front, i.e., from the

sacral promontory to the symphysis. It should be noted particularly that the baby's head enters the inlet with its longest diameter (anteroposterior) in the transverse diameter of the pelvis. In other words, as shown in Figure 2-5, the greatest diameter of the head accommodates itself to the greatest diameter of the inlet. As the inlet is entirely surrounded by bone, it cannot be measured directly with the examining fingers in a living woman. However, the measurements of its anteroposterior diameter can be estimated on the basis of the diagonal conjugate diameter (see Figs. 2-21, 22).

The measurements of these diameters are very important, since variations from the normal (e.g., smaller in size or flattened) may cause grave difficulty at the time of labor (see p. 492).

Pelvic Outlet. When viewed from below, the pelvic outlet is a space bounded in front by the symphysis pubis and the pubic arch, at the sides by the ischial tuberosities, and behind by the coccyx and the greater sacrosciatic ligaments (Fig. 2-6). It requires only a little imagination to see that the front half of the outlet resembles a triangle, the base of which is the distance between the ischial tuberosities, and the other two sides of which are represented by the pubic arch. From an obstetric point of view, this triangle is of great importance, since the baby's head must make use of this space to gain exit from the pelvis and the mother's body (Fig. 2-6). For this reason Nature has provided a wide pubic arch in females, whereas in males it is narrow (see Fig. 2-14). If the pubic arch in women were as narrow as it is in men, natural childbearing would be extremely difficult, since the baby's head, unable to squeeze itself into the narrow anterior triangle of the outlet, would be forced backward against the coccyx and the sacrum, where its progress would be impeded.

As has been stated, the greatest diameter of the inlet is the transverse (from side to side), whereas the greatest diameter of the outlet is the anteroposterior (from front to back) (Fig. 2-7). Moreover, the baby's head, as it emerges from the pelvis, passes through the outlet in the anteroposterior position, again accommodating its greatest diameter to the greatest diameter of the passage. Since the baby's head enters the pelvis in the transverse position and emerges in the anteroposterior, it is obvious that the head must rotate some 90° as it passes through the pelvis. This process of rotation of the baby's head is one of the most important phases of the mechanism of labor and will be discussed in more detail later on pages 221 and 222.

Pelvic Cavity. This is the space between the inlet above, the outlet below and the anterior, the posterior and the lateral walls of the pelvis. The pelvic canal is practically cylindric in shape in its upper portion and curved only in its lower half. It is important to note the axis of the cavity when viewed from the

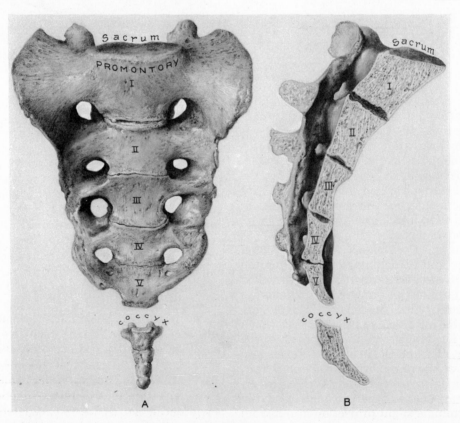

FIG. 2-3. Sacrum and coccyx. (A) Front view. (B) Median section. Note how promontory of sacrum juts forward.

Fig. 2-4. False and true pelves, sagittal section, in erect position.

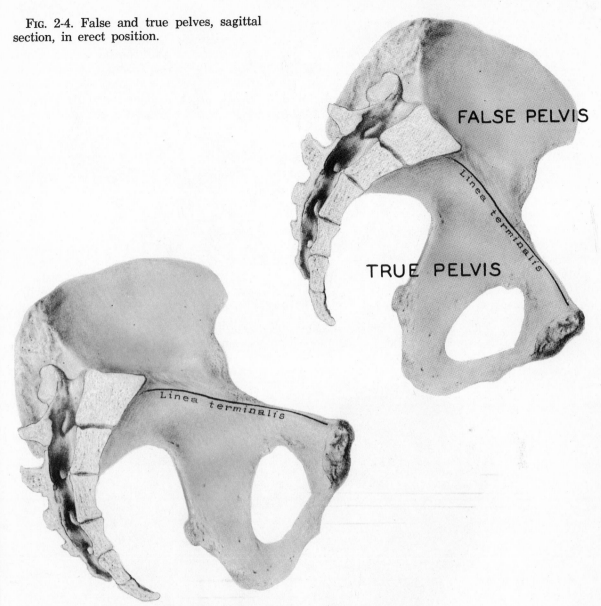

side (Fig. 2-9). It is apparent that during the delivery the head must descend along the downward prolongation of the axis until it nearly reaches the level of the ischial spines and then begins to curve forward. The axis of the cavity determines the direction which the baby takes through the pelvis in the process of delivery. As might be expected, labor is made more complicated by this curvature in the pelvic canal, because the baby has to accommodate itself to the curved path as well as to the variations in the size of the cavity at different levels.

Pelvic Variations

The pelvis presents great individual variations—no two pelves are exactly alike. Even those patients with normal measurements may present differences in contour and muscular development which influence the actual size of the pelvis. These varying differences are due in part to heredity, disease, injury and development. Heredity may be responsible for passing on many racial and sexual differences. Such diseases as tuberculosis and rickets cause malformations. Accidents and injuries during

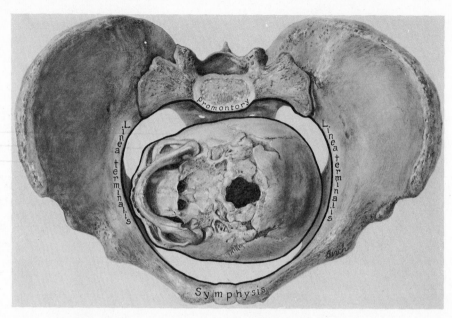

Fig. 2-5. Largest diameter of baby's head entering largest diameter of inlet (as viewed from above). Therefore it enters transversely.

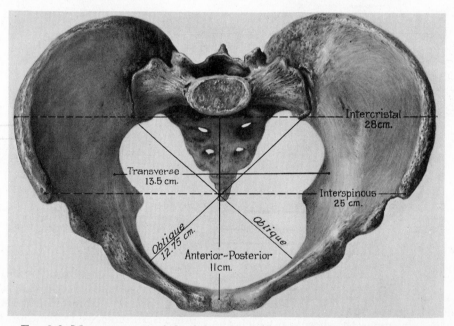

Fig. 2-6. Measurements of the inlet of a normal female pelvis, showing the 4 diameters: the anteroposterior, the transverse, and the 2 oblique diameters. The diameters shown with broken lines indicate transverse measurements of the false pelvis.

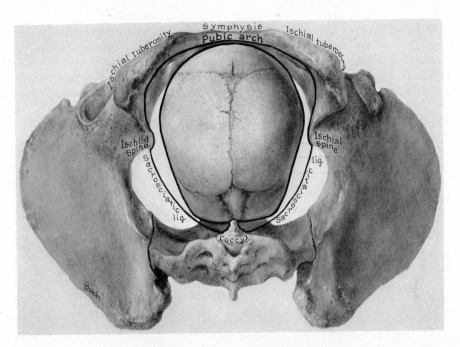

FIG. 2-7. Largest diameter of baby's head passing through largest diameter of outlet (as viewed from below). Therefore it passes through outlet anteroposteriorly.

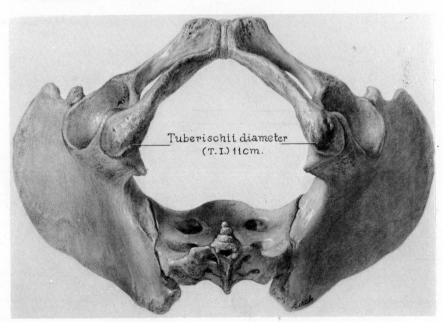

FIG. 2-8. Measurement of the outlet, showing transverse diameter in a normal female pelvis.

childhood or at maturity result in deformities of the pelvis or other parts of the body which affect the pelvis. Adequate nutrition and well-formed habits related to posture and exercise have a very definite influence on the development of the pelvis.

It must be remembered also that the pelvis does not mature until between the ages of 20 and 25 years, and until that time complete ossification has not taken place.

There are many so-called borderline cases of abnormal pelvic development. Such pregnant patients should be supervised closely. At periodic intervals the size of the fetus is estimated (by palpation of the abdomen), and definite arrangements are made for the type of delivery indicated.

There are several **types of pelves.** Even pelves whose measurements are normal differ greatly in the shape of the inlet, in the proximity of the greatest transverse diameter of the inlet to the sacral promontory, in the size of the sacrosciatic notch, and in their general architecture. Dr. H. C. Moloy and the late Dr. W. E. Caldwell, of the Sloane Hospital for Women, New York City, have utilized these characteristics in establishing a classification of pelves which has been of great interest and value to obstetricians. The four main types, according to this classification, are shown in Figures 2-10 to 13. The manner in which the baby passes through the birth canal and, consequently, the type of labor vary considerably in these pelvic types.

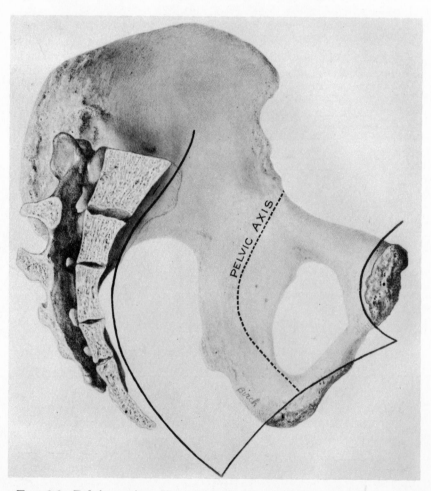

FIG. 2-9. Pelvic cavity. Heavy black line indicates location of soft parts, vagina, etc.

In addition, of course, there are many pelvic types which result from abnormal narrowing of one or the other diameters. These contracted pelves will be described in a subsequent chapter (see p. 492).

In comparing the male and the female pelves, several differences will be observed (Fig. 2-14). As already emphasized, the most conspicuous difference is in the pubic arch, which has a much wider angle in women. The symphysis is shorter in women, and the border of the arch probably is more everted. Although

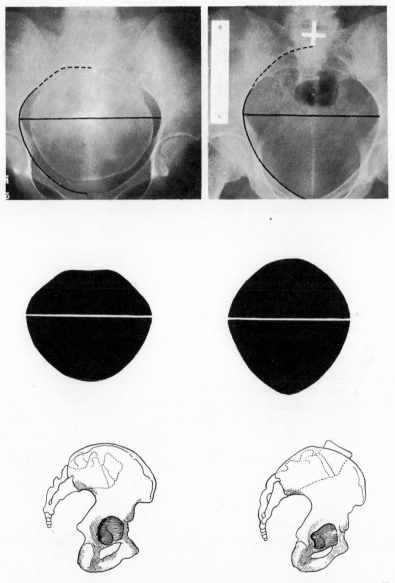

Fig. 2-10. (*Left*). Gynecoid (normal female) pelvis. Inlet is well rounded in hind- and fore-pelvis (A, B). Sacrosciatic notch is curved, moderate in width and depth (C).

Fig. 2-11. (*Right*). Anthropoid pelvis. Inlet is deep in hind- and fore-pelvis, increased in anteroposterior diameter (A, B). Sacrosciatic notch is broad, shallow (C).

(Roentgenograms from W. E. Caldwell, M.D., and H. C. Moloy, M.D., Sloane Hospital for Women, New York)

the female pelvis is more shallow, it is more capacious than the male, much lighter in structure and smoother. The male pelvis is deep, compact, conical and rougher in texture, particularly at the site of muscle attachments. The findings of Drs. Daniel G. Morton and Charles T. Hayden, of San Francisco, indicate that both males and females start life with pelves which are identical in type, and that the major differences observed in adult male and female pelves do not appear until puberty and are therefore due to the influence of the sex hormones. (For definition and description of the sex hormones, see pp. 56-58, 63.)

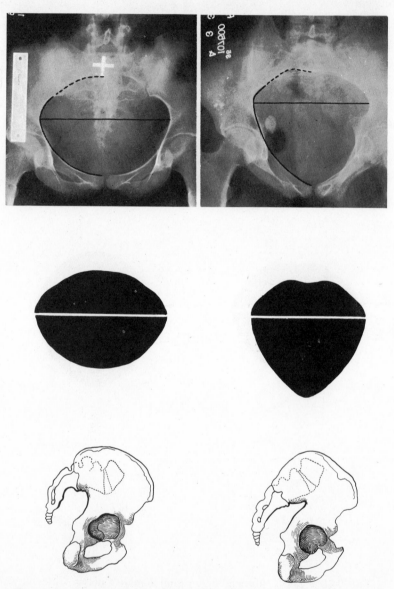

Fig. 2-12 (*Left*). Platypelloid pelvis. Inlet is a transverse oval, well-curved but decreased in anteroposterior diameter (A, B). Sacrosciatic notch is curved, small (C).

Fig. 2-13 (*Right*). Android pelvis. Inlet is wedged-shaped with shallow hind-pelvis and pointed fore-pelvis (A, B). Sacrosciatic notch is narrow, deep, pointed (C).

(Roentgenograms from W. E. Caldwell, M.D., and H. C. Moloy, M.D., Sloane Hospital for Women, New York)

Pelvic Measurements

Importance of Pelvic Measurements. The entire problem in childbirth centers on the safe passage of the fully developed fetus through the pelvis of the mother. Slight irregularities in the structure of the pelvis may delay the progress of labor, while any marked deformity may render the delivery by the natural passages impossible. For these reasons the pelvis of every pregnant woman should be measured accurately in the antepartal period to enable the physician to determine before labor begins whether or not there is anything in the condition of the mother's pelvis that may complicate the delivery. This examination is a part of the antepartal examination. In addition to a general physical examination, the pelvic measurements are made and compared with the dimensions of the normal pelvis.

Types of Pelvic Measurements. Physicians rely chiefly on internal and external pelvic measurements, made manually, as a means of estimating the size of the pelvis. In occasional instances, however, x-ray pelvimetry may be desirable (see p. 38). In the majority of abnormal pelves the most marked deformity affects the anteroposterior diameter of the inlet. It has long been a practice to determine a number of external measurements of the pelvis (intercristal diameter, interspinous diameter, intertrochanteric diameter, external conjugate) with an instrument called a pelvimeter, in the belief that they permit an approximate estimation of the size of the inlet (Figs. 2-15

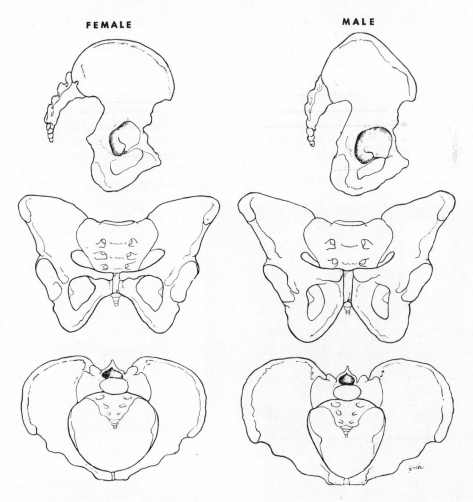

FEMALE   MALE

FIG. 2-14. Female pelvis contrasted with male in lateral, front and inlet views.

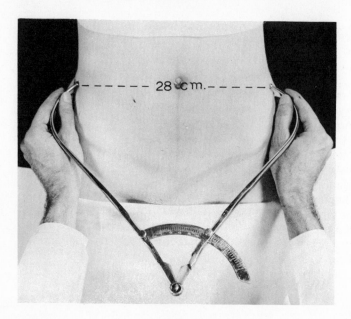

Fig. 2-15. Method of measuring inter-cristal diameter.

to 20). Authorities today (among them Green-hill, Thoms, Eastman) consider the transverse external measurements to be of dubious value as methods of measuring the true pelvis. Nevertheless, these measurements are still required on the records in many hospitals and clinics and are used by many experienced obstetricians in the belief that they do possess some value.

The EXTERNAL PELVIC MEASUREMENTS which are used to obtain an approximate idea of the size of the pelvic inlet are taken with a pelvimeter. Those measurements most commonly made are: (1) the intercristal diameter or the distance between the lateral edges of the iliac crests (average, 28 cm.); (2) the interspinous diameter or the distance between the external aspects of the anterosuperior iliac spines (average, 25 cm.); (3) intertrochanteric diameter or the distance between the external aspects

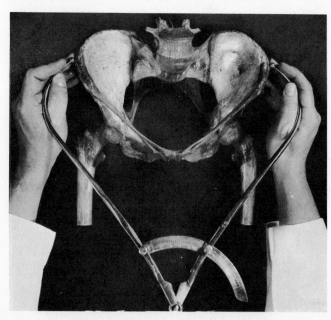

Fig. 2-16. Intercristal diameter measured on bony pelvis.

FIG. 2-17. Method of measuring interspinous diameter.

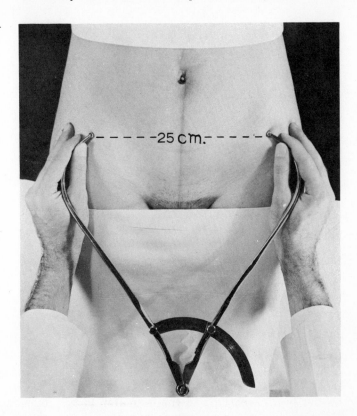

of the trochanters of the femurs (average, 31 cm.); (4) the external conjugate (Baudelocque's diameter) or the distance between the anterior aspect of the symphysis pubis in front and the depression below the spine of the 5th lumbar vertebra behind (average, 18 to 20 cm.). In addition, some physicians measure the right and the left oblique external

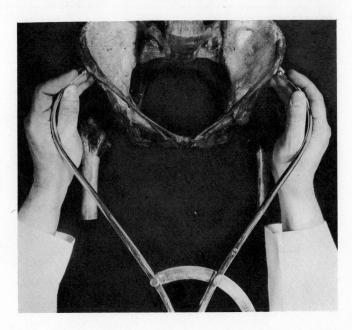

FIG. 2-18. Interspinous diameter measured on bony pelvis.

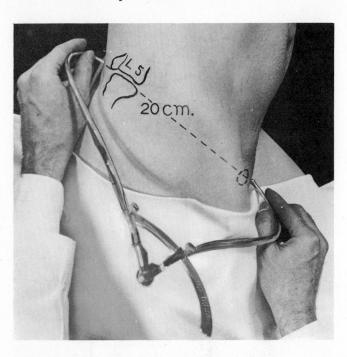

FIG. 2-19. Method of measuring external conjugate diameter (Baudelocque's diameter).

diameters. For all the pelvic measurements just described, the patient lies on her side or on her back, according to the diameter to be measured, with the abdomen exposed.

The INTERNAL PELVIC MEASUREMENTS are made to determine the actual diameters of the inlet. The chief internal measurement taken is the *diagonal conjugate, or the distance between the sacral promontory and the lower margin of the symphysis pubis*. The patient should be placed on her back on the examining table with her knees drawn up and her feet supported by stirrups. Two fingers are introduced into the vagina, and, before measuring

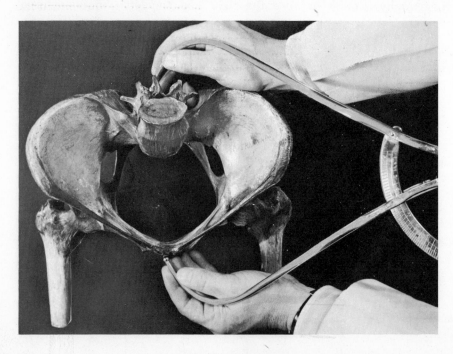

FIG. 2-20. External conjugate diameter measured on bony pelvis.

FIG. 2-21. Method of obtaining diagonal conjugate diameter (solid line). The upper broken line represents the conjugata vera, and the lower broken line represents the obstetric conjugata.

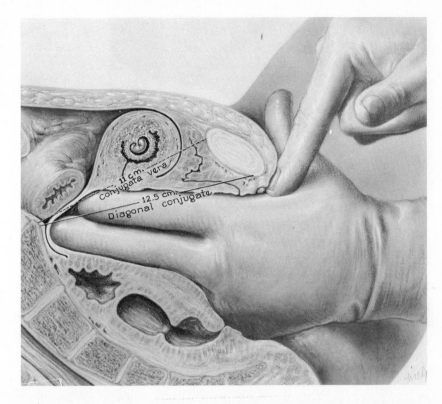

the diagonal conjugate, some evaluation of the pelvis is made by palpation: the height of the symphysis pubis and the shape of the pubic arch, the motility of the coccyx, the inclination of the anterior wall of the sacrum and the side walls of the pelvis and the prominence of the ischial spines.

In order to obtain the length of the diagonal conjugate, the 2 fingers passed into the vagina are pressed inward and upward as far as pos-

sible until the middle finger rests on the sacral promontory. The point on the back of the hand just under the symphysis is then marked by putting the index finger of the other hand on the exact point (Fig. 2-21), after which the fingers are withdrawn and measured. The distance from the tip of the middle finger to the point marked represents the *diagonal conjugate measurement*. This distance may be measured with a rigid measuring scale attached to

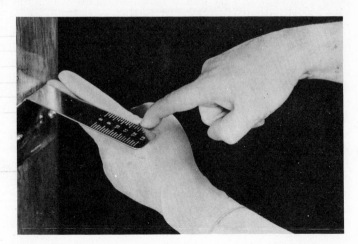

FIG. 2-22. Method of measuring diagonal conjugate diameter as obtained in Figure 2-21, using wall bracket.

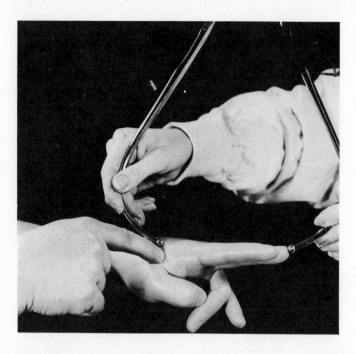

Fig. 2-23. Method of measuring diagonal conjugate diameter as obtained in Figure 2-21, using pelvimeter.

the wall (Fig. 2-22) or with a pelvimeter (Fig. 2-23), but the former is preferred because there is less chance of error. If the measurement is greater than 11.5 cm., it is justifiable to assume that the pelvic inlet is of adequate size for childbirth. In common medical parlance this measurement is often referred to as the "C.D." (conjugata diagonalis).

An extremely important internal diameter is the *true conjugate* or, in Latin, the conjugata vera (C.V.), which is the distance between the posterior aspect of the symphysis pubis and the promontory of the sacrum. However, direct measurement of this diameter cannot be made except by means of a roentgenogram; consequently, it has to be estimated from the diagonal conjugate measurement. It is believed that if 1.5 to 2 cm., according to the height and the inclination of the symphysis pubis, is deducted from the length of the diagonal conjugate, the true conjugate is obtained. For example, if the diagonal conjugate measures 12.5 cm., and the symphysis pubis is considered to be "average," then the conjugata vera may be estimated as being about 11.0 cm. In this method the problem consists of estimating the length of one side of a triangle, the conjugata vera; the other two sides, the diagonal conjugate and the height of the symphysis pubis, are known. If the symphysis

pubis is high and has a marked inclination, the physician takes this into consideration and may deduct 2 cm. The length of the true conjugate, or conjugata vera, is of utmost importance, since it is about the smallest diameter of the inlet through which the baby's head must pass. Indeed, the main purpose in measuring the diagonal conjugate is to give an estimate of the size of the conjugata vera.

Students sometimes are confused when they are confronted with the term "obstetric conjugate." This term identifies a diameter which begins at the sacral promontory and terminates just below the conjugata vera on the inner surface of the symphysis pubis, a few millimeters below its upper margin (Fig. 2-21). The *obstetric conjugate* is in reality the shortest diameter through which the infant's head must pass as it descends into the true pelvis. A distinction is rarely made between the *conjugata vera* and the *obstetric conjugate*, except in x-ray pelvimetry (pp. 38, 39).

Next to the diagonal conjugate measurement the most important clinical dimension of the pelvis is the transverse diameter of the outlet, the diameter between the ischial tuberosities. This is sometimes called the *tuberischii diameter* (often abbreviated T.I.), or biischial diameter, or intertuberous diameter (Fig. 2-8). This measurement is taken with the patient in

FIG. 2-24. Method of measuring tuberischii or intertuberous diameter of outlet, using the Williams' pelvimeter. The measurement is made on a line with the lower border of the anus.

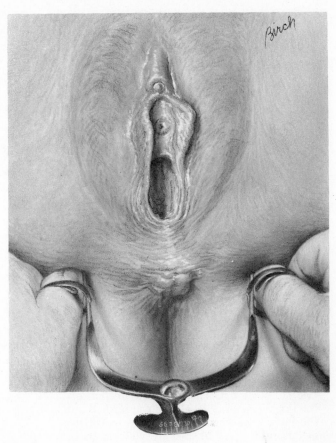

the lithotomy position, well down on the table and with the legs widely separated. The measurement is taken from the innermost and lowermost aspect of the ischial tuberosities, on a level with the lower border of the anus. The instruments usually employed are the Williams' pelvimeter (Figs. 2-24, 25) or the Thoms' pelvimeter. A diameter in excess of 8 cm. is considered average.

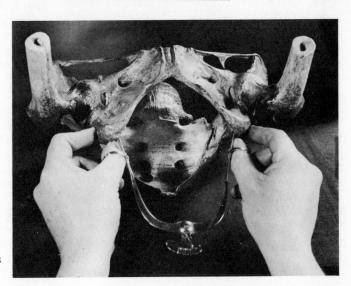

FIG. 2-25. Tuberischii or intertuberous diameter measured on bony pelvis.

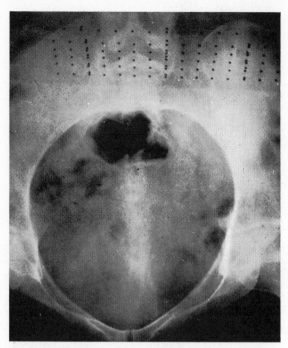

FIG. 2-26. Pelvic inlet roentgenogram. The scale represents corrected centimeters for various levels of the pelvic canal. The top line is used for measuring the diameters of the inlet. The other levels are established on the lateral roentgenogram. Pelvic morphology is readily established by viewing both lateral and inlet views. (Herbert Thoms, M.D., Yale School of Medicine)

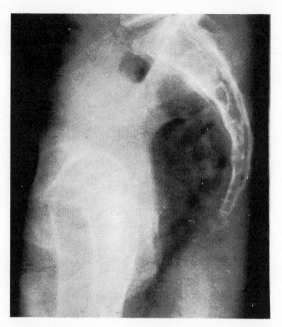

FIG. 2-27. Lateral roentgenogram. The scale represents corrected centimeters in the mid-plane of the body. By means of calipers the various diameters may be measured. The lateral morphologic aspects are readily visualized. (Herbert Thoms, M.D., Yale School of Medicine)

X-ray Pelvimetry

The most accurate means of determining pelvic size is x-ray pelvimetry. But this subjects the maternal ovaries and the fetal gonads to a certain amount of irradiation. Although the amount involved is minimal, exposure of pregnant women to irradiation should be avoided unless this procedure is really necessary. Hence x-ray pelvimetry never is used routinely but only in cases in which there are sound reasons for suspecting pelvic contraction, such as small manual measurements or a history of difficult labor in the past.

Possibly the most widely used method, and one of the simplest, is that of Dr. Herbert Thoms, of New Haven, Conn., a pioneer worker in this field. For a complete study two roentgenograms are made as follows:

1. The patient is placed on the x-ray table in a semirecumbent position so that her pelvic inlet is horizontal and as nearly parallel as possible with the plate beneath her (Fig. 2-26). The exact plane in which the patient's inlet lies, both front and back, is now determined and recorded. After an exposure of the film has been made, the patient is removed from the table, and a lead plate or grid containing perforations a centimeter apart is placed in the plane previously occupied by the inlet of the patient. Another exposure now is made on the same film. When the latter is developed, the outline of the inlet is shown, as are also the dots produced by the perforations in the lead plate. Since the projected dots on the film represent centimeters in the plane of the inlet, the diameters of the inlet can be read off directly as centimeters.

2. A somewhat similar procedure is carried out with the patient standing and from the lateral view (Fig. 2-27). Here, however, an upright lead and iron rod, with a centimeter scale notched on its edge, is placed posterior to the

Fig. 2-28. External organs of reproduction.

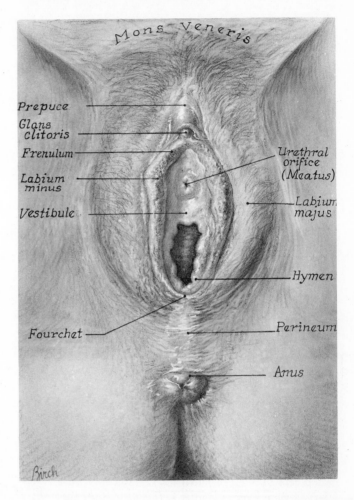

Mons Veneris

Prepuce

Glans clitoris

Frenulum

Labium minus

Vestibule

Fourchet

Urethral orifice (Meatus)

Labium majus

Hymen

Perineum

Anus

Birch

patient and close to the gluteal fold. After an exposure has been made, the developed film will show a lateral view of the symphysis pubis, the sacral promontory, other bony landmarks and, in addition, of course, the notched centimeter scale for establishing the distance between important points. Diameters which may be measured by x-ray pelvimetry are the obstetric conjugate, posterior sagittal at the inlet, midpelvis and outlet, and the anteroposterior diameter at the midpelvis and outlet.

Other technics entail the use of stereoscopic procedures which allow the physician to view the films with 3-dimensional vision and thus gain a clear image of all pelvic relationships.

When roentgenograms are made late in pregnancy by any of these methods, it is possible to secure also an impression of the size of the baby's head. When this is considered in relation to the pelvic picture, helpful information may be obtained in forecasting whether or not this particular pelvis is large enough to allow this particular baby to pass through.

Preventive Care Based on Pelvimetry. The importance of the knowledge gained through skillful performance of external and internal pelvimetry cannot be overestimated. Especially it should never be neglected in the case of a woman pregnant for the first time, or in any case in which the patient has suffered previously from difficult or tedious labors.

FEMALE ORGANS OF REPRODUCTION

The female organs of reproduction are divided into two groups—the external and the internal (Figs. 2-28 to 33).

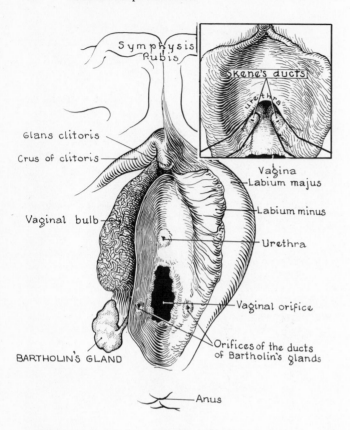

Glans clitoris

Crus of clitoris

Vaginal bulb

BARTHOLIN'S GLAND

Symphysis Pubis

Skene's ducts

urethra

Vagina

Labium majus

Labium minus

Urethra

Vaginal orifice

Orifices of the ducts of Bartholin's glands

Anus

FIG. 2-29. The vestibule, showing the urethra, the vaginal orifice and Bartholin's glands. Insert shows the orifices of the ducts of Skene's glands, which open just within the urethral meatus.

External Organs

The external female reproductive organs are called the *vulva* (L., covering). This includes everything which is visible externally from the lower margin of the pubis to the perineum, namely, the mons veneris, the labia majora and minora, the clitoris, the vestibule, the hymen, the urethral opening and various glandular and vascular structures (Fig. 2-28). The term "vulva" often has been used to refer simply to the labia majora and minora.

The mons veneris is a firm, cushionlike formation over the symphysis pubis and is covered with crinkly hair.

The labia majora are 2 prominent longitudinal folds of adipose tissue covered with skin which extend downward and backward from the mons veneris and disappear in forming the anterior border of the perineal body. These 2 thick folds of skin are covered with hair on their outer surfaces after the age of puberty but are smooth and moist on their inner surfaces. At the bottom they fade away into the perineum posteriorly, joining together to form

a transverse fold, the posterior commissure, situated directly in front of the fourchet. This fatty tissue is supplied with an abundant plexus of veins which may rupture as the result of injury sustained during labor and give rise to an extravasation of blood or hematoma.

The labia minora are 2 thin folds of reddish tissue covered entirely with thin membrane and situated between the labia majora, with their outer surfaces in contact with the inner surfaces of the labia majora; the labia minora extend from the clitoris downward and backward on either side of the orifice of the vagina. In the upper extremity each labium minus separates into two branches which when united with those of the opposite side enclose the clitoris. The upper fold forms the prepuce and the lower the frenum of the clitoris. At the bottom the labia minora pass almost imperceptibly into the labia majora or blend together as a thin fold of skin forming the anterior edge of the perineum or perineal body. This thin edge is known as the fourchet.

The clitoris is a small, highly sensitive projection composed of erectile tissue, nerves and

FIG. 2-30. Muscles of the pelvic floor. (After Dickinson)

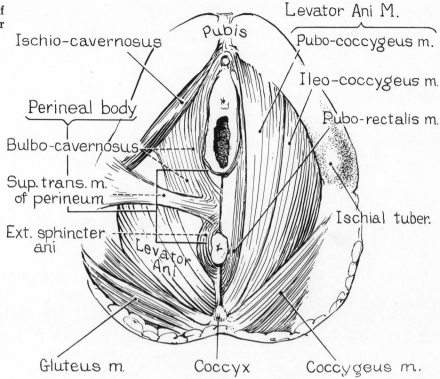

blood vessels and is covered with a thin epidermis. It is analogous to the penis in the male and is regarded as the chief seat of voluptuous sensation. The clitoris is so situated that it is partially hidden between the anterior ends of the labia minora.

The vestibule is the almond-shaped area which is enclosed by the labia minora and extends from the clitoris to the fourchet. It is perforated by 4 openings: the urethra, the vaginal opening, the ducts of Bartholin's glands and the ducts of Skene's glands. Bartholin's glands are 2 small glands situated beneath the vestibule on either side of the vaginal opening. During sexual excitement varying amounts of mucoid material are secreted by these glands. In women infected with gonorrhea, these ducts sometimes harbor gonococci, which may cause the glands to suppurate, so that the entire labia become distended by pus. Skene's ducts open upon the vestibule on either side of the urethra (Fig. 2-29).

The hymen marks the division between the internal and the external organs. It is a thin fold of mucous membrane situated at the ori-

fice of the vagina. It may be entirely absent, or it may form a complete septum across the lower end of the vagina. In women who have had children the irregularity of torn edges remains. The hymen presents marked differences in shape and consistency. In the newborn child it projects beyond the surrounding parts. In adult virgins it is a membrane of varying thickness which closes the vaginal opening more or less completely and presents an aperture which varies in size from a pinpoint to one which will readily admit 1 or even 2 fingers. The opening is circular or crescentic in shape. In rare instances the hymen may be imperforate and cause retention of menstrual discharge if it occludes the vaginal orifice completely.

The perineum consists of muscles and fascia of the urogenital diaphragm, which lies across the pubic arch, and the pelvic diaphragm, which consists of the coccygeus and the levator ani muscles. The levator ani is the larger and consists of 3 portions: the iliococcygeus, the pubococcygeus and puborectalis. These muscles form a slinglike support for the pelvic structure, and between them pass the urethra, the

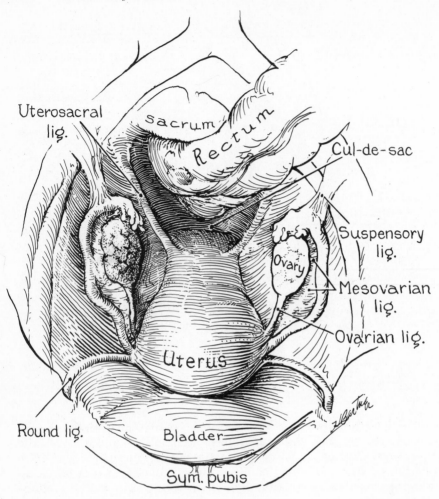

Uterosacral
lig.

sacrum

Rectum

Cul-de-sac

Ovary

Suspensory
lig.

Mesovarian
lig.

Ovarian lig.

Round lig.

Uterus

Bladder

Sym. pubis

Fig. 2-31. Pelvic contents from above, showing the position of the pairs of ligaments and the relationship to the uterus, the tubes and the ovaries. (After Dickinson)

vagina and the rectum (Fig. 2-30). Between the anus and the vagina the levator ani is reinforced by a central tendon of the perineum to which 3 pairs of muscles converge: the bulbocavernosus, the superficial transverse muscles of the perineum and the external sphincter ani. These structures constitute the perineal body and form the main support of the perineal floor. They often are lacerated during delivery.

Internal Organs

The internal organs of reproduction are the vagina, the uterus, the fallopian tubes and the ovaries.

Ovaries. The ovaries are 2 small almond-shaped organs situated in the upper part of the pelvic cavity, one on either side of the uterus. Their chief functions are the develop-

ment and the expulsion of ova and the provision of certain internal secretions (hormones). These organs correspond to the testes in the male. They lie embedded in the posterior fold of the broad ligament of the uterus (Fig. 2-31) and are supported by the suspensory, the ovarian and the mesovarian ligaments.

Each ovary contains in its substance at birth a large number of germ cells or ovules (primordial ova) (p. 54). This huge store of primordial follicles present at birth more than suffices the woman for life. It is usually believed that no more are formed, and that this large initial store is gradually exhausted during the period of sexual maturity. Beginning at about the time of puberty, 1 (or possibly 2) of the follicles which contain the ovules enlarges each month, gradually approaches the surface of the ovary and bursts (Fig. 3-1). The

FIG. 2-32. Pelvic contents in median section with the subject on her back. (Robert L. Dickinson, M.D., New York)

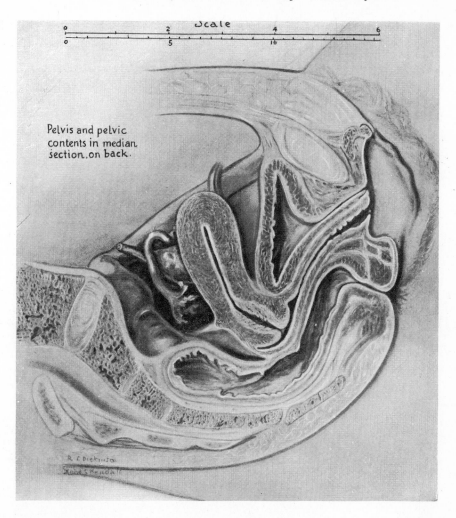

Pelvis and pelvic contents in median section, on back.

ovum and the fluid content of the follicle are liberated on the exterior of the ovary into the abdominal cavity; then they are swept into the tube and so pass into the uterus. The development and the maturation of the follicles (containing the ova) and the ova continue from puberty to menopause.

The arteries which supply the ovary are 4 or 5 branches that arise from the anastomosis of the ovarian artery with the ovarian branch of the uterine (Fig. 2-34). The veins proceeding from the ovary become tributary to both the uterine and the ovarian plexus.

The nerves supplying the ovaries are derived from the craniosacral and the thoracolumbar sympathetic systems. The postganglionic and visceral afferent fibers form a plexus surrounding the ovarian artery, which in turn is formed by contributions from the renal and the aortic plexuses and corresponds to the spermatic plexus in the male.

Fallopian Tubes. The fallopian tubes (Figs. 2-31, 34, 36, 3-1, 4-5) are 2 trumpet-shaped, thin, flexible, muscular tubes, about 4½ inches long and somewhat thinner than a lead pencil. They extend from the upper angles of the uterus, the cornua, in the upper margin of the broad ligament, toward the sides of the pelvis. They have 2 openings: one into the uterine cavity and the other into the abdominal cavity. The opening into the uterine cavity is minute and will admit only a fine bristle. The abdominal opening is somewhat larger and is surrounded by a large number of fine fringes; hence the term "fimbriated end." The fimbriated extremity lies in the neighborhood of the ovary, but it is not necessarily in direct contact with it. It is generally believed that the cilia upon the fimbriated end of the tube give rise to a current in the capillary layer of fluid lying between the various pelvic organs. The fallopian tubes convey the discharged ova by peristaltic action from the ovaries to the cavity of the uterus; by their tentaclelike processes the fimbriated ends of the tube draw the escaped ova into the tube. Thus, the function of the fallopian tube is to conduct the ovum along the canal by peristaltic action until it reaches the uterus.

The tubes are lined with mucous membrane containing ciliated epithelium. The muscular layer is made up of longitudinal and circular fibers which provide peristaltic action. The serous membrane covering the tubes is a continuation of the peritoneum, which lines the whole abdominal cavity.

The fallopian tubes receive their blood supply from the ovarian and the uterine arteries (Fig. 2-34). The veins of the tubes follow the course of these arteries and empty into the uterine and the ovarian trunks. The nerves which supply the uterus supply the tubes.

Uterus. The uterus is a hollow thick-walled, muscular organ (Figs. 2-31, 32, 33). It serves two important functions: (1) it is the organ of menstruation and (2) during pregnancy it receives the fertilized ovum and retains and nourishes it until it expels the products of conception at the time of labor.

The uterus varies in size and shape according to the age of the individual and whether or not she has borne children. The uterus of the adult nullipara weighs approximately 60 Gm. and measures 5.5 to 8 cm. in length. It resembles a flattened pear in appearance and has two divisions: the upper triangular portion, the corpus, and the lower constricted cylindric portion, the cervix, which projects into the vagina. The fallopian tubes extend from the cornu (L., horn) of the uterus at the upper outer margin on either side. The upper rounded portion of the uterus between the points of insertion of the fallopian tubes is called the fundus (Fig. 2-33).

The nonpregnant uterus is situated in the

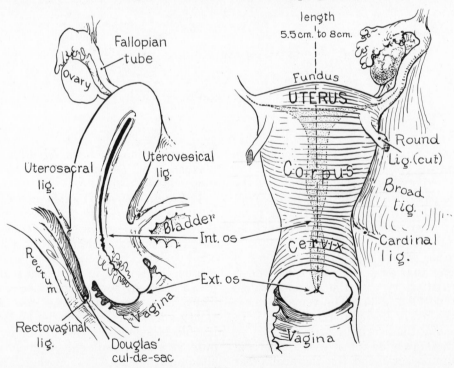

Fig. 2-33. Lateral and anterior views of the uterus. The ligaments which support the uterus in the pelvic cavity are the broad ligaments (2), the round ligaments (2), the uterosacral ligaments (2).

pelvic cavity between the bladder and the rectum. Almost the entire posterior wall and the upper portion of the anterior wall is covered by peritoneum. The lower portion of the anterior wall is united to the bladder wall by a thick layer of connective tissue. The lower posterior wall of the uterus and the upper portion of the vagina are separated from the rectum by an area called Douglas' cul-de-sac. Due to its

muscular composition, the uterus is capable of enlarging to the size of a pumpkin; at the termination of pregnancy it weighs about 2 pounds. It is made up of involuntary muscle fibers arranged in all directions, making expansion possible in every direction to accommodate the products of conception. Due to the nature of this arrangement of the muscle, the uterus is able to expel its contents at the ter-

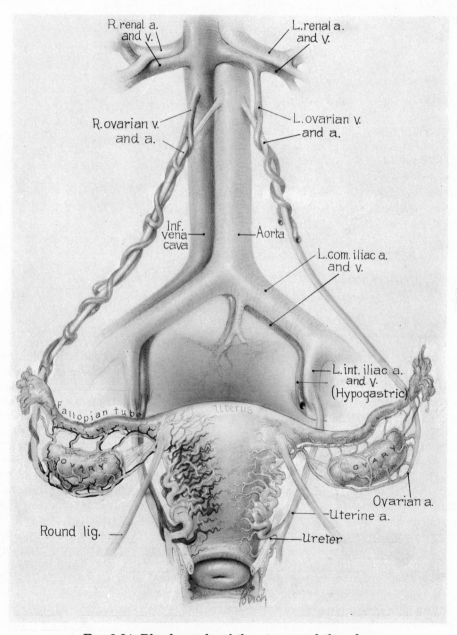

Fig. 2-34. Blood supply of the uterus and the adnexa.

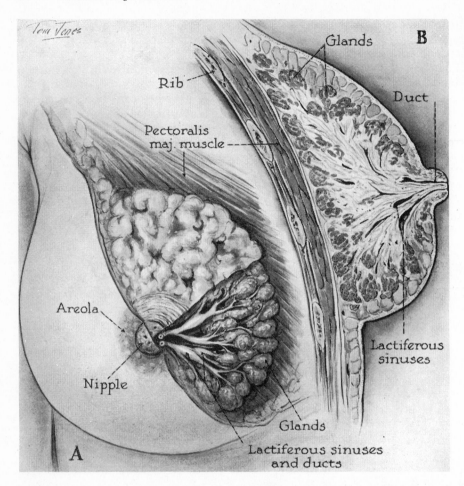

Rib

Pectoralis
maj. muscle

Areola

Nipple

A

Glands

Glands

Lactiferous sinuses
and ducts

Glands   B

Duct

Lactiferous
sinuses

FIG. 2-35. (A) Mammary gland, showing the lactiferous ducts and sinuses. (B) Cross section of the breast.

mination of normal labor (Fig. 6-7). Arranged between these muscular layers are many blood vessels, lymphatics and nerves.

The cavity of the uterus is very small and somewhat triangular in shape, being widest at the fundus, between the very small openings into the canals of the fallopian tubes, and narrowest below at the opening into the cervix. The anterior and the posterior walls lie almost in contact, so that if a cross section of the uterus could be examined, the cavity between them would appear as a mere slit. The uterus is lined with mucous membrane (endometrium) and is divided into 2 parts: the cavity of the body of the uterus and the cavity of the cervix.

The cervix is less freely movable than is the body of the uterus. Its muscular wall is not so thick, and the mucous membrane lining its cavity (cervical endometrium) is different in

that it is much folded and contains more glands, which produce mucus and are the chief source of the mucous secretion during pregnancy. The cervix has an upper opening called the internal os, leading from the cavity of the uterine body into the cervical canal, and a lower opening called the external os, opening into the vagina. The cervix is very small in the nonpregnant woman, barely admitting a probe, but at the time of labor it dilates to a size sufficient to permit the passage of the fetus (Fig. 10-6).

LIGAMENTS. The uterus is supported in two ways: by ligaments extending from either half of the uterus (Fig. 2-33) and by the muscles of the pelvic floor (Fig. 2-30). The ligaments which support the uterus in the pelvic cavity are the broad ligaments (2) (Fig. 2-33), the round ligaments (2), and the uterosacral (2). The broad ligaments are 2 winglike structures which extend from the lateral margins of the uterus to the pelvic walls and serve to divide the pelvic cavity into an anterior and a posterior compartment. Each consists of folds of peritoneum which envelop the fallopian tubes, the ovaries and the round and the ovarian ligaments. Its lower portion, the *cardinal ligament* (Fig. 2-33), is composed of dense connective tissue which is firmly united to the supravaginal portion of the cervix. The median margin is connected with the lateral margin of the uterus and encloses the uterine vessels. The round ligaments are 2 fibrous cords which are attached on either side of the fundus just below the fallopian tubes. They extend forward through the inguinal canal and terminate in the upper portion of the labia majora. These ligaments aid in holding the fundus forward. The uterosacral ligaments are 2 cordlike structures which extend from the posterior cervical portion of the uterus to the sacrum. These aid in supporting the cervix. The uterovesical ligament is merely a fold of the peritoneum which passes over the fundus and extends over the bladder. The rectovaginal ligament is a fold of the peritoneum which passes over the posterior surface of the uterus and is reflected upon the rectum.

UTERINE BLOOD SUPPLY. The uterus receives its blood supply from the ovarian and the uterine arteries (Fig. 2-34). The uterine artery, the principal source, is the main branch of the hypogastric, which enters the base of the broad ligament and makes its way to the side of the uterus. The ovarian artery is a branch of the aorta. It enters the broad ligament and on reaching the ovary breaks up into smaller branches which enter that organ, while its main stem makes its way to the upper margin of the uterus, where it anastomoses with the ovarian branch of the uterine artery.

The uterovaginal plexus returns the blood from the uterus and the vagina. These veins form a plexus of exceedingly thin-walled vessels which are embedded in the layers of the uterine muscle. Emerging from this plexus, the trunks join the uterine vein, which is a double vein. These veins follow on either side of the uterine artery and eventually form one trunk, emptying into the hypogastric vein, which makes its way into the internal iliac.

UTERINE NERVE SUPPLY. The uterus possesses an abundant nerve supply derived principally from the sympathetic nervous system but partly from the cerebrospinal and parasympathetic system. Both the sympathetic and the parasympathetic nerve supplies contain motor and a few sensory fibers. The functions of the nerve supply of the 2 systems are in great part antagonistic. The sympathetic causes muscular contraction and vasoconstriction; the parasympathetic inhibits contraction and leads to vasodilatation.

Since the uterus is a freely movable organ suspended in the pelvic cavity between the bladder and the rectum, the position of the uterus may be influenced by a full bladder or rectum, which pushes it backward or forward (see Figs. 2-32, 36). The uterus also changes its position when the patient stands, lies flat or turns on her side. Also, there are abnormalities such as anteflexion, in which the fundus is tipped too far forward (Fig. 2-36); retroversion, in which it is tipped too far backward (Fig. 2-36); and prolapse, due to the relaxation of the muscles of the pelvic floor and the uterine ligaments.

LYMPHATIC VESSELS. The lymphatic vessels drain into the lumbar lymph nodes.

Vagina. The vagina is a dilatable passage lined with mucous membrane situated between the bladder and the rectum. The vaginal opening occupies the lower portion of the vestibule and in the virgin appears almost completely closed by the hymen. The vagina is from 3 to 5 inches in length, and at the upper end is a blind vault, commonly called the fornix, into which the lower portion of the cervix projects. The fornices (plural of fornix) are divided into 4 parts for convenience of description. The lateral fornices are the spaces between the vaginal wall on either side and the cervix; the anterior fornix is between the anterior vaginal wall and the cervix; the posterior fornix is between the posterior vaginal wall and the cervix. The posterior fornix is considerably deeper than the anterior since the vagina is attached higher up on the posterior than the anterior wall of the cervix. The fornices are important because the physician is usually able to palpate the internal pelvic organs through their thin walls. The vagina serves 3 important functions: it represents the excretory duct of the uterus through which its secretion and the menstrual flow escape, it is the female organ of copulation, and it forms part of the birth

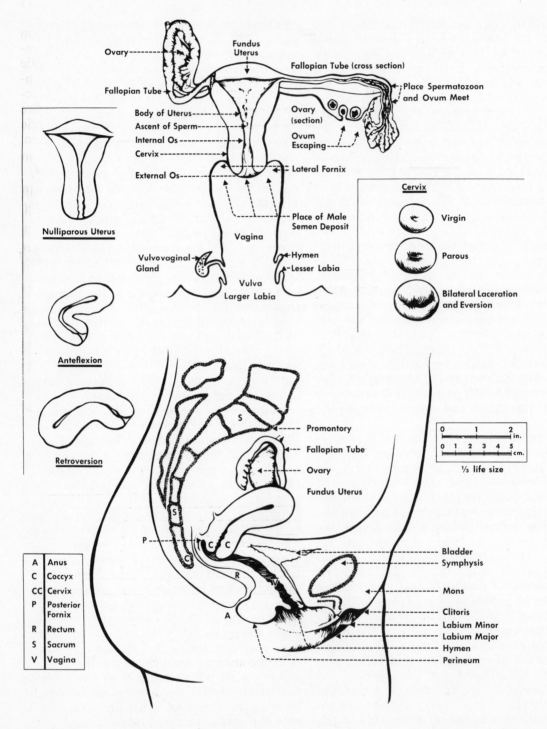

FIG. 2-36. Female anatomy. (Dickinson, Robert L.: Human Sex Anatomy, Baltimore, Williams & Wilkins)

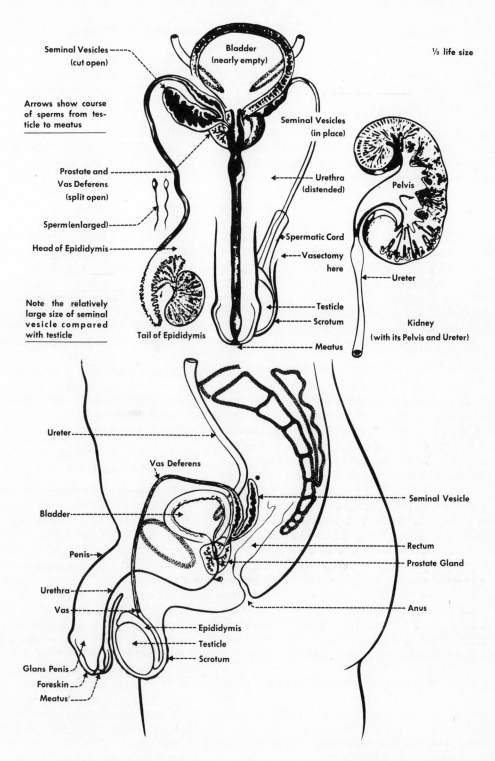

FIG. 2-37. Male anatomy. (Dickinson: Human Sex Anatomy, Williams & Wilkins)

canal during labor. Its walls are arranged into thick folds, the columns of the vagina, and in women who have not borne children, numerous ridges or rugae extend outward and almost at right angles to the vaginal columns and give the surface a corrugated appearance. Normally, the anterior and the posterior walls of the vagina lie in contact, but they are capable of stretching to allow marked distention of the passage, as in the process of childbirth. The vagina is kept moist by a small amount of secretion from the uterus.

The vagina receives its abundant blood supply from branches of the uterine, the inferior vesical, the median hemorrhoidal and the internal pudic arteries. The passage is surrounded by a venous plexus; the vessels follow the course of the arteries and eventually empty into the hypogastric veins. The lymphatics empty into the inguinal, the hypogastric and the iliac glands.

Related Pelvic Organs

Bladder. The bladder is a thin, muscular sac which serves as a reservoir for the urine. It is situated in front of the uterus and behind the symphysis pubis. When empty or only moderately distended, it remains entirely in the pelvis, but if it becomes greatly distended, it rises into the abdomen. Urine is conducted into the bladder by the ureters, 2 small tubes which extend down from the basin of the kidneys over the brim of the pelvis and open into the bladder at about the level of the cervix. The bladder is emptied through the urethra, a short tube which terminates in the meatus (Fig. 2-28). Lying on either side of the urethra and almost parallel with it are 2 small glands, less than 1 inch long, known as Skene's glands. Their ducts empty into the urethra just above the meatus. Often in cases of gonorrhea, Skene's glands and ducts are involved (see Fig. 2-29).

Anus. The anus is the entrance to the rectal canal. The rectal canal is surrounded at the opening or anus by its sphincter muscle, which binds it to the coccyx behind and to the perineum in front. It is supported by the muscles passing into it (see Fig. 2-30).

The muscles involved are those that aid in supporting the pelvic floor. The rectum is considered here because of the proximity to the field of delivery.

MAMMARY GLANDS

The *breasts*, or mammary glands, are 2 highly specialized cutaneous glands located on either side of the anterior wall of the chest between the 3rd and the 7th ribs (Fig. 2-35). Because they are abundantly supplied with nerves, formerly it was believed that direct nervous system connection existed between the uterus and the breasts. But the demonstration that lactation can be established after excluding the spinal nervous mechanism by severing all nerves supplying the breasts clearly indicated that some other factor must be involved in the explanation of mammary changes in pregnancy. It is evident that the stimulation to growth of the mammary gland is hormonal and not nervous in origin.

The internal mammary and the intercostal arteries supply the breast gland, and the mammary veins follow these arteries. Also, there are many cutaneous veins which become dilated during lactation. The lymphatics are abundant, especially toward the axilla. These breast glands are present in the male, but only in the rudimentary state, and are not connected by the sympathetic system to the male generative organs.

Internal Structure

The breasts of a woman who never has borne a child are, in general, conic or hemispheric in form, but they vary in size and shape at different ages and in different individuals. In women who have nursed one or more babies they tend to become pendulous. At the termination of lactation, certain exercises aid in restoring the tone of the breast tissue.

The breasts are made up of glandular tissue and fat. Each organ is divided into 15 or 20 lobes, which are separated from each other by fibrous and fatty walls. Each lobe is subdivided into many lobules, and these contain numerous acini cells. The acini are composed of a single layer of epithelium, beneath which is a small amount of connective tissue richly supplied with capillaries. By the process of osmosis the products necessary for the milk are filtered from the blood, but the secretion of the milk really begins in the acini cells. As the ducts leading from the lobules to the lobes and from the lobes approach the nipple, they are dilated to form little reservoirs in which the milk is stored; they narrow again as they pass into the nipple. The size of the breast is dependent on the amount of fatty tissue present and in no way denotes the amount of lactation possible.

External Structure

The external surface of the breasts is divided into 3 portions. The first is the white, smooth and soft area of skin extending from the circumference of the gland to the areola. The second is the areola, which surrounds the nipple and is of a delicate pinkish hue in blondes and a darker rose color in brunettes. The surface of the areola is more or less roughened by small fine lumps of papillae, known as the glands of Montgomery (Plate 3, *right, bottom*). These enlarged sebaceous glands, white in color and scattered over the areola, become more marked during pregnancy. Under the influence of gestation, the areola becomes darker in shade, and this pigmentation, which is more marked in brunettes than in blondes, in many cases constitutes a helpful sign of pregnancy (Plate 4). The nipple or third portion is largely composed of sensitive, erectile tissue and forms a large conic papilla projecting from the center of the areola and having at its summit the openings of the milk ducts. These openings may be from 3 to 20 in number. The care of the breasts (see Chap. 8) constitutes one of the important phases of the nursing care of the maternity patient throughout pregnancy and the puerperium.

MALE ORGANS OF REPRODUCTION

The male reproductive system consists of the testes and a system of excretory ducts with their accessory structures (Fig. 2-37).

External Organs

The scrotum and the penis are called the external genitalia. The scrotum contains the testes and may be considered as an evagination of the body wall or a continuation of the abdominal cavity. In the adult male the testes have descended into the scrotal sac, and the canal connecting the sac with the abdominal cavity has closed, although it is open in the fetus.

The penis, the male organ of copulation, consists of the cavernous bodies (erectile parts) and a urethra through which the seminal fluid is brought to the female generative tract. The cavernous bodies contain blood spaces which are usually quite empty, and the organ is flaccid. When these spaces fill with blood, the organ becomes turgid. The flow of blood is controlled by the autonomic nervous system (vasodilator fibers) and varies with sexual activity. The enlarged conic structure at the free end of the penis which contains the external orifice of the urethra is called the glans penis. The glans is almost completely enclosed by a fold of skin called the prepuce or foreskin. At circumcision this part of the skin is removed.

Internal Organs

The internal organs consist of the testes and a canal system with accessory structures. Each testis is a compound gland, divided into lobules. These contain the terminal portions of the seminiferous tubules which join repeatedly and eventually form the single much-coiled tube of the epididymis. The epithelium lining the tubules consists of supporting cells and spermatogenetic cells which produce the spermatozoa. In the human testes, spermatogenesis begins at the age of puberty and continues throughout life. However, the seminiferous tubules undergo gradual involution with advancing age.

The blood supply to the testes is derived from the internal spermatic arteries. The arteries and the veins form a part of the spermatic cords.

The lymphatic vessels accompany the blood vessels in the spermatic cord, and eventually the lymphatics empty into the lumbar lymph nodes.

The efferent nerves which supply the testes are derived from the thoracolumbar and sacral divisions of the autonomic system. They are distributed chiefly to the walls of the blood vessels. Afferent fibers convey impulses from these structures to the central nervous system.

The canal system consists of the epididymis (which is made up of numerous seminiferous tubules), the ductus deferens (which passes from the epididymis to the ejaculatory duct), the ejaculatory duct (formed by the union of the ductus deferens and the duct of the seminal vesicle) and the urethra, which is surrounded by the prostate gland and terminates in the penis.

The accessory structures consist of the seminal vesicles (sacculated structures located behind the bladder and in front of the rectum), the prostate gland (which surrounds the base of the urethra and the ejaculatory duct) and the bulbo-urethral glands or Cowper's glands (which lie at the base of the prostate and on either side of the membranous urethra).

SUGGESTED READING

Anthony, C. P.: Textbook of Anatomy and Physiology, ed. 6, St. Louis, Mosby, 1963.

Caldwell, W. E., and Moloy, H. C.: Anatomical variations in the female pelvis and their effect in labor with a suggested classification, Am. J. Obstet. Gynec. 26:479, 1933.

Eastman, N. J., and Hellman, L. M.: Williams Obstetrics, ed. 12, New York, Appleton, 1961.

Greisheimer, E. M.: Physiology and Anatomy, ed. 8, Philadelphia, Lippincott, 1963.

Netter, F. H.: Reproductive System, Summit, N. J., Ciba Pharmaceutical, 1954.

Chapter 3

Physiology in Relation to Human Reproduction

Only a brief statement of the most elementary facts of physiology, the science dealing with the functions of the organs and the tissues of the body, can be attempted here, but such a review is essential so that the nurse may better understand the special relation of physiology to the problems in obstetrics.

SEXUAL MATURITY

Evidences of sexual maturity in the female begin at the time of puberty with the establishment of the specific reproductive functions of ovulation and menstruation. At puberty certain well-defined changes take place; the establishment of the menses, the monthly bloody discharge from the uterus, is an indication that the internal organs have matured. Changes in the external organs, such as an increase in size and the appearance of axillary and pubic hair are other evidences of this period of development; the breasts at this time also become larger and more prominent. Along with these physical changes are emotional changes as well.

Puberty

Puberty usually occurs between the ages of 12 and 16, although heredity, race, climate and environment may influence its early or late appearance; for example, maturity tends to appear earlier in warm climates and later in cold regions. The reproductive period covers about 30 years, from the beginning of menstruation at or about the age of 12 until its cessation during the menopause at about the age of 45 to 50.

Ovulation and Menstruation

Ovulation. Each month, with considerable regularity, a blisterlike structure about half an inch in diameter develops on the surface of one or the other ovary. Inside this bubble, almost lost in the fluid about it, lies a tiny speck, scarcely visible to the naked eye; a thimble would hold 3 million of them. This little speck is the human ovum—a truly amazing structure. It not only possesses within its diminutive compass the potentialities of developing into a human being with all the complicated physical organization entailed, but also embodies the mental as well as the physical traits of the woman and her forebears: perhaps her own brown eyes or her father's tall stature; possibly her mother's love of music or her grandfather's genius at mathematics. These and a million other potentialities are all wrapped in this little speck, or ovum, so small that it is about one fourth the size of the period at the end of this sentence.

With the exact periodicity which characterizes so many of Nature's works, one blister on one ovary bursts at a definite time each month and discharges an ovum, a process known as *ovulation.* The precise day on which ovulation occurs is a matter of no small importance. For instance, since the ovum can be fertilized (or impregnated by the male germ cell) only within the 36-hour period after its escape from the ovary, this is the only time when a woman is really fertile. During the rest of the monthly cycle, theoretically at least, it is impossible for her to conceive. Evidence of various sorts indicates that ovulation usually occurs between the 10th and the 16th days of the menstrual cycle, counting from the day on which bleeding begins. Ordinarily, then, the most fertile time is a week to 10 days after the cessation of menstruation. While this is the rule, there are many exceptions, and ovulation may take place at any time between the 9th and the 18th days of the cycle. The fact that ovulation rarely occurs during the last 10 days of a 28-day cycle has given rise to the birth-control doctrine of the "safe period," or "rhythm," according to which it is impossible to conceive after the 18th day. Theoretically, this claim is altogether sound; practically, not a few women appear to have conceived during this period, so that it would seem that occasionally ovulation may take place later than theory would indicate.

Graafian Follicle. In delving further into this process of ovulation, we find that at birth each ovary contains a huge number of undeveloped ova, probably more than 100,000. These are rather large round cells with clear cytoplasm and a good-sized nucleus occupying the center. Each of these ova is surrounded by a layer of a few small, flattened or spindle-shaped cells. The whole structure—ovum and surrounding cells—is spoken of as a "follicle," while in its underdeveloped state at birth it is referred to as a "primordial follicle." It is the consensus that the manufacture of these primordial follicles ceases at birth or shortly after, and that the large number contained in the ovaries of the newborn represents a lifetime's supply. Nevertheless, the majority of these disappear before puberty, so that there are then perhaps 30,000 or so left in each ovary. This disintegration of follicles continues throughout the reproductive period, with the result that usually none is found after the menopause.

Meanwhile, from birth to the menopause a certain few of these primordial follicles show signs of development. The surrounding granu-

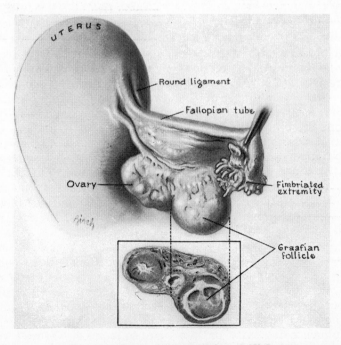

Fig. 3-1. Ovary with graafian follicle.

lar layer of cells begins to multiply rapidly until they are several layers deep, at the same time becoming cuboidal in shape. As this proliferation of cells continues, a very important fluid develops between them, the follicular fluid. After puberty this accumulates in such quantities that the multiplying follicle cells are pushed toward the margin, and the ovum itself is almost surrounded by fluid, being suspended from the periphery of the follicle by only a small neck or isthmus of cells. The structure is now known as the *graafian follicle*, after the famous Dutch physician who in 1672 first described it (Figs. 3-1, 2). While increasing in size so enormously, the graafian follicle naturally pushes aside other follicles, forming each month, as has been said, a very noticeable, blisterlike projection on the surface of the ovary. At one point the follicular capsule becomes thin, and as the ovum reaches full maturity, it breaks free from the few cells attaching it to the periphery and floats in the follicular fluid. The thinned area of the capsule now ruptures, and the ovum is expelled into the peritoneal cavity.

Changes in the Corpus Luteum. After the discharge of the ovum, the ruptured follicle undergoes a change. It becomes filled with large cells containing a special yellow colored matter called lutein. The follicle then is known as the corpus luteum or yellow body. If pregnancy does not occur, the corpus luteum reaches full development in about 8 days, then retrogresses and is gradually replaced by fibrous tissue, corpus albicans. If pregnancy does occur, the corpus luteum enlarges somewhat and persists throughout the period of gestation, reaching its maximum size about the 4th or 5th month and retrogressing slowly thereafter. The corpus luteum secretes an extremely important substance, *progesterone*, which will be considered in a later section of this chapter.

MENSTRUAL CYCLE

Menstruation in Relation to Pregnancy

Menstruation is the periodic discharge of blood, mucus and epithelial cells from the uterus. If the individual is normal, it occurs throughout the reproductive period at fairly regular intervals of about 28 days, except during pregnancy and lactation, when usually it is suppressed entirely. Accordingly, the span of years during which childbearing usually is possible—that is, from the age of about 12 to 45—corresponds to the period during which menstruation occurs. In general, moreover, a woman who menstruates is able to conceive, whereas one who does not is probably sterile. There is good reason for believing, therefore, that these two phenomena are closely interlinked, and since no process of Nature is purposeless, that menstruation must play some vital and indispensable role in childbearing. What is this role?

If day by day we were privileged to watch the endometrium or lining membrane of the

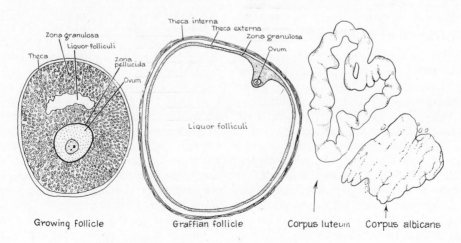

Fig. 3-2. Development of the graafian follicle.

uterus, we would observe some remarkable alterations. Immediately following the termination of a menstrual period, this membrane is very thin, measuring perhaps a twentieth of an inch in depth. Each day thereafter it becomes a trifle thicker and harbors an increasing content of blood, while its glands become more and more active, secreting a rich nutritive substance that used to be called "uterine milk." About a week before the onset of the next expected period this process reaches its height; the endometrium is now of the thickness of heavy, downy velvet and has become soft and succulent with blood and glandular secretions. At this time the egg, if one has been fertilized, embeds itself into this luxuriant lining.

All these changes have only one purpose: to provide a suitable bed in which the fertilized ovum may rest, secure nourishment and grow. If an egg is not fertilized, these alterations are unnecessary; accordingly, through a mechanism which even today is obscure, the swollen endometrium disintegrates, and the encased blood and glandular secretions escape into the uterine cavity; passing through the cervix, they flow out through the vagina, carrying the egg with them. In other words, menstruation represents the abrupt termination of a process designed to prepare board and lodging, as it were, for a fertilized ovum; it betokens the breakdown of a bed which was not needed because the "boarder" did not materialize; its purpose then is to clear away the old bed so that a new and fresh one may be created the next month.

Hormonal Control of Menstruation

The menstrual cycle is regulated primarily through the highly coordinated function of the pituitary, the ovaries and the uterus. If, while watching the changes in the endometrium during the menstrual cycle, as described above, it were possible to inspect the ovaries from day to day, it would be noted that the uterine alterations are related directly to certain phenomena that take place in the ovary. If it were possible to look further, one might see that the alterations which occur regularly in the ovarian cycle are related directly to certain phenomena which take place in the anterior pituitary gland. Thus, the whole sequence represents the harmonious, integrated reactions of several processes within the human organism, all of which are necessary to maintain proper relationships in the menstrual cycle.

Proliferative Phase. Immediately following menstruation, it will be recalled, the endometrium of the uterus is very thin. During the subsequent week or so it proliferates markedly. The cells on the surface become taller, while the glands which dip into the endometrium become longer and wider. As the result of these changes, the thickness of the endometrium increases 6-fold or 8-fold. During this phase of the menstrual cycle (from the 5th to the 14th days, approximately) a graafian follicle each month is approaching its greatest development and is manufacturing increasing amounts of follicular fluid. This fluid contains a most important substance, the estrogenic hormone, so-called *estrogen*. The word "hormone" comes from a Greek word which means "I bring about," and in the case of estrogen it brings about (among other things) the thickening of the endometrium described. Each month, then, after the cessation of menstruation, a developing graafian follicle produces this hormone, estrogen, as an ingredient of the follicular fluid; and estrogen acts on the endometrium to build it up. For this reason this phase of the menstrual cycle is more commonly referred to as the *proliferative phase*, although it is still sometimes referred to as the *follicular* or *estrogenic phase*. The first 4 or 5 days of this phase sometimes are called the resting or postmenstrual phase.

Secretory Phase. Following rupture of the graafian follicle (ovulation), the cells which form the corpus luteum begin to secrete, in addition to estrogen, another important hormone, *progesterone*. This supplements the action of estrogen on the endometrium in such a way that the glands become very tortuous or corkscrew in appearance and are greatly dilated. This change is due to the fact that they are swollen with a secretion containing large amounts of glycogen and mucin. Meanwhile, the blood supply of the endometrium is increased, with the result that it becomes very vascular and succulent. Since these effects are directed at providing a bed for the fertilized ovum, it is easy to understand why the hormone which brings them about is called "progesterone," meaning "for gestation." It is also clear why this phase of the cycle (from the 14th to the 28th days, approximately) is more commonly called the *secretory phase*, and why occasionally it is referred to as the *progestational, luteal* or *premenstrual phase*.

Menstrual Phase. Unless the ovum is fertilized, the corpus luteum is short-lived, and its activity ceases after about 10 days (or around the 25th day of the cycle). Since corpus luteum cells secrete not only progesterone but also estrogen, cessation of corpus luteum activity means a withdrawal of both of these hormones which have been responsible for building up the endometrium. As a result, the endometrium degenerates. This is associated with rupture of

countless small blood vessels in the endometrium with innumerable minute hemorrhages. Along with the blood, superficial fragments of the endometrium, together with mucin from the glands, are cast away, and all this constitutes the menstrual discharge (Fig. 3-3). Naturally, this phase of the cycle (the 1st to the 5th days, approximately) is called the *menstrual phase*.

Role of the Pituitary Gland. The pituitary gland is of considerable importance in the function of the reproductive system. The *anterior lobe* of the pituitary, the "master clock," secretes, among other hormones, two hormones whose function is to produce these ovarian alterations at fairly regular monthly

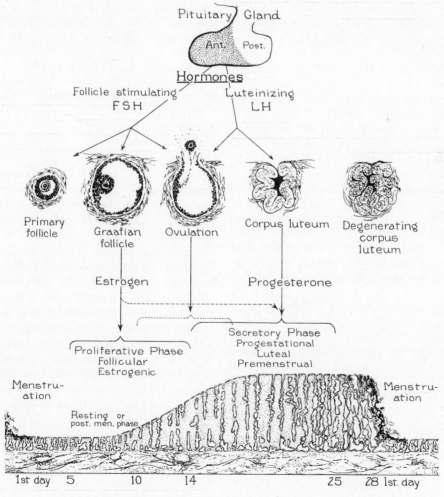

Fig. 3-3. Hormonal control of the normal menstrual cycle.

intervals during the reproductive years. One is called the *follicle-stimulating hormone* (sometimes abbreviated as *FSH*), active from the 5th to the 15th days of the cycle, and the other is the *luteinizing hormone* (*LH*), active during the luteal phase. A third pituitary gonadotrophic hormone, *luteotrophin*, is less often referred to in the context of menstruation. Its function in the ovarian cycle is to initiate and to maintain the secretion of progesterone from the corpus luteum (though it does not prolong its life-span). During the normal menstrual cycle, *LTH*, as it is abbreviated, is excreted in increasing amounts as urinary prolactin. This same hormone, described earlier as *prolactin*, is more commonly referred to in relation to lactation (see Chap. 6).

The *posterior lobe* of the pituitary gland produces *oxytocin*, a hormone that has an important role in obstetrics but one that differs altogether from the purposes of the present discussion (see Chaps. 12 and 13).

Other Functions of Estrogen and Progesterone. In addition to their role in controlling menstruation, these two ovarian hormones, estrogen and progesterone, have other far-reaching and important functions. Estrogen is responsible for the development of the secondary sex characteristics, that is, all those distinctive sex manifestations which are not directly concerned with the process of reproduction. Thus, the growth of the breast at puberty, the distribution of body fat, the appearance of pubic hair, the size of the larynx and its resulting influence on the quality of the voice, as well as mating instincts, are all the result of estrogenic action. We may almost say, therefore, that a woman is a woman because of estrogen.

Often this hormone is used therapeutically. Estrogen is available in ampules for intramuscular administration; usually it is distributed by the several pharmaceutical companies under various brand names, such as Theelin or Delestrogen. During more recent years the medication has been available also in tablet form for oral administration, e.g., Premarin, a naturally occurring estrogen extracted from pregnant mare's urine. In addition, synthetic compounds having estrogenic activity have been widely used, e.g., diethylstilbestrol or chlorotrianisene (Tace). The effects of these synthetic compounds are essentially the same as those achieved with the administration of estrogen.

Aside from its action on the endometrium, progesterone plays a most important role in preserving the life of the embryo during the first 2 or 3 months of pregnancy. It also has a relaxing action on the uterine muscle. For these two reasons, sometimes it is employed therapeutically in cases in which there is a tendency to abort (see p. 459). In this connection it is available as intramuscular progesterone or under the proprietary names, such as Delalutin or Proluton.

Clinical Aspects of Menstruation

From what has been said concerning the underlying mechanism of menstruation, it is clear that the monthly flow of blood is only one phase of a marvelous cyclic process which not only makes childbearing possible but also profoundly influences both body and mind. For this reason the time of the onset of menstruation is a critical period in the life of a young woman. The term "menarche" is used to indicate the onset of the first menstruation. The term "puberty" has a much broader connotation and refers to the whole transitional stage between childhood and maturity. During this time the appearance of secondary sex characteristics and the development of sex consciousness are other equally important manifestations. Not only do notable bodily changes occur, but a radical transformation takes place in the mental attitude of the girl. She matures rapidly in mind, and her interests broaden. Nevertheless, her emotions are often unstable, with the result that she may laugh or cry without reason. This transition period from girlhood to womanhood is sometimes a most trying one; but a good foundation in sex education from early childhood, so that knowledge of the physical bodily changes supplements careful observance of the rules of general hygiene, together with tolerance, sympathy and understanding on the part of parents and those closely associated with the adolescent, will do much to secure a normal adjustment.

The average age of the onset of menstruation is between 13 and 14 years. It may be as early as the 10th year or as late as the 17th year and still be within normal limits. Although the interval of the menstrual cycle, counting from the beginning of one period to the onset of the next, averages 28 days, there are wide variations even in the same woman. Indeed, there is scarcely a woman who menstruates exactly every 28 or 30 days. This question has been the subject of several studies on normal young women, chiefly student nurses, who have conscientiously recorded the time and the nature of each period. These investigations show that the majority of women (almost 60%) experience variations of at least 5 days in the length of their menstrual cycles; differences in the same woman of even 10 days are not uncommon and may occur without explanation or apparent detriment to health. For reasons which even today are obscure, menstrual blood does not clot.

Normal menstruation should not be accompanied by pain, although quite often there is some general malaise, together with a feeling of weight and discomfort in the pelvis. Frequent, also, are such disturbances as a sense of fatigue, headache, backache, sensitivity in the breasts and unstable emotional reactions. If there is great irregularity or extremely profuse flow or marked pain, a pathologic condition may be present. Painful menstruation is known as *dysmenorrhea*. Absence of the menses is known as *amenorrhea*. The most common cause of amenorrhea is pregnancy, but sometimes it is brought about by emotional disturbances, such as fear, worry or fatigue, or disease (anemia, tuberculosis), and occasionally it may be the result of a decided change in climate.

The cessation of menstrual function usually occurs between the ages of 45 and 50. The period over which this alteration takes place is known as the *menopause*, or *climacteric*, but generally it is referred to by the laity as the "change of life." About one half of all women cease menstruating between these years, about one fourth stop before 45, and another quarter continue to menstruate until past 50.

Variations in Basal Body Temperature

Beginning about the first year of life, slight daily variations in body temperature occur normally in all human beings. These temperature variations have relation to the time of the day and the nature of the circumstances surrounding the individual. For example, the body temperature is lowest in the morning before breakfast after a good night's rest in bed and prior to assuming activity. Then after a day of normal activity the body temperature is usually highest toward afternoon and early evening. The fact that physiologic variations in basal body temperature occur also in relation to the menstrual cycle is important here, because it can be useful in assessing ovarian activity and in establishing the time of ovulation. Such an index becomes extremely important in studies of fertility and sterility.

There is a slight rhythm of variation in the basal body temperature curve of a healthy woman in relation to the menstrual cycle. Her basal temperature is *lower* during the first part of the menstrual cycle, the proliferative phase. It is *lowest* just about the time of ovulation, but then it *rises* to a peak within 24 hours and thereafter is *higher* during the latter half of the cycle, the luteal phase (Fig. 3-4).

Each month after the cessation of menstruation, as was explained on page 56, the graafian follicle secretes estrogen (the basal temperature is lower at this time). At about the time of ovulation estrogen secretion reaches a peak of production (the basal temperature drops and then rises immediately). If fertilization occurs, the levels of estrogen and progesterone are maintained (the basal temperature remains high). However, when fertilization does not occur, the corpus luteum reaches full development in about a week, then regresses, and the secretion of progesterone ceases (the basal temperature falls—prior to the next menstrual period).

If the woman's basal body temperature curve is studied over a period of several consecutive months, the physician can assess her characteristic menstrual cycles. One must understand that ovulation does not occur with clocklike precision. Thus, only an approximate date of ovulation can be established in advance. The established day of ovulation becomes most important in family planning, for the woman's becoming pregnant or not becoming pregnant may depend largely on whether or not at a particular time ovulation has occurred, and the ovum is fertilized (see p. 61 and in Chap. 14, Family Planning).

BASAL TEMPERATURE RECORD

NAME _Jane Doe_   ADDRESS _10 Main St._   PHONE _24107_

FOR DR. _Wm. Smith_   ADDRESS _8 State St._   PHONE _25621_

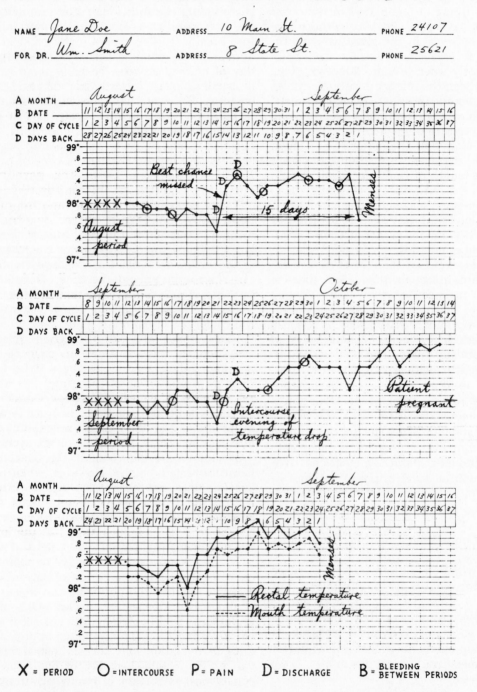

X = PERIOD   O = INTERCOURSE   P = PAIN   D = DISCHARGE   B = BLEEDING BETWEEN PERIODS

PUBLISHED UNDER THE AUSPICES OF THE MEDICAL COMMITTEE OF THE PLANNED PARENTHOOD FEDERATION OF AMERICA, INC.

FIG. 3-4. Directions for using this chart are given on the 2 following pages.

THE USE OF THE BASAL TEMPERATURE GRAPHS

The taking of basal body temperatures is proving to be a valuable procedure in determining the probable ovulation and in planning a pregnancy. Pregnancy is most likely to occur if intercourse takes places shortly before or after ovulation. In most women ovulation occurs about 14 days before menstruation. It is difficult for patients whose menstrual interval is irregular to calculate the date of ovulation. The use of a temperature graph for a record of body temperatures may help to determine the probable time of ovulation and hence the time when intercourse is mostly likely to result in pregnancy. Temperature may vary slightly from day to day from one tenth to one half a degree, and so it is essential that the temperature be taken and recorded accurately according to the following directions:

Directions

1. Take the temperature *rectally* with a well-lubricated blunt-tipped rectal thermometer for *five* (5) *minutes by the clock immediately after* waking in the morning and *before* getting out of bed, talking, eating, drinking or smoking. Take the temperature at about *the same time every morning.*

2. Read the thermometer to within one tenth of a degree and record the reading accurately.

3. Any known cause for temperature variation should be noted on the chart, for example, interrupted or shortened sleep, a cold, grippe, indigestion, a severe emotional disturbance or even indulgence in alcohol.

4. Some women can recognize ovulation by a characteristic pain in the lower abdomen. Others have slight vaginal bleeding or increased clear, slippery vaginal discharge around the time of ovulation. If any of these manifestations is present, note it on the chart on the day of occurrence. If the pain occurs on more than one day, record the exact hour when it is greatest.

Plotting the Temperature

1. The menstrual cycle is counted from the first day of one period to the first day of the next period. Start a new graph at the beginning of the period. The first day of menstruation is marked as the first day of the cycle.

2. (A) MONTH—Write the month on this line.

(B) DATE—Put the day of the month on this line.

Write down the day of the month of the first day of menstruation above 1 on the line for "day of cycle" and continue with the days to the end of the line.

(C) DAYS OF CYCLE—This line shows the days of the menstrual cycle.

(D) DAYS BACK—When the next menstrual period starts, fill in this line beginning with the day the period starts, and from then on number the days backward to the first day of the past period. This serves to show the number of the day at which ovulation occurred in the cycle and the length of the cycle.

3. Chart the temperature daily with a dot, and with a line connect this temperature dot with the dot of the day before. If intercourse occurs in the morning, encircle the dot. If it takes place at night, mark a circle on the line between that dot and the temperature dot of the next morning.

4. It is necessary to continue the graph for at least 3 menstrual cycles before the probable time of ovulation can be judged. Sexual abstinence for several days before ovulation allows time for the male to store up sperm and probably increase the chance of fertilization.

5. The temperature will fall and rise within a range of $\frac{1}{2}$ to 1 degree. Watch for a drop in temperature about 15 days before the expected period. The last drop in the cycle (usually the largest) is the important one, and intercourse should take place that day or evening if the couple is planning a pregnancy.

Oral Temperature

If for one reason or another it seems more desirable for the woman to take her temperature orally, she may be permitted to do so. However, she should be instructed that the route of taking her daily temperature should be consistent; i.e., the temperatures should be either all rectal or all oral. Temperature may be taken by mouth immediately upon awakening, *before getting out of bed and before talking, eating, drinking or smoking.* The variations in oral temperatures are similar to the variations in temperatures taken rectally. However, the variations in temperatures taken by mouth usually are not as marked as the variations in temperatures taken rectally—a factor of some importance in interpreting the temperature graph.

INFERTILITY

Although the problem of infertility is considered to be in the field of gynecology, it is a factor which has complicated the childbearing of many women. Thus, the obstetric nurse needs to be aware of its implications.

Dr. Abraham Stone stated that the United States Census Bureau's records show that more than 15 per cent of all married women never bear any children, and most of this childlessness is involuntary. Within the last quarter of a century many very important scientific advances have been made in the field of human infertility. Two newer concepts are of particular significance. One is that impaired fertility is due most often not to a single cause but to a multiplicity of factors. Systemic, local, nutritional, glandular and emotional conditions affect both the husband and the wife; therefore, in each instance it is necessary to make a complete study of the history of the health situation and the mode of life of the couple. The second concept is that the husband bears a far greater responsibility as a factor in sterile matings than had been recognized previously. Indeed, modern investigations indicate that about 40 per cent of cases of sterility are attributable to deficiencies on the part of the husband.

A few of the causes in women may be failure of ovulation, obstructions in the genital tract, especially in the cervix or the fallopian tubes, or disturbances in the development of the uterus and its lining which interfere with the implantation and the growth of the fertilized ovum. In the male the causes may be deficiency in the seminal fluid and particularly in the quantity and the quality of the spermatozoa, or obstructions in the seminal ducts which prevent the spermatozoa from passing through. Lack of sperm production may be caused by developmental anomalies, glandular disturbances, local injuries or infections and constitutional diseases.

Due to modern developments in the field of human infertility, about 30 per cent of the barren marriages can be rendered fertile. Today there is continued research in the physiologic and the psychological aspects of reproduction, and physicians have available better technics and methods for the diagnosis and the treatment of infertility.

MENOPAUSE

The term "menopause" refers to the cessation of menstruation which usually occurs during a woman's middle years, somewhere in the neighborhood of the age of 45 and 50. It has been said that, in general, the earlier puberty occurs in the child, the later the menopause will occur in womanhood. Conversely, the later puberty is experienced, the earlier the menopause will begin. The menopause, which is a normal consequence of aging, takes place as a gradual process. The periods first become scanty, then one may be missed, and finally they cease altogether.

The cause of the natural menopause is due to cessation of ovarian activity. As one considers the normal life cycle of the woman and focuses on the reproductive years, an analogy can be made that as the menarche is associated with puberty, so the menopause is associated with the climacteric. Often the terms "menopause" and "climacteric" are used synonymously, but one can readily understand that this usage is not accurate. The climacteric, a word derived from the Greek, meaning "rung of ladder, critical time in human life," is defined as "the syndrome of endocrine, somatic and psychic changes occurring at the termination of the reproductive period in the female. . . ."[1] Consider briefly the implication that these endocrine changes have for the ovaries. Having for some 30 years performed the function of providing a mature ovum each month with some degree of regularity, the ovary now regresses and gradually shrivels up into a small, flat organ composed mostly of scar tissue. As a consequence of this, estro-

[1] Dorland's Illustrated Medical Dictionary, ed. 24, Philadelphia, Saunders, 1965.

gen no longer is produced. This permanent and complete withdrawal of estrogen results in atrophy of the uterus, the fallopian tubes, the vagina and the vulva. Furthermore, the withdrawal of estrogen is likely to produce other symptoms, such as "hot flashes," vague muscle and joint pains, headache, edema, and manifestations of emotional instability—for example, irritability, sudden outbursts of tears, etc. Other evidences of the climacteric may be observed in the dryness of the skin and the hair, which makes the fact that she is aging more apparent to the woman.

"Hot flashes" is a familiar term to most people. Mentioned in association with the menopause down through the years, the expression has been passed along for generations almost like an old wives' tale. But "hot flashes" are no old wives' tale; they are the result of vasomotor instability, just as sweating or sensations of cold are during this time. The term "hot flashes" is descriptive; it says what the patient feels—an abrupt sensation of being very hot that seems momentarily to sweep upward from the body to envelop her to the very top of the head, and most particularly about the face and the neck. The face suddenly becomes very flushed, and she may break out in a sweat, manifestations that will be quite apparent to others. The women so affected may have "hot flashes" at any time and in varying degrees, from very mild to severe.

The menopause may result from other than the natural physiologic alterations of the climacteric. Artificial menopause relates to the cessation of menstruation produced by some artificial means, such as irradiation of the ovaries or surgical operation for the removal of the ovaries (oophorectomy) or the uterus (hysterectomy). Each of these brings about one manifestation in common, i.e., the woman will no longer menstruate. But beyond this the manifestations in the patient are not identical.

Certain misunderstandings based on incorrect interpretation of terminology are rather widespread and should be clarified. The fact that a woman has had a hysterectomy and ceases to menstruate does not mean that her healthy ovaries will now cease to function, because the hysterectomy involves only the removal of the uterus. On the other hand, if the ovaries are removed surgically or are treated by irradiation, the source of estrogen is withdrawn abruptly, and thus the symptoms relating to the sudden withdrawal of this hormone will occur.

When severe symptoms are produced by lack of ovarian function resulting from either the normal climacteric or artificial menopause, the patient may find them intolerable and may require hormone therapy to control the symptoms. Estrogen, either as the pure hormone or as one of the several synthetic estrogens, finds its greatest usefulness in alleviating these menopausal disorders (see p. 58). It can be said that the better the woman's general health is as she approaches her middle years, the more she can look forward to an uneventful menopause.

SUGGESTED READING

Corner, G. W.: The Hormones in Human Reproduction, rev. ed., Princeton, N. J., Princeton Univ. Press, 1952.

Eastman, N. J., and Hellman, L. M.: Williams Obstetrics, ed. 12, New York, Appleton, 1961.

Greenhill, J. P.: Obstetrics, ed. 13, Philadelphia, Saunders, 1965.

Greisheimer, E. M.: Physiology and Anatomy, ed. 8, Philadelphia, Lippincott, 1963.

Guyton, A. C.: Textbook of Medical Physiology, ed. 2, Philadelphia, Saunders, 1961.

Hytten, F. E., and Leitch, I.: The Physiology of Human Pregnancy, Philadelphia, Davis, 1963.

Lammert, A. C.: The menopause . . . a physiologic process, Amer. J. Nurs. 62, No. 2:56-57, February, 1962.

McLane, C. M. (ed.): Symposium on infertility, Clin. Obstet. Gynec. 8, No. 1:11-141, March, 1965.

Tyler, E. T.: Semen studies and fertility, J.A.M.A. 146:307, 1951.

Maturation of Ovum and Sperm Cells • Determination of Sex • Fertilization and Changes Following Fertilization • Implantation of the Ovum • Decidua • The Three Germ Layers • Amnion, Chorion and Placenta • Size and Development of the Fetus • Duration of Pregnancy • Calculation of the Expected Date of Confinement • Physiology of the Fetus • Periods of Development • Maternal Impressions

Chapter 4

Development and Physiology of the Fetus

In all Nature's wide universe of miracles there is no process more wonderous, no mechanism more incredibly fantastic, than the one by which a tiny speck of tissue, the human egg, develops into a 7-pound baby. So miraculous did primitive peoples consider this phenomenon that they frequently ascribed it all to superhuman intervention and even overlooked the fact that sexual intercourse was a necessary precursor. Throughout unremembered ages our own primitive ancestors doubtless held similar beliefs, but now we know that pregnancy comes about in only one way: from the union of a female germ cell, the egg or ovum, with a male germ cell, the spermatozoon (Fig. 4-1). These two gametes, ovum and spermatozoon, become fused into one cell or zygote, which contains the characteristics of both the female and the male from which these gametes originated.

MATURATION OF OVUM AND SPERM CELLS

The maturation of the ovum takes place about the time of ovulation and is probably complete before the ovum is discharged from the graafian follicle. The spermatozoon also is fully matured before it is discharged from the tubules. By the time the two gametes or sex cells, the ovum and the spermatozoon, in humans are matured or ready for union,

a number of peculiar changes already have occurred, as shown in Figure 4-2.

Typical cells of the testes and the ovary are shown at the top of Figure 4-2. On the left are shown the steps as a typical testes cell changes into 4 motile sperm cells or spermatozoa. On the right are seen the stages leading to the development of a single mature ovum. Beside the changes in appearance, very important internal changes also have taken place.

Chromosomes

In all human cell tissues there are normally 46 chromosomes (*chroma*, color; *soma*, body). Within each somatic cell there are normally 22 pairs of homologous autosomes (*auto*, self) and 1 pair of sex chromosomes. The sex chromosomes of the female germ cell are always the X type, and the male germ cells are dependent on the presence of the Y chromosome.

The cells of the human body develop from a fertilized ovum that has 46 chromosomes. To maintain genetic balance, the 46 chromosomes characteristic for the general somatic (body) cells of the species are reduced in gametogenesis to half the number (meiosis), so that each gamete normally receives only one chromosome of each pair. Thus, each motile spermatozoon has 23 chromosomes in its nucleus and each mature ovum also contains 23 chromosomes (haploid). The chromosomes of the ovum have been reduced, not by division as in the sperm, but by extrusion of chromosome material, so-called "polar bodies" because they are observed at one pole of the developing ovum (Fig. 4-2). Upon fertilization a new diploid set of 46 chromosomes is conceived, the chromosomes of the fertilized ovum being derived from both germ cells, i.e., half from the ovum and half from the male germ cell that fertilized the ovum.

The chromosomes differ in form and size, ranging from small spherical masses to long rods. More recently it was discovered that human cells could be photographed and examined by the application of cytologic technics (Figs. 4-3, 4). "Karyotype" is the technical term for an arrangement of chromosomes of a single cell according to the relative length and the position of the centromere. Figures 4-3 and 4 show the chromosomes at metaphase, the most convenient stage of cell division for the examination of somatic chromosomes. The

46 chromosomes (greatly magnified) appear as rod-shaped structures split longitudinally into two chromatids, lying side by side and

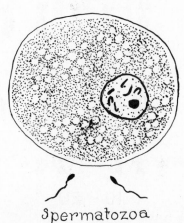

FIG. 4-1. Relative size of spermatozoa and ovum. (After Eastman)

FIG. 4-2. Diagram of gametogenesis. The various stages of spermatogenesis are indicated on the left; 1 spermatogonium gives rise to 4 spermatozoa. On the right the various stages of oogenesis are indicated. From each oogonium 1 secondary oocyte and 3 polocytes arise. An ovum reaches maturity only if it is fertilized. In gametogenesis the chromosomes are reduced to one half the number characteristic for the general body cells of the species. In man the number in the body cells is 46, and that in the mature spermatozoon (and secondary oocyte) is 23. (Greisheimer, E. M.: Physiology and Anatomy, ed. 8, p. 766, Fig. 401, Philadelphia, Lippincott, 1963)

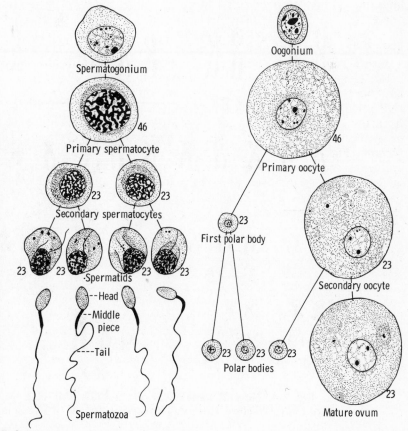

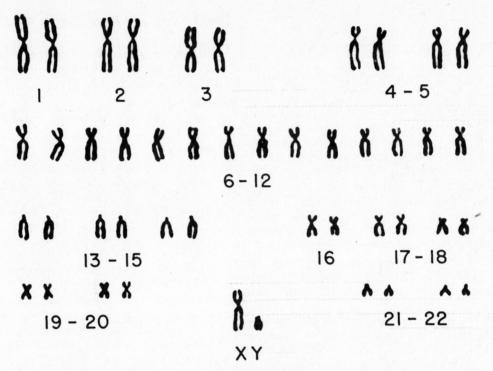

Fig. 4-3. Normal male karyotype. (Dr. M. Neil Macintyre, Department of Anatomy, Western Reserve Univerity School of Medicine)

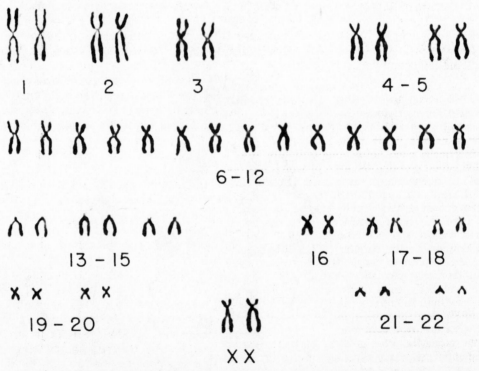

Fig. 4-4. Normal female karyotype. (Dr. M. Neil Macintyre, Department of Anatomy, Western Reserve University School of Medicine)

held together at the constricted region, the centromere.

Only as a preparation for reproduction, i.e., for the fertilization of the ovum by a spermatozoon, does the number of chromosomes vary. After fertilization occurs, the fertilized ovum has its full complement of 46 chromosomes. In every cell division thereafter until adulthood, throughout the differentiation of all tissues, each cell will have 46 chromosomes. Preparation for the passing on of the requisite number of chromosomes to each of the 2 daughter cells resulting from the splitting of the original cell is accomplished by an internal change in the cell before division. Each of the chromosomes splits in half, and each of the 2 new cells (daughter cells) receives its half of the halved chromosomes. This splitting and halving is continued in all dividing cells until growth ceases.

Within the chromosomes, distributed along the chromosomal threads, are the ultramicroscopic self-perpetuating bodies called genes. When the cell divides into 2 daughter cells, each daughter cell is an exact duplicate of the other and of the mother cell before division. For the daughter cells to be identical, each must have the same complement of genes in its chromosomes; thus there must be a duplication of genes before cell division occurs. This is accomplished by mitosis.

It is now known that the genes are duplicated in the interphase. . . . Accordingly, each chromosome of a cell that enters the prophase of mitosis has a double set of genes. However, the 2 sets of genes do not lie in the same thread, for in the interphase each splits longitudinally into 2 threads called chromatids, each of which has one full set of genes. The 2 chromatids of each chromosome remain close to each other along their lengths and firmly attached to each other at one point, the centromere, until, at one step in the process of mitosis, the centromere of each chromosome divides so that its two chromatids become individual entities. When this happens, each chromatid is called a chromosome. . . .[1]

As division proceeds, then, the mother cell will have identical sets of 46 chromosomes for each daughter cell.

Now consider briefly what happens when conception takes place, and the ovum from

[1] Ham, A. W.: Histology, ed. 5, pp. 73-74, Philadelphia, Lippincott, 1965.

the woman is fertilized by the sperm from her mate. Each gamete, ovum and spermatozoon, comes from a different person with a different ancestral history—and with different genes in its 23 chromosomes. To these genes are attributed such differences as color of hair and eyes, facial characteristics, body build, etc. Since a single gene may carry more than one character, there may be numerous variable results in the offspring of any two parents. The hereditary possibilities discarded or retained in the mature gametes is a matter of chance, but the nature of the combination of the germ plasm which occurs in each generation when two gametes fuse in fertilization is of great significance. If either parent brings defective germ plasm, the result may affect the zygote and later the characteristics of the child.

Biologists have estimated that at the time of the reduction division some 17 million different combinations are possible due to the interchange of genes. Apparently, there is sufficient stability produced during this intricate interchange process to ensure perpetuation of the characteristics of the progenitors.

Chromosomal Aberrations. The normal development of the embryo depends on the normal complement of chromosomes in the zygote, as well as the proper genetic balance. When this is not the case, developmental abnormalities occur. Malformations may result from alterations in a single gene, or in a number of genes, and from chromosomal abnormalities involving whole chromosomes. Some of these abnormalities are determined before fertilization takes place (during gametogenesis), almost certainly due to nondisjunction in the first reduction division in meiosis. For example, this aberration is now known to be the cause of Down's syndrome (mongolism). Here the zygote has 3 homologous autosomes, and it is trisomic; thus it is sometimes referred to as "trisomy 21."

Table 4 presents a summary of the various chromosomal aberrations which can occur in humans, involving the total number of chromosomes, both autosomes and sex chromosomes. Because this subject is highly specialized, the student is referred to the current literature on genetics for elaboration on it. A number of excellent references are included in the suggested readings for this chapter.

Table 4. Chromosomal Aberrations in Man*

I. In all cells of body (presumed to be due to an error occurring prior to conception).
  A. Anomalies of number. (Normal male:−(46) 44 + X + Y; normal female:−(46) 44 + X + X.)
    1. Involving individual chromosomes (aneuploidy).
      (*a*) Autosomes.
        α Monosomy (45) ♂ 43 + X + Y; ♀ 43 + X + X.
        β Trisomy (47) ♂ 45 + X + Y; ♀ 45 + X + X (mongolism). (Trisomy may involve more than one chromosome. Thus 49 chromosomes in an abnormal child have been interpreted as 46 + X + X + Y; i.e., trisomy of two autosomes and an extra X chromosome.)
      (*b*) Sex chromosomes (gonosomes).
        α Y absent (45) ♀ 44 + X + O (Turner's syndrome).
        β One X deficient (46) ♀ 44 + X + x (primary amenorrhoea).
        γ Extra X (47) ♀ 44 + X + X + X (sometimes called superfemale).
        δ Extra X (47) ♂ 44 + X + X + Y (Klinefelter's syndrome).
        ε Two extra X (48) ♂ 44 + X + X + X + Y (? Klinefelter's syndrome).
        (Y + O has not been observed; it would almost certainly be lethal.)
    2. Involving chromosome sets. (Normal—two sets diploid.)
      (*a*) Monoploidy (23) 22 + X; 22 + Y (not known).
      (*b*) Triploidy (69) ♂ 66 + X + X + Y (one case reported by Böök and Santeson (1960); male with multiple abnormalities). The condition could be regarded as trisomy of every chromosome pair which results in a triploid individual.
      (*c*) Higher degrees of polyploidy. (Not known.)
  B. Translocations.

II. In certain cells only of body. *Mosaicism* (presumed to be due to error occurring subsequent to conception).
  A. Anomalies of number.
    1. Mosaic of XO and XX (45/46) ♀ 44 + X + O/44 + X + X (Turner's syndrome).
    2. Mosaic of XO and XXX (45/47) ♀ 44 + X + O/44 + X + X + X.
    3. Mosaic of XX and XXY (46/47) ♂ 44 + X + X/44 + X + X + Y (Klinefelter's syndrome).
  B. Translocations.

* Hamilton, W. J., Boyd, J. D., and Mossman, H. W.: Human Embryology, ed. 3, p. 144, Cambridge, England, W. Heffer & Sons Ltd., 1962.

The Ovum

As described in Chapter 3, ova normally are discharged from the human ovary at the rate of 1 a month. The ovum at this time is a relatively large cell, measures about 0.2 millimeters (1/125 of an inch) and is just visible to the naked eye. The nucleus is small in comparison with the amount of cytoplasm and contains many strands or filaments of deeply staining material. These minute particles are called chromosomes and are the all-important links in the endless chain of heredity; they were discussed in more detail earlier in this chapter. The large amount of cytoplasm surrounding the nucleus of the ovum contains a small quantity of nutritive material in the form of yolk granules. The surface of the ovum is immediately surrounded by a thick membrane, the zona pellucida (translucent belt).

Transport Through the Fallopian Tube

After the ovum has been discharged from the ovary, it faces a 10-day journey. Its goal is the cavity of the uterus, more than 3 inches away (Fig. 4-5). The only pathway of approach is the tortuous fallopian tube, whose lining is wrinkled unevenly by the folds of tubal epithelium, and whose passageway at the inner end is no larger than a bristle. Moreover, the ovum has no means of locomotion but must depend on extraneous forces for propulsion through the fallopian tube. Offhand, it would seem to be impossible; actually, the ovum is not only able to make this journey with apparent ease but has been known to reach its destination after the most unbelievable meanderings. For instance, if one fallopian tube has been removed by an operation, the ovum may migrate to the opposite side of the uterus and enter the other tube. This whole "transportation system" is made possible, it seems, through two factors. In the first place, currents in the film of fluid which bathes the lining of the tube waft the ovum downward. If this lining were inspected with a microscope, there would be observed little hairlike projections, called cilia, which wave or beat in such a manner as to direct any overlying fluid (as well as any particle afloat thereon) in the direction of the uterine cavity. Once the ovum has been expelled from the ovary, it is drawn by these currents into the funnellike opening of the tube and is then propelled down the tube by these same currents. The second factor responsible for the migration of the ovum down the tube is found in the peristaltic action of the tubal musculature. But the ovum is scarcely a third of the way down the tube when the supreme event happens: it meets a spermatozoon, and a new human being is created. As Margaret Shea Gilbert has so happily expressed it in her book, *Biography of the Unborn*, "Life begins for each of us at an unfelt, unknown, and unhonored instant when a minute wriggling sperm plunges headlong into a mature ovum or egg."

Spermatozoa

These minute, wriggling spermatozoa are in some respects even more remarkable than the ova which they fertilize. In appearance they resemble microscopic tadpoles, with oval heads and long, lashing tails about 10 times the length of the head. The human spermatozoon consists of 3 parts: the head, the middlepiece (or neck) and the tail (Fig. 4-6). The nucleus, and consequently the chromatin material, is in the head; the tail serves for propulsion. Spermatozoa are much smaller than ova, their over-all length measuring about one quarter the diameter of the egg, and it has been estimated that the heads of 2 billion of them—

enough to regenerate the entire population of the world—could be placed, with room to spare, in the hull of a grain of rice. As a result of the wriggling motion of the tails, spermatozoa swim with a quick vibratory motion and have been "timed" under the microscope at rates as fast as one seventh of an inch a minute. In ascending the uterus and the fallopian tube they must swim against the same currents that waft the ovum downward; nevertheless, they seem to be able to reach the outer part of the tube within 1 or 2 hours. Perhaps the most amazing feature of spermatozoa is their huge number. At each ejaculation, the climax of intercourse in the male, about 300 million are discharged; if each of these could be united with an ovum, the babies which would thus be created would exceed the total number born in the United States during the past hundred years—all from a single ejaculation. So lavish is Nature in her effort to perpetuate the species! Although many million spermatozoa die in the vagina as the result of the acid secretion there, myriads survive, penetrate the neck of the uterus and swarm upward to the uterine cavity and into the fallopian tube. There they lie in wait for the ovum (Fig. 4-5).

DETERMINATION OF SEX

In the human being, age, state of health and natural physical strength have nothing to do with the determination of the sex of the offspring. The sex is determined at the time of fertilization by the spermatozoon—not by the ovum. All spermatozoa and ova have 46 chromosomes originally. Each spermatozoon has 44 regular chromosomes and an X and a Y chromosome, whereas each ovum contains 44 regular chromosomes and two X sex chromosomes. When maturation occurs, each spermatozoon and ovum divides into 2 cells. Each of the 2 ovum cells contains 22 regular chromosomes and an X chromosome; but one half of the spermatozoon cells contain 22 regular chromosomes and an X chromosome, and the other half of the spermatozoon (or sperm) cells contain 22 regular chromosomes and a Y chromosome. If a sperm cell containing

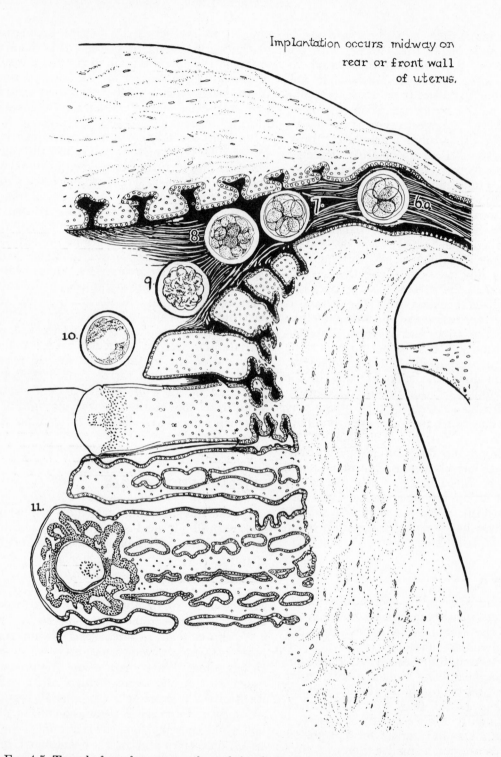

Implantation occurs midway on rear or front wall of uterus.

FIG. 4-5. Travel of egg from ovary through implantation, with alterations en route: 3 days in tube, 4 days in uterus before implantation. (Robert L. Dickinson, M.D., New York, adapted from Sellheim, with suggestions from Streeter, Frank and Hartman)

70

1. Follicle bursts.
2. Ovum with adhering granulosa cells.
   First polar body.
   2nd. maturation spindle.
3. Sperm enters egg.
   2nd. maturation division
4. Male and Female pronuclei

5. Pronuclei fusing
   Fertilization accomplished
5a. First cleavage division
6-7 Early cleavage
8. Morula.
9-10 Early and later gastrula
11 Fully implanted growing embryo. (Miller.)

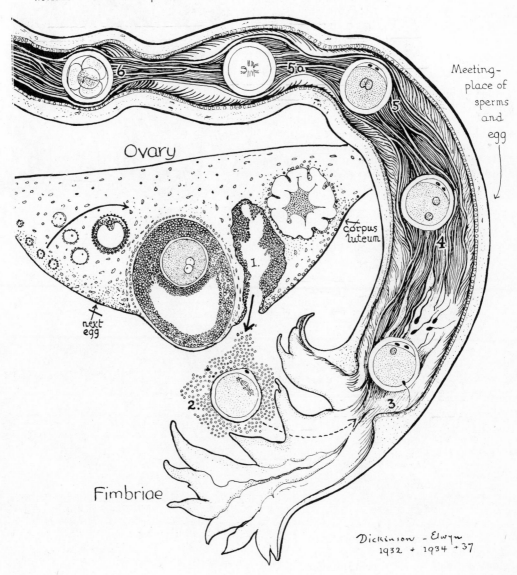

Ovary

Meeting-place of sperms and egg

corpus luteum

next egg

Fimbriae

Dickinson - Elwyn
1932 + 1934 + 37

Fig. 4-6 (*Left*). Spermatozoa.

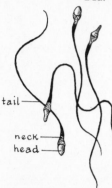

tail

neck

head

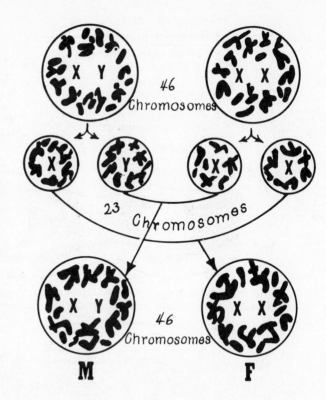

Fig. 4-7 (*Right*). The sex of the offspring is determined at the time of fertilization by the combination of the sex chromosome of the spermatozoon (either X or Y) and that of the ovum (X). The ovum fertilized by a sperm cell containing the X chromosome produces a female (44 regular chromosomes + 2 X chromosomes). If it is fertilized by a spermatozoon containing the Y chromosome, the union produces a male (44 regular chromosomes + X + Y).

Note: The structures depicted as chromosomes are diagrammatic only. In this illustration it was not possible to include the total correct number.

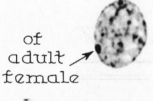

sex chromatin

of infant female

of adult female

not seen in male

Fig. 4-8. Photomicrographs of epithelial cells from the oral mucosa stained with cresyl-echt violet (× 2,000). The upper 2 nuclei have Barr bodies, which are indicated by arrows. (Moore, K. L., and Barr, M. L.: Lancet 2:57, July 9, 1955, *in* Ham, A. W.: Histology, ed. 5, p. 69, Philadelphia, Lippincott, 1965)

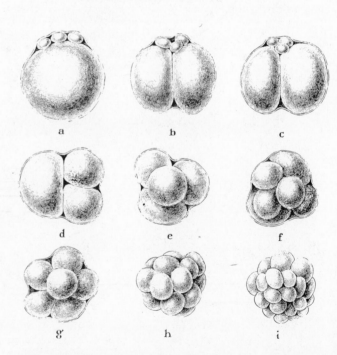

Fig. 4-9. Cleavage of the fertilized ovum. The ovum divides into 2, each of the 2 into 2, making 4, and so on to form a solid mass of cells, called a *morula*. (Modified from Sobotta)

22 chromosomes and an X chromosome fertilizes an ovum, a female will result, because in the union of the sperm and the ovum there will be 44 regular chromosomes and an X chromosome from the ovum and an X chromosome from the spermatozoon. If, on the other hand, a sperm cell containing 22 regular chromosomes and a Y chromosome fertilizes an ovum, a male will result, because in the union there will be 44 regular chromosomes and an X chromosome from the ovum and a Y chromosome from the spermatozoon (Fig. 4-7). It is definitely a matter of chance, as far as is known today, whether a sperm with an X or a Y chromosome will fertilize an ovum. This is evidenced by the fact that almost universally about 94 female babies are born to every 100 male babies in single births. Although many attempts have been made to influence Nature's roulette wheel of sex, to the end of having a child of a desired sex, no success has been met. Nor can a physician predict with any degree of assurance, even late in pregnancy, whether the baby will be a girl or a boy.

Sex Chromatin. In females most nuclei of the somatic (body) cells contain a small mass of material which stains red with suitable dyes, known as sex chromatin. This is probably formed by fusion of the two X chromosomes, since it is not usually present in the body cells of males. This sex chromatin has proved to be useful in determining the sex of the embryo or fetus in early abortions and under other circumstances in which the generative organs are too immature for the determination of sex (Fig. 4-8).

FERTILIZATION AND CHANGES FOLLOWING FERTILIZATION

The process of union of ovum and spermatozoon is known as fertilization. It usually takes place in the outer third of the fallopian tube. As soon as the ovum comes near the army of spermatozoa, the latter, as though they were tiny bits of steel drawn by a powerful magnet, fly at the ovum. One penetrates, but only one. It appears that the entrance of one sperm into an egg causes a change in the surface of the egg which prevents entrance of other spermatozoa. The union of ovum and spermatozoon is followed at once by profound changes in the nuclei, which result in cell division and multiplication and the development of a new being. Seemingly electrified, all the particles which make up the ovum (now fused with the sperm) exhibit vigorous agitation, as though they were being rapidly churned about by some unseen force; this becomes more and more violent until it amounts to

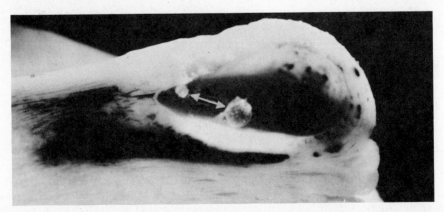

FIG. 4-10. Monochorionic twin embryos of about 17 days, at present the earliest known twin embryo. As seen in the opened chorion one embryo is smaller than the other. It is in fact somewhat retarded, but the apparent smallness is partly due to folding, and the sections show it to be similar in all essentials to its sibling. (Dr. George W. Corner, Sr., Department of Embryology, Carnegie Institution of Washington)

such an upheaval that the fertilized ovum divides into two cells. Before division the male and the female chromosomes and their genes are mingled and finally split, forming two sets of 46 chromosomes, one set of 46 going to each of the 2 new cells. This process is repeated again and again, until masses containing 16, 32 and 64 cells are produced successively, and so on endlessly. These early cell divisions produce a solid ball of cells called the "morula," because they resemble a mulberry (Fig. 4-9). It is believed that the 16-cell stage is reached about 96 hours after ovulation. Meanwhile, this growing aggregation of cells is being car-

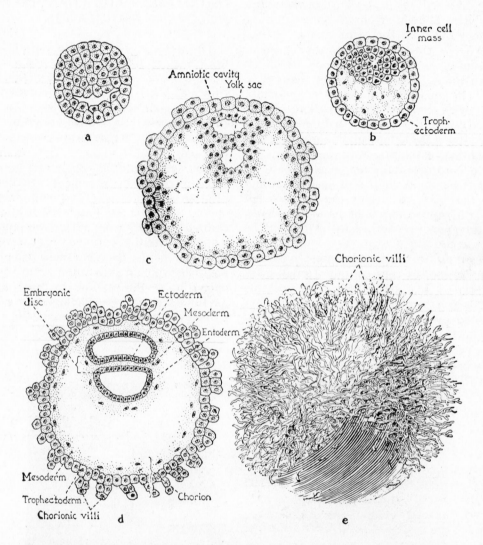

FIG. 4-11. Early stages of development. (a, b) The cells are separated into a peripheral layer and an inner cell mass; the peripheral layer is called the trophoblast or trophectoderm; the entire structure is called a blastodermic vesicle. (c) The formation of the amniotic cavity and yolk sac is indicated. The former is lined by ectoderm; the latter, by entoderm. (d) The location of the embryonic disk and the three germ layers are shown, together with the beginning of the chorionic villi. (e) The external appearance of the developing mass is shown; the chorionic villi are abundant. (Greisheimer: Physiology and Anatomy, Philadelphia, Lippincott)

Fig. 4-12. Various stages in the process of implantation; the relation of the uterine mucosa to the embryonic vesicle during implantation is shown: (s) decidua basalis, (v) decidua vera, (c) decidua capsularis, and (o) the ovum or embryonic vesicle. (Greisheimer: Physiology and Anatomy, Philadelphia, Lippincott)

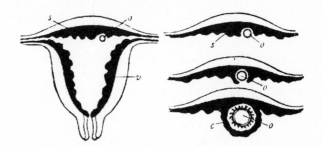

ried down the fallopian tube in the direction of the uterine cavity.

The journey of the ovum down the fallopian tube is believed to require about 3 days, and then it spends a period of some 4 days in the uterine cavity before actual embedding takes place, a total interval of some 7 days between ovulation and implantation. Meanwhile, important changes are taking place in the internal structure of the fertilized ovum. The cells in the center of the mulberry mass secrete a fluid which pushes the remaining cells to the periphery of the sphere. At the same time it becomes apparent that this external envelope of cells is actually made up of two different layers, an inner and an outer. A specialized portion of the inner layer, after some 260 days, will develop into the long-awaited baby. The outer layer is a sort of foraging unit, called the trophoblast (trophectoderm), which means "feeding" layer; it is the principal function of these cells to secure food for the embryo (Figs. 4-10, 11).

While the ovum is undergoing these changes, the lining of the uterus, it will be recalled, is making preparations for its reception. Considering that ovulation took place on the 14th day of the menstrual cycle and that the tubal journey and the uterine sojourn required 7 days, 21 days of the cycle will have passed before the ovum has developed its trophoblastic layer of cells. This is the period when the lining of the uterus has reached its greatest thickness and succulence. In other words, the timing has been precisely correct; the bed is prepared, and the ovum has so developed that it is now ready to embed itself.

IMPLANTATION OF THE OVUM

The embedding of the ovum is the work of the outer "foraging" layer of cells, the trophoblast, which possesses the peculiar property of being able to digest or liquefy the tissues with which it comes into contact. This process is carried out by means of enzymes. In this manner these cells not only burrow into the uterine lining and eat out a nest for the ovum but also digest the walls of the many small blood vessels that they encounter beneath the surface. The mother's blood stream is thus tapped, and presently the ovum finds itself deeply sunk in the lining epithelium of the uterus, with tiny pools of blood around it (Fig. 4-12). Sprouting out from the trophoblastic layer, quivering, fingerlike projections now develop and extend greedily into the blood-filled spaces. Another name for the trophoblast, and one more commonly employed as pregnancy progresses, is the chorion, and the fingerlike projections mentioned above become known as chorionic villi (Fig. 4-11). These chorionic villi contain blood vessels connected with the fetus and are extremely important, because they are the sole means by which oxygen and nourishment are received from the mother. The entire ovum becomes covered with villi, which grow out radially and convert the chorion into a shaggy sac.

DECIDUA

The thickening of the uterine endometrium, which occurs during the premenstrual phase of menstruation, has been described already. If pregnancy ensues, this endometrium becomes even more thickened, the cells enlarge, and the structure becomes known as the decidua. It is simply a direct continuation in exaggerated form of the already modified premenstrual mucosa.

For purposes of description, the decidua has

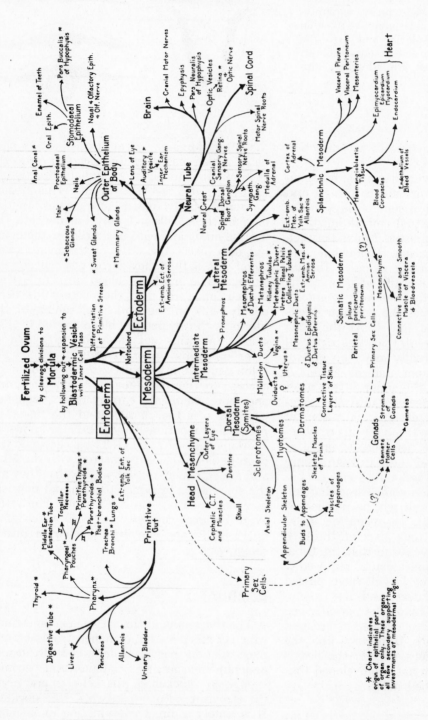

Fig. 4-13. Derivation of various parts of the body by progressive differentiation and divergent specialization. Note especially how the origin of all the organs can be traced back to the 3 primary germ layers. (Patten, B. M.: Human Embryology, New York, Blakiston)

FIG. 4-14. Amniotic cavity, placenta and membranes (amnion and chorion).

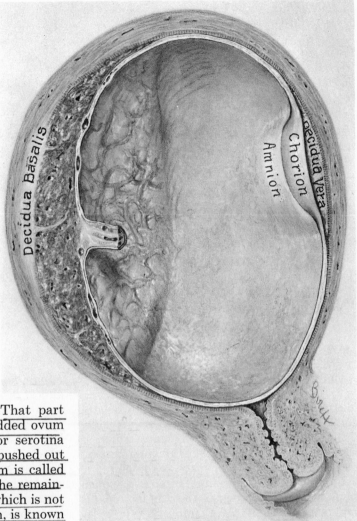

been divided into three portions. That part which lies directly under the embedded ovum is known as the decidua basalis, or serotina (Fig. 4-12). That portion which is pushed out by the embedded and growing ovum is called the decidua capsularis or reflexa. The remainder of the decidua, or that portion which is not in immediate contact with the ovum, is known as the decidua parietalis or vera. As pregnancy advances, the decidua capsularis expands rapidly over the growing embryo and at about the 4th month lies in intimate contact with the decidua vera.

THE THREE GERM LAYERS

With nutritional facilities provided, the cells which are destined to form the baby grow rapidly. At first they all look alike, but soon after embedding, groups of cells here and there assume distinctive characteristics and differentiate into 3 main groups: an outer covering layer, a middle layer and an internal layer. These are called, respectively, the ectoderm, the mesoderm and the entoderm.

From the *ectoderm* the following structures arise: epithelium of skin, hair, nails, sebaceous glands, sweat glands, epithelium of the nasal and the oral passages, salivary and mucous glands of the mouth and the nose, enamel of the teeth, and the nervous system. From the *mesoderm* are derived: muscles, bone, cartilage, dentin of teeth, ligaments, tendons, areolar tissue, kidneys, ureters, ovaries, testes, heart, blood, lymph and blood vessels, and lining of pericardial, pleural and peritoneal cavities. From the *entoderm* arise: the epithelium of the digestive tract, of glands which pour their secretion into the tract, of the respiratory tract and of the bladder, the urethra, the thyroid and the thymus (Fig. 4-13).

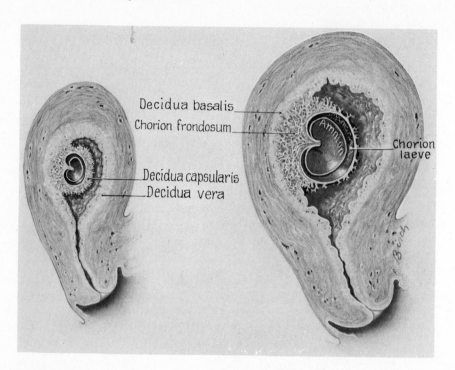

FIG. 4-15. Development of decidua basalis, capsularis and vera; chorion frondosum.

In figure labels:
- Decidua basalis
- Chorion frondosum
- Decidua capsularis
- Decidua vera
- Amnion
- Chorion laeve

AMNION, CHORION AND PLACENTA

Amnion. Even before these structures become evident, however, a fluid-filled space develops about the embryo, a space which is lined with a smooth, slippery, glistening membrane, the amnion. The space is the amniotic cavity; being filled with fluid, often it is spoken of as the bag of waters; in this the fetus floats and moves (Fig. 4-14). At full term this cavity normally contains from 500 to 1,000 cc. of liquor amnii, or the "waters." The amniotic fluid has a number of important functions: it keeps the fetus at an even temperature, cushions it against possible injury and provides a medium in which it can move easily; furthermore, it is known that the fetus drinks this fluid. At the end of the 4th month of pregnancy the bag of waters has enlarged to the size of a large orange and, with the fetus, occupies the entire interior of the uterus.

Chorion. As explained, the early ovum is covered on all sides by shaggy chorionic villi, but very shortly those villi which invade the decidua basalis enlarge and multiply rapidly. This portion of the trophoblast is known as the chorion frondosum (leafy chorion) (Fig. 4-15). Contrariwise, the chorionic villi covering the remainder of the fetal envelope degenerate and almost disappear, leaving only a slightly roughened membrane. This latter is called the chorion laeve (bald chorion). The chorion laeve lies outside of the amnion, of course, with which it is in contact on its inner surface, while its outer surface lies against the decidua vera. The fetus is thus surrounded by two membranes, the amnion and the chorion, and in ordinary clinical discussions these are usually referred to simply as "the membranes."

Placenta. By the 3rd month another important structure has formed, the placenta. This is a fleshy, disklike organ; late in pregnancy it measures about 8 inches in diameter and 1 inch in thickness. It receives its name from a Latin word meaning cake, which this structure resembles somewhat in shape. The placenta is formed by the union of the chorionic villi and the decidua basalis. An analogous situation is seen when a tree or a plant sends down its roots into a bed of earth for nourishment; when the plant is removed a certain amount of the earthy bed clings to the interlocking roots. Similarly, a thin layer of the uterine bed clings to the branching projections of chorionic villi, and together they make up this organ which supplies food to the fetus, as the roots

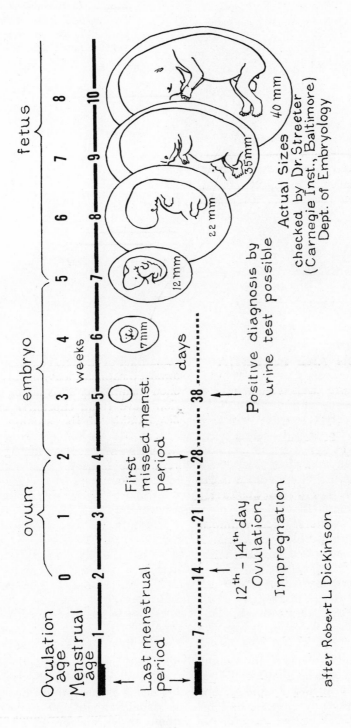

Fig. 4-16. Growth of ovum, embryo and fetus during the early weeks of pregnancy.

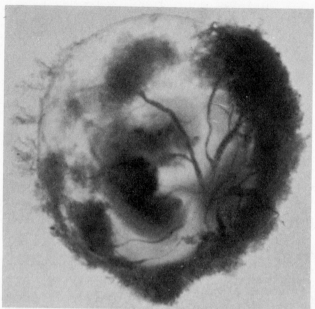

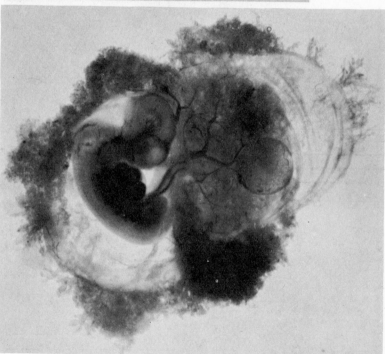

Fɪɢ. 4-17. Human embryo. Length, 7 mm. C. R. Estimated age, 35 days. (*Top*) In the closed sac. (*Bottom*) In the open sac. (Photos by Wesley Kaswell, University Hospitals of Cleveland)

and the earth provide nourishment for a plant. At term the placenta weighs about 500 Gm., or 1 pound. Its fetal surface is smooth and glistening, being covered by amnion, and beneath this membrane may be seen a number of large blood vessels (Plates 1 and 2). The maternal surface is red and fleshlike in character and is divided into a number of segments, about an inch in diameter, called cotyledons.

The placenta and the fetus are connected by means of the *umbilical cord*, or funis, which is usually about 20 inches in length and about three quarters of an inch in diameter. The cord leaves the placenta near the center and enters the abdominal wall of the fetus at the umbilicus, a trifle below the middle

Fig. 4-18. Human embryo photographed by Chester F. Reather. This specimen represents about 40 days' development and is shown in the opened chorion. It is reproduced at a magnification of 1.7. (Carnegie Institution, Washington, D. C.)

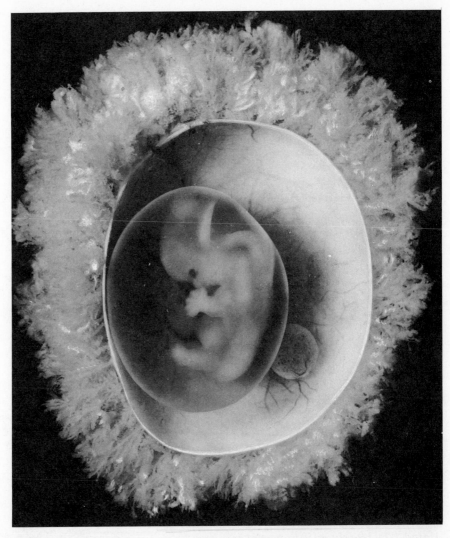

of the median line in front. It contains 2 arteries and 1 large vein, which are twisted upon each other and are protected from pressure by a transparent, bluish-white, gelatinous substance called Wharton's jelly.

SIZE AND DEVELOPMENT OF THE FETUS

Size at Various Months

The physician, as well as the nurse, is sometimes called upon to estimate the intra-uterine age of a fetus which has been expelled prematurely.

In general, the length affords a more accurate criterion of the age of the fetus than its weight. Haase's rule suggests that for clinical purposes the length of the embryo in centimeters may be approximated during the first 5 months by squaring the number of the month to which the pregnancy has advanced; in the second half of pregnancy, by multiplying the month by 5. Conversely, the approximate age of the fetus may be obtained by taking the square root of its length in centimeters during the first 5 months, and thereafter by dividing its length in centimeters by 5. For instance, a fetus 16 cm. long is about 4 months old; a 35-cm. fetus is about 7 months old.

Development Month by Month

Most women consider themselves 1 month

pregnant at the time of the first missed menstrual period, 2 months pregnant at the second missed period, and so on. Since conception does not ordinarily take place until some 14 days after the onset of menstruation, it is obvious that an embryo does not attain the age of 1 month until about a fortnight after the first missed period (assuming a 28-day cycle), and its "birthday" by months regularly falls 2 weeks or so after any numerically specified

FIG. 4-19. Actual size of fetus at approximately 1 month, 2 months and 3 months, respectively. (Eastman: Expectant Motherhood, Boston, Little)

missed period. This should be remembered in reading the month-by-month development of the fetus. Thus, in speaking of the age of a pregnancy in "months," physicians refer to "lunar months," that is, periods of 4 weeks. Since a lunar month corresponds to the usual length of the menstrual cycle, they find it easier to "figure" in this way (Fig. 4-16).

Month by month the development of the fetus is something as follows:

End of First Lunar Month. The embryo is about one quarter of an inch long if measured in a straight line from head to tail—for it does have a tail at this early stage—and recognizable traces of all organs have become differentiated. The backbone is apparent but is so bent upon itself that the head almost touches the tip of the tail. At one end of the backbone the head is extremely prominent, representing almost one third of the entire embryo. (Throughout intra-uterine life the head is always very large in proportion to the body, a relationship which is still present, although to a lesser degree, at birth.) The rudiments of the eyes, the ears and the nose now make their appearance. The tube which will form the future heart has been formed, producing a large, rounded bulge on the body wall; even at this early age this structure is pulsating regularly and propelling blood through microscopic arteries. The rudiments of the future digestive tract are also discernible—a long, slender tube leading from the mouth to an expansion in the same tube

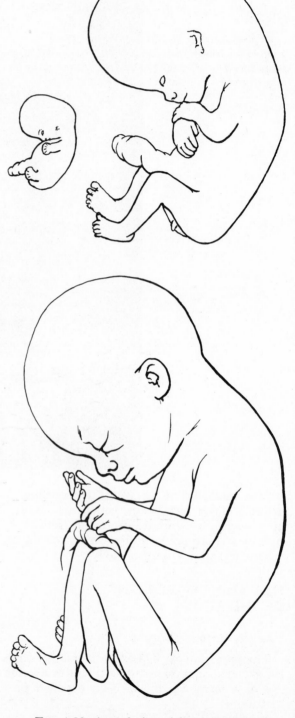

FIG. 4-20. Actual size of fetus at approximately 4 months.

which will become the stomach; connected with the latter the beginnings of the intestines may be seen. The incipient arms and legs are represented by small nubbins that resemble buds.

End of Second Lunar Month. The fetus, the term used to refer to the product of conception after the 5th week of gestation, now begins to assume human form (Fig. 4-18). Due to the development of the brain, the head becomes disproportionately large so that the nose, the mouth and the ears become relatively less prominent. It has an unmistakably human face and also arms and legs, with fingers, toes, elbows and knees. During the past 4 weeks it has quadrupled in length and measures about

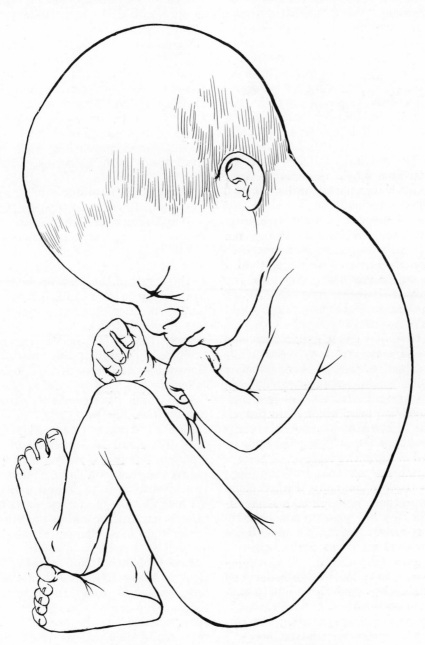

FIG. 4-21. Actual size of fetus at approximately 5 months.

1 inch from head to buttocks; its weight is approximately one thirtieth of an ounce. The external genitalia become apparent, but it is difficult to distinguish between male and female. During the 2nd month the human tail reaches its greatest development, but by the end of the month it is less prominent and then undergoes retrogression.

End of Third Lunar Month. The fetus now measures somewhat over 3 inches in length and weighs almost an ounce. The sex can now be distinguished because the external genitalia are beginning to show definite signs of sex. Centers of ossification have appeared in most bones; the fingers and the toes have become differentiated, and the fingernails and the toenails appear as fine membranes. Early in this month buds for all the temporary "baby" teeth are present, and sockets for these develop in the jawbone. Rudimentary kidneys have developed and secrete small amounts of urine into the bladder, which in all probability escape later into the amniotic fluid. Movements of the fetus are known to occur at this time, but they are too weak to be felt by the mother (Fig. 4-19).

End of Fourth Lunar Month. The fetus from head to toe is now 6½ inches long and about 4 ounces in weight. The sex as evidenced by the external genital organs is now quite obvious (Fig. 4-20).

End of Fifth Lunar Month. The length of the fetus now approximates 10 inches, while its weight is about 8 ounces. A fine downy growth of hair, *lanugo, appears on the skin* over the entire body. Usually, about this time the mother becomes conscious of slight fluttering movements in her abdomen, which are due to movements of the fetus. Their first appearance is referred to as *quickening,* or the perception of life. At this period the physician often is able to hear the fetal heart for the first time. If a fetus is born now, it may make a few efforts to breathe, but its lungs are insufficiently developed to cope with conditions outside the uterus, and it invariably succumbs within a few hours at most (Fig. 4-21).

End of Sixth Lunar Month. The length of the fetus is 12 inches, and its weight is 1½ pounds. It now resembles a miniature baby, with the exception of the skin, which is wrinkled and red with practically no fat beneath it. At this time, however, the skin begins to develop a protective covering called *vernix caseosa,* which means "cheesy varnish." This fatty, cheesy substance adheres to the skin of the fetus and at term may be an eighth of an inch thick. Although a few cases are on record in which fetuses of this size have survived, the outlook must be regarded as practically hopeless.

End of Seventh Lunar Month. The fetus measures about 15 inches in length and weighs approximately 2½ pounds. If born at this time, it has some chance of survival, perhaps 1 in 10. There is a widespread notion, quite incorrect, that infants born at the 7th month are more likely to survive than those born at the 8th month. This is another of those old superstitions which have descended through more than 2,000 years from the time of the ancient Greek physicians. They believed that the fetus is born by means of its own effort; that is, it pushes with its legs against the upper part of the womb and wriggles out into the world. It was their opinion that the fetus first attempts to escape from the uterus at the 7th month and, if strong, it succeeds. If the attempt fails, it is repeated at the 8th month. However, if it now succeeds, it is so exhausted as the result of the previous attempt that it is more likely to die than if it had been successful in the prior attempt a month earlier. We now know, of course, that the fetus is entirely passive, that it is expelled from the mother's body solely through the muscular action of the uterus, and that this old belief is wholly fallacious. The fetus born at the 8th month stands a much better chance of survival than one born at the 7th.

End of Eighth Lunar Month. The fetus measures about 16.5 inches and weighs some 4 pounds. Its skin is still red and wrinkled, and vernix caseosa and lanugo are still present. In appearance it resembles a little old man. With proper incubator and good nursing care, infants born at the end of the 8th month have better than even chances of survival, possibly as high as 2 chances in 3.

End of Ninth Lunar Month. For all practical purposes the fetus is now a mature infant, measures some 19 inches and weighs around 6 pounds. Due to the deposition of subcutaneous fat, the body has become more rotund and the skin less wrinkled and red. As though to improve its appearance before mak-

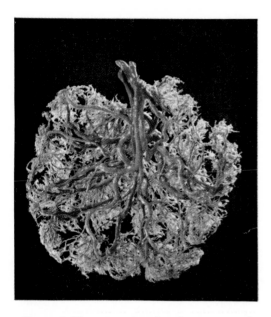

PLATE 1. Placenta stripped to the main vessels. Arteries are red; veins, blue. (Life Magazine. Picture taken by Rudolph Skarda Research Anatomist, University of California, San Francisco, Calif.)

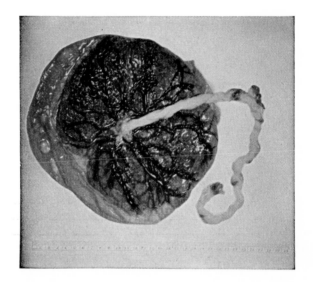

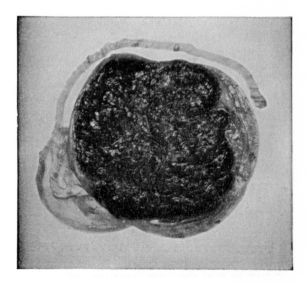

PLATE 2. (*Top*) Fetal surface of placenta. (*Bottom*) Maternal surface of placenta.

ing its debut into the world, the fetus devotes the last 2 months in the uterus to putting on weight and during this period gains ½ pound a week. Its chances of survival are now quite as good as though born at full term.

Middle of Tenth Lunar Month. Full term has now been reached, and the fetus weighs on an average about 7 pounds if a girl and 7½ if a boy; its length approximates 20 inches. Its skin is now white or pink and thickly coated

with the cheesy vernix. The fine, downy hair which previously covered its body has largely disappeared. The fingernails are firm and protrude beyond the end of the fingers (Fig. 4-22).

DURATION OF PREGNANCY

The length of pregnancy varies greatly; it may range, indeed, between such wide ex-

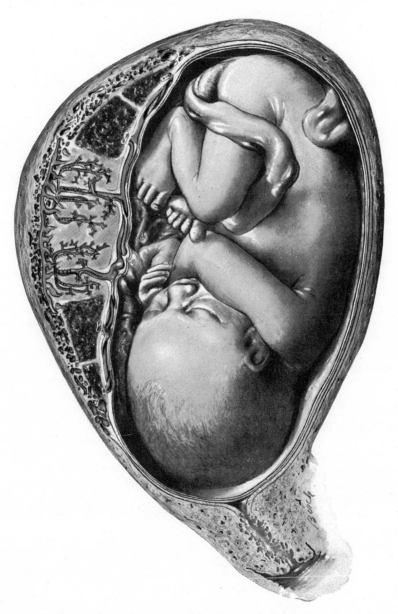

FIG. 4-22. Full-term fetus in utero, with placental circulation shown in color.

TABLE 5. DEVIATION FROM CALCULATED DATE OF CONFINEMENT, ACCORDING TO NAEGELE'S RULE, OF 4,656 BIRTHS OF MATURE INFANTS*

DEVIATION IN DAYS	EARLY DELIVERY	DELIVERY ON CALCULATED DATE	LATE DELIVERY
0	....	189 (4.1)†	....
1– 5	860 (18.5)†	....	773 (16.6)†
6–10	610 (13.1)	....	570 (12.2)
11–20	733 (15.7)	....	459 (9.9)
21–30	211 (4.5)	....	134 (2.9)
31 and over	75 (1.6)	....	42 (0.9)

The menstrual cycles of the mothers were 28 ± 5 days. The infants were at least 47 cm. in length and 2,600 Gm. in weight (Burger and Korompai).

* Eastman, N. J.: Williams Obstetrics, ed. 11, p. 216, New York, Appleton, 1956.

† Numbers in parentheses represent per cent of cases considered.

tremes as 240 days and 300 days and yet be entirely normal in every respect. The average duration from the time of conception is 9½ lunar months, that is, 38 weeks or 266 days. From the first day of the last menstrual period its average length is 10 lunar months, that is, 40 weeks or 280 days. That these average figures mean very little, however, is shown by the following facts. Scarcely one pregnancy in 10 terminates exactly 280 days after the beginning of the last period. Less than one half terminate within 1 week of this 280th day. In 10 per cent of cases birth occurs a week or more before the theoretical end of pregnancy, and in another 10 per cent it takes place more than 2 weeks later than we would expect from the average figures cited above. Indeed, it would appear that some fetuses require a longer time, others a shorter time, in the uterus for full development.

CALCULATION OF THE EXPECTED DATE OF CONFINEMENT

In view of the wide variation in the length of pregnancy, it is obviously impossible to predict the expected day of confinement (often abbreviated EDC) with any degree of precision. The time-honored method, based on the above "average figures," is simple. Count back 3 calendar months from the first day of the last menstrual period and add 7 days (Naegele's rule). For instance, if the last menstrual period began on June 10, we would count back 3 months to March and, adding 7 days, arrive at the date of March 17. An easier

way to calculate this is to substitute numbers for the months. Then this example becomes: 6/10 minus 3 months equals 3/10, plus 7 days equals 3/17. Athough it may be satisfying to the curiosity to have this date in mind, it must be understood that less than 5 per cent of all pregnant women go into labor on the estimated date of confinement, and in 35 per cent a deviation of from 1 to 5 days before or after this date may be expected (Table 5).

Yet, whether pregnancy terminates a week before or 2 weeks later than the day calculated, the outlook for mother and baby is usually as good as though it had ended at "high noon" on the due date. Actually, women seldom go "overterm"; in most of these cases it is the system of calculation and not Nature which has erred. For example, ovulation and hence conception may have occurred some days later than calculated; this error would make the beginning and the end of pregnancy that many days later. If, in addition to this circumstance, we were dealing with a baby which required a slightly longer stay in the uterus for complete development, it would be clear that the apparent delay was quite normal and for the best.

PHYSIOLOGY OF THE FETUS

Nutrition; Placental Transmission

During the period when the ovum lies unattached in the uterine cavity, its nutriment is provided by an endometrial secretion which is rich in glycogen and has been called "uterine

FIG. 4-23. Roent-genogram showing fetal and placental circulation at 11 weeks gestation, injected with Thorotrast (a contrast medium) by Charles H. Hendricks, M.D., and Frederick P. Zuspan, M.D. (Department of Obstetrics and Gynecology, Western Reserve University)

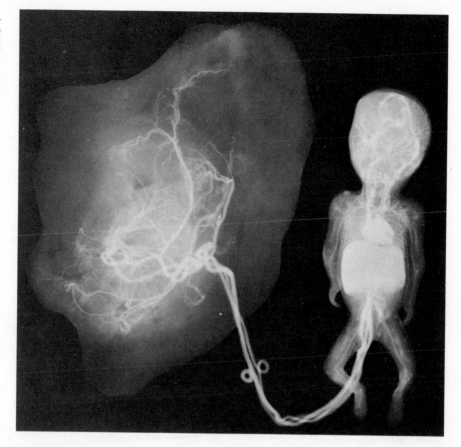

milk." With the burrowing of the ovum into the endometrium, it lies in a lake of fluid representing the broken-down product of endometrial cells and obtains nourishment from this source (Fig. 4-12).

Very early in pregnancy, certainly by the 3rd or the 4th week, the chorionic villi have blood vessels within them (connected with the fetal blood stream), and since these villi have already opened up the maternal blood vessels, nourishment is available from the maternal blood by the process of osmosis. In this connection it must be clearly understood that the maternal and the fetal bloods are never in contact and never intermingle. Indeed, even such substances as oxygen and glucose in the maternal blood must diffuse through several layers of tissue of the chorionic villi to reach the fetus. These layers are the cellular epithelium covering the villus, the loose connective tissue within it and finally the endothelium of the capillary blood vessel in the center of the villus. In this manner oxygen passes into the fetal cir-

culation, while the fetal waste product, carbon dioxide, diffuses in the opposite direction. The placenta thus serves as the "lungs" of the baby in utero. Simple food substances, such as glucose, salt, calcium, phosphorus, iron, amino acids and fatty acids, all diffuse through the chorionic villus to the fetus by this process of osmosis.

It is particularly important to note that most drugs pass readily to the fetus and, if given to the mother very shortly before birth, may affect the behavior of the newborn baby (p. 227). In addition, it is interesting to observe that estrogen is transmitted to the fetus and produces certain effects in the newborn which may be very striking. First, as the result of the action of this hormone, the breasts of both boy and girl babies may become markedly enlarged during the first few days of life and even secrete milk—the so-called "witch's milk" (Chap. 15, Breast Engorgement). Second, estrogen causes the endometrium of the female fetus to hypertrophy, as it does that of an adult woman. After birth, when this hormone is suddenly withdrawn, the endometrium breaks down, and sometimes bleeding occurs. For this reason perhaps 1 girl baby in every 15 manifests a little spotting on the diaper during the first week of life. This is entirely normal and clears up of itself within a few days.

Fetal Circulation

Since the placenta acts as the intermediary organ of transfer between the mother and the fetus, the fetal circulation differs from that required for extra-uterine existence. The fetus receives oxygen through the placenta, since the lungs do not function as organs of respiration in utero. To meet this situation the fetal circulation contains certain special vessels (they may be regarded as "bypasses" or "detours") which shunt the blood around the lungs, with only a small amount circulating through them for nutritional purposes (Fig. 4-23).

The oxygenated blood flows up the cord through the umbilical vein and passes into the inferior vena cava; on the way to the inferior vena cava, part of the oxygenated blood has gone through the liver, but most of it has passed through a special fetal structure, the *ductus venosus*, which connects the umbilical vein and the inferior vena cava (Fig. 4-24). The liver is proportionately so large in a newborn infant because it receives a considerable supply of freshly vitalized blood directly from the umbilical vein.

From the inferior vena cava the current flows into the right auricle and goes directly on to the left auricle through a special fetal structure, the *foramen ovale*, passing thence into the left ventricle and out through the aorta. The blood which circulates up the arms and the head returns through the superior vena cava to the right auricle again, but instead of passing through the foramen ovale, as before, the current is deflected downward into the right ventricle and out through the pulmonary arteries, partly to the lungs (for purposes of nutrition only), but mainly into the aorta through the special fetal structure, the ductus arteriosus.

The blood in the aorta, with the exception of that which goes to the head and the upper

extremities (this blood has been accounted for), passes downward to supply the trunk and the lower extremities (Fig. 4-24). The greater part of this blood finds its way through the internal iliac, or hypogastric arteries, and so back through the cord to the placenta, where it is again oxygenated; but a small amount passes back into the ascending vena cava to mingle with fresh blood from the umbilical vein and again make the circuit of the entire body.

Circulation Change at Birth

The fetal circulation is so arranged that the passage of blood to the placenta through the umbilical arteries and back through the umbilical vein is possible up to the time of birth, but it ceases entirely the moment the baby breathes and so begins to take its oxygen directly from its own lungs. During intra-uterine life the circulation of blood through the lungs is for the nourishment of the lungs and not for the purpose of securing oxygen (Figs. 4-24, 25).

In order to understand, even in a general way, the course of the blood current and how it differs from the circulation after birth, it must be borne in mind that in infants after birth, as in the adult, the venous blood passes from the 2 venae cavae into the right auricle of the heart, thence to the right ventricle and through the pulmonary arteries to the lungs, whence it gives up its waste products and takes up a fresh supply of oxygen. After oxygenation the so-called arterial blood flows from the lungs, through the pulmonary veins to the left auricle, thence to the left ventricle and out through the aorta, to be distributed through the capillaries to all parts of the body and eventually collected, as venous blood, in the venae cavae and discharged again into the right auricle.

Circulation Path After Birth

As soon as the baby is born and breathes, the function of the lungs is established, and the placental circulation ceases (the baby no longer is dependent on his mother's blood for oxygen but is a separate being and breathes to oxygenate his own blood). This change not only alters the character of the blood in many vessels but also makes many of these vessels

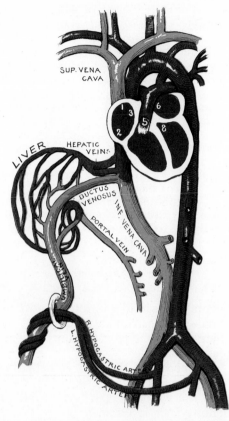
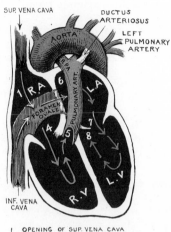

1 OPENING OF SUP. VENA CAVA
2 OPENING OF INF. VENA CAVA
3 FORAMEN OVALE
4 TRICUSPID VALVE TO R.VENTRICLE
5 PULMONARY VALVE
6 OPENING FROM PULMONARY VEINS
7 BICUSPID OR MITRAL VALVES
8 AORTIC VALVE

Fɪɢ. 4-24 (*Left*). Fetal circulation before birth. The material needed for the nourishment and the development of the fetus is brought to it from the placenta by way of the umbilical vein. Since the lungs do not function in the exchange of gases, the placenta serves as the respiratory organ in supplying oxygen to the fetus and also serves as an excretory organ for waste products. After the blood is purified in the placenta, it is sent with its nutritive material to the fetus by way of the umbilical vein; this vein divides into two branches after entering the abdominal wall. One of these branches joins directly to the portal vein which empties its blood into the liver, from which it is carried to the inferior vena cava by way of the hepatic veins. The other branch, the ductus venosus, joins directly the inferior vena cava, from which the blood is then carried to the right auricle of the heart. From the right auricle it goes through the foramen ovale to the left auricle and then to the left ventricle to the upper extremity by way of the aorta.

The blood returning from the upper extremity through the superior vena cava enters the right auricle, then the right ventricle, and then goes to the lungs by way of the pulmonary artery. Since the lungs do not function before birth, only a small portion of this blood gains access to them. Most of the blood from the pulmonary artery is diverted through the ductus arteriosus to the aorta and is then carried to the trunk and lower extremities.

Fɪɢ. 4-25 (*Right*). Fetal circulation after birth. Pulmonary circulation becomes established with birth. The umbilical cord circulation ceases. The arteries and the vein become obliterated immediately at the body junction. Shortly the hypogastric arteries, which are a continuance of the umbilical arteries after entrance into the body, become obliterated at their distal ends, followed by occlusion and obliteration of the umbilical vein and ductus venosus. The ductus arteriosus and the foramen ovale undergo a slower metamorphosis, finally occluding the circulation through the ductus arteriosus and closure of the foramen ovale. (Philips J. Carter, M.D., Louisiana State University, New Orleans)

TABLE 6.   CHANGES IN FETAL CIRCULATION AFTER BIRTH*

STRUCTURE	BEFORE BIRTH	AFTER BIRTH
Umbilical vein	Brings arterial blood to liver and heart	Obliterated. Becomes the round ligament of liver
Umbilical arteries	Bring arteriovenous blood to the placenta	Obliterated. Become vesical ligaments on anterior abdominal wall
Ductus venosus	Shunts arterial blood into inferior vena cava	Obliterated. Becomes ligamentum venosum
Ductus arteriosus	Shunts arterial and some venous blood from the pulmonary artery to the aorta	Obliterated. Becomes ligamentum arteriosum
Foramen ovale	Connects right and left auricles (atria)	Obliterated usually. At times open
Lungs	Contain no air and very little blood	Filled with air and well supplied with blood
Pulmonary arteries	Bring little blood to lungs	Bring much blood to lungs
Aorta	Receives blood from both ventricles	Receives blood only from left ventricle
Inferior vena cava	Brings venous blood from body and arterial blood from placenta	Brings venous blood only to right auricle

* Williams, J. F.: Anatomy and Physiology, ed. 7, Philadelphia, Saunders.

of no use as such; the umbilical arteries within the baby's body become filled with clotted blood and ultimately are converted into fibrous cords, and the umbilical vein within the body, after occlusion of the vessel, becomes the round ligament of the liver. After the umbilical cord is tied and separated, the large amount of blood returned to the heart and the lungs, which are now functioning, causes more or less equal pressure in both of the auricles—this pressure causes the foramen ovale to close. The foramen ovale remains closed and eventually disappears, and the ductus arteriosus and the ductus venosus finally shrivel up and are converted into fibrous cords or ligaments in the course of 2 or 3 months. The instantaneous closure of the foramen ovale changes the entire course of the blood current and converts the fetal circulation into the adult type.

The changes in the fetal circulation after birth may be tabulated as given in Table 6.

PERIODS OF DEVELOPMENT

Human life may be divided into periods. The successive periods, with the duration of each, are indicated below.

The period of the ovum extends from fertilization to implantation, about the close of the 2nd week of prenatal life. (The term "ovum" is used in a strict sense to denote the female germ cell and also to indicate the developing zygote [fertilized ovum] previous to implantation.)

The period of the embryo extends from the 3rd to the 5th weeks of gestation, during which time the various organs are developed, and a definite form is assumed.

The period of the fetus extends from after the 5th week to the time of birth.

The period of the newborn (neonatal) extends from birth to the close of the 1st month of postnatal life.

The period of infancy extends from the close of the 1st month to the close of the 2nd year of life (Nelson's Textbook of Pediatrics, Saunders, 1959).

The period of childhood extends from the close of the 2nd year to about the 14th year in females and to about the 16th year in males. Puberty ends the period of childhood.

The period of adolescence extends from puberty to the last years of the 2nd decade (late teens) in females and to the first years of the 3rd decade (early 20's) in males.

The period of maturity extends from the end of the adolescent period to senility (old age).

Development goes on throughout life; during senility, retrogressive or degenerative changes occur.

MATERNAL IMPRESSIONS

One of the commonest superstitions relating to childbearing is the old belief that the mental condition of the mother may modify the development of the unborn infant or, as people used to say, "mark it." For instance, if a pregnant woman were frightened by some ugly beast, let us say, it used to be thought that when the baby was born, it might be "marked" or distorted in the likeness of the animal. Very often the "marking" took the form of reddish blotches on the skin of the infant, which in the mother's imagination seemed to resemble the beast. Or, sometimes it was thought that the blotch resembled some article of food that the pregnant woman particularly craved.

This belief, like most obstetric superstitions, is of hoary antiquity. The Biblical story of Jacob and the "speckled and spotted" cattle and goats and the "brown" sheep reflects it, and dramatists and novelists from Shakespeare to Dickens have perpetuated the idea in stirring plots. The facts are these: There is no nervous connection between mother and fetus —in other words, no possible pathways along which any such impulses, pleasant or otherwise, could travel. The blood of the mother is likewise separate and distinct from that of the fetus. Furthermore, the anlagen for the various organs of the fetus are developed by the 6th week of pregnancy, that is, at a period when most women scarcely realize that they are pregnant; and, almost without exception, the causative mental shock or experience which is alleged to have brought about the "marking" occurred much later, long after the organ in question was in its final state of formation. Finally, all modern experience refutes the belief. Obstetricians of vast experience, as well as maternity hospitals with thousands of deliveries annually, never have reported an authentic case.

How, then, is this age-old superstition to be explained? A number of factors probably contribute to it, chiefly coincidence. Approximately 1 baby in every 200 is born with some kind of blemish. In the event that such a blemish is present—let us say a reddish blotch on the buttocks of the baby—would it not be easy for an introspective mother, who had been told of this legend, to think finally of some object, some animal, or possibly some article of diet that she craved during pregnancy and, in her imagination, correlate it with the little red blotch?

SUGGESTED READING

Corner, G. W.: Ourselves Unborn; An Embryologist's Essay on Man, New Haven, Yale Univ. Press, 1944.

Ferguson-Smith, M. A.: The techniques of human cytogenetics, Am. J. Obstet. Gynec. 90, No. 7, Part 2:1035-1054, 1964.

Flanagan, G. L.: The First Nine Months of Life, New York, Simon and Schuster, 1962.

Greisheimer, E. M.: Physiology and Anatomy, ed. 8, Philadelphia, Lippincott, 1963.

Ham, A. W.: Histology, ed. 5, Philadelphia, Lippincott, 1965.

Hamilton, W. J., Boyd, J. D., and Mossman, H. W.: Human Embryology, Baltimore, Williams & Wilkins, 1962.

Honegger, W., *et al.*: Genetics, New York, Dell Books, 1962.

Miller, O. J.: The sex chromosome anomalies, Am. J. Obstet. Gynec. 90, No. 7, Part 2:1078-1139, 1964.

Osborne, R., and DeGeorge, F. V.: Sex determination and development, Am. J. Nurs. 59:213, 1959.

Patten, B. M.: Human Embryology, ed. 2, New York, Blakiston Division of McGraw-Hill, 1953.

Potter, E.: Fundamentals of Human Reproduction, New York, McGraw-Hill, 1947.

Scheinfeld, A.: You and Heredity, Philadelphia, Lippincott, 1950.

Smith, D. W.: Autosomal abnormalities, Am. J. Obstet. Gynec. 90, No. 7, Part 2:1055-1077, 1964.

Sohval, A. R.: Recent progress in human chromosome analysis and its relation to the sex chromatin, Am. J. Med. 31:397, 1961.

Thuline, H., *et al.*: Chromosomal sex test, Am. J. Dis. Child. 94:130, 1957.

Chapter 5

Presentations and Positions

FETAL HABITUS

By habitus, or attitude, of the fetus is meant the relation of the fetal parts to one another. The most striking characteristic of the fetal habitus is flexion. The spinal column is bowed forward, the head is flexed with the chin against the sternum, and the arms are flexed and folded against the chest. The lower extremities also are flexed, the thighs on the abdomen and the calves of the lower legs against the posterior aspect of the thighs. In this state of flexion the fetus assumes a roughly ovoid shape, occupies the smallest possible space and conforms to the shape of the uterus. In this attitude it is about half as long as if it were completely stretched out. However, there are times when the fetus assumes many other positions.

FETAL HEAD

From an obstetric viewpoint the head of the fetus is the most important part. If it can pass through the pelvic canal safely, there is usually no difficulty in delivering the rest of the body, although occasionally the shoulders may cause trouble.

The cranium, or skull, is made up of 8 bones. Four of the bones—the sphenoid, the ethmoid and the 2 temporal bones—lie at the base of the cranium, are closely united and are of little obstetric interest. On the other hand, the 4 bones forming the upper part of the cranium are of great importance; these are the frontal, the occipital and the 2 parietal bones. These bones are not knit closely together at the time of birth but are separated by membranous interspaces called *sutures*. The intersections of these sutures are known as *fontanels* (Fig. 5-1).

By means of this formation of the fetal skull the bones can overlap each other somewhat during labor and so diminish materially the size of the head during its passage through the pelvis. This process of overlapping is called "molding," and after a long labor with a large baby and a snug pelvis, the head often is so definitely molded that several days may elapse before it returns to its normal shape.

The most important sutures are: the sagittal, between the 2 parietal bones; the frontal, between the 2 frontal bones; the coronal, between the frontal and the parietal bones; and the lambdoid, between the posterior margins of the parietal bones and the upper margin of the occipital bone. The temporal sutures, which separate the parietal and the temporal bones on either side, are unimportant in obstetrics because they are covered by fat parts and cannot be felt on the living baby.

The fontanels of importance are the anterior and the posterior. The anterior fontanel, large and diamond-shaped, is at the intersection of the sagittal and the coronal sutures, while the

92

small triangular posterior fontanel lies at the junction of the sagittal and the lambdoid suture. The sutures and the posterior fontanel ossify shortly after birth, but the anterior fontanel remains open until the child is over a year old, constituting the familiar "soft spot" just above the forehead of an infant. By feeling or identifying one or another of the sutures or fontanels, and considering its relative position in the pelvis, the physician is enabled to determine accurately the position of the head.

PRESENTATION

The term "presentation" or "presenting part" is used to designate that portion of the infant's body which lies nearest the internal os, or, in other words, that portion which is felt by the examining fingers of the physician when they are introduced into the cervix. When the presenting part is known, by abdominal palpation, it is possible to determine the relation between the long axis of the baby's body and that of the mother.

Head or *cephalic presentations* are the most common, being present in about 97 per cent of all cases at term. Cephalic presentations are divided into groups, according to the relation which the infant's head bears to its body. The most common is the *vertex presentation*, in which the head is sharply flexed so that the chin is in contact with the thorax; then the vertex is the presenting part. The *face presentation*, in which the neck is sharply extended so that the occiput and the back come in contact, is more rarely observed.

Next to the cephalic presentation, *the breech presentation* is the most common, being present, however, in only about 3 per cent of all cases. In breech presentations the thighs may be flexed and the legs extended over the anterior surface of the body (*frank breech presentation*), or the thighs may be flexed on the abdomen and the legs on the thighs (*full*

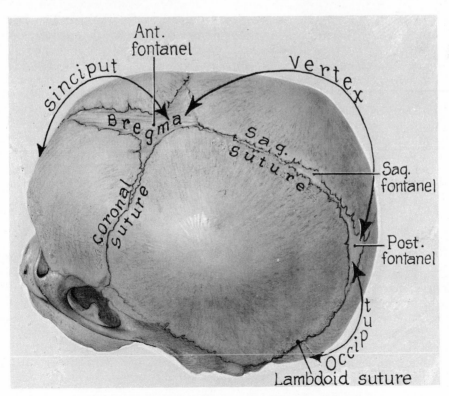

FIG. 5-1. Fetal skull, showing sutures and fontanels.

breech presentation), or one or both feet may be the lowest part (*foot or footling presentation*).

When the fetus lies crosswise in the uterus, the shoulder is the presenting part—*shoulder presentation*. The common causes of a "transverse lie" are: (1) abnormal relaxation of the abdominal walls due to great multiparity, (2) pelvic contraction, and (3) placenta previa. Shoulder presentations are relatively uncommon, and, with very rare exceptions, the spontaneous birth of a fully developed child is impossible in a "persistent transverse lie."

POSITIONS

Beside knowing the presenting part of the baby, it is important to know the exact position of this presenting part in relation to the pelvis. This relationship is determined by finding the position of certain points on the pre-

POSITIONS OF PRESENTING PARTS

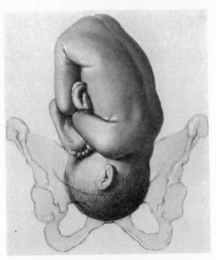

Fig. 5-2. Left-occipito-anterior (L.O.A.).

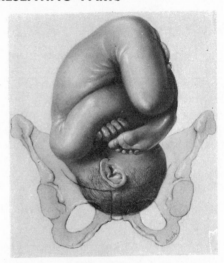

Fig. 5-4. Right-occipitotransverse (R.O.T.).

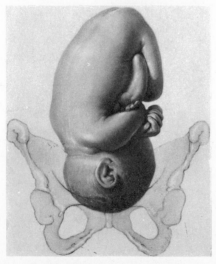

Fig. 5-3. Right-occipito-anterior (R.O.A.).

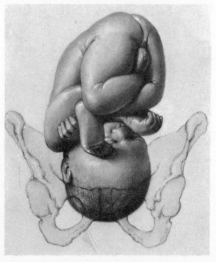

Fig. 5-5. Right-occipitoposterior (R.O.P.).

senting surface with regard to the four imaginary divisions or regions of the pelvis. For this purpose the pelvis is considered to be divided into quadrants: left anterior, left posterior, right anterior and right posterior. These divisions aid the physician in indicating whether the presenting part is directed toward the right or the left side and toward the front or the back of the pelvis. Certain points on the presenting surface of the baby have been arbitrarily chosen as points of direction in determining the exact relation of the presenting part to the quadrants of the pelvis. In vertex presentations the occiput is the guiding point; in face presentations, the chin (mentum); in breech presentations, the sacrum; and in shoulder presentations, the scapula (acromion process).

Position, then, has to do with the relation of some arbitrarily chosen portion of the fetus to the right or the left side of the mother's pelvis. Thus, in a vertex presentation, the back of the head (occiput) may point to the front or to the back of the pelvis. The occiput rarely points directly forward or backward in the median line until the second stage of labor, but usually is directed to one side or the other.

The various positions are usually expressed by abbreviations made up of the first letter of each word which describes the position. Thus, left-occipito-anterior is abbreviated L.O.A. This means that the head is presenting with the occiput directed toward the left side of the mother and toward the front part of the pelvis. If the occiput were directed straight to the left with no deviation toward front or back of the pelvis, it would be termed left-occipitotransverse, or L.O.T. The occiput might also be

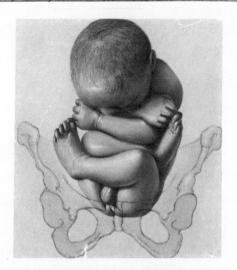

FIG. 5-6. Left-sacroposterior (L.S.P.).

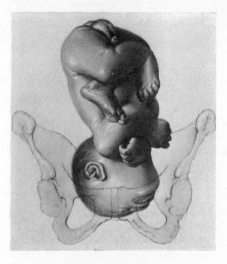

FIG. 5-7. Left-mento-anterior (L.M.A.).

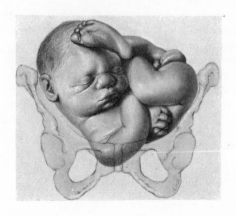

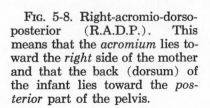

FIG. 5-8. Right-acromio-dorso-posterior (R.A.D.P.). This means that the *acromium* lies toward the *right* side of the mother and that the back (dorsum) of the infant lies toward the *posterior* part of the pelvis.

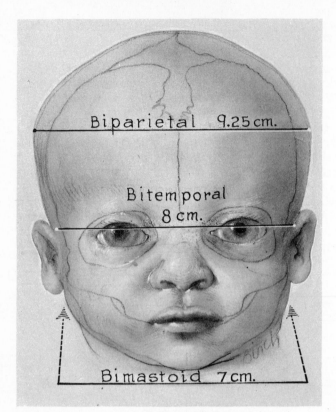

FIG. 5-9. Fetal head, showing transverse diameters.

directed toward the back or posterior quadrant of the pelvis, in which case the position would be left-occipitoposterior, or L.O.P. There are also three corresponding positions on the right side: R.O.A., R.O.T. and R.O.P.

The occipital positions are considered the most favorable for both mother and baby, and of these, the L.O.A. position is preferred. The same system of terminology is used for face, breech and shoulder presentations, as indicated in the following list of abbreviations (S indicating breech; M, chin or face; and A, shoulder).

Although it is customary to speak of all "transverse lies" of the fetus simply as shoulder presentations, the examples of terminology sometimes used to express position in the shoulder presentation are listed. Left-acromio-dorso-anterior (L.A.D.A.) means that the acromion is to the mother's left and the back is anterior.

POSITIONS—VERTEX PRESENTATION

L.O.A.—Left-occipito-anterior (Fig. 5-2)
L.O.T.—Left-occipitotransverse
L.O.P.—Left-occipitoposterior
R.O.A.—Right-occipito-anterior (Fig. 5-3)
R.O.T.—Right-occipitotransverse (Fig. 5-4)
R.O.P.—Right-occipitoposterior (Fig. 5-5)

POSITIONS—BREECH PRESENTATION

L.S.A.—Left-sacro-anterior
L.S.T.—Left-sacrotransverse
L.S.P.—Left-sacroposterior (Fig. 5-6)
R.S.A.—Right-sacro-anterior
R.S.T.—Right-sacrotransverse
R.S.P.—Right-sacroposterior

POSITIONS—FACE PRESENTATION

L.M.A.—Left-mento-anterior (Fig. 5-7)
L.M.T.—Left-mentotransverse
L.M.P.—Left-mentoposterior
R.M.A.—Right-mento-anterior
R.M.T.—Right-mentotransverse
R.M.P.—Right-mentoposterior

POSITIONS—SHOULDER PRESENTATION

L.A.D.A.—Left-acromio-dorso-anterior
L.A.D.P.—Left-acromio-dorso-posterior

FIG. 5-10. Fetal head, showing anteroposterior diameters.

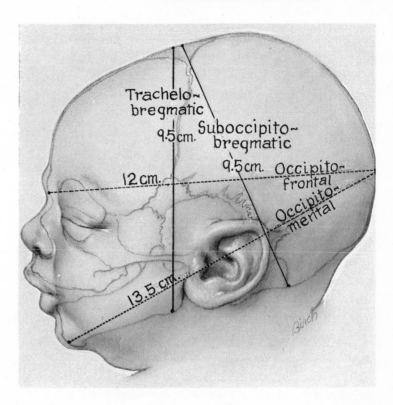

R.A.D.A.—Right-acromio-dorso-anterior
R.A.D.P.—Right-acromio-dorso-posterior
(Fig. 5-8)

Figures 5-9 and 10 show the principal measurements of the fetal skull. The most important transverse diameter is the biparietal; it is the distance between the biparietal protuberances and represents the greatest width of the head. It measures, on an average, 9.25 cm. There are three important anteroposterior diameters: the suboccipitobregmatic, which extends from the undersurface of the occiput to the center of the anterior fontanel and measures about 9.5 cm.; the occipitofrontal, which extends from the root of the nose to the occipital prominence and measures about 12.0 cm.; and the occipitomental, which extends from the chin to the posterior fontanel and averages about 13.5 cm.

In considering these three anteroposterior diameters of the fetal skull, it is important to note that with the head in complete flexion and the chin resting on the thorax, the smallest of these, the suboccipitobregmatic, enters the pelvis, whereas if the head is extended or bent back (with no flexion whatsoever), the greatest anteroposterior diameter presents itself to the pelvic inlet. Herein lies the great importance of flexion; the more the head is flexed, the smaller is the anteroposterior diameter which enters the pelvis. Figures 5-11 to 13 show this basic principle in diagrammatic form.

DIAGNOSIS OF FETAL POSITION

Diagnosis of fetal position is made in four ways: (1) abdominal palpation; (2) vaginal and rectal examination; (3) combined auscultation and examination; (4) in certain doubtful cases, the roentgenogram.

Inspection

Nurses thus should be able to determine whether a presentation is normal or otherwise, as work in rural, sparsely settled localities often may require of her knowledge not demanded in her hospital experience. Only under

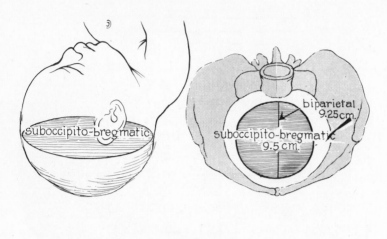

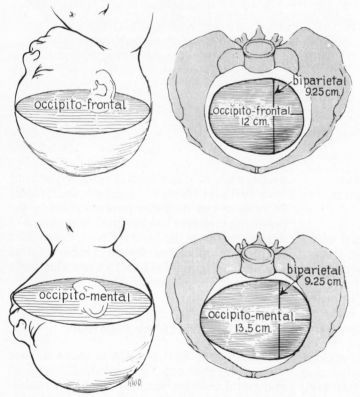

Fig. 5-11 (*Top*). Complete flexion allows smallest diameter of head to enter pelvis.

Fig. 5-12 (*Center*). Moderate extension causes larger diameter to enter pelvis.

Fig. 5-13 (*Bottom*). Marked extension forces largest diameter against pelvic brim, but it is too large to enter.

most unusual conditions would she be expected to ascertain this in any other way than by palpation.

Palpation

The nurse should familiarize herself thoroughly with this method. She will find it extremely helpful to palpate the abdomen before listening to the fetal heart tones. The region of the abdomen in which the fetal heart is heard most plainly varies according to the presentation and the extent to which the presenting part has descended. The location of the fetal heart sounds by itself does not give very important information as to the presentation and the position of the child, but it sometimes reinforces the results obtained by

Fig. 5-14. Palpation: (*top, left*) first maneuver; (*top, right*) second maneuver; (*bottom, left*) third maneuver; (*bottom, right*) fourth maneuver.

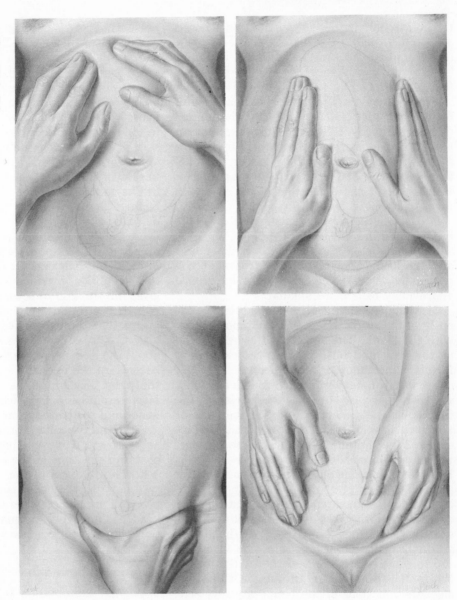

palpation. In order to obtain satisfactory information by abdominal palpation for the determination of fetal position, the examination should be made systematically by following the four maneuvers suggested by Leopold, often called the _Leopold maneuvers._

The nurse should make certain that the patient has emptied her bladder before the procedure is begun. This will not only contribute to the patient's comfort but also will aid the nurse to gain more accurate results in the latter part of the examination. During the first three maneuvers the nurse stands at the side of the bed facing the patient; during the last one she faces the patient's feet. Although a diagnosis should not be made on the basis of inspection, actual observation of the patient's abdomen should precede palpation. For the examination the patient should lie flat on her back, with her knees flexed, to relax the abdominal muscles; the nurse should lay both hands gently, and at first, flat upon the abdomen. If done in any other manner than this, or if her hands are not warm, the stimulation of her fingers will cause the abdominal muscles to contract. She should accustom herself to palpate the uterus in a definite, methodical way, and it will be found best to carry out successively the following four maneuvers .

First Maneuver. The nurse should ascertain, facing the patient, what is lying at the fundus of the uterus by feeling the upper abdomen with both hands; generally she will find there a mass, which is either the head or the buttocks (breech) of the fetus. She must decide which pole of the fetus this is by observing three points (Fig. 5-14):

1. Its relative consistency: the head is harder than the breech.

2. Its shape: if the head, it will be round and hard, and the transverse groove of the neck may be felt. The breech has no groove and usually feels more angular.

3. Mobility: the head will move independently of the trunk, but the breech moves only with the trunk. The ability of the head to be moved back and forth against the examining fingers is spoken of as ballottement.

Second Maneuver. Having determined whether the head or the breech is in the fundus, the next step is to locate the back of the fetus in relation to the right and the left sides of the mother. Still facing the patient, the nurse places the palmar surfaces of both hands on either side of the abdomen and makes gentle but deep pressure. If the hand on one side of the abdomen remains still to steady the uterus, a slightly circular motion with the flat surface of the fingers on the other hand can gradually palpate the opposite side from the top to the lower segment of the uterus to feel the fetal outline. Then, to palpate the other side, the functions of the hands are reversed, i.e., the hand which was used to palpate now remains steady, and the other hand palpates the opposite side of the uterus. On one side is felt a smooth, hard, resistant plane, the back, while on the other, numerous angular nodulations are palpated, the small parts; these latter represent the knees and the elbows of the fetus.

Third Maneuver. This maneuver consists in an effort to find the head at the pelvic inlet and to determine its mobility. It should be conducted by gently grasping the lower portion of the abdomen, just above the symphysis pubis, between the thumb and the fingers of one hand and then pressing together. If the presenting part is not engaged, a movable body will be felt, which is usually the head.

Fourth Maneuver. In this maneuver the nurse faces the feet of the patient and places the tips of her first three fingers on both sides of the midline about 2 inches above Poupart's ligament. Pressure is now made downward and in the direction of the birth canal, the movable skin of the abdomen being carried downward along with the fingers. It will be found that the fingers of one hand meet no obstruction and can be carried downward well under Poupart's ligament; these fingers glide over the nape of the baby's neck. The other hand, however, usually meets an obstruction an inch or so above Poupart's ligament; this is the brow of the baby and is usually spoken of as the "cephalic prominence." This maneuver gives information of several kinds:

1. If the findings are as described above, it means that the baby's head is well flexed.

2. Confirmatory information is obtained about the location of the back, as naturally the back is on the opposite side from the brow of the baby, except in the uncommon cases of face presentation, in which the cephalic prominence and the back are on the same side.

3. If the cephalic prominence is very easily palpated, as if it were just under the skin, a posterior position of the occiput is suggested.

4. The location of the cephalic prominence tells how far the head has descended into the pelvis. This maneuver is of most value if the head has engaged and may yield no information with a floating, poorly flexed head.

Vaginal Examination

Vaginal examination is done by the physician and consists in identifying the fontanels and the suture lines of the fetal skull. During pregnancy the vaginal examination gives limited information concerning the position of the fetus because the cervix is closed. However, during labor, after more or less complete dilatation of the cervix, important information about the position of the baby and the degree of flexion of its head can be obtained.

Auscultation

The location of the fetal heart sounds, as heard through the stethoscope, yields helpful confirmatory information about fetal position but is not wholly dependable. Certainly, it never should be relied on as the sole means of diagnosing fetal position. Ordinarily, the heart sounds are transmitted through the convex portion of the fetus, which lies in intimate contact with the uterine wall, so that they are heard best through the infant's back in vertex and breech presentations, and through the thorax in face presentation. In cephalic presentations the fetal heart sounds are heard loudest midway between the umbilicus and the anterior superior spine of the ilium. In general, in L.O.A. and L.O.P. positions the fetal heart sounds are heard loudest in the left lower quadrant. A similar situation applies to the R.O.A. and R.O.P. positions. In posterior positions of the occiput (L.O.P. and R.O.P.) often the sounds are heard loudest well down in the flank toward the anterosuperior spine. In breech presentation the fetal heart sounds usually are heard loudest at the level of the umbilicus or above (see Fig. 7-3).

Roentgenograms

Roentgenograms are of particular value in diagnosis of fetal position in doubtful cases, particularly in obese women or in those with abdominal walls so rigid that abdominal palpation is difficult. In such situations the roentgenogram enables the physician to recognize the existence of conditions which might otherwise have escaped detection until late in labor. They give accurate information concerning position, presentation, flexion and descent of the fetal head (see Fig. 7-5).

SUGGESTED READING

Beck, A. C., and Rosenthal, Alexander: Obstetrical Practice, ed. 8, Baltimore, Williams & Wilkins, 1965.
Eastman, N. J., and Hellman, L. M.: Williams Obstetrics, ed. 12, New York, Appleton, 1961.
Greenhill, J. P.: Obstetrics, ed. 13, Philadelphia, Saunders, 1965.
The books listed above are among the standard American works on obstetrics. One of these, at least, will be found in any nurses' library and all in most medical libraries. The nurse will do well to augment her reading by consulting one or another of these volumes from time to time.

CONFERENCE MATERIAL

1. What would be your responsibility to a friend who is pregnant and yet has not registered for delivery with either a doctor or a clinic?
2. How would you present the subject of human reproduction to a group of Girl Scouts or junior high school students?
3. What illustrative material and reference readings would you select for a group conference of young parents or those about to be married?
4. How would you go about looking up the costs of obstetric care in your community?
5. If a patient appealed to you to secure information about the best obstetric care available in a certain city in the United States, how would you get this information for her?
6. What authentic sources are available for obtaining maternal and infant mortality statistics?
7. What is the status of the midwife in this country? How does this situation compare with that in other countries?
8. What forces are in operation to improve the quality of maternity care?
9. How can you stimulate the interest of a lay group in the community which is willing to give time and some financial support to help with an educational program for the less fortunate?

SELF-EXAMINATION QUESTIONS FOR THE STUDENT

After each unit of this book some objectively scorable test questions are provided to aid you in making immediate *use* of the information and the knowledge that you have gained through studying each of these units. The questions are planned to enable you to see how some of the important facts function in the nursing care of patients, and how knowledge of the facts enables you to (1) recognize, analyze and interpret the nursing needs of maternity patients, (2) plan to meet these needs, (3) carry out the plan and (4) evaluate both the plan and the results.

These questions represent only a few sample instances in which information, facts and principles presented in the units function in nursing care. If you are successful in these samples, you may be in many more instances, but you should not assume that success here guarantees success in all. Likewise, failure on many of these items does not necessarily mean complete lack of understanding, but it is a rather good indication that you need to restudy the unit more carefully.

Use these tests as a study device. After you believe that you have mastered the important points in the unit, fill out the objectively scorable test questions at the end of the unit. Think through each question and response carefully. Complete the entire unit test and then (and not until then) turn to the key on page 597, where you will find the right answers. See how many you had correct. Look up the answers to those that you answered incorrectly.

You will observe that many of the questions demand that you use your previously acquired knowledge of anatomy and physiology, bacteriology, chemistry, pharmacology, psychology, nursing arts and nutrition, together with maternity nursing knowledge, for all nursing care demands the simultaneous functioning of facts and principles from many of these fields, along with those of the special clinical field.

In some judgments on debatable questions the answer given in the key may conflict with the current practice in your institution or locality. Ask your teacher how she thinks you should evaluate yourself on this knowledge.

Since the purpose of these self-scoring tests is to aid you in learning, you will be defeating that purpose and penalizing yourself if you misuse them. Carefully think through the question. *No one but you is interested in how well or how poorly you do on these tests.* When you have discovered how well or how poorly you have done, you will know better what you need to study again, and how much more study is necessary.

Your teacher's evaluation of your ability to use the material presented in each unit may sample some of these and many other points presented in the unit. Your best preparation for your teacher's appraisal in classroom and in the practice of nursing is your own evaluation of your attainment and study in light of your accomplishment. But, more important, your best preparation for giving skilled professional nursing care to maternity patients is to have a complete understanding of and ability to use the important principles that relate to that care, an understanding that is largely within your own power to obtain through your own efforts.

Study Questions

UNIT ONE: HUMAN REPRODUCTION

Read through the entire question and place your answer on the line to the right.

1. Which of the following complications of pregnancy are responsible for the greatest toll in maternal mortality?
   A. Cardiac complications
   B. Toxemia
   C. Hemorrhage
   D. Infection
   E. Diabetes

   Select the number corresponding to the correct letters.
   1. A and B
   2. A, C and E
   3. B, C and D
   4. B, C and E

   _3_

2. What improvement is believed to be the greatest single factor for decreasing maternal deaths during the past half century?
   A. Antepartal care
   B. Management of labor
   C. Analgesia during delivery
   D. Nursing care during delivery
   E. Care by the physician during delivery
   F. Care during the puerperium

   _A_

3. A patient in the clinic, who was in the latter part of her pregnancy, reported to the nurse that she was suffering from backache and wanted to know the cause. What would be the most likely reason that the nurse could give her?
   A. The larger size of the fetus tires her more easily.
   B. Increased mobility of joints throws greater weight on surrounding muscles.
   C. She must have some abnormality in pelvic structures.
   D. The descent of the presenting part into the pelvic cavity prior to labor increases pressure against the sacrum.

   _B_

4. In each of the following write the term or the phrase by which the pelvic measurement described is commonly called.
   A. Between the symphysis pubis and the depression below the 5th lumbar vertebra   A. _external conjugate_
   B. From the lower margin of the symphysis pubis to the sacral promontory   B. _diagonal conjugate_
   C. Between the lateral edges of the iliac crests   C. _intercristal_
   D. The posterior portion of the symphysis pubis to the promontory of the sacrum   D. _conjugate vera_
   E. From the inner aspects of the ischial tuberosities   E. _intertuberous diameter_

5. By using the letter or letters of the measurements described in Question 4 indicate:
   A. The one which must be estimated rather than measured directly   A. _D_
   B. The one which represents the most important diameter   B. _D_
   C. The one which represents the largest diameter   C. _C_

6. A patient's chart shows pelvic measurements of 11 cm. for the diagonal conjugate and 9.5 cm. for the true conjugate; therefore, the nurse caring for the patient in the labor room should anticipate that the patient might have:
   A. An easy, rapid delivery
   B. A delivery of reasonable duration
   C. A protracted labor with difficult delivery

   _C_

7. To give adequate care to the patient during and after delivery, the nurse should fully understand the structure of the uterus. Which of the following are true of the uterus?
A. Its muscular tissue is:
   1. Chiefly striated
   2. Chiefly nonstriated
   3. Entirely striated
   4. Entirely nonstriated   *4*
B. Its muscle fibers are arranged to run:
   1. Circularly
   2. Longitudinally
   3. In all directions
   4. In three layers, the inner and the outer circularly, the other longitudinally   *3*
C. Its blood is supplied directly from:
   1. Ovarian and uterine arteries
   2. Abdominal aorta and uterine arteries
   3. Internal iliac and ovarian arteries
   4. Internal iliac and uterine arteries   *1*
D. Normally, it is:
   1. Attached anteriorly to the bladder wall
   2. Suspended freely movable in the pelvic cavity
   3. Suspended between the bladder and the rectum
   4. Attached posteriorly to the anterior wall of the sacrum   *2*

8. The perineum lies between the vagina and the rectum. This structure has:
A. A single, strong elastic muscle
B. A strong elastic tendon
C. A tendon to which 5 muscles are attached
D. Two strong muscles, the anal and the transverse perineal   *C*

9. Every effort is made to prevent the tearing of the perineum during childbirth. The chief hazard to the patient from laceration of the perineum would likely be:
A. Incontinence
B. Postpartal hemorrhage
C. Perineal abscess
D. Prolapsed uterus   *B*

10. A patient with small breasts in her first pregnancy was worried about her ability to feed her baby.
A. The nurse could respond correctly to the patient by telling her that:
   1. She probably would be unable to feed her baby.
   2. The size of the breasts does not influence the amount of lactation possible.
   3. Mothers with small breasts usually have less difficulty feeding their babies.
   4. Her baby would be fed better by means of a formula.   *2*
B. Milk is produced by the process of:
   1. Dialysis
   2. Osmosis
   3. Secretion   *2*
C. The structures most directly involved in the production of milk are:
   1. Papillae
   2. Glands of Montgomery
   3. Acini cells
   4. Lactiferous sinuses
   5. Areola
   6. Lactiferous ducts   *3*

11. What are the ovarian hormones produced by the graafian follicle and the cells of the corpus luteum?
A. Progesterone and gonadotropin
B. Estrogen and progesterone
C. Gonadotropin and FSH
D. FSH and estrogen   *B*

12. A young mother-to-be told a nurse that she was sure that she would have a boy because her husband was such a strong, physicially well-developed man. The nurse could respond correctly by saying:
   A. "It is the female cell which determines the sex of the child."
   B. "It is unlikely because there are more girls born than boys."
   C. "Physical strength does not influence the sex of the child."
   D. "You are probably right."

C

13. A patient expelled a fetus of 16 cm. prematurely. What would be the approximate age of the fetus?
   A. 2 months
   B. 3 months
   C. 4 months
   D. 5 months

C

14. Although the exact date of delivery cannot be predetermined, if a pregnant woman's last menstrual period began on September 10, the estimated due date would be nearest:
   A. May 6
   B. May 10
   C. June 10
   D. June 17

D

15. The only direct connection between the fetus and any other structure is through the umbilical cord. The umbilical cord contains which of these important structures?
   A. Umbilical artery
   B. Umbilical arteries
   C. Umbilical vein
   D. Umbilical veins
   E. Umbilical nerves
   F. Umbilical lymphatic duct
   G. Wharton's jelly

Select the number corresponding to the correct letters.
   1. A, D and F
   2. B, C and G
   3. C, E and G
   4. All of them

2

16. After a protracted labor and a difficult delivery, the mother, upon seeing her baby, was shocked at the elongated appearance of the infant's head. The nurse could correctly reassure the patient by saying:
   A. "The baby's head is molded during delivery and will return to normal in a few days."
   B. "All newborn babies' heads are shaped this way."
   C. "The child's head shape was changed during delivery, and it will take six months for it to return to normal."
   D. "After the 'soft spot' closes, the head will return to normal."

A

17. Indicate the abbreviations that might be used on a patient's chart to represent each of the positions and the presentations described:
   A. Back of head directed straight to the left   A. *LOT*
   B. Back of head directed toward the left side and the front quadrant of the pelvis   B. *LOB*
   C. Back of head directed toward the right side and the back quadrant of the pelvis C. *ROP*
   D. Breech presentation, buttocks at the left back quadrant   D. *LSP*
   E. Face presentation, chin at the right front quadrant   E. *RMA*
   F. Transverse lie, shoulder is to the right of mother's pelvis, back is posterior   F. *RADP*

Note: The key to the correct answers to these questions is given on page 597.

Nursing in Pregnancy

Normal Pregnancy
Signs and Symptoms of Pregnancy
Antepartal Care
Mental Hygiene of Pregnancy and Childbirth

Chapter 6

Normal Pregnancy

INTRODUCTION

This chapter is concerned with the anatomic and the physiologic adaptations of the human organism to pregnancy. Knowledge of human reproduction, presented in the previous unit, is essential to the understanding of this phase of the reproductive process. From a biologic point of view, pregnancy and labor represent the highest function of the female reproductive system and should be considered as a normal process.

The length of human pregnancy varies greatly, but the average duration, if counted from the time of conception, is approximately 267 days or 38 weeks (see Chap. 3).

Many changes in maternal physiology occur during pregnancy. These adaptations to pregnancy, although most apparent in the reproductive organs, involve other body systems as well. Concomitant to these changes, the expectant mother usually has many emotional adjustments to make: sometimes fear, apprehension, worries (financial as well as physical) and family problems are present. The fact that delivery must be "faced," that there is no turning back or "changing the mind," can in itself sometimes create an overwhelming crisis (see Chaps. 8 and 9). However, these are all temporary alterations, and usually they can be expected to regress on a return to a normal nonpregnant status after the birth of the baby (see Chap. 13).

PHYSIOLOGIC CHANGES OF PREGNANCY

By the physiologic changes of pregnancy are meant those alterations, both local and general, which affect the maternal organism as the result of pregnancy but subside at or before the end of the puerperium and leave the patient in practically the same condition in which she was before conception occurred. In other words, the physiologic changes of pregnancy are to be regarded as normal, inevitable and purely temporary; for they are present in varying degrees in every instance, and in the case of a physically healthy woman there should be no traces of them left after convalescence is complete. It must be remembered, however, that after pregnancy the uterus does not return to its normal nulliparous size, though it does return to a normal nonpregnant state. The adult parous uterus is slightly larger and weighs more than that of a woman who has never borne children (Chap. 2).

LOCAL CHANGES

Uterus

The uterus increases in size to make room for the growing fetus. Naturally, the enlargement of the uterus is the most striking change wrought by pregnancy and, moreover, is di-

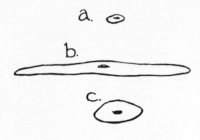

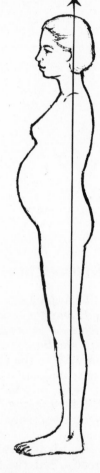

Fig. 6-1 (*Left*). Size of muscle cells. This illustrates the size of the muscle cells of the uterus (a) before pregnancy, (b) during pregnancy, showing the change in the size of these cells, and (c) in the puerperium. (After Stieve)

Fig. 6-2 (*Right*). Pregnancy should and usually does improve posture. The diagram illustrates the correct standing posture showing that a straight line may be drawn from the ear to the ankle. During pregnancy "walk tall, stand tall and sit tall."

rectly responsible for other important alterations. The growth of this organ in gestation is phenomenal. It increases in size from approximately 6.5 cm. long, 4 cm. wide and 2.5 cm. deep to about 32 cm. long, 24 cm. wide and 22 cm. deep. Its weight increases from 50 to 1,000 Gm. The small, almost solid organ which has a capacity of perhaps 2 cc. increases to become a thin-walled muscular sac capable of containing the fetus, the placenta and a large quantity of amniotic fluid. The tremendous growth is due partly to the formation of new muscle fibers during the early months of pregnancy, but principally to the enlargement of pre-existent muscle fibers which are 7 to 11 times longer and 2 to 7 times wider than those observed in the nonpregnant uterus (Fig. 6-1). Simultaneously, fibroelastic tissue develops between the muscle bands and forms a network about the various muscle bundles. This is of great importance in view of the function of the uterus in pregnancy and labor, because it strengthens the uterine walls. During early pregnancy the hypertrophy of the uterus is probably due to the stimulating action of estrogen on muscle fibers, but after the first trimester the increase in size is partly mechanical due to the pressure of the growing fetus (Fig. 6-2). The uterine wall thickens during the first few months of pregnancy from about 1 cm. to almost 2 cm., but thereafter it thins to about 0.5 cm. or less. By the end of pregnancy the uterus becomes a thin, soft-walled muscular sac which yields to the movements of the fetal extremities and permits the examiner to palpate the fetus easily.

The muscle fibers are arranged in three layers: the external hoodlike layer which arches over the fundus; the internal layer of circular fibers around the orifices of the fallopian tubes and the internal os; and the figure-8 fibers in the middle layer which make an interlacing network through which the blood vessels pass. This last group plays an important role in childbearing and will be referred to particularly in the care of the mother during labor and after delivery, for when these muscle fibers contract, they constrict the blood vessels.

Between the 3rd and the 4th months of pregnancy the growing uterus rises out of the pelvis and can be palpated above the symphysis pubis, rising progressively to reach the umbilicus about the 6th month and almost impinging on the xiphoid process at the 9th month (Figs. 6-3 to 6). As the uterus becomes larger, it comes in contact with the anterior abdominal

FIG. 6-3. Changes in abdominal contour in pregnancy. Photographic study of actual patient.

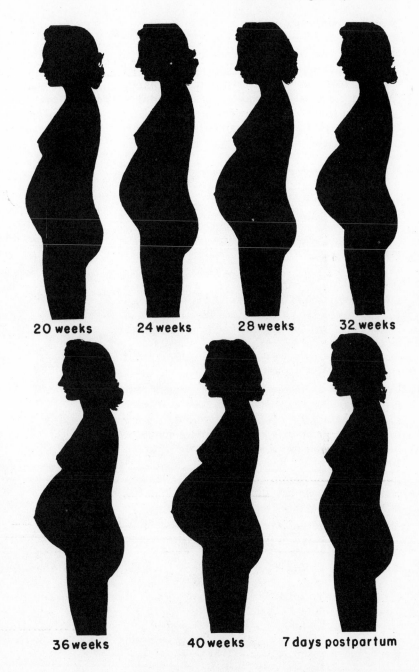

20 weeks 24 weeks 28 weeks 32 weeks

36 weeks 40 weeks 7 days postpartum

wall and displaces the intestines to the sides of the abdomen. About 2 weeks before term, in most primigravidae the fetal head descends into the pelvic cavity. As a result, the uterus sinks to a lower level and at the same time falls forward. Since this relieves the upward pressure on the diaphragm and makes breathing easier, this phenomenon of the descent of the head has been called "lightening" (Fig. 6-7). These changes usually do not occur in multiparas until the onset of labor. By palpating the height of the fundus experienced examiners can determine the approximate length of gestation.

Since the full-term pregnant uterus and its contents weigh about 12 pounds, a gravid woman may be likened to a person carrying a heavy basket pressed against the abdomen. Such a person will instinctively lean backward to maintain equilibrium. This backward tilt of the torso is characteristic of pregnancy. From a practical viewpoint it is important to note that this posture imposes increased strain on the muscles and the ligaments of the back and the thighs, and in this way is responsible for many of the muscular aches and cramps so often experienced in late pregnancy.

The cervix undergoes certain remarkable changes during pregnancy. One of the first physical signs of pregnancy, softening of the cervix, may be apparent as early as a month after conception (see p. 125). The softening of the cervix in pregnancy is due to increased vascularity, edema and hyperplasia of the cer-

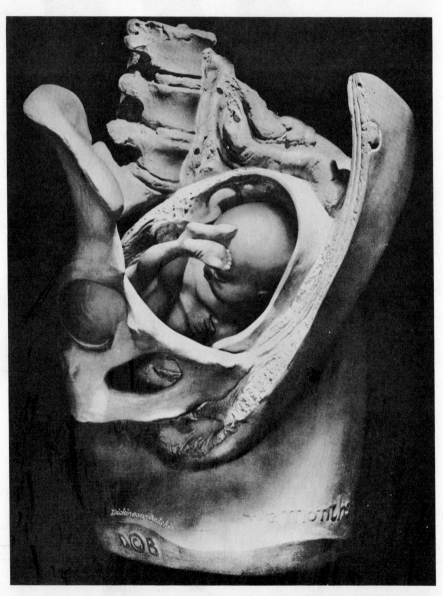

Fig. 6-4. Size and position of the fetus in the pelvis, at 4½ months. At about this time the mother first feels the fetal movements known as "quickening." (Dickinson-Belskie Birth Atlas Series, Maternity Center Association, New York)

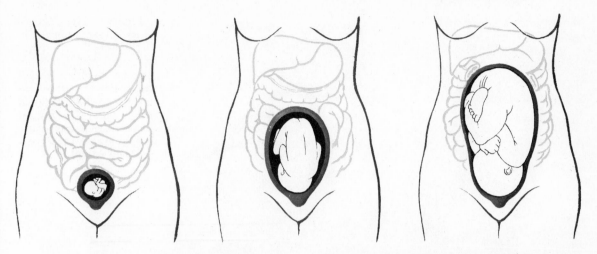

FIG. 6-5. Relative size of the growing uterus (front views), showing the fetus at 4 months, 6½ months and 9 months of gestation. The fundus reaches a height between the symphysis pubis and the umbilicus by the 4th month, is about the level of the umbilicus at 6½ months and almost impinges on the xiphoid process at about the 9th month of gestation.

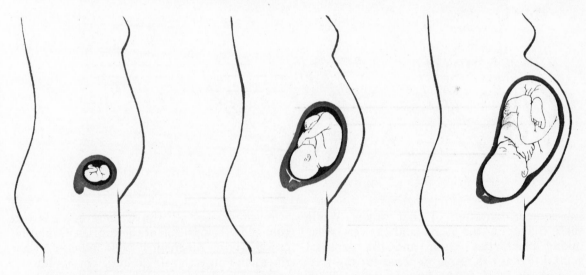

FIG. 6-6. Relative size of the growing uterus (side views), showing the fetus at 4 months, 6½ months and 9 months of gestation. (See the last sentence of the caption for Fig. 6-5.)

vical glands. As shown in Figures 6-8 and 9, the glands of the cervical mucosa undergo marked proliferation and distend with mucus. As a result they form a structure resembling honeycomb and make up about one half of the entire structure of the cervix. This is the so-called "mucous plug" and is of practical importance for a number of reasons. First, it seals the uterus from contamination by bacteria in the vagina. Second, it is expelled at the onset of labor and along with it a small amount of blood; this gives rise to the discharge of a small amount of blood-stained mucus, which is known as "show." Frequently, the onset of labor is heralded by the appearance of show. Third, since the discharge of the mucous plug removes a substantial portion of the interior of the cervix, it is very helpful in preparing for

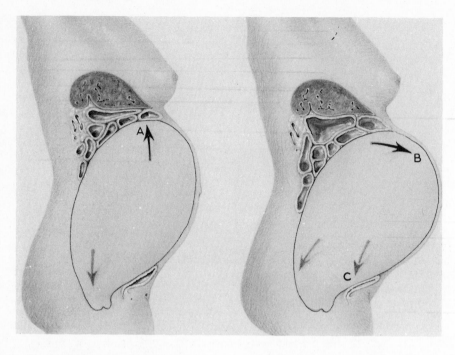

Fig. 6-7. The changes which take place in "lightening." (A) Pressure exerted on diaphragm before lightening. (B) Pressure relieved by falling forward of uterus. (C) Descent of head causes pressure on pelvic structures, particularly bladder.

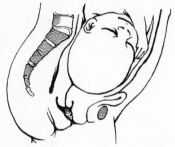

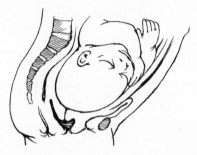

subsequent dilatation of that organ. While these changes in the uterus and the cervix are taking place, the vagina and the external genital organs are being prepared for the passage of the fetus at the time of labor. These parts become thickened and softened, and their vascularity is greatly increased. This increase in the blood supply of the genital canal gives to the tissues a dark violet hue (Chadwick's sign), in contrast with the ordinary pink color of the parts, which is often described as a valuable sign of pregnancy. As the result of the succulence of the parts, the vaginal secretions may be considerably increased toward the end of gestation. The increased vascularity extends to the various structures in the vicinity, i.e., tissues in the perineal region, skin and muscle, and effects changes in preparation for labor.

As pregnancy advances, there is a marked change in the position of the ovaries. Ovulation ceases during pregnancy. New follicles do not ripen, and only the single large corpus luteum can be found on one of the ovaries. The large size of the corpus luteum of pregnancy is due mainly to the increased vascularity of the organ.

Abdominal Wall

The abdomen naturally enlarges to accommodate the increase in size of the uterus. The mechanical effect of this distention of the abdominal wall causes in the later months of pregnancy the formation of certain pink or slightly reddish streaks or striations in the skin covering the sides of the abdomen and the

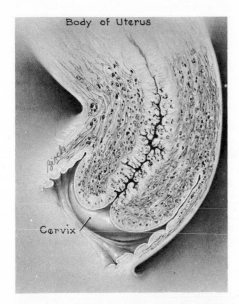

FIG. 6-8. Normal nonpregnant cervix.

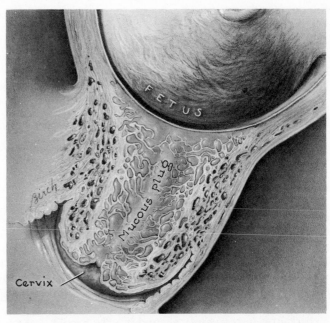

FIG. 6-9. Cervix at full term, showing mucous plug.

anterior and the outer aspects of the thighs. These streaks are known as *striae gravidarum* and are due to the stretching, the rupture and the atrophy of the deep connective tissue of the skin (Plate 3, *left, top and bottom*). They grow lighter after labor has taken place and finally take on the silvery whiteness of scar or cicatricial tissue. In subsequent pregnancies new pink or reddish lines may be found mingled with old silvery-white striae or striations. The number, the size and the distribution of striae gravidarum vary exceedingly in different women, and patients occasionally are seen in whom there are no such markings whatever, even after repeated pregnancies. As the striae are due solely to the stretching of the cutis, they are not peculiar to pregnancy but may be found in other conditions which cause great abdominal distention, such as the accumulation of fat in the abdominal wall or the development of large tumors of rapid growth.

Coincident with the uterine and the abdominal enlargement, the umbilicus is pushed outward until at about the 7th month its depression is completely obliterated, and it forms merely a darkened area in the smooth and tense abdominal wall. Later, it is raised above

SOME IMPORTANT DEFINITIONS

Gravida: a pregnant woman.
Primigravida: a woman pregnant for the first time.
Primipara: a woman who has given birth to her first child. Usage is not uniform.
Multipara: a woman who has had two or more children.
Para I: a primipara.
Para II: a woman who has had two children (and so on up numerically, Para III, Para IV, etc.).

(The plural of these words is usually formed by adding "e," as "primigravidae.")

(The term *gravida* refers to a pregnant woman, regardless of the duration of pregnancy. In reference it includes the present pregnancy. The term *para* refers to past pregnancies which have produced an infant which has been viable, whether or not the infant is dead or alive at birth. The terms *gravida* and *para* refer to pregnancies, not to fetuses.)

the surrounding integument and may project, becoming about the size of a hickory nut.

When the abdominal wall is unable to withstand the tension created by the enlarging uterus, the recti muscles become separated in the median line—so-called *diastasis.*

Breasts

Slight temporary enlargement of the breasts, causing sensations of weight and fullness, is noted by most women prior to their menstrual periods. The earliest breast changes of pregnancy are merely exaggerations of these changes. After the 2nd month the breasts begin to become larger, firmer and more tender; a sensation of stretching fullness, accompanied by tingling both in the breasts and in the nipples, often develops, and in many instances a feeling of throbbing also is experienced. As time goes on, the nipple and the elevated, pigmented area immediately around it—the areola —become darker in color. The areola tends to become puffy, and its diameter, which in virgins rarely exceeds 1½ inches, gradually widens to reach 2 or 3 inches. Embedded in this areola lie tiny sebaceous glands which take on new growth with the advent of pregnancy and appear as little protuberances or follicles. These have been called Montgomery's tubercles, after a famous Irish obstetrician of the 19th century who described them very fully and, in summarizing, created a famous medical pun by saying, "They are, in fact, a constellation of miniature nipples scattered over a milky way" (Plate 3, *bottom, right*). These glands of Montgomery result from hypertrophy of the sebaceous glands. In a few cases it is observed that patches of brownish discoloration appear on the normal skin immediately surrounding the areola. This is known as the secondary areola and is an almost certain sign of pregnancy, provided that previously the woman never has nursed an infant (Plate 4, *center, right*). With the increasing growth and activity of the breasts, it is not surprising that a richer blood supply is needed, and to this end the blood vessels supplying the area enlarge. As a result the veins beneath the skin of the breast, which previously may have been scarcely visible, now become more prominent and occasionally exhibit intertwining patterns over the whole chest wall.

The alterations in the breasts during pregnancy are directed ultimately to the preparation for breast-feeding the baby. After the first few months a thin viscous yellowish fluid may be expressed from the nipples by gentle massage. This is a watery precursor of breast milk called *colostrum.*

METABOLIC CHANGES

Weight Gain

A desirable total weight gain in pregnancy for the average woman is about 20 pounds. During the first 3 months there may be a slight weight loss, or if weight is gained, it is perhaps only a small per cent. About one half of the increment is gained in the second trimester and a similar amount in the last trimester. However, there are wide individual variations observed, even in completely normal patients. The greater part of this 20-pound increment is quite understandable, as shown by the following figures:

Baby	7	pounds
Placenta	1	"
Amniotic fluid	1½	"
Increase in weight of uterus	2	"
Increase in blood volume	1	"
Increase in weight of breasts	1½	"
	14	pounds

The remaining 6 pounds gained by the pregnant woman represent, in part, general accumulation of fat and, in part, the increased amount of fluid that tissues tend to retain at this time. Gains between 15 and 20 pounds are natural and in keeping with good health; usually they are lost after the baby is born.

CHANGES IN THE VARIOUS SYSTEMS

Blood

The total volume of blood in the body increases during pregnancy about 30 per cent. The minimal hematologic values for nonpregnant women apply to pregnant women, namely, 12 Gm. of hemoglobin, 3.75 million erythrocytes, 35 per cent of hematocrit. If there are adequate iron reserves in the body, or if sufficient iron is supplied from the diet, the hemoglobin, the erythrocyte count and the hematocrit values remain normal during pregnancy.

Heart

An important aspect of this increase in blood volume relates to its effect on the heart. As a natural result of this change, the heart has more blood to pump through the aorta— about 50 per cent more blood per minute than it did prior to pregnancy. This augmented cardiac output attains a peak at the end of the second trimester, then declines to the nonpregnant level at the last weeks of gestation. Immediately following delivery there is a sharp rise again. In women with normal hearts this is of no particular concern. However, in women with heart disease this increase in the work that the heart has to do may add to the seriousness of the complication (see Chap. 18).

Palpitation of the heart is not uncommon; in the early months of pregnancy this is due to sympathetic nervous disturbance, and toward the end of gestation to the intra-abdominal pressure of the enlarged uterus.

Respiration

In the later months of pregnancy the lungs are subjected to pressure from the underlying uterus, and the diaphragm may be displaced upward as much as an inch. As a consequence, shortness of breath at that period is common. It might seem that this upward displacement of the diaphragm would decrease the capacity of the lungs, but a concomitant widening of the thoracic cage occurs which more than compensates for the other change. Actually, indeed, the pregnant woman breathes in much more air than the nonpregnant. This is necessary, since the mother is called upon to oxygenate not only her own blood but, by osmosis, that of her baby as well.

Digestion

The function of the digestive organs may be somewhat altered during pregnancy. During the early months the appetite may be diminished, particularly if nausea exists. Since the nutritional requirements to meet the needs of the mother's body and the growing fetus demand quality of the diet rather than an appreciable increase in the quantity of food ingested, this temporary manifestation should not produce injurious effects. As pregnancy advances, and the digestive apparatus seems to become accustomed to its new conditions, the appetite is increased and may be voracious. Heartburn and flatulence may occur at this time, since the majority of pregnant women have a reduction in the total acidity of their gastric juice. Also, the pressure from the diaphragm and the diminished tone may delay the emptying time of the stomach. Constipation is exceedingly common in pregnancy; at least one half of all gravid women suffer from this disorder. This suggests that the entire gastrointestinal tract is limited by diminished tone and pressure of the growing uterus during gestation.

Skin

Striae gravidarum, which have already been discussed in relation to changes in the abdominal wall, often develop in the breasts, the buttocks and the thighs, presumably as the result of deposition of fat in those areas with consequent stretching of the skin. Certain pigmentary changes also are common, particularly the development of a black line running from the umbilicus to the mons veneris, the so-called *linea nigra* (Plate 3, *bottom, left*). In certain cases irregular spots or blotches of a muddy brown color appear on the face. This condition is known as *chloasma* or the "mask of pregnancy" (Plate 3, *top, right*). These facial deposits of pigment often cause the patient considerable mental distress, but her mind may be relieved by the assurance that they will disappear after delivery. However, the increased pigmentation of the breasts and the abdomen never disappears entirely, although it usually becomes much less pronounced. All these pigmentary deposits vary exceedingly in size, shape and distribution and usually are more marked in brunettes than in blondes. Vascular spiders are minute, fiery-red elevations of the skin with branching legs coming out from the central body. They develop more often in white women, are of no clinical significance and will disappear. The skin changes may be associated with hypertrophy of the cortex of the adrenals.

In addition to the above skin changes, there is a great increase in the activity of the sebaceous and the sweat glands and of the hair follicles. The augmented activity of the sweat glands produces an increase in perspiration, an alteration which is helpful in the elimination of waste material.

Urinary System

The urine in pregnancy usually is increased in amount and has a low specific gravity. Pregnant women show a tendency to excrete dextrose in the urine. Although a reduction in the renal threshold for sugar is often associated with pregnancy, the presence of any sugar in the urine should always be reported to the physician. Lactosuria may be observed at times, especially during the latter part of pregnancy and the puerperium. It is of no significance, being due to the presence of milk sugar which is supposed to be absorbed from the mammary glands.

The ureters become markedly dilated in pregnancy, particularly the right ureter. This change apparently is due in part to the pressure of the gravid uterus on the ureters as they cross the pelvic brim and in part to a certain softening which the ureteral walls undergo as the result of endocrine influences. These dilated ureters, the walls of which have now lost much of their muscular tone, are unable to propel the urine as satisfactorily as previously; consequently, stasis of urine is common. Following delivery, the ureters return to normal within 4 to 6 weeks. The stretching and the dilatation do not continue long enough to impair the ureter permanently unless infection has developed, or pregnancies are repeated so rapidly that a subsequent pregnancy begins before the ureters can return to normal.

The bladder functions efficiently during pregnancy. The urinary frequency experienced in the first few months of pregnancy is caused by pressure exerted on the bladder by the enlarging uterus. This is observed again when "lightening" occurs prior to the onset of labor.

EFFECTS ON THE NERVOUS SYSTEM

The effect of pregnancy on the nervous system varies greatly; although many women escape nervous manifestations entirely, some patients present more or less altered mental and emotional characteristics, varying all the way from cravings for unusual foods, fretfulness and peevishness to rare instances of true psychoses. In exceptional cases the change is to the opposite extreme, and a woman who is ordinarily of an irritable disposition becomes exceedingly amiable and agreeable. The more unstable emotionally the patient is, the more likely is her nervous system to be affected by the strain of pregnancy.

ENDOCRINE CHANGES

Placenta

The most important endocrine changes in pregnancy concern the function of the placenta as an endocrine organ, i.e., secreting chorionic gonadotropin, estrogen and progesterone (see Chap. 3).

In Chapter 4 the placenta is considered simply as an organ designed to transmit nutritive substances from mother to fetus and waste products in the reverse direction. The placenta has another highly important function: it is one of the most important organs of internal secretion. The early chorionic villi of the implanted ovum secrete a gonad-stimulating substance derived from chorion, a hormone, so-called *chorionic gonadotropin*, which prolongs the life of the corpus luteum. The result is the continued production of estrogen and progesterone, which are so necessary for the maintenance of the secretory phase of the endometrium. During pregnancy this hormone is excreted in the mother's urine and makes possible the Aschheim-Zondek and the Friedman tests for pregnancy (see pp. 125-126).

In addition to its function in the formation of chorionic gonadotropin, the placenta takes over the production of estrogen and progesterone from the ovaries and after the first 2 months of gestation becomes the major source of these two hormones. The increase in these hormones in the maternal organism is thought to be responsible for many important changes that take place during pregnancy, such as the growth of the uterus and the development of the breast. In the breast, the development of the duct system is promoted by estrogen, and the development of the lobule-alveolar system, by progesterone.

The relatively high levels of estrogen and progesterone during pregnancy suppress the secretion of *luteotrophin*, an anterior pituitary hormone. This substance, sometimes referred to as *LTH, prolactin, lactogenic hormone* or the *mammogenic hormone*, plays a major role in the onset of lactation. With the delivery of the placenta the estrogen and the progesterone levels of the body drop significantly, thereby releasing the factor that inhibits luteotrophin secretion; in turn luteotrophin plays an important part in the onset of milk production. This relationship betwen the ovary and the pituitary hormones and lactation is only one link in the very complicated but beautifully integrated endocrine change that dominates pregnancy, in which the placenta plays a pre-eminent role.

Pituitary Body

The *anterior lobe* of this small gland located at the base of the brain has already been referred to as the "master clock" which controls the menstrual cycle (see Chap. 3). Its role in pregnancy is likewise very important. It secretes a number of hormones, one of which acts on the breasts, producing lactation (the lactogenic hormone, so-called luteotrophin, active only after the placenta has been delivered) (see previous paragraph); another acts on the thyroid, another on the ovaries and still another on the growth process. The last is believed by some observers to be responsible for the rather coarse features which some pregnant women develop.

The *posterior lobe* of the pituitary secretes an oxytocic hormone, which has a very strong stimulating effect on the uterine muscle. That portion of extracts of the pituitary gland which contains this hormone, known as *oxytocin*, is widely employed in obstetrics to cause the uterus to contract after delivery, thereby diminishing postpartal hemorrhage. It is sometimes used also to initiate labor and to stimulate weak contractions during labor. It is marketed under the names Pitocin and Syntocinon, the latter a synthetic product.

Other Endocrine Glands

The pituitary body is thus another important link in the endocrine network of pregnancy. Probably as a result of the far-reaching action of its hormones and those of the placenta, many other endocrine glands show alterations during normal pregnancy, as exemplified below.

The *thyroid* tends to enlarge slightly, due to the moderate degree of hypertrophy that occurs with normal pregnancy. The increased thyroid activity is reflected in the elevated basal metabolic rate that occurs during the last trimester of pregnancy. Likewise, the serum protein-bound iodine concentration (PBI) increases, and this level is maintained until shortly after delivery. This appears to be but is *not* usually a case of hyperthyroidism.

The *parathyroids* also hypertrophy during pregnancy, often to a greater degree than the thyroid. Parathyroid secretion is essential to the normal progress of pregnancy. A deficiency in its secretion may well bear some relationship to the tetany that results when the increased calcium requirements of pregnancy are not met.

The *adrenal cortex* hypertrophies during pregnancy, and it is believed that its activity increases. This increase may bear some relationship to the occurrence of striae gravidarum of pregnancy.

The characteristic changes which develop in the *ovary* during pregnancy have already been discussed. Eastman and Hellman are of the opinion that the telangiectatic nevi, or vascular spiders, which develop on the face and the neck of some pregnant women may be due to the high estrogen level of pregnancy.

SUGGESTED READING

Eastman, N. J., and Hellman, L. M.: Williams Obstetrics, ed. 12, New York, Appleton, 1961.

Gillespie, E. C.: Principles of uterine growth in pregnancy, Am. J. Obstet. Gynec. 59:949, 1950.

Greenhill, J. P.: Obstetrics, ed. 13, Philadelphia, Saunders, 1965.

Holly, R. G.: Anemia in pregnancy, Obstet. Gynec. 5:562, 1955.

Hytten, F. E., and Leitch, I.: The Physiology of Human Pregnancy, Philadelphia, Davis, 1963.

Nesbitt, R. E. L., Jr.: Prolongation of pregnancy; a review, Obstet. Gynec. Survey 10:311, 1955.

Potter, Edith: Fundamentals of Human Reproduction, New York, McGraw-Hill, 1947.

Chapter 7

Signs and Symptoms of Pregnancy

CLASSIFICATION OF SIGNS AND SYMPTOMS

The first visit of the expectant mother to her physician is usually prompted by the query, "Am I really pregnant?" Oddly enough, this is the one question which the physician may answer equivocally, because even the most careful examination rarely will reveal clear-cut evidence of pregnancy until 2 menstrual periods have been missed, and occasionally the diagnosis may remain uncertain for a longer time. Some of the signs and symptoms of pregnancy can be recognized readily by the nurse, whereas others can be determined accurately only by one who has had a thorough medical or technical training.

Certain signs are absolutely indicative of pregnancy, but even these may be absent or lacking if the fetus has died in the uterus. Some so-called "positive" signs are not present until about the middle of gestation, and at that time the physician usually can make a diagnosis without them by the "circumstantial evidence" of a combination of earlier and less significant symptoms.

The signs of pregnancy are usually divided into 3 groups, as indicated in the following classification:

A. Presumptive signs
  1. Menstrual suppression
  2. Nausea, vomiting, "morning sickness"
  3. Frequency of micturition
  4. Tenderness and fullness of the breasts, pigmentation, etc.
  5. "Quickening"
  6. Dark blue discoloration of the vaginal mucous membrane (Chadwick's sign)
  7. Pigmentation of the skin and abdominal striae
  8. Fatigue
B. Probable signs
  1. Enlargement of the abdomen
  2. Fetal outline, distinguished by abdominal palpation
  3. Changes in the uterus—size and shape and consistency (Hegar's sign)
  4. Changes in the cervix
  5. Braxton Hicks contractions
  6. Positive pregnancy tests
C. Positive signs
  1. Fetal heart sounds
  2. Fetal movements felt by examiner
  3. Roentgenogram—outline of fetal skeleton

PRESUMPTIVE SIGNS

Menstrual Suppression

In a healthy married woman who previously has menstruated regularly, cessation of menstruation strongly suggests that impregnation has occurred. However, not until the date of

121

the expected period has been passed by 10 days or more can any reliance be put on this symptom. When the second period is also missed, the probability naturally becomes stronger.

Although cessation of menstruation is the earliest and one of the most important symptoms of pregnancy, it should be noted that pregnancy may occur without prior menstruation and that occasionally menstruations may continue after conception. An example of the former circumstance is noted in certain Oriental countries, where girls marry at a very early age; here pregnancy frequently occurs before the menstrual periods are established. Again, nursing mothers, who usually do not menstruate during the period of lactation, often conceive at this time; more rarely, women who think they have passed the menopause are startled to find themselves pregnant. Conversely, it is not uncommon for a woman to have 1 or 2 periods after conception; but almost without exception these are brief in duration and scant in amount. In such cases the first period ordinarily lasts 2 days instead of the usual 5, and the next only a few hours. Although there are instances in which women are said to have menstruated every month throughout pregnancy, these are of questionable authenticity and are probably ascribable to some abnormality of the reproductive organs. Indeed, vaginal bleeding at any time during pregnancy should be regarded as abnormal and reported to the physician at once.

Absence of menstruation may result from a number of conditions other than pregnancy. Probably one of the most common causes of delay in the onset of the period is psychic influence, particularly fear of pregnancy. Change of climate, exposure to cold, as well as certain chronic diseases such as anemia, likewise may suppress the menstrual flow.

Nausea and Vomiting

About one half of pregnant women suffer no nausea whatsoever during the early part of pregnancy. About 50 per cent experience waves of nausea; of these perhaps one third experience some vomiting. "Morning sickness" usually occurs in the early part of the day and subsides in a few hours, although it may persist longer or may occur at other times. When this "morning sickness" occurs, it usually makes its appearance about 2 weeks after the first missed menstrual period and subsides spontaneously 6 or 8 weeks later. Since this symptom is present in many other conditions, such as ordinary indigestion, it is of no diagnostic value unless associated with other evidence of pregnancy. When the vomiting is excessive, when it lasts beyond the 4th month, when it begins in the later months, or when it affects the general health, it must be regarded as pathologic. Such conditions are termed "hyperemesis gravidarum" or "pernicious vomiting" and will be discussed with complications of pregnancy in Chapter 18.

Frequent Micturition

Irritability of the bladder with resultant frequency of urination may be one of the earliest symptoms of pregnancy. It is attributed to the fact that the growing uterus stretches the base of the bladder, so that a sensation results identical with that felt when the bladder wall is stretched with urine. As pregnancy progresses, the uterus rises out of the pelvis, and the frequent desire to urinate subsides. Later on, however, the symptom is likely to return, for during the last weeks the head of the fetus may press against the bladder and give rise to a similar condition. Although frequency of urination may be somewhat bothersome, both at the beginning and at the end of pregnancy, it never should constitute a reason for reducing the quantity of fluid consumed, which should be not less than 6 or 8 glasses a day.

Breast Changes

The breast changes of pregnancy have already been described (p. 116). In primigravidae (women pregnant for the first time) these alterations are helpful adjuncts in the diagnosis of pregnancy, but in women who have already borne children, particularly if they have nursed an infant within the past year, they naturally are of much less significance.

"Quickening"

This is an old term derived from an idea prevalent many years ago that at some particular moment of pregnancy life is suddenly infused into the infant. At the time this notion was in vogue, the first tangible evidence of intra-uterine life lay in the mother's feeling the baby move, and the conclusion was only natural that the infant "became alive" at the moment these movements were first felt. As is reflected in the Biblical reference to "the quick and the dead," the word "quick" used to mean "alive," and the word "quickening" meant "becoming alive." Hence, our forebears were accustomed to say that when fetal movements were first felt, "quickening" or "coming to life" of the baby had occurred. We now know that the infant is a living organism from the moment of conception, but the old term "quickening" is still used in obstetric terminology, whereas among the laity "feeling life" is the common synonym. As used today, quickening refers only, of course, to the active movements of the fetus as first perceived by the mother.

Quickening is usually felt toward the end of the 5th month as a tremulous fluttering low in the abdomen. The first impulses caused by the stirring of the fetus may be so faint as to raise some doubt as to their cause; later on, however, they grow stronger and often become disturbingly active.

Many fetuses, although alive and healthy, seem to move about very little in the uterus, and, not infrequently, a day or so may pass without a movement being felt. Inability to feel the baby move does not mean that it is dead or in any way a weakling but, in all probability, that it has assumed a position in which its movements are not felt so readily by the mother. Moreover, it is a well-established fact that the fetus sleeps in the uterus, and it seems likely that the periods of active movement and quiescence which the mother notices correspond to the phases of somnolence and wakefulness. Should 3 or 4 days pass without movements, the physician should be asked to listen for the fetal heart sounds. If these are heard, it means beyond doubt that the fetus is alive and presumably in good condition. It might seem that the sensations produced by the baby's movements would be so characteristic as to make this a positive sign of pregnancy, but, oddly enough, women occasionally misinterpret movements of gas in the intestines as motions of a baby and on this basis imagine themselves to be pregnant. Therefore, the patient's statement that she feels the baby move cannot be regarded as absolute proof of pregnancy.

Vaginal Changes

On inspection of the vagina, the physician is able to observe discoloration of the vaginal mucous membrane due to the influence of pregnancy. The mucosa about the vaginal opening and the lower portion of the anterior wall frequently becomes thickened and of a dark bluish or purplish congested appearance instead of its customary pinkish tint in the nonpregnant state. This sign, known as *Chadwick's sign,* is of no special value in women who have borne children; and, as it may be due to any condition leading to the congestion of the pelvic organs, it can be considered only as a presumptive sign of pregnancy.

Skin Changes

The changes in the skin which may accompany pregnancy, i.e., striae gravidarum, linea nigra, chloasma, pigmentation of the breasts, etc., have been referred to in the previous chapter. These manifestations often are observed in pregnant women but vary exceedingly in different persons, often being entirely absent. The pigmentation changes in particular are frequently absent in decided blondes and exceptionally well marked in pronounced brunettes. As already mentioned, this pigmentation may remain from former pregnancies and cannot be depended on as a diagnostic sign in women who have borne children previously.

Fatigue

During the early months of pregnancy the expectant mother becomes easily fatigued and experiences periods of lassitude and drowsiness. This condition frequently accompanies pregnancy and usually disappears after the first few months of gestation.

PROBABLE SIGNS

Abdominal Changes

The size of the abdomen in pregnancy corresponds to the gradual increase in the size of the uterus, which at the end of the 3rd month is at the level of the symphysis pubis. At the end of the 5th month it is at the level of the umbilicus, and toward the end of the 9th month, at the ensiform cartilage (Figs. 6-3 to 5). Mere abdominal enlargement may be due to a number of causes, such as accumulation of fat in the abdominal wall, edema, or uterine or ovarian tumors. However, if the uterus can be distinctly felt to have enlarged progressively in the proportions stated above, pregnancy may properly be suspected.

Fetal Outline

After the 6th month the outline of the fetus (head, back, knees, elbows, etc.) usually may be identified sufficiently well by abdominal palpation to justify a diagnosis of pregnancy. As pregnancy progresses, the outline of the fetus becomes more and more clearly defined. The ability to outline the fetus makes pregnancy extremely probable. In rare instances, however, tumors of the uterus may so mimic the fetal outline as to make this sign fallible.

Changes in the Uterus

Changes in shape, size and consistency of the uterus which take place during the first 3 months of pregnancy are very important indications. These are noted in the bimanual examination which shows the uterus to be more anteflexed than normal, enlarged and of a soft, spongy consistency. About the 6th week the so-called Hegar's sign, so named for the man who first described it, is perceptible (Fig. 7-1). At this time the lower uterine segment, or lower part of the body of the uterus, becomes

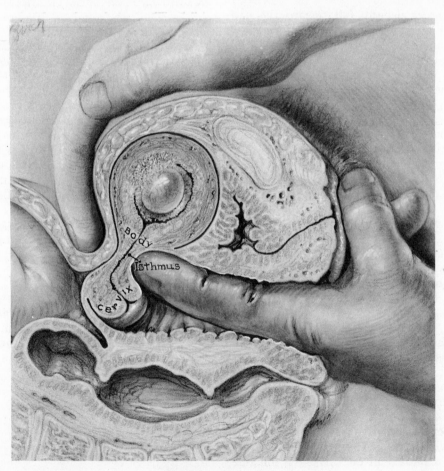

FIG. 7-1. Hegar's sign.

much softer than the cervix. So soft does it become that in its empty state (for it has not yet become encroached upon by the growing embryo) it can be compressed almost to the thinness of paper. This is one of the most valuable signs in early pregnancy. Another valuable sign found on vaginal examination is ballottement (from the French *balloter*, to toss up like a ball). During the 4th and the 5th months of pregnancy the fetus is small in relation to the amount of amniotic fluid present; a sudden tap on the presenting part makes it rise in the amniotic fluid and then rebound to its original position and, in turn, tap the examining finger. When elicited by an experienced examiner, this response is the most certain of the probable signs.

Cervical Changes

Softening of the cervix usually occurs about the time of the 2nd missed menstrual period. In comparison with the usual firmness of the nonpregnant cervix (which has a consistency approximate to that of the cartilaginous tip of the nose), the pregnant cervix becomes softened, and on digital examination the external os feels like the lips or like the lobe of the ear (Goodell's sign) (see page 112).

Braxton Hicks Contractions

Uterine contractions begin during the early weeks of pregnancy and recur at intervals of from 5 to 10 minutes throughout the entire period of gestation. These contractions are painless, and the patient may or may not be conscious of them. They may be observed during the later months by placing the hand on the abdomen and during the bimanual examination. By means of these contractions the uterine muscles contract and relax, thereby enlarging in size to accommodate the growing fetus. These contractions are referred to as the Braxton Hicks sign, after a famous London obstetrician of the last century who first described them.

Pregnancy Tests

Since the very dawn of civilization efforts have been made to devise a satisfactory test for pregnancy. The priest-physicians of an- cient Egypt, in the earliest writings handed down to us, tell of a test then in vogue based on the seeming ability of pregnancy urine to stimulate the growth of wheat and barley seeds. The itinerant physicians of classical Greece employed similar tests, and during the Middle Ages the omniscient physician merely gazed at the urine and claimed in this way to be able to diagnose not only pregnancy but also many other conditions.

Today, interestingly enough, as in the tests of old, urine is used in a large number of tests for pregnancy. The tests are based on the fact that the early chorionic villi of the implanted ovum secrete a hormone, chorionic gonado-tropin, which is excreted in the maternal urine. The method of its detection is dependent on the fact that urine containing this hormone, when injected into specific rodents and amphibia, produces readily visible changes on the rodent ovary and on the gonads of various amphibia. The tests based on this fact, which are used most widely today, are: (1) the Asch-heim-Zondek test, (2) the Friedman test, (3) the Hogben test, (4) the American male frog and toad tests and (5) the Frank-Berman test.

The reactions of such tests are not of real diagnostic value unless 2 weeks have elapsed after the 1st missed menstrual period.

The great value of the endocrine tests lies in the fact that they become positive very early in pregnancy, usually about 10 days after the 1st missed menstrual period, sometimes even a few days earlier than this. If any of the tests has been carried out properly, the results are accurate in more than 95 per cent of cases. They are not, therefore, absolutely positive signs of pregnancy, but very nearly so.

If the diagnostic test for pregnancy is to be of value, the following procedure must be carried out. The patient is instructed to avoid drinking any fluids after the evening meal the night before the test in order to secure a concentrated urine specimen in the morning. She should void at bedtime and discard this urine. On arising the next morning, she should void the specimen to be examined into a clean, dry container. If it is impossible to send the specimen to the laboratory immediately, it should be kept cold.

Aschheim-Zondek Test. Five immature female white mice are injected with minute amounts of the urine specimen on 6 different occasions over a period of 2 days, each mouse receiving a total of 2.4 cc. of urine. Ordinarily, of course, the ovaries of these very immature animals (6 to 8 Gm. in weight) would be quiescent, but when the hormone is present in the urine injected, the follicles manifest very rapid development, so much so that several of them rupture or ovulate within a few days after the injection. Accordingly, if the urine of a pregnant woman has been injected into these animals, when the ovaries are inspected after a suitable interval (100 hours) they will reveal hemorrhagic follicles or corpora lutea. Even if only 1 mouse has an ovary which exhibits either a ruptured follicle and/or corpus luteum, the test is said to have a positive reaction. If the woman is not pregnant, the immature ovaries of the mice will remain in their quiescent condition and no points of follicle rupture will be seen—a negative test.

The Aschheim-Zondek test is the original endocrine test from which all others have been developed. From a practical viewpoint, the Aschheim-Zondek test has certain drawbacks: first, the difficulty of securing immature female mice of the correct weight for the procedure; second, the long 4-day wait before the result can be obtained; last, the many injections required by the procedure itself.

Friedman Test. In order to circumvent the difficulties of the Aschheim-Zondek test, Dr. M. H. Friedman, of the University of Pennsylvania, introduced an important modification of the test, using adult female rabbits instead of mice. Ten cc. of urine specimen is injected into the marginal vein of the rabbit's ear, and 24 hours later the animal is anesthetized, the abdomen is opened, and the ovaries are inspected. The presence of ruptured follicles means that the test is positive.

For the reason stated, the Friedman test is used in the United States much more widely than the original Aschheim-Zondek test and was long regarded as the standard laboratory test for pregnancy in this country, although now it has been superseded to a great extent by one or another of the frog tests. Its accuracy is about the same as that of the Aschheim-Zondek test.

Hogben Test. Another laboratory procedure that has gained wide popularity in the diagnosis of pregnancy is the South African toad or frog test, more properly called the Hogben

test after the British physician who first described it in 1930. The test is based on the fact that female South African toads, when injected with the urine of a pregnant woman, extrude a large number of eggs within 8 to 12 hours. The particular toad employed in any given test is kept in a small glass aquarium with a black paper or cardboard beneath it, and, against this background, the myriad of eggs extruded (in the event the test is positive) are very plainly seen. The accuracy of this test is about the same as that of the Aschheim-Zondek and the Friedman tests, and it possesses the additional advantage that the result of a test can be ascertained much sooner than with the other procedures. It owes its popularity in part also to the fact that the toads are easier and more economical to keep than are mice or rabbits.

Male Frog Test. The American male frog is injected with a pregnant woman's urine. If the test produces positive results, spermatozoa will appear in the frog's urine and can be readily detected microscopically within 2 to 4 hours.

Male Toad Test. Two natice species of the male toad have recently been employed as test animals in the same manner as the male frog.

Frank-Berman Test. This test has the advantage that results can be demonstrated within 8 to 24 hours. Two immature female rats (50 Gm. weight) are injected with urine. Pregnancy urine produces characteristic changes in the ovaries.

Immunologic Tests. The above tests depend on characteristic changes produced on the genital organs of laboratory animals when chorionic gonadotropin (present in pregnancy urine) is injected. But since chorionic gonadotropin is an antigen capable of producing specific antibodies when injected into an animal, such as the rabbit, the serum of the animal so injected will contain an antibody or antihormone specific for chorionic gonadotropin. This serum then can be used by reliable immunologic methods to establish the presence or absence of chorionic gonadotropin in pregnancy urine. Since such serum, properly standardized, can be bought and stored in the laboratory, immunologic tests have two main advantages over the tests described in the foregoing paragraphs: (1) they provide an answer within a few minutes rather than after many, many hours, as is true of the other methods, and (2) <u>they eliminate the need for maintaining an animal colony</u>. These tests appear to be accurate, but since they are relatively new (1962), further observations are necessary to establish their complete dependability.

POSITIVE SIGNS

Although certain of the signs mentioned above—notably, the hormone tests, ballottement and palpating the fetal outline—are nearly positive evidences of pregnancy, they are not 100 per cent certain; errors in technic occasionally invalidate the hormone tests, and on rare occasions the other signs may be simulated by nonpregnant pathologic states. If the term "positive" is used in the strict sense, there are only 3 positive signs of pregnancy, namely, the fetal heart sounds heard, fetal movements felt by the examiner and the x-ray outline of the fetal skeleton.

Fetal Heart Sounds

When heard distinctly by an experienced examiner, the fetal heart sounds can leave no doubt about the existence of pregnancy. Ordinarily, they <u>become audible at about the middle of pregnancy, or around the 20th week.</u> If the abdominal wall is thin, and conditions are favorable, they may become audible as early

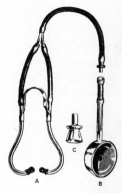

FIG. 7-2. Left stethoscope for use with interchangeable bells (A). Weighted bell used for auscultation of fetal heart sounds (B). Small bell used to determine mother's blood pressure (C). (J. Sklar Manufacturing Co., Long Island City, N. Y.)

as the 18th week, but obesity or an excessive quantity of amniotic fluid may render them inaudible until a much later date. Although the <u>usual rate of the fetal heart is about 140 per minute, it may vary under quite normal conditions between 120 and 160</u>. The use of the ordinary bell stethoscope, steadied by rubber bands, is entirely satisfactory (Figs. 7-2 and 7-3, *left*), but in doubtful cases the head stethoscope is superior, since the listener receives bone conduction of sound through the headpiece in addition to that transmitted to the eardrum (Fig. 7-3, *right*).

The nurse will find it advantageous to determine the fetal position by abdominal palpation before attempting to listen to the fetal heart tones, since ordinarily the heart sounds are best heard through the infant's back (see

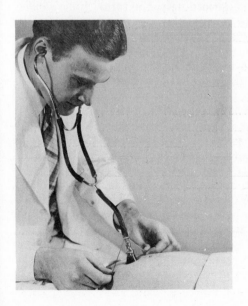

FIG. 7-3. (*Left*) Listening to fetal heart sounds with ordinary stethoscope. (*Right*) Listening to fetal heart sounds with "head" stethoscope. The head stethoscope gives bone conduction of sound in addition to otic (by ear) and also possesses the advantage that it can be used when hands are sterile.

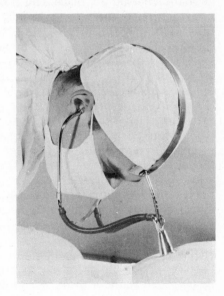

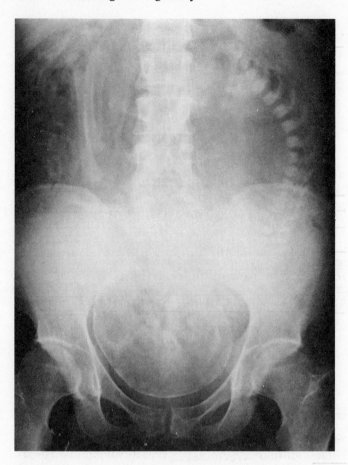

Fig. 7-4. Normal vertex position. (Bonner, K. P.: Radiography and Clinical Photography, Eastman Kodak Company, Rochester, N. Y.)

Chap. 5). Also, she will do well, while learning the characteristics of the fetal heart sounds, to accustom herself to place one hand on the maternal pulse and feel its rate at the same time that she hears the fetal heart tones through the stethoscope. Occasionally, the inexperienced attendant, particularly when listening high in the abdomen, may mistake the mother's heart sounds for those of the baby. Since the two are not synchronous (fetal, 140; maternal, 80), the method suggested above will obviate this mistake; in other words, if the rate that comes to the ear through the stethoscope is the same as that of the maternal pulse, it is probably the mother's heart beat; on the other hand, if the rates are different, it is undoubtedly the sound of the fetal heart.

Two additional sounds may be heard in listening over the pregnant uterus: the funic souffle and the uterine souffle. Since the word "souffle" means a blowing murmur, or whizzing sound, the nature of these two sounds is simi-lar, but their timing and causation are quite different. The word *funis* is Latin for umbilical cord, and, accordingly, the term "funic souffle" refers to a soft blowing murmur caused by blood rushing through the umbilical cord. Since this blood is propelled by the fetal heart, the rate of funic souffle is synchronous with that of the fetal heart. It is heard only occasionally, perhaps in 1 case out of every 6. The funic souffle is a positive sign of pregnancy, but it is not usually so listed, because almost always it is heard in close association with the fetal heart sounds. The uterine souffle is produced by blood rushing through the large vessels of the uterus. Since this is maternal blood, propelled by the maternal heart, it is synchronous with the rate of her heart beat. In other words, the rate of the funic souffle is ordinarily around 140 per minute (or the same as that of the fetal heart rate); the rate of the uterine souffle, near 80 (that of the maternal heart rate).

FIG. 7-5. Normal breech position. (Bonner, K. P.: Radiography and Clinical Photography, Eastman Kodak Company, Rochester, N. Y.)

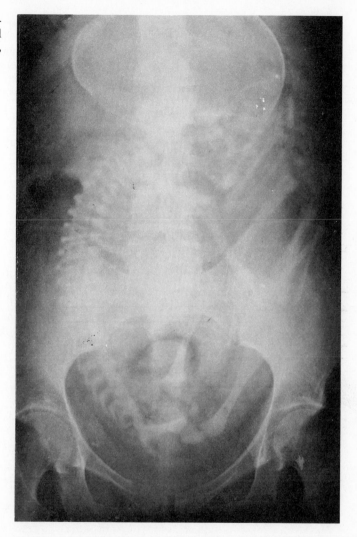

Fetal Movements Felt by Examiner

As already noted, fetal movements supposedly felt by the patient may be very misleading in the diagnosis of pregnancy. However, when an experienced examiner feels the characteristic thrust or kick of the baby against his hand, this is positive evidence of pregnancy. Often this can be felt after the end of the 5th month.

Roentgenogram

A roentgenogram showing the outline of the fetal skeleton is, of course, undeniable proof of pregnancy. How early the fetal skeleton will show in the roentgenogram depends on the thickness of the abdominal wall, the x-ray equipment and other factors. It has been demonstrated as early as the 14th week and is quite easily demonstrated as a rule after the 20th week (Figs. 7-4, 5).

SUGGESTED READING

Bruel, F.: Development of pregnancy tests, Am. J. Obstet. Gynec. 63:591, 1952.

Eastman, N. J., and Hellman, L. M.: Williams Obstetrics, ed. 13, New York, Appleton, 1966.

Foote, E. C., and Jones, G. E. S.: An evaluation of the Hogben pregnancy test, Am. J. Obstet. Gynec. 51:672, 1946.

Galloway, C. E.: The cervix in pregnancy, Am. J. Obstet. Gynec. 59:999, 1950.

Greenhill, J. P.: Obstetrics, ed. 13, Philadelphia, Saunders, 1965.

Mayo, R. W., *et al.*: Comparison of Pregnancy Tests, Obstet. Gynec. 25:699-704, May, 1965.

Merkel, R. L.: A comparative study of chemical tests for the early diagnosis of pregnancy, Am. J. Obstet. Gynec. 60:827, 1950.

Reifenstein, E. C., Jr., Rosenthal, M., and Hartzell, R. A.: Oral Hormone (Geltest) Diagnostic Test for Early Pregnancy, Fertil. Steril. 14: 85-143, January-February, 1963.

Southam, A. L., Sultzer, B. M., and Cohen, H.: Evaluation of a rapid immunologic test for pregnancy, Am. J. Obstet. Gynec. 84:495-499, February 15, 1963.

Tietz, N. W.: Comparative study of immunologic and biologic pregnancy tests in early pregnancy, Obstet. Gynec. 25:197-200, February, 1965.

The Importance of Preventive Care • Medical Care • Nursing Care •
Nutrition in Pregnancy • General Hygiene • Minor Discomforts •
Preparation for Parenthood • Psychophysical Preparation for Childbearing
• Preparations for the Baby • Plans for After-Care of Mother and Baby

Chapter 8

Antepartal Care

INTRODUCTION

Within the last decade there has appeared a rising tide of comment about what constitutes "adequate antepartal care." In the literal sense antepartal* care refers to the medical supervision and the care given to pregnant women during the period between conception and the onset of labor. Opinions vary, but generally in current practice adequate antepartal care is that care which considers the physical and the emotional needs of the woman and her unborn baby, her husband and their other children. It provides the best of medical science to protect the life and the health of the mother and the fetus, and it takes into consideration the social conditions under which the family lives, i.e., its economic status, educational level, housing, nutrition, etc. (see Chap. 1), so that the mother may pass through pregnancy and labor with a maximum of mental and physical fitness. It also aims to increase the knowledge of the mother-to-be, so that she and her infant may be kept healthy and happy after the delivery. These aims are accomplished through the combined efforts of the expectant parents, the obstetrician, the nurse and the other members of the health team.

Antepartal care may be considered as the foundation for the normal development, the adequate growth and the good health of the

baby. During this formative period the teeth, the bones and the various systems of the body have their beginnings, as well as the foundations for his future health. Adequate antepartal care also aids in stabilizing the daily health of the mother. As pregnancy advances, the demands of the fetus increase. Since individuals react differently to pregnancy, this supervision is of the utmost importance in detecting these reactions, for it not only helps to relieve discomforts and to prevent accidents and complications but also aids in ensuring a more rapid convalescence and continued good health.

THE IMPORTANCE OF PREVENTIVE CARE

Prior to the rise of present-day obstetrics, the physician usually had only one interview with his patient before he saw her in labor, and often at this interview he merely sought to compute the expected date of confinement. When he next saw her, she might be in the throes of an eclamptic convulsion or striving vainly to overcome the resistance offered by a contracted pelvis. It is in the prevention of such calamities as these that care and supervision of the pregnant mother have been found to be of such value. Indeed, antepartal care is an absolute necessity if a substantial number

---

* Derived from Latin, *partus* means birth and *ante*, before; i.e., before labor.

131

of women are to avoid disaster; and it is helpful to all.

From a biologic point of view, pregnancy and labor represent the highest function of the female reproductive system. As has been mentioned previously, this should be considered to be a normal process. But the numerous physiologic changes which occur in the mother's body during pregnancy (see Chap. 6) demonstrate that the borderline between health and illness is less distinctly marked during pregnancy than during the nonpregnant state. A slight variation in bodily function, which might be of but little significance if the woman

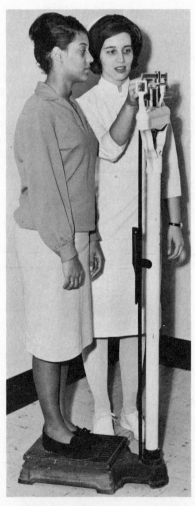

FIG. 8-1. Clinic nurse weighing pregnant patient.

were not pregnant, may be a warning signal of a potential pathologic condition in pregnancy which could seriously threaten the health of the mother or the child or both. Examples of such symptoms might be a weight gain of several pounds during 1 week or a persistent headache. Health supervision and teaching begun early in pregnancy are often the means of avoiding complications of pregnancy; and in the event that symptoms do occur, their early detection and prompt treatment may avert serious problems.

The importance of early and continued medical supervision during pregnancy cannot be overemphasized. If it were possible, care should begin as early as the patient conceives or perhaps even earlier than that, not only at the very beginning of her pregnant period but ideally with her own mother's antepartal state, which likewise had everything to do with the patient's health. In recent years much has been accomplished through premarital and prepregnancy examinations to determine the patient's fitness for pregnancy. More and more physicians are offering this care and encouraging this plan toward positive health.

MEDICAL CARE

Today the emphasis is on positive health, to determine the health status of those anticipating parenthood. Every patient should be under the care of her obstetrician during the entire period of her pregnancy. She should be seen as early in pregnancy as possible and at least every 4 weeks thereafter until the 7th month. Then she should make her visits every 2 weeks until the last month of pregnancy, during which time it is most important that she be seen every week. The therapy of all patients should be individualized. In the case of an expectant mother who has some abnormal condition, the visits should be spaced according to the demands of the situation. Each physician has his own system. Some prefer to see their patients in groups in order to facilitate discussions of common concerns, some utilize nurse midwives, and some prefer to maintain a one-to-one relationship with their patients. Whatever the approach, at the first examination the history of the patient is taken, then a general medical examination is carried out, and finally the obstetric examination, which includes an examination *per vaginam*, is given. The examination may be carried out according to the following outline.

The History

The name and the address of the patient, her age and parity and the date of the latest menstrual period are recorded, and the date of delivery is estimated. Inquiries are made regarding the family history, with special reference to any condition likely to affect childbearing, such as hereditary disease, tuber-culosis or multiple pregnancy. The personal history of the patient then is reviewed not only in regard to previous diseases and operations but particularly in relation to any difficulties experienced in previous pregnancies and labors, such as miscarriages, prolonged labor, death of infant, hemorrhage and other complications. Inquiry then is made into the history of the present pregnancy, especially in relation to nausea, edema of the feet or the face, headache, visual disturbance, vaginal bleeding, constipation, breathlessness, sleeplessness, cramps, heartburn, lower abdominal pain, vaginal discharge, varicose veins, etc. Usually a suitable form for recording these particulars is em-

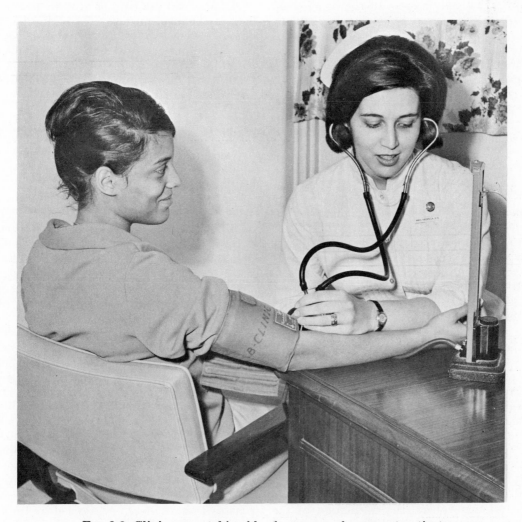

Fig. 8-2. Clinic nurse taking blood pressure of pregnant patient.

ployed. As a rule, obstetricians, hospital clinics and other community health agencies have their own forms for recording these details.

General Medical Examination

The general medical examination includes weighing the patient, taking the blood pressure, inspecting the teeth and the throat and making an examination by auscultation and percussion of the heart and the lungs. Opportunity is taken at this time to inspect the breasts and the nipples, particularly in relation to their suitability for subsequent nursing. From an obstetric viewpoint, one of the important details of the general medical examination is the measurement of the blood pressure (Fig. 8-2). This is usually carried out first and always should be done when the patient is seen on subsequent visits. As will be explained subsequently, any substantial increase in blood pressure indicates one of the most serious complications in pregnancy—toxemia. A fact for the nurse to keep in mind is that any sudden or gradual rise in the systolic or the diastolic blood pressure is significant and may be alarming.

Obstetric Examination

The obstetric examination is comprised of 3 parts: (1) palpation and auscultation of the abdomen; (2) estimation of pelvic measurements; and (3) vaginal examination. Palpation and auscultation of the abdomen yield valuable information concerning the size and the position of the fetus and the rate of the fetal heart. The great importance of careful pelvic measurements has already been emphasized, and the purpose of the vaginal examination (aside from its use in the diagnosis of pregnancy) is to rule out abnormalities of the birth canal (particularly those which might impede labor) and to take the diagonal conjugate measurement.

Laboratory Tests

The laboratory tests carried out in antepartal care are the urine examination, the blood test for syphilis, the estimation of the hemoglobin, tests for the Rh factor and blood type. At the first and subsequent examinations the urine is tested for albumin and sugar. The patient should be instructed to collect a part of the first urine voided in the morning before breakfast. The reason for this is that glucose may spill into the urine of a normal pregnant woman due to a decreased kidney threshold for glucose. Hence, it is more likely to appear in the urine after a meal. The test for sugar is the same as that used to test a diabetic's urine; several simple tests are available today and may be completed quickly and accurately in a matter of minutes. A positive reaction to sugar should be reported to the physician so that the possibility of diabetes or a prediabetic condition can be ruled out.

The test for albumin also is simple. The principle involved here is the application of heat in chemical form, which solidifies any albumin present and causes a whitish precipitate. The presence of albumin in the urine is another symptom of possible toxemia and should be reported immediately. The sudden appearance of albuminuria is regarded as a symptom of preeclampsia (see p. 445).

The blood for the Wassermann or other serologic test for syphilis is usually obtained by venipuncture. A sufficient quantity of blood should be drawn at this time so that a portion may be employed for the Rh factor and hemoglobin estimation. Since many pregnant women develop anemia, the latter examination is highly important. A metabolism test is routine in the practice of some obstetricians.

If the test for the Rh factor shows the patient to be Rh negative, it may be necessary to check the husband. It is also a wise precaution for the doctor to have the husband's blood type (see Chap. 18).

In many antepartal and postpartal clinics the secretions in the cervix and the vagina are examined microscopically to ascertain whether the cells contained therein exhibit certain changes suggestive of incipient uterine cancer. A drop of the cervical or the vaginal fluid is placed on a glass slide, and after this has been spread out in a very thin layer, it is stained for microscopic study. This is called a Papanicolaou smear or Papanicolaou spread. According to the cellular picture seen, it is classified by number from Class 1 to Class 5. Smears in Classes 1 and 2 are characterized by the complete absence of malignant or "suspicious" cells. They are regarded as normal. Smears in

Classes 3, 4 and 5 contain cells that either are suggestive of malignancy or actually malignant. These call for further investigation and, in some cases, intensive treatment. The rationale of this procedure is that it provides a method whereby incipient uterine cancer can be detected in its earliest stages. Since the success of treatment in any form of cancer depends on early diagnosis and early treatment, the use of the Papanicolaou smear promises to

prevent many fatalities from uterine cancer, one of the most common causes of death in women.

Weight

The routine estimation of weight at regular intervals during pregnancy is an important detail of antepartal care. Any *marked gain* or *loss* in weight will be discussed by the obstetri-

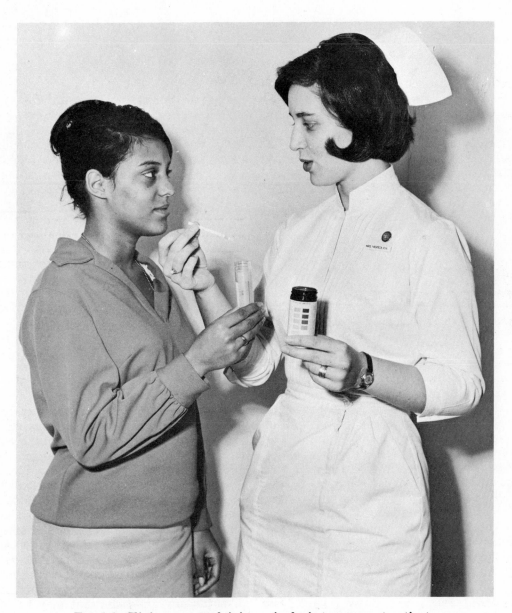

FIG. 8-3. Clinic nurse explaining urinalysis to pregnant patient.

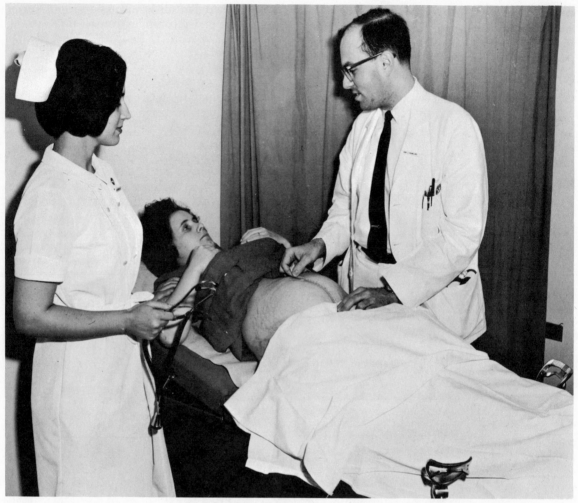

Fig. 8-4. Patient on examining table. Doctor is measuring the height of the fundus.

cian. At first the average gain in weight of the fetus is 1 Gm. daily; nine tenths of the weight is gained after the 5th month, and one half of the weight of the fetus is acquired during the last 8 weeks. A desirable weight gain is about 20 pounds during the entire pregnancy. In any excessive weight gain, or for a patient who is markedly overweight, one of the low caloric diets may be prescribed in an effort to control the weight. Weight gain should be considered in relation to the patient's general physical condition.

Return Visits

At return visits careful inquiry is made into the general well-being of the patient, and questions are asked concerning any untoward signs and symptoms, such as edema of the fingers or the face, bleeding, constipation and headache. The patient then is weighed, her blood pressure is taken, and the urine is analyzed for albumin and sugar. An abdominal examination is usually carried out at this time. Abdominal, vaginal and rectal examinations should be done at regular intervals to determine that pregnancy is progressing at the expected rate and, following quickening, that the fetus is living. During these visits the patient should avail herself of the opportunity of asking the physician any questions that may be of concern to her.

Instructions to Patients

After the routine examination the doctor or the nurse may instruct the patient regarding diet, rest and sleep, daily intestinal elimination, proper exercise, fresh air and sunshine, bathing, clothing, recreation and dental care.

It is usually possible and always desirable to assure the patient that the findings on examination were normal, and that barring complications, she may anticipate an uneventful pregnancy followed by an uncomplicated delivery. At the same time, however, she is tactfully instructed regarding certain danger signals which demand immediate report to the physician. These symptoms are as follows:

1. *Vaginal bleeding, no matter how slight*
2. *Swelling of the face or the fingers*
3. *Severe continuous headache*
4. *Dimness or blurring of vision*
5. *Flashes of light or dots before the eyes*
6. *Pain in the abdomen*
7. *Persistent vomiting*
8. *Chills and fever*
9. *Sudden escape of fluid from the vagina*

In addition to this detailed supervision the patient needs an explanation of the changes that are taking place within her body. This point cannot be stressed enough. Intelligent exploration with the patient regarding her concerns about these changes and appropriate instruction will give her greater reassurance and self-confidence. An understanding and empathic attitude on the part of the doctor and the nurse will do much to buoy the patient's morale and to diminish unnecessary anxiety.

As the patient approaches full term, she should be instructed also about the signs and symptoms of oncoming labor, so that she may know when the process is beginning and when to notify the physician. At this time the physician will want to know the frequency of contractions and any other pertinent symptoms.

Most hospitals conduct routine tours of the maternity division for the registered maternity patients and their husbands. It is advisable to encourage the expectant parents to take advantage of this opportunity sometime during the pregnancy. Becoming familiar ahead of time with the surroundings where the mother-to-be will be delivered reduces the anxiety that may be experienced in going to a strange hospital for the first time after labor has begun. The details of the hospital admission routine should be explained, so that she is familiar with this procedure before being admitted for delivery.

NURSING CARE

In spite of the fact that adequate antepartal care is becoming more readily available throughout the nation, health workers find that although most women want this care, they often do not utilize available services, or they may discontinue their care at some point in the pregnancy. This is particularly true of those who attend clinics. There are many reasons for this, as a review of the literature will indicate. The reason that most concerns us here is that many pregnant patients are often discouraged in either seeking or continuing antepartal care. One of the deterrents frequently cited for patient dissatisfaction is that members of the staff are too impersonal in their attitudes.

If those who provide care merely focus on a maintenance type of physical care and make no attempt to discover and help the expectant mother to satisfy her needs as she perceives them, the patient does not really receive good nursing care. Those who attend her must recognize that the pregnant woman is an individual involved in one of life's most important experiences. When the atmosphere of the hospital, the clinic or the doctor's office is such that a patient encounters regard for her human dignity and worth, and her concerns are listened to with interest and respect, she returns for care and profits by it. Therefore, one of the most important activities of the nurse who attends antepartal patients is to establish a relationship with the patient that conveys regard for her as a human being and permits free and frank discussion. This type of relationship not only will enable the nurse to instruct and counsel the mother more effectively about the various aspects of her pregnancy but also will allow the patient to express the more covert concerns and nuances of the pregnancy that are troublesome to her. The nurse then will be in a better position to deal with these herself or to refer them, as the occasion warrants, to the other members of the health team.

The nurse involved in antepartal care will find herself in one of three settings, a private doctor's office, a clinic or the community. Whatever the setting, the nurse should be skilled in communication technics, since these are basic to establishing a productive nurse-patient relationship. The nurse must be able to notice what goes on in the interaction between herself and the patient, to interpret what she observes, and to determine appropriate nursing intervention accordingly. In conferring with patients, the nurse not only should teach and give information; she also should be able to get information as well. Hence, she must be able to *listen* to what the patient is saying, to make nonjudgmental responses, to question and to elicit significant information from the patient when it is appropriate, e.g., to increase the nurse's understanding.

The nurse who *listens actively* to what the patient is saying will discern the covert as well as the overt cues. In conversation she must be able to reflect the gist of the patient's remarks so that the patient, as well as the nurse, may gain insight into the topic under discussion. The skilled nurse can probe gently but effectively to get at the crux of the problem or the concern. In helping the patient to separate fact from fiction in the situation and eventually to see what alternatives she has for action, the nurse helps the patient to confront her problems more realistically.

The nurse's understanding of human behavior will guide her in choosing the appropriate time and circumstances to help the patient in this way. The skillful nurse focuses her attention on the mother and listens, reflects and questions to learn more about the mother-to-be as an individual, her usual methods or ways of coping with problems, whether she needs help, and how she reacts to advice.

The Office and Clinic Settings

The Problem of Limited Time. The nurse who is accustomed to caring for patients on the inpatient hospital service, where she has rather continuous contacts with the same patient for days, or even weeks at a time, often finds the initial adjustment to an office or especially a clinic service difficult because of the limited time that the schedule usually permits for contacts with each patient. During the patient's brief appointment period in these last two settings the nurse must evaluate the present and the continuing nursing needs of the individual and plan to meet these needs effectively. The nurse who recognizes and understands this problem of limited time will find the orientation period less frustrating, and as she becomes more skilled in communication and observation of nonverbal as well as verbal behavior, she will enjoy the satisfactions of giving patient care and guidance in these types of settings.

Teaching the Patient. In addition to assisting the physician with examinations and performing various procedures, the nurse in the office or the clinic should devote much of her nursing care to health teaching and anticipatory guidance, i.e., informing mothers about what to expect regarding their pregnancy, delivery, postpartal and child-rearing periods before they begin to worry or to make mistakes. Therefore, the nurse should have broad knowledge and understanding about the physiology of pregnancy and childbearing, general hygiene, nutrition, the emotional, psychological and sociologic-economic aspects of family living, and the part played by a family in the larger community. Her teachings must be individualized for each patient, and it should include instruction in ways of maintaining good health habits in daily living, interpretation of the reasons that these practices are important, and suggestions of ways in which undesirable habits may be changed or modified. It is important to remember that health teaching and anticipatory guidance in any setting involve motivating the patient—and consequently influencing the degree of her interest and her desire to change or to continue present patterns of behavior. To accomplish the desired end, the nurse first must identify the level of knowledge and understanding of the patient through exploration of what the patient knows and feels about the topic in question. Second, the nurse should clarify any misinformation or misconceptions. Finally, she should add to the base of knowledge and understanding, when indicated, through reinterpretation, clarification, re-emphasis and reinforcement.

THE INITIAL CONTACT with the patient is

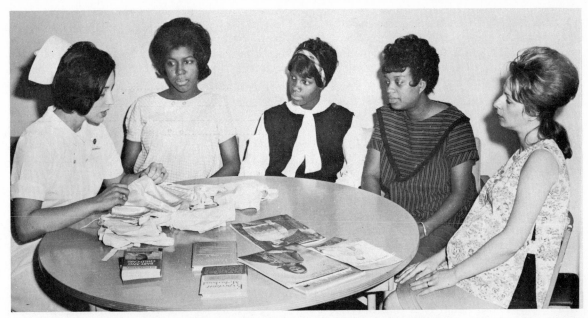

Fig. 8-5. Group counseling by the nurse in the clinic.

particularly important. By her pleasant greeting and professional manner the nurse can initiate a productive relationship that conveys her interest and concern for the patient. In making a patient comfortable who is waiting for her appointment with the physician, the nurse can utilize the opportunity to find out any questions, symptoms or problems that the mother may have and deal with them or report them to the proper person. This is an example of one way that the nurse can utilize limited contacts with the patient constructively.

Referrals. The problems that come to light are not always of a physical nature; emotional and social problems also may interfere with the patient's ability to derive full benefit from health services. It is the responsibility of the nurse to find out in what ways the patient needs help and to make appropriate referrals when they are indicated, e.g., to the nurse in the community, to allied community services or to other members of the extended health team. This is one of her most important nursing activities, since through the use of referrals she can keep lines of communication open between her particular health agency, the community and the members of the health team. Thus comprehensive care for the patient is assured.

Visual Aids; Teaching Groups. In hospitals and offices where the appointment system is used, the waiting time for the patient is minimized. In others the patient may have to wait longer periods. Waiting time in any setting may be utilized advantageously by providing reading material that will contribute to the patient's knowledge of her condition. Visual aids such as posters and charts may be both instructive and diverting. Flannelboard posters are excellent in this respect, since they can be changed frequently. These visual aids also provide an outlet for the creative ideas of the staff. Some offices and clinics use a group approach for discussion, teaching and guidance. These groups may be under the leadership of the nurse and provide a maximum amount of instruction and discussion for a large number of patients in a short period of time.

The Physical Examination. When the nurse assists the physician with the physical examination, she has an opportunity to learn more about the patient's condition. She should be alert to the cues and the events that transpire during this time, since she may be questioned afterward by the patient regarding her condition, or she may have to interpret the physician's instructions to make certain that they are understood. Often a patient is hesitant to discuss some matter with the physician, because she considers it too trivial, but she may feel comfortable in talking about it with the nurse. In turn, the nurse may consider this a problem of some importance, and on reporting it to the physician, she finds that it has a bearing on the course of treatment that he prescribes.

Another of the nurse's responsibilities is to prepare the patient for the physical examination. Since the initial examination is thorough, it is desirable that the patient disrobe completely and wear a gown that opens easily. In addition, the expectant mother should be covered with a small sheet to prevent unnecessary exposure and chilling. The nurse will want to instruct the mother to empty her bladder, since a full bladder is uncomfortable for the mother and may interfere with the physician's manipulations. A good footstool is imperative if the patient is to mount the table in safety and comfort. Many patients move somewhat awkwardly, especially as they near term, and the nurse can contribute a great deal to their safety as well as to the alleviation of embarrassment by assisting the mother, as she changes her position, to move slowly but steadily. For the patient's physical and emotional comfort and for the doctor's protection the nurse should be present during the entire examination.

THE PELVIC EXAMINATION. One aspect of the physical examination, the vaginal or pelvic examination, deserves special consideration, because often it is the most stressful part of the experience for the patient. This examination is carried out with the patient in the dorsal recumbent position. In this position the patient lies on her back with the lower limbs flexed and rotated outward. Her heels are supported in stirrups, which are level with the table, perhaps a foot in front of her buttocks. In this position the anxious patient, already under stress during the physical examination, is likely to tense her abdominal, pelvic and thigh muscles, attempting to adduct her thighs. Moreover, if the patient arches her back as her tension increases, her pelvis will be tilted downward, a position that makes the pelvic examination almost impossible to achieve.

The nurse can be most effective in assisting the patient to relax if she encourages her to keep breathing naturally, reminds her to breathe if she holds her breath, and helps her to let the small of her back press down on the table. Merely telling the anxious patient to relax is of no avail; thus the nurse needs to give the patient rather direct guidance, often step by step. For example, if the patient is clenching her fists, the nurse may say, "See, your wrist and hands are tense. Try to let them go limp—very limp—like a rag doll's. That's it—very limp." And a moment later, "Keep breathing naturally." Such short, explicit requests and instruction give the mother in each instance a simple task that she can do with guidance. This diverts her attention from the anticipated discomfort and promotes relaxation.

Since the doctor must see the cervix clearly, he will need a stool to sit on and a good light to focus into the vagina. Any equipment that he may need, such as the vaginal speculum, swabs, cotton balls, slides, lubricating jelly, etc., should be close at hand, so that he can reach them readily.

The pelvic examination will begin with an examination of the external genitalia and will include the urethra, Skene's and Bartholin's glands. If any unusual discharge is present, a specimen may be obtained for culture or microscopic examination. Usually, the doctor will next insert a speculum into the vagina to distend the folds so that he may observe the cervix. If a Papanicolaou smear is to be taken, no lubricating jelly will be used; instead, the speculum may be rinsed under *tepid* running water to facilitate the ease of insertion. Occasionally, the dilatation of the vagina by the speculum may cause an unpleasant sensation of stretching. Unfortunately, the mother already may be tense from the effect of strange surroundings and experiences, and the intrusion of this instrument may contribute to her discomfort, increasing her tenseness.

The fear, tension, pain syndrome in labor, described by Dr. Grantly Dick Read (see Suggested Reading), can affect the mother-to-be under these circumstances as well. Her fear of the examination increases her tenseness, which enhances the discomfort; hence a vicious circle is established. The nurse can do much to break this circle by encouraging the mother to breathe naturally while she is being examined.

Allowing the patient to squeeze or to hold her hand is often very helpful, although the nurse should recognize that not all patients want or need this physical contact. It is wise to be readily available to the patient but to let her initiate the contact. In our culture it is important that people "control themselves"; this is difficult to do when one's privacy is invaded, as it is by these intrusive procedures. It becomes especially important, then, to help the patient to preserve a positive concept of herself in this obstetric situation, since these early encounters all help to form an integral part of the mosaic that determines her self-concept as a mother.

As the examination proceeds, the cervix is visualized, and the doctor will note its color and character. Normally, the cervix of the primigravida is pink or bluish and smooth, with a dimple for the os. The cervix of a multigravida may have an irregular os due to lacerations from previous deliveries. If erosions of the cervix are present, they may be treated with silver nitrate swabs. Any discharge, such as a purulent, a greenish or a frothy discharge, is considered to be abnormal, and a specimen may be secured for microscopic examination or culture.

After the cervix has been examined, the doctor will withdraw the speculum and proceed with the bimanual examination to evaluate the uterus and the adnexa. He will determine the size, the consistency and the contour of these organs as well as the relationship of the uterus to the pelvis. At this time he will take the internal measurements to determine the diameters of the pelvic inlet (see Chap. 2). The physician usually completes the pelvic examination with an examination of the rectum to ascertain the presence of hemorrhoids, polyps or other abnormalities.

At the completion of this examination, disposable tissues should be offered the patient so that she may wipe the perineum adequately. Optimally, further activity and demands should be kept at a minimum, so that the mother may recoup the energy which has been dissipated through trying to absorb all the new experiences and information. Further specific health teaching and counseling is better postponed until a subsequent visit, when the patient is not so overloaded with new stimuli and fatigue.

The Patient and Her Family. In a program which emphasizes family-centered service, the health problems of the individual patient and their relationship to other members of the family are of major importance. An example of a situation might be the case of Mrs. Brown, the wife of a laborer and the mother of a small toddler and a 4-year-old boy. Her physician has advised her that she needs more rest in the course of the day. Her husband is at work, and the older boy is in nursery school until noon. In order to provide more rest for the mother, she needs help to make plans for the safety and the care of the children during these rest periods; otherwise the physical rest would not accomplish its purpose. Even the consideration of meeting the nutritional needs for this family with a limited income may require guidance. To give real help at this point requires some knowledge of nutrition and entails extra planning so that the meals supply the nutritional requirements for a pregnant woman, a father who performs hard physical labor and 2 small children.

The nurse in the office or the clinic who is alert to such actual or potential health problems that affect both the patient and her family recognizes that a home visit by a public health nurse often is very helpful. If such a situation arises, she should tell the patient about available public health services and explain what a public health nurse might do while making a home visit and how such a visit could benefit the patient. With the doctor's knowledge and the patient's permission, she can institute a referral through the proper channels. Each institution, agency, etc., will have its particular method and procedure. Real value may be derived from a visit in which the nurse is able to see the patient in her usual surroundings. For instance, if the patient has the problem of excessive weight gain and is not responding to clinic therapy, the public health nurse, visiting the patient in her home, may gain some insight into the basis of the problem during her visit. In her report to the clinic or the office staff she would relate information that would contribute both to the medical and the nursing management of this pregnancy. In situations in which the clinic program is limited in educational opportunities, such as parents' classes and/or individual guidance, the public health nurse's visit to the home may be necessary to supplement the health teaching and anticipatory guidance done in the clinic.

The Community Setting

The extensive adoption of early antepartal care by various institutions, both lay and medical, is doing much to improve obstetric standards; and, in connection with this movement, the public health nurse has proved to be an invaluable asset. During the period before antepartal care was fully accepted, a case-finding program was a part of the work done by some organizations; i.e., the nurse would canvass the district for pregnant mothers. In recent decades the demand for hospital deliveries has increased rapidly; thus the present trend is toward hospital care. This has resulted in an increased demand for hospital beds, and some hospitals, especially those in congested areas or those with limited facilities, have requested that patients register early in their pregnancy to be assured of adequate accommodations for their deliveries. This early registration has resulted in more mothers getting adequate antepartal supervision early in pregnancy. In some isolated rural areas the public health nurse does case finding in the course of her usual activities and can assist the local practitioner in the antepartal care of maternity patients in the community.

Ideal Role of the Public Health Nurse Serving in an Agency. The nurse in the community is "home-based" in either an official or a voluntary agency. The official health agency may have an antepartal clinic offering complete antepartal services for those families who are having financial crises that may or may not be a result of the pregnancy. Many agencies have recognized that the public health nurse is not being utilized to her fullest potential when she is responsible for the administrative aspects of the clinic. When the professional nurse is caught up in the mechanics of record work, room preparation, directing traffic, assisting with procedures, etc., she can barely reinforce the physician's orders and perhaps clarify information relative to the obstetric condition. To utilize the time of the professional nurse more efficiently, so that she is free to counsel

patients in depth in any matters relative to health, many agencies are employing registered nurses for clinic management who do not have the public health credential, i.e., formal preparation in public health and public health certification. In addition, to maximize patient care, various types of other auxiliary personnel may be utilized, e.g., lay volunteers, licensed vocational nurses, nursing aides, etc. The clinic managers together with other nonprofessional personnel may be responsible for all of the clinic activities with the exception of patient counseling. Similarly, more hospital clinics throughout the nation are beginning to utilize a public health nurse for the health teaching and the anticipatory guidance aspects of patient care. As has been described already, most clinic schedules are very full, and the distribution of activities in such a manner results in more comprehensive patient care.

If the patient and/or her family has a problem that the public health nurse in the clinic thinks needs follow-up in the home between clinic visits, she will contact her district counterpart and communicate the necessary information. In turn, the district public health nurse will inform the clinic personnel of any pertinent findings. If complete comprehensive care is to be given to patients, open lines of communication and an expeditious interagency referral system are basic to the best service of all members of the health team, whatever their level of responsibility.

Home Visits. The district public health nurse does not follow a stereotyped routine when she makes her home visits, since each visit involves an individual patient in her own home setting. She does not have the "captive audience" that the hospital nurse does; rather she is a guest in her patient's home, and this involves a somewhat different approach and orientation. In such a situation it is especially important to orient the visit to what the patient wants and needs to know. Repeated visits based on the *nurse's* needs (to impart certain information, instruction, etc.) may very well result in a firmly closed door and a consequent severing of the nurse-patient relationship. Astute assessment of the situation at each visit includes, first of all, finding out what the patient needs to know. Communication and observation skills previously mentioned are, of course, of paramount importance here. It is the wise nurse who takes her cues from the mother and handles each need as it arises without feeling compelled to "teach" a certain amount of material each visit. If the visits are managed in this way, topics may include basic information about pregnancy, hygiene and nutrition, specific preparations for the baby, how to handle sibling rivalry, and so on. These subjects may come up naturally in the course of the visits, or the nurse can guide conversation around to them as she explores with the mother certain areas of need. By the end of the antepartal supervision period all necessary counseling usually can be accomplished.

OPPORTUNITIES FOR FAMILY HEALTH SUPERVISION. During the course of antepartal care the nurse has many opportunities for family health supervision. In her observation of other children in the home, she may be the first person to notice a neglected orthopedic condition, to suspect a need for a chest roentgenogram or to observe a possible vision or hearing difficulty. In addition observation of the mother's interaction with her children may give valuable clues to the patient's mothering patterns. This will aid the nurse in planning more effective anticipatory guidance and health teaching.

Comprehensive antepartal care, then, is a quality of patient care that is goal-directed toward the total health and the well-being of the pregnant woman. With this as the central objective, the combined efforts of several disciplines, in addition to those of medicine and nursing, may be required in the cooperative plan to achieve the ultimate goals. The practitioner-patient relationship is reciprocal, involving one giving and the other receiving care, and, to be meaningful, it must be a positive interaction. This type of interaction can be achieved only if the patient and her problems are understood and viewed with respect. The patient, in turn, must be helped to understand the goals of the health practitioners. A positive effort on the part of the health team becomes possible if each member has a clear understanding of his own role, appreciates and understands the contribution of the other professions represented on the team, knows something of the processes involved in the differing approaches, recognizes commonality of interest and skill, and has the intellectual and the

emotional capacity to enter into a team relationship.

The Medical Social Worker

Although nursing care is the primary consideration in this section, one member of the extended health team will be mentioned specifically since she works so closely with the nurse in the care of the pregnant woman. Most hospitals today have a substantial Social Service Department; it is hoped that more public health agencies will be able to take advantage of this service as more funds and personnel make this possible.

The function of Social Service workers is to help people to meet and to cope with problems that interfere with social functioning. These problems may include the problems of unmarried parenthood, divorce, desertion, placing older children during the mother's hospital stay, arranging for a working housekeeper, planning convalescent care for the mother, or arranging financial or material assistance. In their professional role social workers are called on to evaluate these problems. Then, with the patient's cooperation they help her to mobilize her resources and assist her, when necessary, through referral and counseling to alleviate the condition. They may make home visits and interview the patient, and perhaps other family members, to aid them in diagnosing the extent of the problems. Social problems may seem overwhelming if the patient's physical condition is affected, and these concerns in turn may interfere with the benefit that the patient may derive from medical services. The social worker may act as an understanding counselor between the family and the patient during her hospital stay. In many hospitals the need for a social service referral is apparent when the patient is registered early in pregnancy. In that event the patient is interviewed after the initial medical examination, and from both the physical and the social findings plans are made with the patient to mobilize her resources.

By her observation, counseling and liaison work, the social worker combines her efforts with the other members of the health team to see the patient not only as an individual maternity patient but also as an important mem-

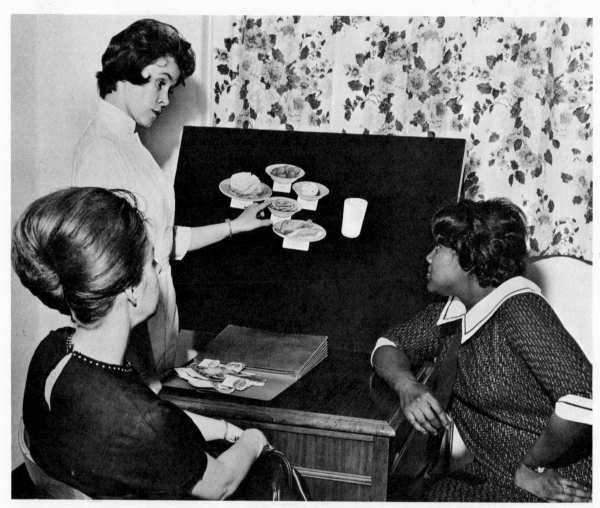

FIG. 86. Nutritional counseling by the dietitian in the clinic (with 2 patients).

TABLE 7. RECOMMENDED DAILY DIETARY ALLOWANCES*

NUTRIENTS	NONPREGNANT WOMAN (25 YEARS OLD, 5'4", 128 LBS.)	PREGNANT WOMAN (LATTER PERIOD)	LACTATING WOMAN	MAN (25 YEARS OLD, 5'9", 154 LBS.) MODERATELY ACTIVE
Calories	2,100	+200	+1,000	2,900
Protein (Gm.)	58	+20	+40	70
Calcium (Gm.)	0.8	+0.5	+0.5	0.8
Iron (mg.)	15	+5	+5	10
Vitamin A (I.U.)	5,000	+1,000	+3,000	5,000
Thiamine (mg.)	0.8	+0.2	+0.4	1.2
Riboflavin (mg.)	1.3	+0.3	+0.6	1.7
Niacin (mg.)	14	+3	+7	19
Ascorbic acid (mg.)	70	+30	+30	70
Vitamin D (I.U.)	x	400	400	x

* Recommended Dietary Allowances (Revised 1963), Publication No. 1146, National Academy of Sciences –National Research Council, Washington, D. C.

ber of the family, and the family as an integral part of the community.

NUTRITION IN PREGNANCY

A very important activity of the nurse is that of nutritional counseling. Much attention has been given to the diet of the pregnant mother in recent years, since studies have shown that the improved nutritional status of the mother promotes not only her well-being but also that of her baby. For instance, a significant relationship has been found between the protein intake of the mother and the physical condition of the infant. Mothers who had a high protein intake gave birth to infants who had high ratings of physical excellence. Other studies have demonstrated that prematurity is associated with poor nutritional status of the mother, as well as other factors (see Suggested Reading). Thus, an appropriate diet promotes the mother's health and provides essential building materials for the growth and the development of her offspring.

General Factors in Planning the Diet

Quality rather than quantity is the main consideration in planning the diet. During the first part of pregnancy the daily energy requirements for the average pregnant woman will be about the same as usual, in the neighborhood of 2,100 to 2,300 calories a day if she is moderately active, unless her weight needs to be regulated. It is important to consider the patient's activity in relation to her diet. In the latter part of pregnancy, if the patient maintains moderate activity, the daily caloric intake may be augmented because of the increased metabolic rate. If, however, activity slows down, as is often the case, and an inappropriate weight gain ensues, then caloric intake may be reduced. The physician will prescribe specifically for each mother to meet her individual needs, and the nurse then will follow through with counseling and planning as necessary. The Food and Nutrition Board of the National Research Council recommends daily allowances of specific nutrients for pregnancy and lactation, as shown in Table 7.

During the early months the appetite may be affected, and there may be phases of dislike for certain foods and beverages. Then, later, there may be an increase in the desire for all food or certain types of food. The mother may need help to discipline her appetite in accord with the amount of food needed and the desirable weight gain. Thoughtful and cooperative meal planning with the patient, with specific and thorough direction as to quantity and quality of nutrients, do much to help the mother to maintain motivation and discipline during these difficult times.

One patient who had been told that she could eat "all the cottage cheese and tomatoes that she wanted" tearfully watched her weight climb each visit. When the matter finally was pursued, it was found that she had taken the words quite literally and was eating a pint of creamed cottage cheese and 6 medium-sized tomatoes for lunch each day. The quantity made up for the low calorie content of the food!

Also, it is well to counsel the mother early in her pregnancy to avoid sweets and high caloric desserts, as well as the habit of frequent nibbling, since these interfere with appetite for the more essential foods and only add additional weight. Early pregnancy is a good time to institute health teaching of this sort, since many mothers are motivated to attain good health for themselves and their impending child at this time and hence are very receptive to anything that will bring this about. Appetite tends to be diminished, and therefore appropriate choosing of the quantity of food may be easier; later, when the "newness" of the pregnancy has worn off, and the appetite is unleashed, self-discipline is much harder, especially without previous reinforcement. Occasional "cravings" for unusual articles of food may occur. These sometimes indicate the lack of a certain element in the diet that the body demands. Any desires of this nature may be granted with safety if they agree with the patient and are not exceptional in amount or content. If the diet supplies all the needs of the patient and the growing fetus, such cravings may not occur.

Salt Restriction. Another important point should be emphasized here, the necessity for salt restriction during pregnancy. If there is any one substance that should be curtailed in any pregnancy, it is salt. First, the amount of salt consumed by the average person is far in excess of human requirements. Second, even if no salt were added to foods either in the kitchen or at the table, this mineral is distributed so widely in food materials that the likelihood of shortage would be exceedingly remote. Finally, there is a definite relationship between the amount of salt eaten and the amount of water retained by the body; that is, the greater the salt intake, the greater is the tendency of tissues to absorb water. The tissues of the pregnant woman manifest a particular avidity for water, as is evidenced by the tendency of the face and the fingers to become puffy, and if, superimposed on this tendency, there is an excess of salt in the diet, the tissues may become actually water-logged, with dire consequences.

Many physicians advise their patients early in pregnancy to watch their salt intake by avoiding salty foods, using salt judiciously in cooking, and avoiding the use of the saltshaker at the table. During the last trimester salt restriction is especially necessary, and it is important that the patient be so advised.

The Balanced Diet

The physician will regulate the patient's diet according to her condition, and the nurse will follow through with planning with the mother how best to implement his orders. If the patient's previous diet has been nourishing and well balanced, few changes will be necessary except to provide for the adjustment in protein, mineral and vitamin intake.

Counseling and Planning Sessions. To provide appropriate guidance for the mother and to assess better her level of understanding and knowledge about her diet, a brief diet history can be taken to find out her present eating patterns. The nurse may ask the mother to write down her usual daily and/or weekly meal pattern and any "extras" that she is likely to consume. These menus then are checked for an adequate intake of those foods that provide a substantial amount of the essential nutrients. As the nurse and the mother plan together, the patient's likes and dislikes are recognized, and those foods that provide the essential nutrients are encouraged. Suggestions may be given for the addition of certain foods or the modification of existing methods of selection and/or preparation. During these planning sessions it is im-

portant to remember that the mother is a member of a family, and although she plans the meals, many of her choices are dictated by the likes and dislikes of her family. The young teen-age bride who has just learned to fry cheeseburgers and french fries for her spouse may not be persuaded easily to broil and to bake instead; furthermore, she deserves recognition for accomplishing something as important as preparing a meal that is pleasing to her husband.

THE RELIGIOUS, RACIAL AND ETHNIC BACKGROUND of the patient and her family is another important consideration in counsel regarding nutrition, as well as in other aspects of care. Many families are fond of their regional or national diet and prefer it to the American "meat and potatoes" regimen. Whenever possible, the preferred diet should be considered and planned through the use of "exchanges" for food groups (see Suggested Reading). Many nutrition books give a "basic national" diet for the various countries, which provides a springboard for planning.

In considering the diet of persons of a different ethnicity, the nurse also should consider the degree of *acculturation* of the patient. This term refers to the acquisition by a group or an individual of the traits of another culture. In this case, it should not be assumed, for instance (without first exploring), that beans and tortillas are a staple in the diet of a bilingual patient with the name of Munoz. She may be a third-generation American and very familiar with and accepting of North American nutrition and eating patterns (i.e., she is acculturated).

PSYCHOLOGICAL ASPECTS OF NUTRITION. Other aspects to be considered are the stage of growth and development of the patient and the psychological factors involved in nutrition; e.g., the meaning that food has for the mother. We are aware, for instance, that foods enjoyed by adolescents are different from the the foods enjoyed by older people; the hamburger-coke-french-fry "typical" teen-age diet has received wide publicity. It seems to meet some need in much the same way as peanut butter sandwiches do for the preschooler. More and more persons are marrying younger and becoming parents at an earlier age, and, of course, they carry their eating patterns into marriage with them. In addition, adolescence is a time for developing independence, and this is healthy. However, many foods are rejected (milk, vegetables, cereal, etc.), because they are associated with "home" and a dependency period. The desire to be free and to select the "forbidden" foods is very strong. Permitting assertion of independence is important if the overall developmental task is to be accomplished, and the patient is to make a healthy adjustment in roles from that of the child to that of the adult; yet limits often must be set if the health of the mother and the health of the baby are to be safeguarded. Therefore, incorporating the mother into the planning and allowing her choices whenever possible, helping her to increase her knowledge of nutrients, encouraging and reinforcing correct choices or willing adaptations, and giving firm guidance when indicated, all help the patient and the nurse to achieve their respective goals.

The psychological aspects of nutrition lend themselves less well to clear-cut analysis. It has been said that people can survive a state of celibacy, however uncomfortably, but no one has been able to survive without food. Food is a basic need, according to the survival criterion, more basic even than the need for sex. We know that hunger is the most fundamental of all sensations. Related to hunger, but of a very different origin, is appetite. Appetite is Nature's primary defense for the prevention of hunger. Based on the anticipation of eating, the impulse is determined by the person's previous experience. Only by coincidence and training does appetite become associated with health-giving foods. Factors affecting food-seeking behavior are the main determinants of eating, i.e., hunger, appetite and custom. The great deterrents to normal appetite are worry, fear, and preoccupation with troublesome or difficult problems—and these may be reflected in either an increase or a decrease of appetite. Some of the positive emotional stimulants include a situation of calm contentedness, a feeling of mild elation or a condition of ego-stimulation.

Present-day cuisine is a potpourri of heritage, superstition, custom, knowledge and opportunity. Subtle cravings are passed along from one generation to the next by the process of training and imitation. Unique methods of food preparation as well as food selection, combinations, and prejudices are embodied in this training. Congeniality and hospitality among normal people are enhanced by the serving of good food; and it has become the custom to serve food at practically all functions, business as well as social.

From infancy onward, food and closeness have been associated with love and security. Food and eating, in and of themselves, are looked upon as symbolizing interpersonal acceptance, warmth and sociability. Throughout all societies this symbolic undertone is unmistakable; from the "breaking of bread" in antiquity to the modern banquet the serving of food is a vehicle for expressing honor, joy or mutual bonds. It is easy to see why food has become associated with the symbolism of motherliness. Feeding is not only kindly and warm in its emotional meaning to those who receive food, but it is also essential to growth and well-being; hence it has become bound up with the idea of the mother, the one who originally nurtured, loved and supported.

The pregnant woman makes a close identification with the concept of the mother, and selections and choices may be influenced profoundly by these symbolic meanings of food. She may respond to worry, frustration or anxiety by overeating—either by nibbling or gorging. Conversely, another patient may develop anorexia. Or she may crave certain foods and reject others, and not because of physiological factors. For instance, she may feel that certain foods will "mark" her baby or will give him strength. It is crucial that the meaning which food has for the patient be explored, and that her feelings and attitudes be respected. Care must be taken not to make her feel deprecated or deprived as she is helped to understand the dynamics involved in hunger and appetite.

In summary, if counseling is to be effective and the results lasting, the nurse should strive to elicit wholehearted cooperation from the patient through involving her in the planning; considering her and her family's needs, background, preferences and attitude; encouraging and reinforcing appropriate choices and preparation; providing gentle but firm limit-setting, when indicated, and careful, thorough explanation regarding the rationale behind the advice.

The following discussion should provide some guidelines in helping patients to plan their diet. Foods have been grouped according to four general classifications: dairy foods, meat group, vegetables and fruits, and breads and cereals.

Dairy Foods. The expectant mother should have at least a quart of milk daily; milk is Nature's most nearly perfect food and is invaluable as a nutrient. It contains all the different kinds of mineral elements that are needed for fetal development. The high content of calcium and phosphorus in milk makes it almost indispensable for good growth of bone and teeth; it provides these minerals in exactly the correct proportions and in a digestible form which permits their complete utilization by both mother and fetus. It is not only an excellent source of protein or tissue-building material but also the most readily digested and easily absorbed of all food proteins. Milk is also rich in energy-providing values, so that 1 quart a day alone furnishes almost one fourth of the total energy requirements. Finally, milk contains some of the most important vitamins, particularly vitamin A, which increases resistance to infection and safeguards the development of the fetus.

An effort should be made to have the mother drink 2 glasses of milk a day; the remainder may be taken in some other form, such as soups, custards, etc. If this is done, then total calories should be watched, since these other dishes involve additional nutrients. Evaporated milk and the instant dried milks are acceptable and may be substituted if fresh cow's milk is not available.

For some patients, milk may be constipating, or it may be distasteful. If it is found to be constipating, it is preferable to treat the constipation in some way other than by omitting the milk. If the milk is distasteful, it may be disguised in other foods, as has been mentioned. The instant nonfat and whole dry milks may be used in a quantity that provides an adequate intake. Approximately 5 tablespoons of dried skim milk will equal 1 pint of fluid milk. The milk may be used dry and worked into meatloaf, mashed potatoes, cereals, sandwich spreads, baked articles, etc. Reconstituted with less than the usual amount of water, it has a richer taste than the regular liquid skim milk. Certain condiments and flavorings (vanilla, nutmeg, instant coffee, cinnamon, etc.), when mixed with the milk, will enhance the flavor.

Some patients complain that milk is "fattening." In most instances the weight gain is due to the consumption of more food than is needed or an excess of such foods as bread, potatoes and desserts. These should be the articles that are restricted, and not the milk. Occasionally, however, it will be necessary to substitute skimmed milk or churned buttermilk for whole milk. This is acceptable and will reduce calories. Most dairies nowadays reinforce skim milk with vitamins A and D, which otherwise would be deficient. Many companies now have another variety of skim milk, one that is fortified by the addition of nonfat milk solids, 400 USP units of vitamin D and 4,000 USP units of vitamin A per quart. It has a standardized 2 per cent butter fat, so that the butter fat content in general is 1½ per cent less than that of whole milk.

American, Cheddar cheese and other dairy-made foods may be used occasionally as a substitute for a part or all of the milk allotment; one ounce of cheese contains approximately the same minerals and vitamins as a large glass of whole milk. However, the total protein and fat content of the diet then needs to be considered, since they may be altered.

If the mother can be helped to realize the importance of this one article of food in relation to the development of her baby, any sacrifices or modifications that may be involved can be made more willingly.

Meat Group. This is a rich source of one of the most essential nutrients, proteins. Two or more servings of beef, pork, lamb, veal, organ meats, fish, poultry, eggs or cheese are recommended daily. Legumes (dried beans, peas) or nuts may be used occasionally as alternates. In addition, these foods contain vitamins and valuable minerals, but their main value is in their amino acids or "building stones," as they sometimes are called. These are the elements that are needed not only by the mother but also by the fetus for the development of all the delicate and intricate systems of his body. Meat, eggs and fish contain complete proteins, with all the 10 amino acids that are necessary to maintain life and support growth. Oftentimes the family's budget restricts the quantity and the variety of these proteins, especially with respect to meat. The substitution of cheese, peanut butter, poultry, fish or legumes then may be suggested. The mother

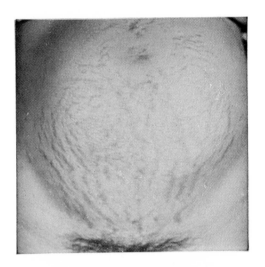
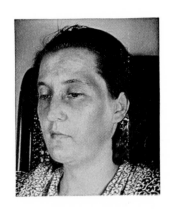
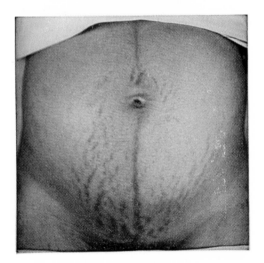
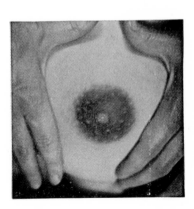

PLATE 3. (*Left, top*) Striae gravidarum.
(*Left, bottom*) Linea nigra and also striae gravidarum.
(*Right, top*) Mask of pregnancy (chloasma).
(*Right, bottom*) Montgomery's tubercles.

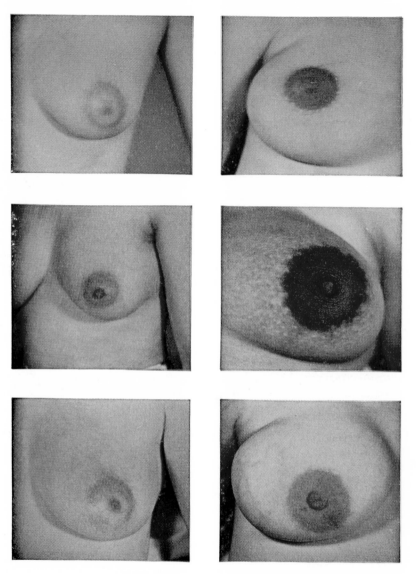

PLATE 4. (*Left, top*) Breast in nonpregnant blonde.
(*Right, top*) Breast in pregnant blonde, showing pigmentary changes.
(*Left, center*) Breast in nonpregnant brunette.
(*Right, center*) Breast in pregnant brunette, showing pigmentary changes
and marked secondary areola.
(*Left, bottom*) Breast in nonpregnant red-haired woman.
(*Right, bottom*) Breast in pregnant red-haired woman.

may need advice also regarding the preparation and the utilization of the organ meats that are so rich in protein, vitamins and minerals. Because some of these are relatively inexpensive, many women do not realize their nutritional worth and further avoid them because of the aesthetics that may be involved in the preparation—skinning, soaking, etc. Taste also is sometimes a factor. Nevertheless, with a little ingenuity and suggestions from a good nutrition and/or cook book, the nurse can do much to help the family to utilize this valuable and inexpensive source of protein. Liver, for instance, can be *lightly* broiled, ground and incorporated into a meatloaf or ground meat patties. The taste and looks are disguised, the nutritional value is retained, and the meat goes further.

Vegetables and Fruits. Four or more servings should be included from this group, especially the leaf, stem, green and yellow varieties of vegetables as well as the citrus fruits and tomatoes. It is desirable to serve at least one portion of each vegetable and fruit raw.

VEGETABLES, particularly, are rich sources of iron, calcium and several vitamins. At mealtimes there is no reasonable limit to the amount of lettuce, tomatoes, celery, string beans, carrots, beets and asparagus which may be eaten, provided that they are not heavily salted, sauced, buttered or served with a rich dressing. By increasing the quantity of such foods to several times the amount ordinarily taken, it is usually possible to satisfy the appetite without gaining abnormally in weight.

Fresh frozen vegetables are a good alternate. Canned vegetables may be used if fresh are not available. If a good brand is obtained, the vitamin content often is higher than that of vegetables cooked at home. Careful preparation and cooking of vegetables will help to retain the maximum vitamin and mineral content. Some vegetables contain several incomplete proteins which add to the total protein intake.

In addition to their value as nutrient agents, these vegetables deserve an important place in the diet as laxative agents, since their fibrous framework increases the bulk of the intestinal content and thereby stimulates the muscular, eliminative action of the intestines.

FRUITS. Citrus fruits—oranges, lemons and grapefruit—are the best sources of vitamin C. Most of these fruits also supply vitamins A

and B. Tomatoes are also an excellent source of vitamin C; the amount, however, must be twice that of the citrus fruits to supply the same amount of vitamin. Other fruits, raw and cooked, such as prunes, raisins, apricots, contain important minerals (iron and copper) as well as vitamins. Fruits may stimulate a lagging appetite and counteract constipation. They may be used in many ways: as juices, combination salads, additions to cereals or in-between meal refreshments and in desserts, such as gelatins and puddings. Fruits contain some incomplete proteins but only supplement the other proteins.

Bread and Cereals. Four or more servings should be included from this group. In the past it has been the practice to counsel patients to eliminate white bread and cereals and to substitute the darker and whole wheat varieties. This is no longer necessary, since almost all breads and cereals are enriched with vitamins, minerals and protein. A careful perusal of the label is usually all that is necessary. However, the darker varieties do provide a welcome change and, of course, are nutritious. When cereals are supplemented by milk, they become adequate for growth as well as for maintaining life. Bread that is buttered increases the vitamin A intake. The coarse cereals and the dark breads add roughage to the diet. Vitamin B and roughage both help to counteract constipation.

In addition to the four basic food groups, special attention should be given to the following:

Fluids. Fluids should be taken freely, averaging 6 to 8 glasses daily. Water aids in the circulation of the blood, body fluids, and the distribution of mineral salts, as well as in stimulating the digestion and the assimilation of foods. Fluids help to increase perspiration and to regulate elimination from intestines and kidneys. Tea and coffee may be included in the daily fluid quota if not found to be constipating or sleep-disturbing. Alcohol should be used sparingly, particularly if the mother must watch her weight, since beverages containing alcohol have a high caloric content. The use of alcohol by the pregnant woman has not shown a tendency to produce any pathologic changes in the mother or the fetus, and no effect on the course of pregnancy or labor has been demonstrated.

Vitamins. Vitamins are the *live* elements in food and are essential to life. The best sources are the natural foods. To retain the vitamin value in foods, they must be fresh, carefully prepared and not overcooked. During pregnancy and lactation the vitamin needs are increased, and so it is apparent that a well-balanced diet containing all the vitamins is of first importance. Some physicians add vitamin preparations to the diet to be sure that an adequate requirement has been met.

Vitamin A is essential in the diet for the maintenance of body resistance to infection. Foods which are good sources of this vitamin include whole milk, fortified skimmed milk, dairy products containing butter fat, eggs, green leafy and yellow vegetables and liver.

The vitamin B complex is essential to good nutrition. During pregnancy, thiamine (B_1) is necessary in increased amounts, as the fetus readily depletes the mother's reserve. Milk, eggs, lean meat and whole grain or enriched bread and cereal are good sources of thiamine. Riboflavin and nicotinic acid, absolute essentials in the diet, are found in such foods as meat, milk, eggs and green vegetables.

Vitamin C is necessary for the proper development of the fetus. Since an adequate reserve of this water-soluble vitamin is not stored in the body, an abundant supply of this vitamin is needed daily throughout pregnancy and lactation. Fresh citrus fruits, berries and green leafy vegetables (with the exception of lettuce) are foods which are a good source of vitamin C. These foods should be eaten raw as often as possible, since cooking destroys about half of their vitamin content.

Vitamin D is of great importance in safeguarding the mother and the fetus during pregnancy, since it bears some relationship to calcium and phosphorus metabolism. Liver, eggs, fortified sweet milk and fish (particularly Atlantic herring and mackerel) are food sources of vitamin D. The National Research Council recommends a daily intake of 400 I.U. for the pregnant and lactating woman. This amount, the Council says, will protect all normal growing individuals from deficiency with an adequate margin of safety. In evaluating vitamin D intake, all fortified foods in the diet should be taken into account, since large doses of either vitamin A or D may be toxic to humans.

Minerals. Studies indicate that 13 or more mineral elements are essential for good nutrition. It is believed that if calcium, phosphorus, iron and iodine are provided in adequate amounts, the others also will be present in sufficient quantities.

CALCIUM. Although two thirds of the calcium in the fetus is deposited during the last month of pregnancy, the mother's daily requirement of calcium is increased during the entire course of pregnancy to prepare adequate storage for this demand. The principal foods from which calcium is obtained are cheese, eggs, oatmeal, vegetables and milk. A quart of milk alone supplies 1.2 Gm. of calcium.

PHOSPHORUS. This element is an essential constituent of all the cells and the tissues of the body. Milk provides an abundant source of phosphorus. Actually, since phosphorus is an almost invariable constituent of protein, a diet which includes sufficient protein-rich foods, such as eggs, meat, cheese, oatmeal and green vegetables, will provide also an adequate amount of phosphorus.

IRON. During the first two trimesters of pregnancy iron is transferred to the fetus in moderate amounts, but during the last trimester, when the fetus builds up its reserve, the amount transferred is accelerated about 10 times. Therefore, the diet should be balanced and nutritious as well as rich in iron-containing foods. It is believed that certain amino acids and vitamin C may be essential to normal iron absorption. If the daily diet contains egg yolk, lean meat (particularly liver), vegetables, fruit and whole grain cereals, the problem of anemia is less likely to occur. Recent studies indicate that expectant mothers who were in good health prior to pregnancy can maintain their hemoglobin concentration at known levels of health by eating a balanced diet (see Suggested Reading). However, most physicians prescribe additional iron in the form of such preparations as ferrous sulfate and ferrous gluconate. These preparations should be administered 3 times a day, following the meals, to allow for maximum absorption and to eliminate much of the intolerance for iron which would occur if the daily prescription for iron were administered in one dose.

IODINE. Only very small amounts of iodine are needed for the health of the mother and the fetus. This mineral is obtained very readily from seafoods; cod liver oil is another good source. In certain localities around the Great Lakes and in parts of the Northwest the water supply and the vegetables grown are poor in iodine. Hence, daily use of iodized salt ensures an adequate intake and prevents deficiency.

Other Information on Nutrition. There will be times when consultation with a nutritionist is advisable; if there is no nutritionist on the hospital staff, one may be found in the area through the local public health department or a home economist's office. Publications and visual aids, charts, etc., may be secured from city, county and state health departments. The U. S. Government Printing Office is another invaluable source of publications. Certain professional organizations offer additional resources: Food and Nutrition Board, National Research Council, Council on Foods and Nutrition, American Medical Association, American Home Economics Association, American Public Health Association, etc. The above associations serve to illustrate only a few of the resources that the nurse and the physician have to assist their patients in planning for adequate nutrition.

Weight Control

An aspect of health closely associated with nutrition is weight control; this topic will be considered briefly before the other facets of counseling are outlined. A weight gain during pregnancy of 20 pounds is desirable and usually in keeping with good health. Irrespective of the mother's gain, the infant generally will weigh from 6 to 8 pounds, the amniotic and other body fluids from 2 to 3 pounds, and the placenta from 1 to 1½ pounds; therefore an increase in total pounds beyond the above amount is undesirable for a number of reasons. First, they represent unnecessary poundage for the muscles of the legs and the back to carry about, and this suddenly imposed strain is a common cause of backache, pain in the legs and also easy fatigability. Second, certain serious complications of pregnancy, preeclampsia and eclampsia (see p. 446), are less common in patients whose weight increment is moderate. Third, excessive weight gain in pregnancy is likely to be a permanent acquisition, especially with successive pregnancies; thus, if the mother is interested in retaining her figure

and health, she should be interested also in limiting weight gain at this time.

Obstetricians are emphasizing more and more the importance of weight control in pregnancy; some insist on as little as a gain of 15 pounds. If the patient's weight gain after the 3rd month is of the order of 3 pounds a month, it may be regarded as satisfactory; but if it exceeds 4 pounds a month, steps should be taken to control it. Here a nurse can be of the utmost help in advising expectant mothers about certain simple steps that may be taken, particularly in regard to the curtailment of certain nonessential foods.

Some of the **specific suggestions** which may be made are as follows:

1. The patient should be acquainted with the amazing fattening potentialities of certain common nonessential foods—foods which, in many people's minds, scarcely deserve that term at all, because most of them are likely to be regarded as mere snacks without perceptible effects on total caloric intake. Actually, these little extras taken between meals or at bedtime constitute one of the most common causes for excessive weight gain in pregnancy and at other times. Even a glass of ginger ale or Coca-Cola averages 100 calories. A chocolate bar approximates more than 300 calories. A single cocktail or highball has 200 calories. A doughnut (without icing) plus a cup of cocoa yields 400 calories, and the average malted milk served at soda fountains contains some 500 calories. Pie à la mode approximates 600 calories. When it is recalled that 2,100 to 2,300 calories per day generally is recognized as a satisfactory (and generous) allowance for pregnancy, it is plain that these "little snacks" loom tremendously large in relation to the total caloric allotment. They simply must be eliminated if the patient is gaining excessively. If she is hungry between meals, she may take the glass of milk scheduled for dinner, omitting it from her evening meal. Raw vegetables and fruit also are helpful in assuaging hunger pangs.

2. The patient should be reminded that the way in which a food is prepared may affect its caloric or fattening value almost as much as the nature of the food itself. Failure to heed this fact has resulted in many women gaining weight on diets which should cause them, theoretically at least, to lose. Perhaps the simplest

way to show how the preparation of a food affects its caloric value is to be found in fried foods. Although the caloric content of a poached or boiled egg is about 80 calories and is so calculated in dietary lists, once that egg is fried, its caloric value jumps to around 120 calories because of the fat absorbed by the egg in cooking. A level tablespoon of fat, let it be emphasized, yields approximately 120 calories. In regard to soups and desserts, it is common knowledge that those made with milk are of much less caloric content than those made with cream, and that those made with skimmed milk are still lower. When flour or cheese in addition to cream is used, as in escalloped or au gratin dishes, the calories soar to unbelievable heights; in general, for this group of foods, the smoother and the more delicious the taste, the higher is the caloric value.

The intrinsic caloric value of foods of the same type varies widely. Fruits show considerable variation according to their degree of sweetness. For instance, canned fruit can be very high in calories because of the sugar in the syrup. Therefore, the mother can be reminded to use fresh fruits regularly, and if for some important reason canned fruit must be served, the unsweetened varieties or those packed in light syrup are the only ones that should be taken. It might be added that these varieties are more economical than those packed in the rich heavy syrups. Likewise, meats vary greatly in their caloric contents, lean meats being low and those with much fat in their substance being high. As an example of the latter, an average serving of linked country sausage may exceed 600 calories. To summarize this aspect of weight control in pregnancy, the patient should be reminded that fried foods invariably possess a high caloric content and must be curtailed or eliminated altogether; that milk, preferably skimmed milk, should be substituted for cream in preparing soups and desserts; and that lean meat rather than fatty meat must be chosen, and fresh fruit rather than canned.

3. The next suggestion to make to the patient is to substitute skimmed milk for the whole milk included in the recommendation about diet in pregnancy. This reduces forthwith the caloric content of the diet by about 300 calories—no small sum. Fat-free or skimmed milk contains the same nutrients as whole milk, except for fat and vitamins A and D, but fortified fat-free milk contains much greater amounts of these two vitamins than does whole milk. However, be sure that the patient is taking this quart of milk every day. It provides more proteins, minerals and vitamins for less calories (and money) than any other food; and skimmed milk contains, of course, as much protein and minerals (including calcium) as does whole milk.

4. The next suggestion is an easy one to carry out, namely, to substitute saccharin for sugar, not only in coffee or tea but also for cereals, fruits and cooking. Improvements in the manufacturing of this product have resulted in both liquid and solid forms, and most, if not all, of the former "bitter" and excessively "sweet" taste has been eliminated. Saccharin now can be used in cooking, and no difference in taste can be detected when it is used according to directions.

5. The salt ordinarily added to foods in the kitchen should be reduced drastically or eliminated altogether for the reasons mentioned previously (see p. 145). It is wise to counsel the mother-to-be to add no salt to the food at the table and in the kitchen to add a little less than she would like. In addition, she should be reminded to read carefully all labels on the foodstuffs that she buys to ascertain what salt and/or sodium content they have. For instance, frozen peas have salt added. Monosodium glutamate (MSG), a substance that brings out the natural flavor in foods, also should be avoided since it has a high sodium content.

As a substitute for flavor, herbs, spices, pepper, paprika, vinegar, lemon juice, vanilla or almond extract may be suggested. In the case of excessive weight gain in pregnancy, it is quite possible that a still further reduction in salt, as recommended above, will reduce superfluous body water and cause a substantial weight loss. At first, this salt-poor diet may seem so bland and tasteless as to constitute something of a hardship; with skillful use of herbs and with motivation and perseverance on the part of the patient, an adjustment can be made. However, it must be remembered that any modification of the meals has an impact on the family as well as the patient. They may need help in understanding and accepting the restrictions. If they cannot, then the patient is put in the position of having to prepare 6 meals a day instead of 3. This can be aggravating, to say the least, if not downright impossible; and certainly it will have implications for her own acceptance of the restrictions and her later follow-through. Thus, in these cases it is especially important to explore with the mother and the family their understanding, feelings and attitudes toward these new alterations rather than merely to issue dictums.

6. If the above recommendations do not serve to curtail weight gain, the patient should eliminate all rich desserts. Fresh fruits can be substituted, sweetened, if necessary, with saccharin.

7. It may be necessary to remind the patient to take servings of average size and only one serving.

Because of the importance of the subject, the nurse must understand that it will not suffice simply to tell the patients to reduce their food consumption or to eat less fattening foods. Directions, to be effective, must be specific as well as rather comprehensive and should be reviewed with the patients in an empathic and understanding way. Above all, it must be emphasized that no curtailment is to be made in food essentials—doubly essential in pregnancy—such as milk, green and yellow leafy vegetables, proteins, minerals and vitamins.

If the suggestions listed above, together with the other counseling mentioned, are not effective, the case is a special one, and the patient may require more meticulous medical supervision and/or the help of a nutritionist. The nurse is in the best position to keep the physician apprised of the dietary situation, and her follow-through is essential for proper referral.

GENERAL HYGIENE

The remainder of the counseling that the physician and nurse will want to give the mother falls under the heading of general hygiene. Pregnancy should be a normal, happy, healthy experience for a woman. During the months preceding labor the physician and the nurse will advise her about her mode of life. She will be encouraged to continue her usual habits with very little change, unless, of course, it is found that she has been leading an existence not conducive to healthy living.

Rest, Relaxation and Sleep

Because rest and sleep are so essential to health, the nurse must emphasize this detail in her teaching during the antepartal period. Pregnant women become tired more readily; therefore, the prevention of fatigue must be stressed very emphatically. The body is made up of various types of cells, each type with a specific function. Depletion of nerve-cell energy results in fatigue, and fatigue causes certain reactions in the body that are injurious. For all body processes, such as digestion, metabolism, working, playing and studying, nerve-cell energy is utilized. Nature has made provision for some reduction in normal energy without injury to health. Beyond this limit the symptoms of fatigue are evidenced in irritability, apprehension, a tendency to worry and restlessness. These symptoms are sometimes very subtle and misleading, but, in contrast, human beings are very conscious of tired muscles. It is more important to avoid fatigue than to have to recover from overfatigue. The pregnant woman should rest to prevent this fatigue. Rest and sleep replenish the cell energy. As Dr. Jastrow says of this code of rest and sleep, they "must be shaped according to the individual's nervous disposition, habits of life, age, and circumstances."

If patients cannot sleep, they should attempt to rest. Rest is the ability to relax. Patients often need to learn how to relax. There is no code so variable, so necessarily adapted to the individual, as that of rest and sleep. The final test is whether the day's work is done with zest and energy to spare. The expectant mother should get as much sleep as she feels she needs. Some people need more than others. In addition to a good night's sleep, it is advisable that the mother take a nap or at least rest for a half hour every morning and afternoon. If this is not possible, then shorter rest periods, taken preferably lying down, several times a day are beneficial.

The nurse must recognize that all mothers are not able to follow the recommended rest periods to the letter. The woman who must work throughout her pregnancy, the mother of several preschool children, all need special attention with respect to planning for adequate rest. Rigid recommendations must be avoided, and the nurse should search with the mother for minutes in her busy day that can be utilized for rest; again, counseling the family may be necessary to maximize the mother's free moments. Although the nurse strives for flexibility, she needs also to emphasize the necessity of this aspect of general hygiene. It can be explained that rest means not only to lie down or perhaps to sleep, but also to lie down or to sit comfortably—to rest the body, the mind, the abdominal muscles, the legs and the back, and to stretch out whenever possible and so make it easier for the heart to pump the blood to the extremities. During the last months of pregnancy a small pillow used for support of the abdomen, while the patient lies on her side, does much to relieve the discomfort common during this period and adds materially to the degree of rest that the patient gets in a given time.

Suggest to the patient that, instead of standing, she sit whenever possible, even while doing her housework. Sitting to rest for other brief periods during the course of the day can be beneficial if the feet and the legs are elevated.

Often the so-called minor discomforts of pregnancy can be overcome by rest. Rest and the right-angle position (see Fig. 8-12) are advised for swelling, edema and varicosities of the lower extremities. Rest and Sims's position (see Fig. 8-15) are advised for varicosities of the vulva and the rectum. Even for the more serious abnormalities, the simple aids included in "diet and rest" may help much until more specific orders from the obstetrician can be obtained. In such instances the nurse must be aware of the mother's interpretation of "rest," and, if indicated, she should provide the necessary guidance to help the mother to understand and to plan for it.

Exercise

Outdoor exercise during pregnancy is usually very beneficial, because it affords diversion in the sunshine and fresh air. However, for each individual patient the obstetrician must decide whether the customary exercise should be increased or diminished. There should be a difference in the amount of exercise for the early and late periods of pregnancy. When pregnancy is advanced, exercise may be limited in comparison with the amount advised previously. Exercise usually means diversion, and, of course, this phase is most important. Exercise also steadies the nerves, quiets the mind, promotes sleep and stimulates the appetite, all of which are valuable aids to the pregnant mother.

Walking in the fresh air is quite generally preferred to every other form of exercise during pregnancy, because it stimulates the muscular activity of the entire body, strengthens some of the muscles used during labor and is available to all women. Exercise of any kind should not be fatiguing; to secure the most beneficial results, it should be combined with fresh air and sunlight, as well as periods of rest.

The woman who does her own housework needs little or no planned exercise from the physical viewpoint. However, she does need fresh air, sunshine and diversion. It is far better for the patient to be occupied than to sit idly, but standing for long periods of time should be avoided. Lifting heavy objects, moving furniture, reaching to hang curtains, any activity which might involve sudden jolts, sudden changes in balance which might result in a fall or the likelihood of physical trauma should be avoided. The more strenuous sports, i.e., horseback riding, skiing, hiking involving long climbs, rough water swimming are subjects that should be discussed with the obstetrician for his opinion and guidance. The pregnant woman who is accustomed to participating in certain sports and finds this participation an enjoyable form of recreation usually will be permitted to continue in moderation and at a mild pace, if it proves harmless.

Employment

The same attitude of moderation should be maintained whether for work or play. Ideally, no work or play should be continued to the extent of even moderate fatigue; however, it is not realistic to expect the mother willingly to discontinue her job because it is tiring, especially if it is essential to the family sustenance. If her employment is influencing her health adversely, then the matter needs conscientious exploration by the health team to see what realistic adjustments can be made. A referral to a social worker may be indicated, the better to ascertain the economic situation of the family and/or the resources in the community that might be helpful. Different job opportunities can be discussed, and the patient's skills, satisfactions and preparation can be considered.

In general, jobs requiring moderate manual labor should be avoided if they must be continued over long hours, if they require delicate balance, or constant standing, or constant working on night shifts. Actually, the woman who has a "desk job" in an office often does less strenuous work than the average homemaker who does not go out to work. Nevertheless, positions which require the worker to sit constantly can be extremely tiring. Adequate rest periods should be provided for all pregnant women employed in such positions.

In some countries the time of discontinuing routine jobs has been regulated by law, and the limits, although arbitrary, are generally from 6 to 8 weeks prior to the expected date of confinement.

Many women are employed in industry, and the problem of pregnancy for the working mother in this type of employment is a most important one. To safeguard the interests of expectant mothers so engaged, the following Standards for Maternity Care and Employment of Mothers in Industry have been recommended by the Children's Bureau of the United States.

1. Facilities for adequate prenatal medical care should be readily available for all employed pregnant women; and arrangements should be made by those responsible for providing prenatal care, so that every woman would have access to such care. Local health departments should make available to industrial plants the services of prenatal clinics; and the personnel management or physicians and nurses within the plant should make available to employees information about the importance of such services and where they can be obtained.

2. Pregnant women should not be employed on a shift including the hours between 12 midnight and 6 A.M. Pregnant women should not be employed more than 8 hours a day nor more than 48 hours per week, and it is desirable that their hours of work be limited to not more than 40 hours per week.

3. Every woman, especially a pregnant woman, should have at least two 10-minute rest periods during her work shift, for which adequate facilities for resting and an opportunity for securing nourishing food should be provided.

4. It is not considered desirable for pregnant women to be employed in the following types of occupation, and they should, if possible, be transferred to lighter and more sedentary work:

a. Occupations that involve heavy lifting or other heavy work.

b. Occupations involving continuous standing and moving about.

5. Pregnant women should not be employed in the following types of work during any period of pregnancy, but should be transferred to less hazardous types of work.

a. Occupations that require a good sense of bodily balance, such as work performed on scaffolds or stepladders and occupations in which the accident risk is characterized by accidents causing severe injury, such as operation of punch presses, power-driven woodworking machines, or other machines having a point-of-operation hazard.

b. Occupations involving exposure to toxic substances considered to be extrahazardous during pregnancy, such as:

Aniline
Benzol and toluol
Carbon disulfide
Carbon monoxide
Chlorinated hydrocarbons
Lead and its compounds
Mercury and its compounds
Nitrobenzol and other nitro compounds of benzol and its homologs
Phosphorus
Radioactive substances and x-rays
Turpentine

Other toxic substances that exert an injurious effect upon the blood-forming organs, the liver, or the kidneys.

Because these substances may exert a harmful influence upon the course of pregnancy, may lead to its premature termination, or may injure the fetus, the maintenance of air concentrations within the so-called "maximum permissible limits" of State codes, is not, in itself, sufficient assurance of a safe working condition for the pregnant woman. Pregnant women should be transferred from workrooms in which any of these substances are used or produced in any significant quantity.

6. A minimum of 6 weeks' leave *before* delivery should be granted, on presentation of a medical certificate of the expected date of confinement.

7. At any time during pregnancy a woman should be granted a reasonable amount of additional leave on presentation of a certificate from

the attending physician to the effect that complications of pregnancy have made continuing employment prejudicial to her health or to the health of the child.

To safeguard the mother's health she should be granted sufficient time off after delivery to return to normal and to regain her strength. The infant needs her care, especially during the first year of life. If it is essential that she return to work, the following recommendations are made:

a. All women should be granted an extension of at least 2 months' leave of absence after delivery.

b. Should complications of delivery or of the postpartum period develop, a woman should be granted a reasonable amount of additional leave beyond 2 months following delivery, on presentation of a certificate to this effect from the attending physician.

Diversion

Recreation is as necessary during pregnancy as it is at any other time in life. The patient is preparing for one of the most important role changes that she will undergo during life, and concomitant with any such change is the production of anxiety. It is to be expected that a certain amount of concern about the impending labor will be present; the additional responsibility of having a helpless new baby in the household, plus caring for and integrating him into the family unit, is also anxiety-provoking. The parents will have occasion to wonder whether they are equal to the enormous responsibility of rearing children, and whether or not they will be "good" parents. Therefore, activities which are diverting, healthful and relaxing help the patient and the family to keep things in their proper perspective. Hence, it is beneficial to discuss with the mother some types of recreation that are most relaxing and pleasing for her and her family. Family group activities still can be enjoyed, even though the mother's energy and dexterity may be somewhat curtailed.

Consideration and understanding on the part of the husband, the family, the doctor and the nurse can do much to relieve any uncertainties or concerns that the mother may have. When the husband, in particular, understands more about the processes involved in the pregnancy (see Suggested Reading), his helpfulness can be increased. If a "blue" day

comes, the husband can make it his particular responsibility to provide a means of counteracting it. On a home visit the nurse might discuss with the family ways in which they might help to diminish the strain in this period. This may necessitate changes in attitudes, understanding and habits; certainly it will mean increased tolerance and forbearance on the part of those involved; yet this is one of the ways that others can make their contribution to a successful pregnancy. The husband's gentleness and tenderness are especially appreciated and therapeutic at this time; the mother, for her part, can help him to maintain his supportive attitude and behavior by letting him know when his actions are helpful and gratifying. This type of "feedback" conveys to the father her appreciation and leads to reinforcement of his positive behavior. The husband is perhaps the key person in helping the mother to secure the kind of social relaxation that she enjoys most.

With respect to the activities themselves, books, radios, music, movies, sporting events, television, sewing clubs, church functions, visiting, drives, walks and entertaining friends are some of the means of providing relaxation and diversion. However, the mother should avoid crowds, chances of infection and all conditions likely to cause a sense of discomfort. Amusements, exercise, rest and recreation at proper intervals help to keep the pregnant mother well and happy in an environment conducive to her well-being and happy anticipation of the baby.

Traveling

This is perhaps a detail of antepartal care which most patients think very little about, unless they have a tendency to become nauseated or have had a previous miscarriage.

The restriction of travel to short trips had been a rule for maternity patients until World War II, when many women found it necessary to follow their husbands regardless of distance or modes of travel. It is now possible to apply the data compiled during that era to show that travel, almost regardless of distance and type of conveyance, has no deleterious effect on pregnancy.

Even though there is little restriction on travel from a medical point of view, this topic should be discussed with the mother, so that any of her concerns or misinformation may come to light. The general information usually given to a pregnant woman is to avoid any trip which will cause undue fatigue, since she is prone to tire easily. For traveling long distances the railway or airplane is safer and provides greater comfort. If travel is by private automobile, rest periods of 10 to 15 minutes should be planned at least every 2 hours. This not only avoids fatigue, but the chance to stretch and walk about also benefits the general circulation.

Although traveling is not usually contraindicated during pregnancy, the expectant mother should consult her physician concerning the advisability of extensive travel at any time during the period of pregnancy.

Care of the Skin

The glands of skin may be more active during pregnancy, and there may be increased or decreased perspiration, resulting in irritation or dryness. Since the skin is one of the organs of elimination, bathing is obviously important, and baths should be taken daily, because they are stimulating, refreshing and relaxing. They not only act as a tonic and a general invigorator but also favor elimination through the skin as well. Elimination through the skin is thought to lessen the strain of elimination by the kidneys.

During pregnancy, showers or sponge baths may be taken at any time. The old idea that tub baths should be avoided because the wash water enters the vagina and thereby carries infection to the uterus now is believed to have little validity. There is only one objection to tub baths during the last trimester of pregnancy. At this period the heavy weight of the large abdomen may put pregnant women off balance and make climbing in and out of the tub awkward. Therefore, the likelihood of slipping or falling in the bathtub is increased. Chilling the body should be avoided; thus, cold baths, sponges or showers should be avoided if they produce this sensation.

Care of the Breasts

Special care of the breasts during pregnancy is one of the important preparations for breast feeding. During the antepartal period the breasts often have a feeling of fullness and weight and in fact do become larger, heavier and more pendulous. A well-fitted supporting brassière which holds the breasts up and in may relieve these discomforts. It may also help to prevent the subsequent tissue sagging so often noticeable after pregnancy due to the increased weight of the breasts during pregnancy and lactation.

There may be sufficient secretion of colostrum from the nipples to necessitate wearing a pad to protect the clothing. The daily care of the nipples and the reason for it, as well as the actual procedure, should be explained to the patient. Early in pregnancy the breasts begin to secrete, and this secretion often oozes out on the surface of the nipple and in drying forms fine imperceptible crusts. If these crusts are allowed to remain, the skin underneath becomes tender; if left until the baby arrives and

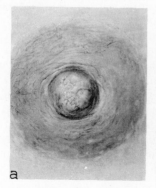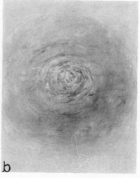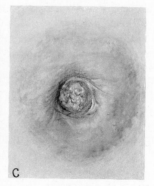

FIG. 8-7. Types of nipples. (a) Normal. (b) Flat. (c) Inverted.

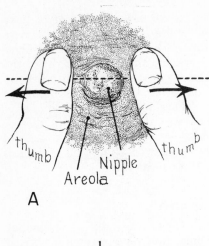

thumb

Nipple

Areola

A

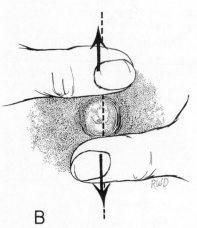

RWD

B

FIG. 8-8. A suggested treatment for inverted nipples. The thumbs are placed close to the inverted nipple, pressed firmly into the breast tissue, then gradually pushed away from the areola. The strokes should be directed horizontally (A) and vertically (B) and be done 4 or 5 times in succession.

nurses, this tender skin area is likely to crack. With this condition there is always a possibility of infection. Nipples that are kept clean and dry do not have a tendency to become sore or cracked.

The breasts should be bathed daily; this may be done at the beginning of the bath, the shower or the sponge. The patient will want to use a clean washcloth and warm water. Some studies have demonstrated that the use of soap, alcohol and other such materials during the antepartal period and puerperium tends to be detrimental to the integrity of the nipple tissue, since they remove the protective skin oils and leave the nipple more prone to damage (see Suggested Reading). Therefore, the patient should discuss the use of these with the doctor. She should begin cleansing each breast by washing the nipple thoroughly with a circular motion, making sure that any dried material has been removed, then gradually continue

working away from the nipple in this fashion until the entire breast is washed. Rinse the breast in this manner and dry with a clean towel. Rubbing the nipples with a rough towel during the last trimester of pregnancy may be helpful in attempting to toughen them. The physician may advise the use of Masse nipple cream, or some similar hydrous lanolin preparation, to prepare the nipples for nursing. This can be applied after the breasts are bathed. First, place a small quantity of cream on the thumb and the first finger, then grasp the nipple gently between the thumb and this finger and, with a kind of rolling motion, work the cream into the tiny creases found on the surface of the nipple. The position of the thumb and finger should be gradually shifted around the circumference of the nipple until a complete circuit has been made. This procedure should be limited to about 30 seconds on each breast.

A nipple which is flat or even slightly inverted in early pregnancy (Fig. 8-7) very probably will become protractile by delivery. If the nipples are inverted, some physicians prefer to start special care in the 5th or the 6th month of pregnancy or earlier. Dr. J. B. Hoffman[1] has suggested a treatment which has proved to be helpful. With the thumbs placed close to the inverted nipple, press firmly into the breast tissue and gradully push the thumbs away from the areola. The strokes should follow an imaginary cross drawn on the breast (see Fig. 8-8) and be done 4 or 5 times in succession on awakening each morning. The nipple will assume an erect, projected position and then can be grasped as a unit and gently teased out a bit further. This should be done daily, so that the nipples may be made more prominent for the baby to grasp. In extreme cases in which the nipples are badly inverted, the obstetrician will give instructions concerning the care needed.

[1] Hoffman, J. B.: A suggested treatment for inverted nipples, Am. J. Obstet. Gynec. 66:346, 1953.

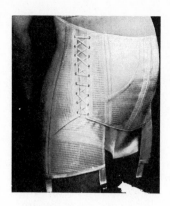

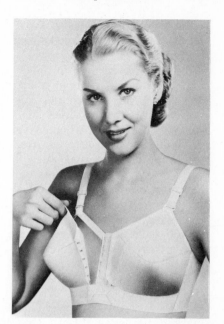

Fig. 8-9 (*Left*). Maternity girdle. (Spencer, Inc., New Haven, Conn.)

Fig. 8-10 (*Right*). Maternity brassière for use during and after the nursing period. Special construction allows for sanitary gauze over the nipples and convenient opening for nursing. (Maiden Form Brassière Co., New York)

Clothing

During pregnancy the clothes should be given the same or perhaps even a little more attention than at other times. The young mother who feels that she is dressed attractively and is well-groomed will reflect this in her manner. Her clothing should be practical, attractive and nonconstricting. Most women are able to dress in the manner to which they are accustomed in the nonpregnant state until the enlargement of the abdomen becomes apparent. Maternity specialty shops and department stores have made maternity fashions available, which has settled the problem of suitable clothing during pregnancy. Today designers and stylists are giving consideration to the pregnant mother's clothing, so that she may dress attractively and feel self-confident about her appearance. The clothes are designed so that they are comfortable and "hang from the shoulders" to avoid any constriction; they are made in a variety of materials. The expectant mother should dress according to the climate and the temperature for her comfort.

Abdominal Support. Women who have been unaccustomed to wearing a girdle will scarcely feel the need of abdominal support, especially during the early months of pregnancy. Later, however, a properly fitted maternity girdle often gives the needed support to keep the mother from becoming fatigued. The natural softening of the pelvic joints which accompanies pregnancy and the increasing weight of the abdomen may encourage a change in posture to such a degree that severe backache results.

If the mother's abdomen is large, or if previous pregnancies have caused her abdomen to become lax or pendulous, a properly made and well-fitting maternity girdle will give support and comfort. The purpose of the garment is support, not constriction of the abdomen (see Fig. 8-9).

Breast Support. It is advisable that every pregnant woman wear a brassière that is well-fitted to support the breasts in a normal uplift position. Proper support of the breasts is conducive to good posture and thus helps to prevent backache (Fig. 8-10).

The selection of a brassière should be determined by individual fitting and influenced by the size of the breasts and the need for support. It is important to see that the cup is large enough, and that the underarm is built high enough to cover all the breast tissue. Wide shoulder straps will afford more comfort for the woman who has large and pendulous breasts. The size of the brassière is, again, a matter to be determined according to the individual being fitted, but in most instances this is about two sizes larger than that usually worn. The mother who is planning to breast-feed will find it practical to purchase nursing brassières which can be worn during the latter months of pregnancy as well as during the postpartal period for as long as she is nursing her baby.

Garters. "Round garters" or any tight bands

(rolled stockings, elastic tops on stockings) that encircle the leg tend to aggravate varicose veins and edema of the lower extremities and should be discarded in favor of suspender garters or some form of stocking supporters attached to an abdominal support. It will be remembered that arteries have muscular tissue in their walls, whereas veins have little or none, so that arteries are able to resist pressure. The external veins lie close to the surface, but the arteries are embedded deeper in the tissues. Hence, any constriction of any extremity affects the veins far more than the arteries. Blood which apparently meets no obstruction whatever in its flow down the extremity through an artery may on its return through the vein find at the point of constriction sufficient closure of the vessel to "dam it back" and so stretch the vein wall that a varicosity is formed. There is already a marked tendency toward this condition, because the enlarged and constantly enlarging uterus tends to impede the return circulation from the lower extremities by compression of the great abdominal vessels, and round garters definitely tend to aggravate the condition. Garters that encircle the leg never should be worn, even by growing children, for the tendency to varicosities always is present; and, when once formed, they never entirely disappear but later may lead to great discomfort.

Shoes. A comfortable, well-fitting shoe is essential for the expectant mother. The postural changes which occur as the mother's abdomen enlarges may be aggravated by wearing high-heeled shoes, with resulting backache and fatigue. It is advisable that only low-heeled shoes be worn during working hours. However, many women do not like to go out on the street without their usual high heels. If they do not develop backache from the increased lordosis induced by the heels, and if they are able to maintain good balance, then a 2-inch heel is permissible. The ingenious and attractive newer styles, however, have taken much of the embarrassment out of wearing lower heels.

The nurse should remember that the height of the heel is but one consideration here, and that the support which the shoe gives the foot adds materially to the mother's comfort. Many of the flat-heeled and ballet-type shoes popular today give little or no support to the feet and thus may be the cause of fatigue and aching legs and backs. A simple method to check the support of a shoe can be done by placing the shoe flat on the floor and then with the thumb pressing down on the inner sole against the shank (the part that would come under the arch of the foot). If the shoe gives under this pressure, it indicates that it will give weak support to the foot.

Care of the Teeth

Good dental care is necessary, because the teeth are important in relation to adequate mastication of food. This care need be little different during pregnancy from what is considered to be good, general mouth hygiene in any person who is not pregnant. The teeth should be brushed carefully on arising, after each meal and before retiring at night. An alkaline mouthwash may be used, if desired. It is advisable for the expectant mother to visit her dentist at the very beginning of pregnancy and to follow his recommendations (Fig. 8-11). However, if he advises any extensive dental work to be done, the patient should consult her obstetrician.

The old saying, "For every child a tooth," based on a belief that the fetus takes calcium from the mother's teeth, has no real scientific basis. It should be carefully explained to the mother that an adequate diet during pregnancy will supply the baby with lime salts and other necessities in sufficient amounts to build his bones and teeth. Therefore, this old adage need not be true if proper attention is given to the care of the teeth and nutrition during pregnancy.

Bowel Habits

The pregnant woman who heretofore has adhered to regular habits of elimination usually experiences little or no change in the daily routine. Those who have a tendency toward constipation become noticeably more irregular during pregnancy due to (1) decreased physical exertion, (2) relaxation of the bowel in association with the relaxation of smooth-muscle systems all over the body, and (3) pressure of the enlarging uterus. Particularly during the latter part of pregnancy, the presenting part of the fetus exerts pressure on the lower bowel.

Personal habits of intelligent daily hygiene are the best resource that the expectant

FIG. 8-11. Dental clinic as part of an obstetric service. Because of the importance of good dental care, some hospitals have a dental clinic in connection with their antepartal supervision. (Margaret Hague Maternity Hospital, Jersey City, N. J.)

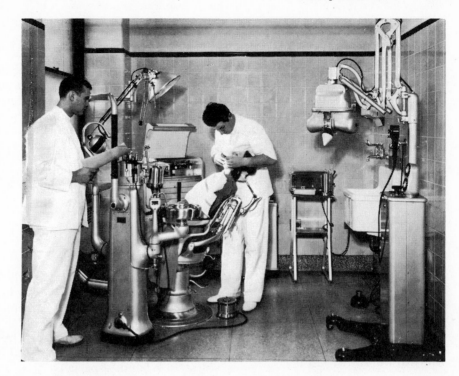

mother has to prevent constipation. The alleviation of this problem in modern society may be attributed to education, more reasonable bowel habits and greater latitude in physical exercise. During pregnancy the mother should pay close attention to bowel habits, drink sufficient quantities of fluid, eat fruits and other foods which add roughage to the diet and get reasonable amounts of daily exercise.

If these simple measures are not effective, the physician should be consulted about the problem. Harsh laxatives and enemas should be avoided unless the physician orders them specifically. He probably will prescribe some mild bulk-producing laxative and/or stool softener. If the mother has been taking a non-absorbable oil preparation, such as mineral oil, she should be advised to take the medication at bedtime, since it has the ability to dissolve and to excrete the oil-soluble vitamins if taken at mealtime, thus depriving her of the vitamins so necessary for good nutrition.

Constipation is conducive to the development of hemorrhoids and may be associated with the incidence of pyelitis. Aside from the discomfort associated with the passage of hard fecal material, this may injure the rectal mucosa and cause bleeding.

Douches

The vaginal douche, for so long considered by most married women to be a requisite of feminine hygiene, is unnecessary in most cases and should be kept at a reasonable minimum. During pregnancy, if it is indicated because of excessive vaginal secretion, the physician will prescribe the kind of douche and the frequency with which it is to be taken.

Specific instructions about douching should be given. The nurse will be able to give more intelligent guidance if she first learns from the patient about the available facilities at home (such as a bathtub), the patient's understanding of proper douching and the reasons for this treatment. It is well to remember that if a woman is not accustomed to douching, she will need guidance in relation to purchasing the necessary equipment or improvising it.

The following precautions require emphasis:

1. *Hand-bulb syringes must be absolutely forbidden,* since several deaths in pregnancy from air embolism have followed their use.

2. Plastic or hard rubber douche nozzles are preferable, since those made of glass may chip or break and injure the walls of the vagina.

3. The physician's order must be followed

as outlined, and the medicated solution prepared according to his instructions, i.e., the quantity of active ingredient and temperature (usually 108° F.), etc.

4. The bathtub should be scrubbed thoroughly before and after the treatment.

5. The external genitalia should be cleansed with soap and water before taking a douche to avoid transmitting bacteria into the vagina.

6. The douche bag should be placed no higher than 2 feet above the level of the hips to prevent high fluid pressure.

7. The nozzle should not be inserted more than 3 inches into the vagina.

For the most effective results, the patient should assume a reclining position with the knees flexed and the thighs slightly separated. The nozzle should be inserted carefully and rotated gently as the solution flows slowly and circulates in the vagina. This usually requires about 10 minutes.

Marital Relations

From the standpoint of both the physician and the nurse, the area of marital relations, perhaps because of its intimate nature, becomes the most difficult in which to give appropriate guidance. Many patients are reluctant to discuss the area of sex in general, especially when the patient-doctor-nurse relationship is new; and yet they are disturbed because of the changes which may be taking place in their feelings and emotions, with consequent influences on their marital relationship. Because of this reluctance, nurses (and doctors) often avoid exploring with the patient the possibility of any existing problem, and the counseling then consists mostly of prohibitions regarding the time and the frequency of intercourse. However, when there is a need, most patients will discuss the subject with a little help, especially when the doctor or the nurse conveys the idea that these are "expected" changes, and that there is nothing "shameful" or unique about them. Some patients prefer to speak only to the doctor regarding this matter, but some patients turn to the nurse at this time, because she is a woman and likely to experience similar feelings and concerns at some time or another. Since she may be utilized as a resource person, the nurse can prepare herself as she would for any other counseling activity. She should know about the anatomic, the physiologic and the psychological aspects involved; she should ascertain the physician's wishes regarding any general restrictions and limitations of the marital relationship during pregnancy, as well as any wishes involving the patient's relationship in particular. She should be aware that her approach here is extremely important and requires adroit use of communication skills, especially with respect to listening, reflecting and gentle probing. Finally, she should examine her own feelings and attitudes regarding sex, femininity, pregnancy and motherhood so that she can understand better and empathize with the patient's predicament.

Early pregnancy has an almost unpredictable effect on the sexual desire of the wife. Some women feel a sense of pleasant release from pregnancy fears, which enhances their desire; others find their ardor distinctly curbed. If this is a gross change from what is usual, concern may be generated in both wife and husband, especially if sexual activity is refused, and misunderstandings ensue. Sudden unexplained aversion to the husband also may occur, which is quite traumatic for both husband and wife. Fortunately, these idiosyncrasies are temporary, and desire and responsiveness soon return. It is important that the couple become aware of this fact before misunderstanding and hurt lead to the establishment of unhealthy and negative mechanisms of antipathy. It is especially gratifying for the husband to realize that these apparent caprices of his wife's are only a temporary accompaniment of the new condition of pregnancy and do not signify any real change in her basic attitude or love for him. Some obstetricians advise that during the first trimester intercourse be avoided during the time of the regular menstrual periods because of the possible danger of abortion. If the patient has had previous abortions, coitus probably will be restricted until about 2 weeks after the third missed menstrual period. This restriction may prove to be burdensome especially for the husband, and since sexual excitement cannot be resolved in the usual way, it is wise to caution the couple to avoid arousing too much sexual interest. Usually the wish to have a happy, healthy pregnancy and a baby helps the parents to accept the restriction.

Abdominal protuberance does not in most cases interfere in any way with sexual activity until about the 5th month. At this time the pressure on the abdomen may create discomfort or impede breathing. Positioning in this case becomes important. The side position for intercourse, placing pillows under the wife's hips and increased flexion of her thighs if she assumes the supine position enhance comfort for a time. By the 7th and the 8th months desire again may diminish, and most women find that they cannot participate very well in coitus in any position. The couple can be encouraged to experiment with positions that allow the wife to play a more passive role. Thus the husband can be satisfied and not feel deprived, and the wife can feel secure in the thought that she can still contribute to his gratification and happiness without exhausting herself in the process.

The physician usually will advise abstinence from intercourse during the last weeks before term in order to avoid possible premature labor or infection. Again, the same counseling as for any other period of restriction during the pregnancy is applicable here. Since relations should not be resumed until after the 6-week examination, or until the doctor can determine that all has returned to normal, many couples feel a genuine deprivation. Recognition and acknowledgment of their sacrifice is one of the most effective ways of reinforcing positive behavior and helping to ease this final limitation on the marital relationship.

Smoking

The Surgeon General's report as well as other studies have indicated that cigarette smoking is a health hazard of sufficient importance in this country to warrant remedial action. Lung cancer and heart disease have been linked significantly with cigarette smoking. With respect to pregnancy, several studies have found a relationship between smoking and a lower birth rate, higher rates of prematurity and higher neonatal mortality. The mechanism is somewhat obscure, but it is thought that the nicotine in the cigarettes causes peripheral vasoconstriction, with subsequent changes in the heart rate, the blood pressure and the cardiac output that appear to have a detrimental effect on the development and the health of the fetus. Carbon monoxide also is found in higher concentrations in smokers, with a consequent decrease of oxygen; this apparently also affects the fetus.

The subject of smoking should be discussed thoroughly with the physician, and his recommendations should be followed. Several "smoking clinics" have been developed around the country, and books and articles have been published on the topic of "how to stop smoking." No one claims to have a sure answer. A combination of motivation, education in the destructive properties of smoking and support seem to be the basic ingredients. The health team certainly can supply the last two and help the patient to achieve the first.

MINOR DISCOMFORTS

The so-called minor discomforts of pregnancy are the common complaints experienced by most expectant mothers, to some degree, in the course of a normal pregnancy. However, all mothers do not experience all of them, and, indeed, some mothers pass through the entire antepartal period without any of these discomforts. They are not serious in themselves, but their presence detracts from the mother's feeling of comfort and well-being. In many instances they can be avoided by preventive measures, or entirely overcome by common sense in daily living, once they do occur.

Frequent Urination

One of the first signs the young woman may notice to make her suspect she might be pregnant is the frequent desire to empty her bladder. This is caused by the pressure of the growing uterus against the bladder and will subside about the 2nd or the 3rd month, when the uterus expands upward into the abdominal cavity. Later, during the last weeks of pregnancy the symptoms will reoccur (see p. 122).

Nausea

Nausea and vomiting of mild degree, the so-called "morning sickness," constitute the most common disorder of the first trimester of pregnancy. For many years it has been thought that this condition has an emotional basis. In all life's encounters, there are probably few experiences which are at first more upsetting, mentally and emotionally, than the realization by a young woman that she is pregnant. At first there is the anxious uncertainty before she can be sure of the diagnosis. Then, there are numerous adjustments that have to be made and responsibilities that may seem to be overwhelming. Emotionally, the implications of pregnancy extend far back into her childhood, long before she met her husband. It is understandable that women who cannot adjust themselves to all these new circumstances could have problems. However, the whole cause of nausea and vomiting should not be attributed to the neurotic factor. Symptoms may be caused by physiologic changes of normal gestation.

Symptoms usually appear about the end of the 4th or 6th week and last until about the 12th week. Nausea occurs in about 50 per cent of all pregnancies; of these, about one third experience some vomiting. Usually, it occurs in the morning only, but a small percentage of patients may have nausea and vomiting throughout the entire day.

The typical picture of morning sickness starts with the patient's experiencing a feeling of nausea on arising in the morning. The mother is unable to retain her breakfast, but by noon she has completely recovered and has no further episodes until the next morning. This does not always occur in the morning but may happen in the afternoon or in the evening. In a small percentage of patients the nausea and the vomiting may persist throughout the day and even be worse in the afternoon. With the majority of patients this problem lasts from 1 to 3 weeks and then suddenly ceases. There may be a slight loss of body weight but no other signs or symptoms.

Treatment. Often this condition can be controlled, and frequently it may be greatly relieved. Various "before breakfast" remedies often are used. If a half hour before rising the patient takes a dry piece of toast or a cracker, relief may be obtained. In some instances sips of hot water (plain or with lemon juice), hot tea, clear coffee or hot milk have been tried, with successful results. However, the dry carbohydrate foods seem to be more effective. After taking any one of these "before breakfast"

remedies, the patient should remain in bed for about a half hour; then she should get up slowly and dress slowly (meanwhile sitting as much of the time as possible). After this she is usually ready for her breakfast.

Greasy foods, and those known to disagree with the patient, should be avoided in the diet. Other suggested remedies include eating an increased amount of carbohydrate foods during this period of disturbance or eating simple and light food 5 or 6 times a day instead of the 3 regular full meals. Unsweetened popcorn during the morning is sometimes advised. The patient may be helped by drinking sweet lemonade, about half of a lemon to a pint of water sweetened with milk sugar. Usually, after vomiting, the patient is quite thirsty, and it is not difficult for her to drink lemonade. Small amounts of ginger ale or Coca-Cola also are often most helpful.

This nausea and vomiting, if once established, are difficult to overcome, and so it is especially desirable to prevent the first attack, or at least to control this condition as soon as possible after it develops. It must be remembered that if the patient is unable to retain most of her food, her system is being depleted when the daily health should be maintained. Pregnancies may differ, and what may help one person may not benefit another. The trial-and-error method often is necessary to obtain results. If persistent vomiting develops, as it does with a small number of these patients, the condition is no longer considered to be a minor discomfort but then may develop into a serious complication. (See Chap. 18, Complications of Pregnancy.)

Heartburn

This is a neuromuscular phenomenon which may occur any time throughout gestation. As a result of the diminished gastric motility, which normally accompanies pregnancy, reverse peristaltic waves cause regurgitation of the stomach contents into the esophagus. It is this irritation of the esophageal mucosa which causes heartburn. It may be described as a burning discomfort diffusely localized behind the lower part of the sternum, often radiating upward along the course of the esophagus. Although referred to as heartburn, it really has nothing to do with the heart. Often it is associated with other gastrointestinal symptoms, of which acid regurgitation, belching, nausea and epigastric pressure are most troublesome. Nervous tension and emotional disturbances may be a precipitating cause. Worry, fatigue and improper diet may contribute to its intensity.

Little or no fat should be included in the diet. Although fatty foods are especially aggravating in this disturbance, strangely enough, the taking of some form of fat, such as a pat of butter or a tablespoon of cream, a short time before meals acts as a preventive, because fat inhibits the secretion of acid in the stomach. However, this will not help if the heartburn is already present.

Home remedies should not be used to relieve this condition. The physician usually will prescribe some alkaline preparation, because it gives the best results. However, *sodium bicarbonate should not be used*, because the sodium ion tends to promote water retention. It is important to make sure that the patient understands this point. Equally effective medications are aluminum compounds, such as aluminum hydroxide gel, or this medication in tablet form with magnesium trisilicate.

Flatulence

This is a somewhat common and very disagreeable discomfort. Usually it is due to undesirable bacterial action in the intestines, which results in the formation of gas. Eating only small amounts of food which are well masticated may prevent this feeling of distress after eating. Regular daily elimination is of prime importance, as is the avoidance of foods that form gas. Such foods as beans, parsnips, corn, sweet desserts, fried foods, cake and candy should be avoided. If these measures fail to relieve the condition, the physician should be consulted.

Constipation

This is not unusual during pregnancy. It is due largely to impaired peristaltic motion of the intestine caused by pressure from the gravid uterus. The patient should understand the importance of good bowel habits (see General Hygiene, p. 160), the influence of drinking adequate fluids and the appropriate diet in avoiding or alleviating this problem. Proper elimination cannot be emphasized too much, and daily regularity of habit aids in preventing constipation. In mild cases of constipation a diet of fruits, vegetables, dark breads and coarse foods, with several glasses of water daily, may relieve the condition.

Enemas, laxatives or cathartics should not be used unless prescribed by the physician. Some obstetricians advise milk of magnesia or cascara for their patients. Cascara is easier to take in the pill form, but it seems to be less effective; when the fluid extract is given, the size of the dose and the frequency of its administration must be determined according to the individual patient's reactions. When the proper dosage has been determined, this drug is generally very satisfactory. The salines are usually reserved for the cases in which they are distinctly indicated, such as certain types of toxemia.

Simple measures, combined with a largely farinaceous diet, are ordinarily all that is necessary, and the obstetrician should be consulted before even these are used.

Diarrhea

Occasionally this occurs during pregnancy, and its onset should be reported at once to the physician. Milk boiled for 2 minutes may be recommended by the nurse, and the patient may be advised to rest. If diarrhea is allowed to persist, it may result in an abortion, either because of severe straining efforts or because of an extension of the existing intestinal contractions. In the latter months of pregnancy, diarrhea may cause premature labor.

Backache

Most pregnant women experience some degree of backache. As pregnancy advances, the woman's posture changes to compensate for the weight of the growing uterus. The shoulders are thrown back as the enlarging abdomen protrudes, and, in order to maintain the body balance, the inward curve of the spine is exaggerated. The relaxation of the sacro-iliac joints, in addition to the postural change, causes varying degrees of backache following excessive strain, fatigue, bending or lifting. The mother should be advised early in pregnancy how to prevent such strain through measures such as good posture and body mechanics in everyday living and avoidance of fatigue. Appropriate shoes worn during periods of activity and a supporting girdle may be helpful (see Clothing, pp. 159 and 160, in General Hygiene).

A woman who has a pendulous abdomen, with a weak abdominal wall which allows the uterus to fall forward, will experience severe back pain, in addition to a "drawing sensation" in the abdomen and general discomfort in walking or standing. The physician will prescribe measures to be taken here or for any persistent complaint.

Dyspnea

Difficult breathing or shortness of breath occasionally results from pressure on the diaphragm by the enlarged uterus and may be sufficient in the last weeks of pregnancy to interfere considerably with the patient's sleep and general comfort. Usually it is not a serious condition, but unfortunately it cannot be wholly relieved until after "lightening" (p. 111) (the settling of the fetus into the pelvic cavity with relief of the upper abdominal pressure) or after the birth of the baby, when it will disappear spontaneously. It is most troublesome when the patient attempts to lie down, so that her comfort may be greatly enhanced by propping her well up in bed with pillows. In this semisitting posture she at least will sleep better and longer than with her head low. It is well for the nurse to demonstrate how these pillows may be arranged comfortably so that the patient's back is well supported.

In patients with known heart disease, shortness of breath, especially of rather sudden onset, may be a sign of oncoming heart failure and should be reported at once to the physician.

Varicose Veins

Varicose veins or varices may occur in the lower extremities and, at times, extend up as high as the external genitals or even into the pelvis itself. A varicosity is an enlargement in the diameter of a vein due to a thinning and stretching of its walls. Such distended areas may occur at short intervals along the course of the blood vessel; they give it a knotted ap-

pearance. Varicosities generally are associated with hereditary tendencies and are enhanced by advancing age, pregnancy and activities which require prolonged standing. During pregnancy the pressure in the pelvis due to the enlarged uterus, which presses on the great abdominal veins, interferes with the return of the blood from the lower limbs. Added to this, any debilitated condition of the patient favors the formation of varicosities in the veins because of the general flabbiness and lack of tone in the tissues.

Naturally, the greater the pressure in the abdomen, the greater will be the tendency to varicose veins of the legs and the vulva. Therefore, any occupation which keeps a patient constantly on her feet, particularly in the latter part of pregnancy, causes an increase in abdominal pressure and so acts as an exciting factor.

Symptoms. The first symptom of the development of varices is a dull, aching pain in the legs due to distention of the deep vessels, and inspection will show a fine purple network of superficial veins covering the skin in a lacelike pattern. Later, the true varicosities appear, usually first under the bend of the knee, in a tangled mass of bluish or purplish veins, often as large as a lead pencil. As the condition advances, the varicosities extend up and down the leg along the course of the vessels, and in severe cases they may affect the veins of the labia majora, the vagina and the uterus.

The treatment consists first and chiefly in the prompt abandonment, at the beginning of pregnancy, of round garters and all other articles of clothing that can cause pressure at any part of the body. If varicosities develop in spite of this precaution, the patient should be

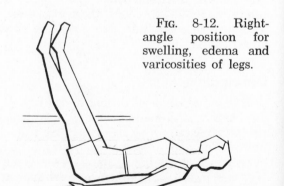

FIG. 8-12. Right-angle position for swelling, edema and varicosities of legs.

taught to take the right-angle position, that is, to lie on the bed with her legs extended straight into the air at right angles to her body, her buttocks and heels resting against the wall (Fig. 8-12). At first this position should be taken for 2 to 5 minutes several times a day, and that will soon demonstrate what can be accomplished. For some patients this position is very uncomfortable at first; but if it is explained, and the discomfort is therefore anticipated, the patient is less likely to discontinue the exercise. Late in pregnancy this position may be too difficult to assume because of pressure against the diaphragm.

In order to give support to the weak-walled veins, either an elastic stocking or elastic bandage often is recommended. The initial cost of elastic stockings is somewhat more than that of bandages, but they are easier to put on, more effective, have a neater appearance and a longer usefulness than bandages. A regular nylon stocking put on over the elastic hose further improves the appearance. Many hosiery companies are manufacturing "support" hose which do not have the strength of the elastic stockings but are very effective in giving a moderate amount of support. This type of stocking is useful in cases in which the vari-

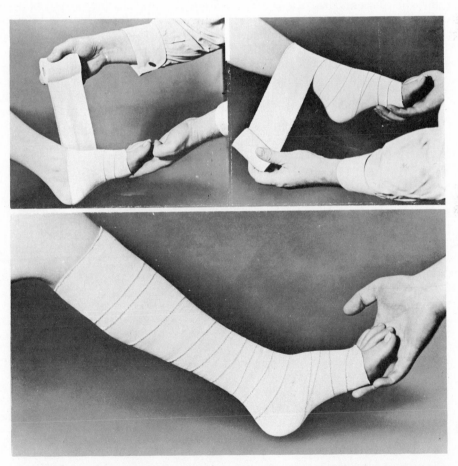

FIG. 8-13. (*Top*) The method of applying the Ace bandage for varicosities or edema of the legs, which are sometimes treated by the application of Ace rubber-elastic bandage (Becton, Dickinson and Company) and Elastoplast bandage (Duke Laboratories).

FIG. 8-14. (*Bottom*) The Elastoplast bandage is applied firmly, adjusting the stretch to produce the amount of compression desired, each turn overlapping to avoid gaps.

cosities are very mild or may not even be apparent peripherally, but may be suspected because of the ache they produce. Many women who must be on their feet a great deal, and do not have the opportunity to rest frequently, wear these stockings during working hours as a "prophylactic" measure. The nurse can be very helpful in apprising mothers of the varieties of hose now available and which will meet the needs of individual patients.

If bandages are used, they should be applied spirally with firm, even pressure, beginning at the foot and continuing up the leg above the varicosities (Figs. 8-13, 14). The nurse can demonstrate the technic of wrapping to the mother and let the patient practice in her presence; this will ensure that the mother understands and is able to wrap the bandages effectively. The patient also must be told that the stocking or the bandage should be removed at night for greater comfort and reapplied in the morning after the legs have been elevated so that the vessels will be less dilated. The longer stocking or bandage is more satisfactory when the varicosities are above the knee. Either the elastic stocking or bandage is washable; indeed, washing helps to maintain the original elasticity of these appliances. However, mild soap rather than detergent should be used.

Varicosities of the vulva may be relieved by placing a pillow under the buttocks and elevating the hips for frequent rest periods or by taking the elevated Sims's position for a few moments several times a day (Fig. 8-15). Patients suffering from this condition should not stand when they can sit, and they should not sit when they can lie down.

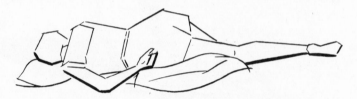

FIG. 8-15. Sims's position for varicosities of vulva and rectum.

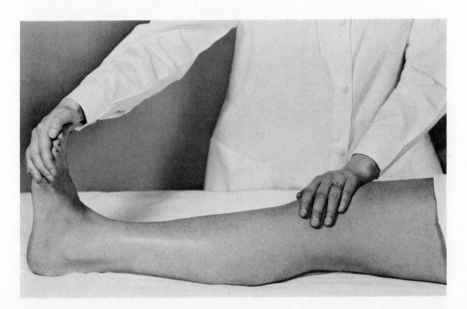

FIG. 8-16. The nurse helping the patient during a leg cramp, forcing the toes upward while making pressure on the knee to straighten the leg.

More important than the treatment of this condition is its prevention. Every pregnant woman should be advised to sit with her legs elevated whenever possible. And when the legs are elevated, care should be taken to see that there are no pressure points against the legs to interfere with the circulation, particularly in the popliteal space. Tight constricting garments, round garters, constipation, standing for long periods of time and an improper amount of rest, all tend to aggravate and also excite this condition.

A varicose vein in the vagina may rupture during the antepartal or intrapartal period, but this is rare. The hemorrhage is venous and can be controlled readily by pressure. The foot of the bed should be markedly elevated.

Hemorrhoids

Hemorrhoids, varicosities of the veins about the lower end of the rectum and the anus, may develop during the antepartal period and may cause rectal bleeding. On the other hand, they may become thrombosed or protrude through the anus. The little bumps and nodules seen in a mass of hemorrhoids are the distended portions of the affected vessels. Like varicosities in other areas, they are due to pressure interfering with return venous circulation and are aggravated by constipation. They often cause great distress to the pregnant patient and, due to pressure at the time of delivery, may cause great distress during the postpartal period.

The first step is the prevention and the treatment of constipation. The guidance that the nurse gives the mother in this respect cannot be stressed enough. In addition, when internal hemorrhoids protrude through the rectum, the mother can be instructed to replace them carefully by pushing them gently back into the rectum. Usually the patient can manage this quite well, after a thorough explanation and/or demonstration. She should lubricate her finger with petrolatum or mineral oil to aid ease of insertion and to avoid trauma to the veins. If the patient wishes, a finger cot can be used to cover her finger. Also taking either the knee-chest position (Fig. 14-25) or elevating her buttocks (Fig. 8-15) on a pillow facilitates replacement through gravity.

The application of an icebag, or cold compresses wet with witch hazel or Epsom salts solution, gives great relief. The physician may order tannic acid in suppositories, or compresses of witch hazel and glycerin. If the hemorrhoids are aggravated the first few days after labor, the same medications usually give relief. Surgery is seldom resorted to during pregnancy.

Cramps

Cramps are painful spasmodic muscular contractions in the legs. These cramps may occur at any time during the pregnancy but more generally during the later months due to pressure of the enlarged uterus on the nerves supplying the lower extremities. Other causes have been attributed to fatigue, chilling, tense body posture and insufficient calcium in the diet. A quart of milk in the daily diet has been generally recommended to meet the calcium needs during pregnancy. However, the studies of Page and Page can leave no doubt that large quantities of milk or dicalcium phosphate predispose to muscular tetany and leg cramps as the result of the excessive amount of phosphorus absorbed from these products (see Suggested Reading). Some authorities suggest that small quantities of aluminum hydroxide gel be taken with the quart of milk as it removes some of the dietary phosphorus from the intestinal tract. Immediate relief may be obtained by forcing the toes upward and by making pressure on the knee to straighten the leg (Fig. 8-16). Elevating the feet and keeping the extremities warm are preventives. Cramps, while not a serious condition, are excruciatingly painful for the duration of the seizure. If the husband has been taught the procedure for immediate relief, much pain will be prevented.

Edema

Swelling of the lower extremities is very common during pregnancy and is sometimes very uncomfortable. It is especially prone to occur in hot weather. Often it may be relieved by a proper abdominal support or by resting frequently during the day. Elevating the feet or taking the right-angle position often gives much relief (Fig. 8-12). If the swelling is persistent, the patient may have to stay in bed, but ordinarily this condition proves to be no more than a discomfort. However, edema is one of the symptoms of toxemia, and it must never be overlooked.

When edema of the lower extremities is observed, careful investigation should be made to see if other parts are affected—the hands or the face, etc. The condition should be reported to the physician at once.

Vaginal Discharge

In pregnancy there is increased vaginal secretion, so that a moderately profuse discharge at this time has no particular significance. However, such a condition always should be brought to the obstetrician's attention, for a profuse yellow discharge may be regarded as a possible evidence of gonorrhea (see Chap. 19), especially when it is accompanied by such urinary manifestations as burning and frequency of urination. A smear may be taken, and the microscopic result will indicate whether or not definite treatment is necessary. If any discharge becomes irritating, the patient may be advised to bathe the vulva with a solution of sodium bicarbonate or boric acid. The application of K.Y. jelly after bathing often relieves the condition entirely. Instructing a patient to wear a perineal pad is sometimes all the advice that is needed. A douche never should be taken unless the obstetrician orders it.

A particularly stubborn form of leukorrhea in pregnancy is caused by the parasitic protozoan known as the *Trichomonas vaginalis*. It is characterized not only by a profuse frothy discharge, white or yellowish in color, but also by irritation and itching of the vulva and the vagina. The diagnosis is easily made by the physician by taking a small quantity of the fresh secretion and putting it under the microscope in a hanging-drop. Here the spindle-shaped organisms, somewhat larger than leukocytes, with whiplike processes attached, can be seen in active motion.

One form of treatment used in this condition is the vinegar douche (3 tablespoons of vinegar in 2 quarts of water), followed by the insertion of 1 Floraquin tablet into the fornix of the vagina. It is imperative that the expectant mother be given specific instructions about douching in pregnancy (see Douches, p. 161, General Hygiene).

Moniliasis, a yeast infection caused by the *Candida albicans,* is another common cause of profuse vaginal discharge. The organism is frequently present in the vaginal canal without producing symptoms, but during pregnancy the physical changes in the vagina produce conditions that foster its development. It is characterized by white patches on the vaginal mucosa and a thick cottage-cheeselike discharge which is extremely irritating, so that burning or pruritus is present. Even the external genitalia often become inflamed, and occasionally extensive edema is observed. Bleeding may accompany the other symptoms if the patches on the mucosa are removed in any way.

It is not necessary to treat patients in whom *Monilia* are found if signs and symptoms are not present. One of the most dependable drugs used to treat this condition is aqueous solution of gentian violet, 1 per cent. Commercial preparations of gentian violet in the form of a gel are available for the patient to use. Although this treatment is effective, the infection is stubborn and likely to recur and require repeated treatment during the pregnancy. When this medication is used, the patient should be advised to wear a perineal pad, because the dye stains clothing permanently. The *pruritus*, or itching of the skin, may be relieved to a marked degree if proper hygienic measures are employed to keep the area free of the irritating material being deposited on the skin surface. The mother who has a monilial infection may transmit it to her infant during the process of delivery. *Thrush* develops when the organisms attack the mucous membrane of the mouth.

PREPARATION FOR PARENTHOOD

Childbirth in modern society reflects the progress brought about by cultural influences, social change, technologic advances and, above all, the progress of medicine. The concept of family-centered care which prevails in all health services today could have no more appropriate application than that to the beginning of a new life in the family unit. Having children is no longer the mother's responsibility alone; it is a joint undertaking of both parents. From the moment of conception, when the baby begins his existence, the husband is encouraged to begin to assume his responsibility as a father. A helpful, understanding and sympathetic husband can do much to make the pregnancy an experience that will contribute to the foundation of a more enriched family life.

Preparation for parenthood actually begins with the mother's own birth or earlier, as was stated in the beginning of this chapter, and its development is influenced by an accumulation of her experiences through infancy, childhood, adolescence and maturity. The father's feelings and attitudes are influenced in like manner by his previous experiences. The addition of courses in sex education and marriage and family living to the high school and the college curricula has had a positive effect on the attitudes of young people. In recent years much has been accomplished also through premarital and prepregnancy examinations and counseling.

The emphasis placed on the education of parents for childbirth has stimulated them to attend antepartal classes, which, in part, have helped further to dispel misunderstandings or lack of knowledge and to increase the understanding of childbirth as a normal physiologic body process. This is not an entirely new approach. In Manchester during the 18th century Dr. Charles White wrote a book that concerns instructions for the supervision of mothers during pregnancy and how to help them in labor and make them comfortable. In our own country the antepartal care programs have influenced the formation of preparation classes which have contributed toward good antepartal care.

Classes

Today there are definite courses offered for mothers and fathers in preparation for childbearing. These classes are included as a part of the programs of the Visiting Nurse Associations, Red Cross Chapters, many State Departments of Health, hospitals and private organizations such as the Maternity Center Association in New York City. Some of these classes are given for expectant mothers or fathers alone; in others the parents attend classes together. In the latter group the classes aid the parents in their mutual appreciation of the value of antepartal preparation and tend to promote the idea of sharing parenthood. The goals set for the parents in any of these classes are similar, namely, to gain increased knowledge about childbearing and increased understanding of ways to promote and to maintain optimum health through the practice of good health habits in daily living.

Several disciplines may be represented in teaching any one group of classes, so that those who teach may be nurses, obstetricians, pediatricians, nutritionists, health educators and, in some courses which include exercise classes, physical therapists. Material related to the physiology of pregnancy and labor, general hygiene and the care of the mother during pregnancy, labor and the puerperium is included, as well as that related to the baby. All of the class content is approved by a medical council or advisory board, but the details of the classes usually are worked out by nurses to suit the conditions under which the courses are conducted.

The classes are attended by individuals from various social, cultural and economic groups, each with his or her own needs and desires. Those who teach must use care to be realistic about their teaching and never forget that although the teacher has set up objectives for the students (in this case, the parents), she must help the parents to attain the goals that they have set up for themselves. For instance, a mother who has the satisfaction of appetite as her goal for family nutrition considers that if her family is not hungry, they are well fed. This goal may astound the nutritionist or the nurse who sees the importance of planning well-balanced meals. In this instance the job of health teaching requires the application of sound educational principles in order not to destroy the mother's goal with one fell swoop. The nurse's teaching can be most effective if she first identifies their common goals, and then, gradually, as she teaches, begins to change the mother's objective without undermining her security.

Conventional Type of Program

This is the most widely used program in this country. It is planned to serve everyone in the community and places its emphasis on a general type of "education for childbirth." The course usually includes the physiology of childbearing, general hygiene, including nutrition, during pregnancy and lactation, preparations for the baby, and the care of the mother and her baby after the delivery. In this type of program a multidisciplinary approach may be used in the teaching, or the nurse may be responsible for giving all of the content.

The material may be covered in a variety of ways: a lecture-type format may be employed, with time allowed for questions and discussion, or a semistructured approach may be used (i.e., no set curriculum is prepared in advance). Group discussion is developed from the contributions of the members. The leader is responsible for guiding the discussion and for opening essential areas not probed by the group members. The group situation demands that the nurse develop a new concept of herself as a leader, and that she acquire new skills. She must have a knowledge and an understanding of what material is relevant, so that she can draw on it as the group needs it; hence she must be totally prepared each time that the group meets, since the discussion may range from nutrition to the physiology of labor. In addition, she also must be skilled in communication technics, in the ability to listen, to probe and to reflect, so that she can help the group to elaborate or to expand on germane comments and statements. She must recognize the importance and the implication of "iceberg questions" (e.g., "How common is going crazy after having a baby?") knowing that such questions may indicate an underlying concern of the questioner. In such instances she should be able to explore and to sift alternatives until the real question can be asked, and appropriate action may be taken. In this instance the patient really was not concerned with how often people became psychotic after childbirth, but rather she wanted to know whether she was likely to experience this malady. Because of a history of mental illness in her family and her own extreme emotional lability during this pregnancy, she was afraid that she might become psychotic after delivery.*

Whatever the approach, the nurse who participates in parent classes is in a favorable position to help her patients and families to develop a better understanding of their immediate situation, together with a balanced view of the physiology of pregnancy and parturi-

* For a more thorough discussion of the group approach to antepartal management see Suggested Reading.

tion, growth and development, and the psychological and emotional aspects of family life.

Natural Childbirth

Childbirth as a normal or natural process has received increasing emphasis during the past decade. The reader will develop more understanding of this broad concept of maternity care from the writings of Read, Thoms and Goodrich (see Suggested Reading).

The interpretation of "labor" as "pain" has been held by women from time immemorial, with the result that today many women still approach childbirth in dread of an ordeal. Much of the misunderstanding, fear and apprehension can be overcome by understanding gained from education. This is no simple way to a painless or easy childbirth, but a means to enable a woman to gain more self-understanding, to help herself in labor and to increase her self-confidence.

Increasing emphasis has been placed on the fact that there is an "emotional labor" which is as definite and important as its physical counterpart. There can be no doubt that the attitude of a woman toward her confinement has a considerable influence on the ease of her labor. This fact was stressed for many years by the British obstetrician, the late Dr. Grantly Dick Read, and has been endorsed by various groups in this country, notably the Maternity Center Association of New York and by Drs. Thoms and Goodrich of New Haven and others. Dr. Read emphasized certain psychological aspects of labor—that "fear is in some way the chief pain-producing agent in otherwise normal labor." The neuromuscular mechanism by which fear exerts a deleterious effect on labor is obscure, but the general validity of Read's contention is in keeping with common clinical knowledge. The mother builds up a state of tensions because she is frightened, and these tensions create an antagonistic effect on the muscular activity of normal labor, with resulting pain. The pain causes more fear, which further increases the tensions, and so on, until a vicious circle is established.

Rather unfortunately, certain overzealous people have inferred that a spontaneous delivery, to be psychologically rewarding, *must* be accomplished entirely without medication of any kind. Furthermore, they have implied that if medication was either requested or required, the parturient somehow had "failed" to accomplish delivery by the natural childbirth method. Thus, the connotation of "painless childbirth" also was injected here, an interpretation that is not accurate.

The family-centered approach to maternity care, which is a fundamental part of the natural-childbirth program, is not basically different from that practiced when deliveries were conducted at home with the father present. But changes are apparent. The current trend to have babies born in the hospital has the advantage of increased safety provided by improved medical technics and modern obstetric practice. For so long women approached childbearing without any real understanding of what to expect or, for that matter, without much knowledge of the anatomy and the physiology of their reproductive organs. The majority of husbands were included insofar as they were present in the household, but they were not actually made to feel that they were really participating in the event. The natural-childbirth program provides an opportunity to help both parents gain more knowledge and the satisfaction of mutual participation.

The program of education during pregnancy is designed to eliminate fear. Facts which concern the anatomy and the physiology of childbearing and the appropriate care of the mother are taught. The mother not only learns how labor progresses but also is helped to gain an understanding of the sensations likely to accompany labor and methods of working cooperatively with them. The exercises which are included are designed for the muscles which will be used in labor, as well as those which will promote the general well-being of the body. In the performance of any skill the individual is more efficient if the muscles involved are in the best condition. The exercises are not strenuous and, for the most part, are ones that will contribute to improved posture, body balance, agility and increased strength and endurance. The mother learns breathing technics that will aid her ability to relax in the first stage of labor, and technics that will help her to work effectively with muscles used in the delivery. To enable the parents to meet better the needs of their baby after he is born, information about his growth and development also is included in these classes.

An important consideration throughout the program is "to help the mother help herself," so that her pregnancy will be a healthy, happy experience, and at the time of labor she will be better able to participate actively in having her baby. In former days when mothers often were given heavy sedation, they were unable to have this satisfying experience.

The encouragement and the support of those about her are particularly important to the expectant mother, especially during labor. Every modern obstetric aid for the mother's safety and comfort is at her disposal. It should be emphasized that the proponents of natural childbirth have never claimed that labor should be conducted without anesthetic aids, or that it can be made devoid of pain (Thoms). The response to pain is individual, and if the mother and/or the physician decides that some assistance in the form of medication is necessary, it is readily available. It would be rather incongruous to suggest that any program would reject medical advances which have made such important contributions to obstetrics. However, many mothers who are "prepared" for natural childbirth often are reluctant to accept any form of medication, feeling that it is rather a personal blow to their integrity. In such a case the mother needs help to understand that this will not detract from her experience, but rather will enhance it. She may need help to remember that the physician is the one person capable of making the final decision as to what is best for her and her baby. The use of medication should not be a criterion in the consideration of "how well the mother did" during labor and delivery. The real measure of success can be determined only by the satisfactions which the mother derives from being able to cooperate with the natural processes of labor to the best of her ability. The new infant is really the important entity and, after he is born, should be the mother's chief concern, not an elaboration of her physical feats.

In summary, satisfactory results in connection with natural childbirth are aided by such factors as attaining good physical health and emotional stability; learning about the baby's development during the antepartal period; understanding the muscular processes that take place during labor and delivery; preparing for labor by attending classes where supervised exercises are practiced and perfected; having empathic understanding and "support" during labor; planning for the postpartal period, the physical and the emotional adjustment of the mother, and the care of the new baby; and the integration of the father into the events of pregnancy and parturition.

Psychoprophylactic Childbirth

Psychoprophylactic preparation for childbirth is a somewhat less permissive version of natural childbirth. The Lamaze method often is cited as an example of this technic. The rationale of the program is based on Pavlov's concept of pain perception and his theory of conditioned reflexes, i.e., the substitution of favorable conditioned reflexes for unfavorable ones. For example, most women have been conditioned since childhood to associate pain with certain functions of the reproductive organs, such as with menstruation and child-bearing. To disprove such beliefs, repeated emphasis is placed on the fact that normal contractions of the uterus need not be any more painful than those of other organs of the body, such as the bladder or the bowel. The teaching in this program consists of combating the fears associated with pregnancy and childbirth by instructing the pregnant woman about the anatomy and the neuromuscular activity of the reproductive system and the mechanism of labor. Nutrition and general hygiene are included during the course. Simple exercises which strengthen the abdominal muscles and relax the perineum are taught, and proper breathing technics to help the process of labor are practiced. These breathing technics differ from the ones taught in the natural-childbirth classes; there is emphasis on rapid, shallow respiration of great intensity and concentration rather than on the slow, deep abdominal type utilized in classes in the so-called natural-childbirth technics.*

The core of this program is the abolition of fear through knowledge, preparation for labor by education and exercise, and peace of mind during labor through cheerful skilled attendance and the creation of a familylike environment.

The psychoprophylactic method and natural childbirth without fear, as practiced by Read or by Thoms, have, in fact, the following 3

points in common: (1) Fear enhances the perception of pain but may diminish or disappear when the parturient knows about the physiology of labor. (2) Psychic tension enhances the perception of pain, but the parturient may relax more easily if childbirth takes place in a calm and agreeable atmosphere, and if good human contacts have been established between her and the nursing personnel. (3) Muscular relaxation and a specific type of breathing diminish or abolish the pains of labor.[2]

Psychoprophylactic-childbirth programs have not been introduced widely into this country but are used more in Russia, parts of China and in various sections of Europe.

PSYCHOPHYSICAL PREPARATION FOR CHILDBEARING

Psychophysical preparation for childbearing is a term applied to concepts and methods of antepartal education used in natural childbirth, psychoprophylaxis and various forms of hypnosis. This last technic is an induced state of extreme suggestibility in which the patient is insensible to all outside impressions except the suggestions of her attendant. In spite of theoretical differences, all have practices in common. Psychophysical preparation aims at helping a mother to manage her body well in activity and rest, to use her natural forces effectively during labor, and to achieve optimal postpartum restoration. Physical methods are only one aspect of preparation and should be correlated with the total program of education and antepartal care. It is important to remember that this method, as well as the others, is not a substitute for pharmaceutical analgesics. However, it often lessens the need for chemical pain relief and sedation during labor and reinforces their effects. Whenever indicated, medication should be given and accepted early enough to enable the mother to stay in control of herself and to achieve the goal of conscious participation, if at all possible.

The authors are indebted to Miss Hazel Corbin, the former General Director of the Maternity Center Association of New York

* For a more thorough description of the breathing technics see Suggested Reading.

[2] de Watteville, P. H.: The use of obstetrical analgesia at the maternity hospital of Geneva, Am. J. Obstet. Gynec. 73:473, 1957.

City, and to Miss Vera Keane, the General Director of the Association, who graciously have permitted us to include here the instructions and the exercises taught by the Association in its course on preparation for childbearing.[3]

Maternity Center chose these particular positions and movements because these exercises achieve their objectives simply, without fatigue, and impose no undesirable strains or pressures. They are intended to promote control of muscle tension for skillful coordination and economy of effort in all the mother's activities, including the management of her body during labor. A mother who has acquired these skills is better able to maintain self-control and to respond to the guidance of her professional attendants.

It goes without saying that the nurse who is responsible for teaching the exercises or assisting a mother at the time of labor must develop her own perception of body position and motion before she can impart "body awareness" to others. In addition, her observations of the effectiveness of what she teaches, in daily living and during labor, can serve as a continuing guideline for the development of the educational program.

To clarify the aims of preparation, the instruction is divided into three sections: avoidance of stress; specific neuromuscular control in preparation for labor; and postpartum restoration. In practice, no arbitrary division is feasible, since many of the same principles apply to all three areas. Considerable flexibility is possible in the sequence, but the section on avoidance of stress should be covered early (before the 6th month of gestation) to promote the formation of desirable habits and to prevent the development of postural faults. The following is a summarization of the focus of instruction and includes some of the various exercises that are illustrative of the psychophysical method of approach.

Avoidance of Stress

Certain positions and movements are aimed

[3] Psychophysical Preparation for Childbearing: Guidelines for Teaching, ed. 2, New York, Maternity Center Association, 1965. Material on this subject as presented on pages 175 to 184 is either a condensation or a direct quotation from this source.

primarily to help the expectant mother to adapt her posture to changes in weight, the shift in the center of gravity and the increased pressure from these changes. Most mothers-to-be need to learn how to make rest periods truly restful and to achieve balanced rest and activity periods in the course of daily living.

General Relaxation. For relaxation to be complete, the environment should be quiet and comfortable; outside stimuli should be kept at a minimum. Clothing should be loosened, and the limbs should be supported with slight flexion of the joints, including the trunk.

A supine position is one of the most useful to promote relaxation. The hips and the knees should be flexed slightly to allow relaxation of the abdominal wall; this is particularly important as pregnancy advances. Pillows can be arranged which provide support for a large area of leg surface without putting pressure on the popliteal space. A side position with the knees slightly flexed or the prone position with one hip and knee flexed to remove pressure from the abdomen can be assumed alternately. In rising from the supine position, the mother first should bend her knees and roll to the side position; then she can help herself to a sitting position by using her upper hand and arm. All such movements should be done slowly, as dizziness can occur if the position is changed too quickly, especially from reclining to the erect position.

Relaxation may be accomplished also while the patient is sitting in an armchair as long as the entire body is well aligned. Small pillows may be used to support the back and/or the head, and the feet should be supported on a footstool if they do not rest flat on the floor. It is helpful if the knees are separated to avoid compressing the enlarging abdomen. The mother also may sit leaning forward, with her arms, head and upper chest supported on a rest surface, e.g., a table or a desk. The surface should be high enough so that the shoulders are comfortable, and the neck relaxed. This position is especially important for working mothers who do not have the opportunity to lie down frequently. In later pregnancy and early labor this position often is more comfortable than lying down.

In helping the mother to practice her breathing and relaxation technics, it is wise for the nurse to establish a cue or signal with her. In tension the breath often is held, and exhaling is associated with relaxation; thus a signal for relaxation might be: *"Breathe in, relax as you breathe out."* This "breathe in, breathe out" cue can be coupled with any of the neuromuscular exercises that are used in labor.

Activity. The mother can maintain her usual work and play activities; however, they should be varied (walking, standing, sitting, etc.), and they should be of shorter duration. Since the major postural changes begin in the second trimester of pregnancy, this is the logical learning time. Body balance is adapted gradually in relationship to the increasing weight and the change in weight distribution. The spinal muscles and joints should be protected from undue strain, and the mother must learn to use her feet efficiently for balance and movement. It is wise for the pregnant woman to stand as little as possible, particularly if it entails prolonged standing in one position. When she stands, her shoulders should be carried back easily, with the chest lifted; her pelvis should be balanced so that the baby is supported in the pelvic girdle; her knees should be straight but not braced.

Exercises. The following exercise is useful in helping the mother *to check for posture.* Standing with her feet about 10 inches from a doorjamb or a flat wall, with the bottom of her spine against the wall, she bends loosely forward from the hips. Then she "uncurls" to assume an erect position until her head reaches as high as it will go, and as she does this, she flattens the lumbar curve to try to make the entire spine touch the wall. This is done 3 times a day until the mother has the feel of an elongated spine.

Another helpful relaxing exercise is that of *pelvic rocking* (Fig. 8-17). It relieves the postural stress and backache resulting from maintaining one position for too long. Pelvic rocking may be done standing, sitting or lying down. To practice, the mother kneels on all fours with her arms and thighs at right angles to her body, and her weight equalized between hands and knees. In this position she tilts the front of the pelvis upward, using the abdominal and the gluteal muscles, and then she relaxes them, allowing the pelvis to drop. There should be no active thrust of the pelvis either upward or downward. This exercise can be done 5 or 6 times a day. When it is combined with proper breathing (*breathe out* as the front of the pelvis is rocked up; *breathe in* as the pelvis is relaxed and dropped), it can be useful for alleviating backache.

Certain principles are applicable to activities in everyday living. For instance, prolonged standing should be avoided, or, if done, it should be done as previously described. Walking back and forth is preferable to standing still. When the mother does housework that requires standing, she should keep one leg forward so that she can shift her weight easily and efficiently from foot to foot (if she is right-handed, she should keep the left leg forward).

As she walks, she should keep her back upright and her chin up and forward.

When she climbs stairs, she should use her "back" foot, which is on the lower step, to

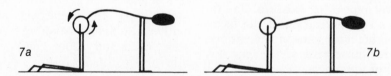

Fig. 8-17. Pelvic rocking. The exercise may be done standing, sitting or lying down. (*Left*) Kneeling on all fours, with arms and thighs at right angles to body and weight evenly distributed between hands and knees, tilt front of pelvis upward, tightening abdominal and gluteal muscles. (Right) Relax abdominal and gluteal muscles; no active downward thrust of pelvis. Avoid hyperextension of lumbar spine. (Psychophysical Preparation for Childbearing: Guidelines for Teaching, ed. 2, p. 24, Fig. 7, New York, Maternity Center Association, 1965)

push off with and plant her front foot firmly on the step, maintaining adequate balance at all times.

Whenever possible, the mother should avoid stooping and lifting. When she must stoop, she should squat, keeping the back straight and the hips flexed. "Use the legs to spare the back" is a good axiom to remember. To reach something in front of her, she squats with her feet level; to reach things to the side, she squats sideways with one leg in front of the other. The legs always should be far enough apart to avoid pressure on the lower abdomen. If lifting is necessary, and the object is at floor level, the mother should squat close to the object, hold it close to her, and use her legs to take the strain as she rises. To lift an object from the side, she advances the leg on the opposite side, squats, holds the object close and rises. Whenever a youngster needs to be lifted, often she can guide him, while he climbs up under his own power, by standing behind him and supporting him with her hands. In carrying, the load should be divided and carried in two hands if it is heavy enough to tilt the shoulders forward. When possible, a cart with wheels that rolls easily should be employed to carry heavy loads.

A good chair, i.e., one that gives proper support, is required for sitting comfortably. Sitting properly, with the knees and the hips flexed, the feet should rest on the floor. The back and the thighs should be supported adequately, and if the chair has arms, they should be at a height to hold the mother's arms without exerting tension on her shoulders. As the mother prepares to sit, she stands in front of the chair with one foot forward and the back of the other leg touching the chair's edge. To sit, she bends her knees and lowers her body slowly, using her leg muscles; her trunk is inclined forward, her back is straight, and her abdominal and gluteal muscles are contracted. She may sit straight in the chair with her feet flat on the floor, or she may want her legs elevated and supported. To rise, she puts one foot slightly ahead of the other and slides her buttocks to the edge of the chair; then she pushes off with her back foot, using her legs to rise. When she is traveling by car, the mother can prevent or alleviate backache by flexing one knee more than the other. On very long trips she should be encouraged to stop and walk every hour. Seat belts, correctly adjusted, should be used.

One final word should be mentioned about the height of work surfaces. These may have to be adjusted for the individual mother to minimize stooping and stretching; e.g., racks may have to be placed in the sink or on tables to heighten the work surface, handles on carts or movable tables may have to be lengthened or shortened, etc. A step stool is an invaluable aid for sitting as well as for reaching high cupboards, etc. An adequate work space is necessary for bathing and changing the baby, and for maximum comfort and efficiency, the work space should be about at the level of the head of the mother's femur.

Relief of Common Minor Discomforts. Certain minor discomforts often accompany pregnancy. Many are temporary, resulting from pressures that can be relieved. As previously mentioned, any persistent complaint, no matter how seemingly trivial, should be reported to the doctor. The following suggestions are helpful in alleviating some of the temporary discomforts.

Backache is one of the more common complaints and often is associated with posture. A modified kneeling position frequently is helpful in relieving the pelvic pressure that gives rise to this condition. (The position also helps to relieve the pain of hemorrhoids and referred pain along the sciatic nerve.) In this position the buttocks and the head should be in a straight line with the back so that there is no exaggeration of the lumbar curve, and the knees are separated to avoid compressing the abdomen. The position can be assumed several times a day but should be maintained only for 1 or 2 minutes, or less if it causes discomfort.

Upper backache, often associated with tingling or numbness in the fingers, can be relieved by improving the posture of the head and the shoulders. Care should be exercised that the breasts are properly supported with an uplift brassière, one with wide nonconstricting straps (see p. 159). Any sustained activities involving sitting and use of the arms should be avoided. Rotating the shoulders upward and backward with the hands placed on the shoulders is useful in improving circulation and strengthening the muscles of the shoulder girdle.

Varicose veins and leg cramps already have been discussed under the section on Minor Discomforts.

Some patients complain of pressure on the rib cage; again, correct posture usually rectifies this. Raising the arm on the affected side and bending to the unaffected side usually brings additional relief.

Sometimes a "stitch" sensation occurs in the lower abdomen. If it is found to be of no medical significance, the mother may obtain relief by lying on the affected side with the knee on the affected side drawn up and the head bent toward the knee. If it occurs when she cannot lie down, then she may squat, with the unaffected leg forward, and bend to the affected side, as though tying her shoe.

Neuromuscular Control

The following exercises can be learned easily with approximately 20 minutes of practice per day. They are focused toward helping the mother to maintain control and to manage her body comfortably and efficiently during labor. They also promote muscle tone, which is helpful in expediting postpartal restoration. It is important that these exercises are learned well, since the mother will not be able to have actual experience before labor. When the threat of labor makes concentration and manipulation of her body difficult, she must be able to call on these technics automatically.

Control of Trunk Muscles and Pelvic Floor. Figures 8-18 and 19 illustrate control of the

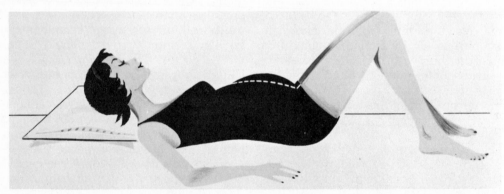

FIG. 8-18. Control of anterior abdominal muscles. Lying on back with knees bent and feet flat on bed or floor, breathe in, relaxing abdominal wall; breathe out, retracting abdominal wall as much as possible without discomfort. (Psychophysical Preparation for Childbearing: Guidelines for Teaching, ed. 2, p. 31, Fig. 23, New York Maternity Center Association, 1965)

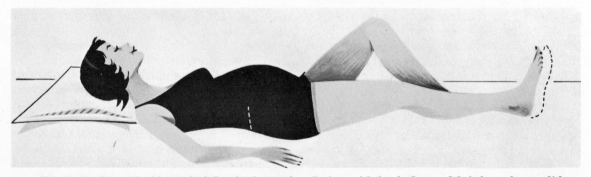

FIG. 8-19. Control of lateral abdominal muscles. Lying with back flat and left knee bent, slide right heel down; then pull it up as far as possible. Do not bend right knee or raise buttocks. Relax; alternate. (Psychophysical Preparation for Childbearing: Guidelines for Teaching, ed. 2, p. 31, Fig. 24, New York, Maternity Center Association, 1965)

abdominal muscles. To control the anterior abdominals the mother lies on her back with her knees bent and her feet flat on the floor; she breathes in, relaxing the abdominal wall, and she breathes out, retracting the wall. This is repeated 6 times (or less); the mother should retract her abdominal wall as much as is possible *without* discomfort. She can place her hand on her lower abdomen to be sure that she is tightening the lower abdominal muscles without elevating the rib cage. To control the lateral abdominals she lies with the back flat and the left knee bent, and slides the right heel down and then back up as far as possible. She should not bend her right knee or raise her buttocks. She relaxes, and then alternates legs.

Figure 8-20 illustrates the arrangements of the muscles of the pelvic floor. A concentric pull (A) is necessary to close the anus, and a forward pull (B), combined with a lateral squeeze (C), is necessary to tighten the vagina and the urethra. The ability to control these muscles is very important if the mother is to cooperate comfortably during rectal and vaginal examinations, help during the second stage of labor and regain muscle tone postpartally.

To learn control of the anal sphincter the mother lies on her side, contracts the sphincter as if controlling a bowel movement, but does not contract the buttocks. She follows this with relaxation. The mother may check her performance by placing her finger over the anus.

After controlled relaxation of the anal

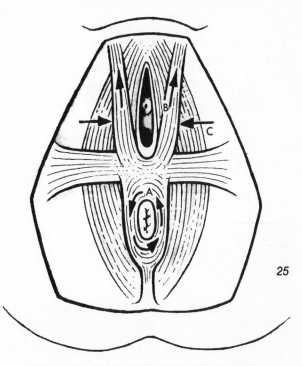

FIG. 8-20. Control of pelvic floor muscles. Concentric pull to close anus (A). Forward pull (B) must be combined with lateral squeeze (C) to tighten vagina and close urethra. (Psychophysical Preparation for Childbearing: Guidelines for Teaching, ed. 2, p. 32, Fig. 25, New York, Maternity Center Association, 1965)

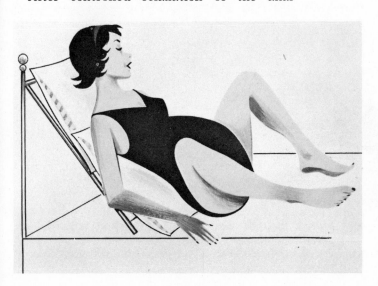

FIG. 8-21. Practice position for delivery table. Tense pelvic floor and inner thigh muscles; then relax them, allowing knees gradually to drop apart. Stay in this relaxed position for a few minutes. (Psychophysical Preparation for Childbearing: Guidelines for Teaching, ed. 2, p. 33, Fig. 27, New York, Maternity Center Association, 1965)

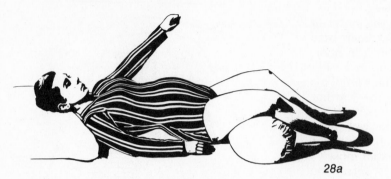

28a

FIG. 8-22. Relaxation of rest of body during uterine contraction; for example, contracting the arm. (Psychophysical Preparation for Childbearing: Guidelines for Teaching, ed. 2, p. 34, Fig. 28a, New York, Maternity Center Association, 1965)

sphincter is achieved, the mother can learn control of the vaginal sphincter. Here she contracts the sphincter as if to control urination without contracting the inner thigh muscles. To practice, she can start and stop in the flow of urine once or twice as she urinates. The third step involves lifting the entire pelvic floor; a contraction is started at the back fibers and is continued through to the front, held for a second and relaxed. This movement is a great help in relieving the sense of pressure in the pelvic area that many women experience and should be practiced several times during the day.

The delivery position is fatiguing if no previous preparation has been done. If the mother-to-be occasionally assumes this position, as illustrated in Figure 8-21, she can possibly alleviate some of the fatigue that otherwise results from the delivery position in the second stage of labor. In this position she

tenses the pelvic floor and inner thigh muscles and then relaxes them, allowing her knees gradually to drop apart and remaining relaxed for several minutes. During practice periods the husband may provide resistance to the outward rotation of the legs with gentle pressure on the outside of the knees. This encourages relaxation of the adductors and inward rotators and facilitates wide separation of the mother's legs.

Selective Relaxation. The emphasis in this section is to help the mother to disassociate the rest of her body from the uterine activity. As she learns relaxation technics during pregnancy, the expectant mother practices contracting the muscles of her arms and legs merely to simulate a uterine contraction; during labor, however, she needs to understand that she must consciously relax the rest of her body while her uterus is contracting.

Relaxation of Rest of Body During Uterine

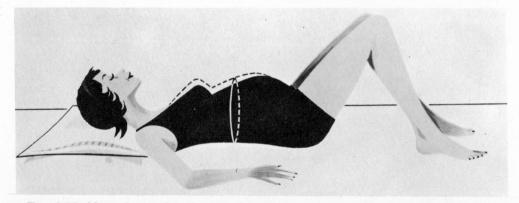

FIG. 8-23. Normal complete breath. Breathe in. Note how abdominal wall rises as diaphragm descends and chest wall rises and expands. Breathe out. Movements of diaphragm and chest wall are in opposite directions. (Psychophysical Preparation for Childbearing: Guidelines for Teaching, ed. 2, p. 35, Fig. 29, New York, Maternity Center Association, 1965)

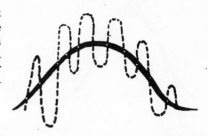

FIG. 8-24. Application of slow deep breathing to labor. At start of contraction, breathe in, relax as you breathe out; then breathe slowly and deeply throughout contraction, maintaining an even rhythm. At end of contraction, resume normal quiet breathing. (Psychophysical Preparation for Childbearing: Guidelines for Teaching, ed. 2, p. 36, Fig. 30, New York, Maternity Center Association, 1965)

Contraction. This can be learned after the mother is able to achieve complete relaxation quickly on the signal, "Breathe in, relax as you breathe out" (see p. 176). Figure 8-22 illustrates the position that is useful for learning this technic. The mother begins by breathing in and contracting her left arm; then she breathes out and relaxes her entire body except her left arm. Following rest she then repeats with the right arm. As each step is mastered, this exercise can be gradually advanced so that there is a progression from the arms to the legs, to the arm and the leg on one side of the body, and so on. The exercise should be repeated 3 times daily for each combination, and sufficient relaxation periods between each combination should be allowed.

Control of Respiration. Although there is rather general agreement that conscious control of respiration during the first stage of labor gives the mother a calming rhythmic activity on which to concentrate, there is no definitive proof pro or con for theories of the mechanical relief of pressure by depression of the diaphragm to expand the abdominal wall (abdominal breathing) or by limiting the downward movement of the diaphragm through restriction of breathing to the upper chest (shallow breathing). Since everyone has a natural breathing pattern, it is more expeditious to adapt the control of respiration to the person's natural pattern than to impose a new pattern. Figure 8-23 illustrates the movements of the chest wall and the diaphragm during a normal complete breath. The mother breathes in through her nose and out through her mouth. She should do this 5 or 6 times during the day, preferably in the fresh air to ensure complete aeration of the entire lung.

Application of Slow Deep Breathing to Labor. Figure 8-24 shows a slow deep breath applied during a contraction. At the beginning of the contraction the mother breathes in and relaxes as she breathes out; then she breathes slowly and deeply throughout the contraction, keeping an even rhythm. At the end of the contraction she resumes regular breathing. This type of breathing is the most

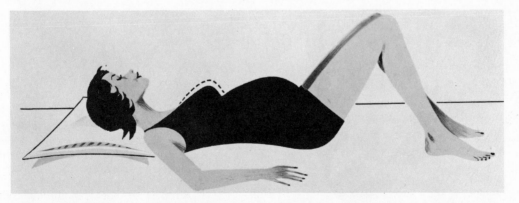

FIG. 8-25. Shallow breathing. Lips relaxed and barely parted. The breathing is very light and shallow: only the upper chest moves. Care must be taken that inhalation and exhalation remain equal, and that the respiratory rate is individually comfortable. (Psychophysical Preparation for Childbearing: Guidelines for Teaching, ed. 2, p. 36, Fig. 31, New York, Maternity Center Association, 1965)

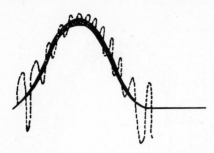

Fig. 8-26. Application of shallow breathing to labor (accelerated breathing). Start slow deep breathing: breathe in; relax as you breathe out. Gradually decrease depth so that shallow breathing is done over peak of contraction. Gradually resume deeper pattern as contraction wanes. (Psychophysical Preparation for Childbearing: Guidelines for Teaching, ed. 2, p. 37, Fig. 32, New York, Maternity Center Association, 1965)

Fig. 8-27. Further adaptation of shallow breathing to transition breathing. Start off as for shallow (accelerated) breathing (see previous Fig.). At the urge to hold breath and bear down, blow out lightly through parted lips, without contracting abdomen, and maintain this pattern until urge to push disappears. (Psychophysical Preparation for Childbearing: Guidelines for Teaching, ed. 2, p. 37, Fig. 33, New York, Maternity Center Association, 1965)

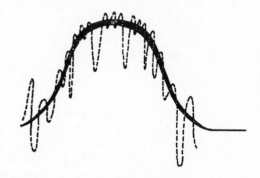

comfortable for women in early labor and can be done in any position. If backache is present, it can be combined with gentle pelvic rocking (Figs. 8-17, 20). To relate this type of breathing more realistically to labor, the mother can tighten the muscles of her arm to simulate a contraction and then correlate her controlled breathing with the increased tension of the contracting muscles.

Shallow Breathing. Here the lips are relaxed and barely parted; the breathing is very light and shallow, and only the upper chest moves. Inhalation and exhalation should be equal, and the *rate should be comfortable* for

the mother, neither too rapid nor too slow. This exercise is basic to learning the accelerated breathing used later in the first stage. The mother should maintain the desired depth and the rhythm of the respiration for at least 30 seconds, although at first she probably will be able to manage only 15 to 20 seconds. Figure 8-25 shows one of the resting positions for practice and the movement of the chest wall.

Application of Shallow Breathing to Labor (Accelerated Breathing). Figure 8-26 illustrates this exercise. As labor advances, breathing tends to become more shallow. At the sig-

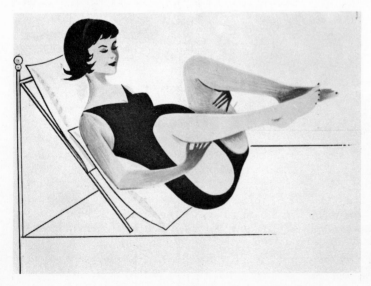

Fig. 8-28. Push position in bed for second stage of labor. Note flexion of head and trunk; position of arms and legs; and absence of pressure on feet. Support of back, shoulders and legs lessens fatigue. (Psychophysical Preparation for Childbearing: Guidelines for Teaching, ed. 2, p. 37, Fig. 34, New York, Maternity Center Association, 1965)

FIG. 8-29. Respiration for second stage of labor. As the contraction starts, breathe in and out through mouth; in once more, close mouth and hold breath, lifting head and legs to pushing position. Maintain this position, holding breath as long as comfortable. Then breathe out in upper part of chest with mouth open, quickly breathe in again; close mouth and again hold breath for as long as the contraction lasts. Abdominal pressure should not be completely relaxed during renewal of breath, which may have to be done more than once during contraction. At end of contraction, breathe out, take a complete breath, and relax. (Psychophysical Preparation for Childbearing: Guidelines for Teaching, ed. 2, p. 38, Fig. 35, New York, Maternity Center Association, 1965)

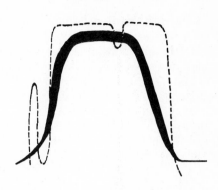

nal of "Breathe in, relax as you breathe out," the mother starts a slow deep breath. In teaching mothers it is well to avoid reference to the rate of respiration to be used in shallow breathing. When mention has been made to increasing the rate of respiration, or when quick breathing was referred to, mothers would pant instead of breathing quickly. There also was a tendency for them to hyperventilate.

TRANSITION BREATHING (Fig. 8-27) is a useful variation of shallow breathing that can be applied in the late active phase of labor. The mother starts off as she would for accelerated breathing, and then, at the urge to bear down, she blows out lightly through her parted lips, without contracting her abdominals. She maintains this pattern until the urge to push diminishes.

Respiration for the Second Stage. The position shown in Figure 8-28 is useful to the mother for pushing before transfer to the delivery table. The support of the back enables the mother to maintain downward pressure of the diaphragm and stabilization of the chest and the abdomen; it also lessens fatigue. Absence of pressure on the feet discourages gluteal tension and thereby contributes to relaxation of the pelvic floor. On the delivery table it is helpful if the legs are positioned in much the same manner. The mother should be encouraged to use the handholds in order to utilize counterforce. Whenever possible, pillows or a backrest should be used to support the back.

In the second stage it will be necessary for the mother to push with a slow, controlled effort in order to make the most of each contraction. Figure 8-29 illustrates the pattern that accomplishes this type of respiration. As the contraction starts, the mother breathes in and out once, inhales once more, closes her mouth, holds her breath, and pushes (after lifting her head and legs to pushing position). She maintains this position and holds her breath as long as is comfortable. Without changing her position, she exhales shallowly, inhales, holds breath, pushes, etc., for as long as the contraction lasts. She should try not to relax her abdominal pressure entirely during breath renewal. She should be coached to relax completely after each contraction.

It should be emphasized that during practice periods the mother actually should *not push*, although she may complete the rest of the exercise. This latter part is very important.

Panting. If the mother suddenly must stop pushing, she breathes in and out deeply—not necessarily rapidly. Care should be taken to help the mother to control the rate and the depth of her breathing to prevent the occurrence of hyperventilation. It is best practiced with the mother lying in the delivery position, with the pelvic floor and the thighs relaxed.

Postpartum Restoration

Regardless of the positive nature of the pregnancy and the labor experience, one can anticipate that the newly delivered mother will have some lessening of muscle tone that can be restored if she utilizes opportunities to contract the important muscle groups so affected. The brief postpartal stay in the hospital affords an opportunity for supervised guidance in a broad scheme of exercises. An individual program for rest, relaxation and practicing the various exercises, based on the mother's particular physical and emotional needs, necessarily will have to be planned with each mother (see Chap. 14).

Early ambulation and the shortened hospital stay for maternity patients create new demands on the mother during the early postpartal period. The physiologic changes of the puerperium alone and the postpartum restoration do not keep pace with the usual sense of well-being that the mother experiences. In general, maternity patients tend to resume normal activity very quickly; thus the newly delivered mother needs to be admonished *never* to continue any activity to the point of fatigue.

The positions and the exercises described in the section on Avoidance of Stress will be helpful (see pp. 175-178).

Before mothers leave the hospital, they should be reminded of the basic principles for the avoidance of stress. If possible, they should continue to practice the exercises for muscle strengthening and toning each day. When the daily routine at home interferes with this, they should be encouraged in the course of daily activities at least to tense the abdominal wall, to contract the pelvic floor muscles from time to time, and to keep in mind what they have

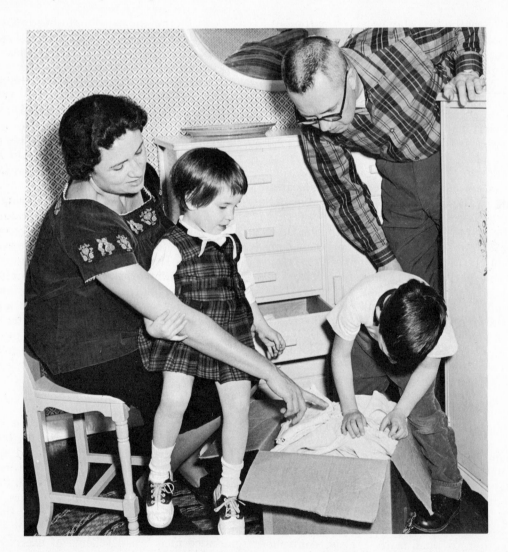

Fig. 8-30. Family group at home. Baby clothes which have been stored away are being made ready for the new baby.

FIG. 8-31. The pullover or slip-on type shirt. The shoulder treatment permits the neck to be opened the full width of the garment when it is slipped on. The pin tab allows the diaper to be pinned to something of a more durable nature than the knitted shirt itself. (The Vanta Company, Inc., Stoughton, Mass.)

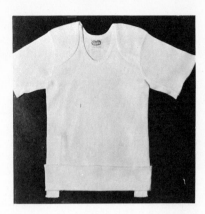

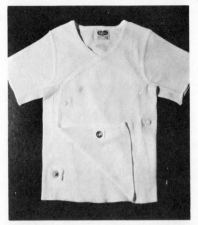

FIG. 8-32. The double-breasted shirt may be fastened with the conventional side-ties or with snap fasteners placed on tabs (as shown above). (The Vanta Company, Inc., Stoughton, Mass.)

learned about standing, sitting, moving—and relaxing.

PREPARATIONS FOR THE BABY

Layette

The baby's layette and equipment are of real interest to all parents—in fact, they are interesting to the majority of people. The cost of the layette should be in keeping with the individual economic circumstances. The entire layette can be purchased ready-made or can be made at home quite inexpensively. Much or little may be spent in its preparation, but nurses who are teaching parents should know why certain types of clothes and equipment are preferable. In the selection of clothing the following points should be considered: comfort; ease in laundering; ease in putting on and taking off; and that it be very light in weight. The new baby's skin is easily irritated by wool. Any clothing which comes in contact with the infant's skin should be made of soft cotton material. Knitted materials have the advantage of ease in laundering and sufficient stretch quality to allow for more freedom in dressing the baby. Garments that open down the full length and fasten with ties or grippers are easier to put on. Ties or grippers are not only less difficult to fasten than buttons but also

are more desirable from the standpoint of safety. The geographic location and climate of the year will greatly influence the selection of the infant's clothing. Size 1 shirts and gowns are recommended, since the infant grows rapidly in the first 6 months and quickly outgrows his garments. It is well to remember that his clothing should not inhibit his normal activities. The complete outfit of clothes that the baby wears should not weigh more than 12 to 16 ounces.

The mother should be advised to prepare a very simple layette. As she sees how fast her baby grows, and what he will need, the additional items can be secured. The complete layettes which can be purchased often contain unnecessary items and are usually costly. Also, many of the articles may be received as baby gifts. Therefore, it is wise to choose only those things which are necessary for immediate use.

Layette necessities are:
5 or 6 shirts
3 to 4 dozen diapers (if diaper service is not used)
4 receiving blankets
3 nightgowns or kimonos
6 diaper pads (11″ x 16″)
2 waterproof protectors for under diaper pads
2 afghans or blankets ⎱ (if climate is cold)
1 bunting ⎰

2 to 4 soft towels (40″ x 40″)
2 to 4 soft washcloths
Nursery equipment should consist of:
basket, bassinet or crib
mattress (firm, flat and smooth)
mattress protector (waterproof)
sheets or pillowcases for mattress
chest or separate drawer
cotton crib blanket
bathtub
diaper pail
toilet tray—equipped
absorbent cotton—or cotton balls
baby soap (bland, white, unscented)
rustproof safety pins
soap dish
bath apron (for mother)
table, for bath or dressing
chair (for mother)

Additional suggestions for layette and equipment are:
sacques
sweaters
kimonos
crib blankets
crib spreads
bibs
clothes drier
chest of drawers
nursery stand
footstool
diaper bag (for traveling)
disposable diapers
nursery light
carriage

Some further suggestions in relation to the selection of specific items are as follows:

Shirts, Gowns, etc. The sleeves should have roomy armholes, such as the raglan-type sleeve. If the pullover-type garments are used, the neck openings should be so constructed that they are large enough to be put on easily from over the feet or the head (Figs. 8-31, 32).

Diapers. Of the several varieties of diapers available, bird's-eye or gauze diapers are the most popular. The selection of diapers should be considered from the standpoint of their comfort (soft and light in weight), absorbency and washing and drying qualities. The mother who plans to use the services of a commercial diaper service should have a dozen diapers of her own.

Receiving Blankets. These should be made of flannelette 1 yard square. This square is used to fold loosely about the baby. If properly secured, the baby may lie and kick and at the same time keep covered and warm. In the early weeks these squares take the brunt of the service and in this way save the fine wool covers from becoming soiled so quickly.

Afghans or Blankets. These should be of very lightweight cotton or wool material. The temperature and the weather will determine the amount of covering needed.

Sheets. Crib sheets are usually 45″ x 72″ and are available in muslin, percale and knitted cotton materials. The knit sheets are practical for bottom sheets and do not need to be ironed. Pillowcases are very usable for the carriage or the basket mattress. Receiving blankets may be used for top sheets.

Waterproof Sheeting. *Various* waterproof materials are suitable to protect the mattress and to be used under the pads. Even though the mattress may have a protective covering, it is necessary to have a waterproof cover large enough to cover the mattress completely—something that can be removed and washed. (Waterproof material should not be dried in the sun.)

Waterproof Pants. These offer protection for special occasions. If the plastic variety is used, they should not be tight at the leg or the waist. For general use, a square of protective material such as Sanisheeting or a cotton quilted pad should be used under the baby next to the diaper.

Bath Apron. This is a protection for both mother and baby and may be made of plastic material covered with terry cloth.

Nursery Equipment

In choosing the equipment, again the individual circumstances should be taken into consideration. Expense, space and future plans all influence the selection. Most nurseries are planned for the satisfaction of the parents. Eventually the baby's room becomes the child's room; and if economy must be considered, furniture should be selected that will appeal to the child as he grows and develops.

The Baby's Room. Preferably, the baby should have his own room. If this is not feasible, a quiet airy place, out of drafts, may be selected.

Bed. The baby should have his own bed. This may be a basket, a bassinet or a crib. The trimming on the basket or the bassinet should be such that it can be removed easily and laundered. A bed may be improvised from a box or a bureau drawer, placed securely on a sturdy table or on chairs which are held together with rope. Many parents may have a carriage that may be used as a bed. However, after about the first 2 months, the baby will need a crib. The crib should be so constructed that the bars are close enough together to prevent the baby's head from being caught between them. If it is painted, a paint "safe for babies" should be used.

Mattress. The mattress should be firm (not hard) and flat. All mattresses, including the waterproof-covered, should be protected by a

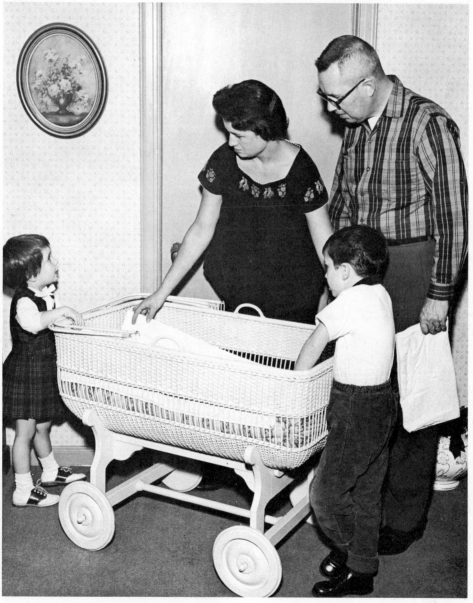

Fig. 8-33. Family group at home, getting the bassinet ready.

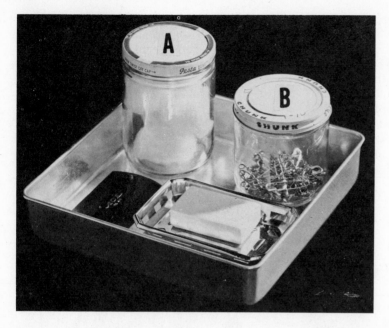

Fig. 8-34. Improvised toilet tray for baby. A household tray or baking pan and miscellaneous jars may be utilized. Comb has fine teeth with smooth rounded edges. Soap dish contains mild, white, unscented soap. (A) Jar for clean absorbent cotton. (B) Jar for safety pins.

waterproof sheeting to prevent the mattress from becoming stained and from absorbing odors. The waterproof sheet is easily washed and dries quickly.

Netting. This will be needed for the carriage, the basket or the crib during the insect season. If the Kiddie-Koop is used, it is screened to protect the baby from insects and animals.

Bathtub. The plastic tub is safe and easy to keep clean.

Bathtub Table. The table on which the tub is placed for the baby's bath should be of convenient height (Fig. 14-21). A kitchen table, or other sturdy table without wheels, may be used for this purpose.

Mother's Chair. The chair also should be a convenient height and comfortable for the individual mother.

Diaper Pail. It should be large enough for the day's supply of soiled diapers. It may be used also for boiling the diapers.

Toilet Tray. This tray should be prepared and ready for use immediately after the delivery of the baby (Fig. 8-34).

PLANS FOR AFTER-CARE OF MOTHER AND BABY

It is always a relief to the mother and her husband when the plans for delivery and the arrangements for the period following have been completed. The parents should make some provision for the mother to be free from other responsibilities until she has regained, in part at least, her physical strength, and until lactation has been established.

The nurse should make an effort to include the father when discussing the details of the mother's care. Often it is only with his help that his wife gets the full care she needs, care that the doctor and the nurse wish her to have (see Chap. 9).

Return to Employment

The expectant mother who is employed may desire to know how early she may return to work after the baby is born. Following delivery, 6 weeks are needed for the obstetrician to determine whether or not the reproductive organs are returning to their approximate normal size and position. Accordingly, no commitments should be made until the baby is from 6 to 8 weeks old. At the time of the postpartal examination, the obstetrician will discuss with the patient her future plans. It always must be kept in mind that the mother-child relationship during the first 6 years of a child's life is most important, and in making these future plans with the mother, this fact must not be ignored because of interest in re-employment. There are, of course, certain unavoidable circumstances within some family units which leave the mother no alternative but to return to work. In such a situation, the mother may require guidance not only from her physician but also from the nurse and the medical social worker to help her plan for this.

SUGGESTED READING

Apgar, V.: Drugs in pregnancy, Am. J. Nurs. 65: 104-106, March, 1965.

————: Health Supervision of Young Children, pp. 47-59, New York, Am. Public Health Assoc., 1960.

Auerback, A. B.: Meeting the needs of new mothers, Children 11:223, November-December, 1964.

Auerback, A. B., and Collier, G. B.: How do nurses take to the "new ways" in leading parent groups?, Nurs. Outlook 6:674-677, December, 1958.

Bagchi, K.: Effect of low nutrient intake during pregnancy on obstetrical performance and offspring, Am. J. Clin. Nutr. 11:586-592, December, 1962.

Barckley, V.: Cigarette smoking—the lag between knowledge and practice, Nurs. Outlook 12:29, March, 1964.

Barnes, A. C.: The clinical approach to the prevention of congenital anomalies, Am. J. Obstet. Gynec. 90, No. 7, Part II:1242, December 1, 1964.

Beaton, G. H.: Nutritional and physiological adaptations in pregnancy, Fed. Proc. 20:196-201, 1961.

Brandl, E.: Cigarette smoking and pregnancy, Nurs. Sci. 3:71-76, February, 1965.

Brown, E. L.: Newer Dimensions of Patient Care, Part 3, New York, Russell Sage Foundation, 1964.

Buxton, C. L.: A Study of Psychophysical Methods for Relief of Childbirth Pain, Philadelphia, Saunders, 1962.

Caplan, G.: Psychological aspects of maternity care, Am. J. Public Health 47:25-31, January, 1957.

————: Concepts of Mental Health and Consultation, Washington, D. C., U. S. Children's Bureau, 1959.

————: The mental hygiene role of the nurse in maternal child care, Nurs. Outlook 2:14-19, January, 1954.

Cashman, Rose: Trends in parent education, Health News 38:4-13, July, 1961.

Chilman, C. S., and Kraft, I.: Helping low-income parents, Children 10:127-136, July-August, 1963.

Committee on Nutrition: The prophylactic requirement and toxicity of vitamin D, Pediatrics 31:512-525, March, 1963.

Dalzell, Irene: Evaluating of a prenatal teaching program, Nurs. Res. 14:160-163, Spring, 1965.

Davis, M. E., and Rubin, R.: DeLee's Obstetrics for Nurses, Philadelphia, Saunders, 1962.

de Watteville, P. H.: The use of obstetric analgesia at the Maternity Hospital of Geneva, Am. J. Obstet. Gynec. 73:473-491, March, 1957.

Donney, E.: Imagination in maternity care, Am. J. Nurs. 60:46-49, January, 1960.

Eastman, N. J.: Williams Obstetrics, ed. 13, New York, Appleton, 1966.

Editors: Behind the cigarette curtain, Trans-Action 2:3-8, January-February, 1965.

Eichenlaub, J. E.: The Marriage Act, New York, Lyle-Stuart, 1961.

Goodrich, F. W., Jr.: Natural Childbirth, New York, Prentice-Hall, 1950.

Hendricks, C. H., and Brenner, W. E.: Patterns of increasing uterine activity in late pregnancy and the development of uterine responsiveness to oxytocin, Am. J. Obstet. Gynec. 90:485-492, October 15, 1964.

Highley, Betty: Antepartal nursing intervention, Nurs. Forum 2, No. 4:62-68, 1963.

Hulka, J. F., and Schasi, J. T.: Obstetrics in adolescents, Obstet. Gynec. 23:678-685, May, 1964.

Kerr, C., et al.: Calcium and phosphorus dynamic in pregnancy, Am. J. Obstet. Gynec. 83:2-8, January, 1962.

LaFever, John: The Lamaze method of natural childbirth—view from the side of the table, Am. J. Nurs. 63:67-69, June, 1963.

LeMat, A. F.: The public health nurse in maternity service, Nurs. Outlook 12:58-61, October, 1964.

Lesser, M. S., and Keane, V. R.: Nurse-Patient Relationships in a Hospital Maternity Service, St. Louis, Mosby, 1956.

Lucey, J. F.: Primates, drugs and fetal safety, Pediatrics 32:953-955, December, 1963.

Madore, C. E., and Deutsch, Y. B.: Talking with parents, Am. J. Nurs. 62:108-111, November, 1962.

Mann, V. R.: Food practices of the Mexican-American in Los Angeles County, Los Angeles County Health Dept., 1963.

Manning, M. L.: The psychodynamics of dietetics, Nurs. Outlook 13:57-59, April, 1965.

Mayer, Jean: Some aspects of the relation of nutrition and pregnancy, Postgrad. Med. 33: 277-282, March, 1963.

Middleton, E., and Hugger, V.: Patients and their obstetricians, Psychosomatics 4:142-149, May-June, 1963.

Morris, Ena: How does a nurse teach nutrition to patients?, Am. J. Nurs. 60:67-70, January, 1960.

Nabatoff, R. A.: Varicose veins of pregnancy, J.A.M.A. 174:1712-1719, 1960.

Newton, M., and Newton, N.: The normal course and management of lactation, Clin. Obstet. Gynec. 5:44-63, March, 1962.

Page, E. W., and Page, E. P.: Leg cramps in pregnancy, Obstet. Gynec. 1:94, 1953.

Parks, John: Premarital Gynecologic Examination, Postgrad. Med. 30:476-478, November, 1961.

Pion, R. P., *et al.*: Prenatal care, a group psychotherapeutic approach, Calif. Med. 97:281-285, November, 1962.

Polk, L. D.: Antepartal care in Philadelphia, Nurs. Outlook 11:822-824, November, 1963.

Psychophysical Preparation for Childbearing: Guidelines for Teaching, ed. 2, New York, Maternity Center Assoc., 1965.

Read, G. D.: Childbirth Without Fear, rev. ed., New York, Harpers, 1953.

Recommended Dietary Allowances, rev. ed., Publication No. 1146, Washington, D. C., National Academy of Sciences, National Research Council, 1963.

Reeder, S. R., and Reeder, L. G.: Some correlates of prenatal care among low income wed and unwed women, Am. J. Obstet. Gynec. 90:1304-1314, December 15, 1964.

Reeder, S. R., and Deck, E.: Nurses' participation in a group psychotherapeutic approach to antepartal management, Nurs. Forum 2, No. 4:82-93, 1963.

Richie, Jeanne: Using an interpreter effectively, Nurs. Outlook 12:27-29, December, 1964.

Rosengren, W. R.: Social instability and attitudes toward pregnancy as a social role, Social Probl. 9:371-378, Spring, 1962.

Rubin, Reva: Behavioral definitions in nursing therapy, conference on Maternal and Child Nursing, Columbus, Ohio, Ross Laboratories, 1964.

Runnerstrom, Lillian: Expectant parent education, Nurs. Sci. 3:57-68, February, 1965.

———: Food iron intake and hemoglobin levels in pregnancy, Nurs. Sci. 1:187-197, August-September, 1963.

———: Food iron intake and hemoglobin levels in uncomplicated pregnancy: implications for nursing, Convention Clinical Sessions No. 11, Am. Nurses Assoc., 1964.

Seide, Diane: Hypnosis—Its Use in Medicine Today, R.N. 23:43-49, April, 1960.

Sterns, G.: Nutrition in preparation for motherhood, Bull. Maternal and Infant Health 9, No. 2:8-11, 1962.

Sturges, S. H.: Opportunities and challenges of the premarital exam, Fertil. Steril. 13:209-219, May-June, 1962.

Thoms, H.: A consideration of childbirth programs, New Eng. J. Med. 255:860-861, October 25, 1956.

Ulin, P. R.: The Lamaze method of natural childbirth—the exhilarating moment of birth, Am. J. Nurs. 63:60-67, June, 1963.

Vellay, Pierre: Childbirth Without Pain, New York, Dutton, 1960.

Wohl, M., and Goodhart, R.: Modern Nutrition in Health and Disease, ed. 3, Philadelphia, Lea & Febiger, 1964.

Chapter 9

The Mental Hygiene of Pregnancy and Childbirth

LEO KANNER, M.D.*

INTRODUCTION

Human pregnancy is a biologic event and an emotional experience. It begins with the relationship between two people and ushers in a new relationship between them and their offspring. The nature of the biologic event depends on anatomic and physiologic conditions; the nature of the emotional experience is determined by the mother's attitude toward herself, her husband and her child. The physical hygiene of pregnancy is directed primarily toward the body of the mother; the mental hygiene of pregnancy addresses itself to her as a thinking, feeling and behaving individual.

It is true of all branches of medicine that a physician's or a nurse's attention should not be limited exclusively and impersonally to the functions and the ailments of the patient's body. The need for sympathy and understanding has been emphasized since the days of Hippocrates. The combination of professional competence and humane interest in the patient has been rightly extolled as the ideal attribute of persons who make themselves responsible for the health of human beings.

The nature of childbearing is such that medical contacts with the parturient mother extend over a period of approximately a whole year. For nearly 12 months the obstetrician and the maternity nurse take over the guidance of an adult woman, supervise her nutrition, regulate her activities, answer her questions, clear up her puzzlements, advise her about the handling of the baby when it comes and generally chart her conduct during the 24 hours of the day. This offers ample opportunity to become acquainted with the mother's personality, the circumstances of her environment, her attitudes and opinions, her outlook on life and the degree of her emotional stability. It is not too difficult to sense and spot genuine happiness over the pregnancy, resentful rebellion against it, stunned acceptance of the conception as an unexpected decree of destiny or disturbing apprehension regarding the outcome.

The present can rarely be understood without reference to the past. Obstetrics cannot possibly dispense with a thoroughgoing evaluation of the patient's past history. Verbal reports, clinical examination and laboratory tests are indispensable as a preparation for the adequate physical hygiene of pregnancy. Needed information is thus obtained about factors of

* Professor Emeritus of Child Psychiatry, The Johns Hopkins University School of Medicine.

pelvic formation, miscarriages and stillbirths, cardiac illness, tuberculosis, syphilis and other conditions which existed before the recent conception and may complicate the course of events and influence the direction of obstetric procedure.

Analogously, a true appreciation of mental health during pregnancy can be obtained only by the ability to trace the mother's present attitudes to those personal experiences which have helped to shape them. In one sense, it is relatively easy to become familiar with such experiences and their effects, because no special or elaborate equipment is required. In another sense, such a study is extremely difficult and complex. Few people are inclined to disclose their most intimate feelings unless they are reasonably assured that the listener has the maturity, the tactfulness and the honest desire to understand, to guard confidences and to alleviate perplexities and anxieties.

THE MOTHER'S ATTITUDE TOWARD HER PREGNANCY

Under ordinary circumstances the discovery of a woman's pregnancy is a happening which is welcome to her and to her husband. It is a source of rejoicing or at least a tranquil acceptance. The temporary discomforts, restrictions and changes of appearance which go with gravidity are awaited and borne with good nature. Even if there is some fear of the delivery, it is richly counterbalanced by the wish to have the baby, the gentleness of husband, relatives and friends, the full confidence in the physician and the nurse, the knowledge of good health and of satisfactory progress of the pregnancy and the ever-shortening distance from the moment of childbirth.

Such an attitude of positive and gratifying anticipation of motherhood, which is the essence of good mental hygiene, is usually predictable, because it is based on a definite constellation of fortunate factors.

1. The mother herself has had a happy childhood and thereby has come to think of a family with children as something desirable and enjoyable. Her vision of a family unit is one of reciprocal satisfactions. Having experienced the benefits of parental fondness, she is prepared to give affection as she has received it.

2. The mother is secure in her relationship with her husband. The child comes to her as the result of intimacy with a man whom she loves and of whose love she is certain. She has no doubt about the safe and unperturbed continuity of her marriage.

3. The mother is not harassed by the drudgeries and the worries which arise from material insecurities, such as the husband's unemployment or protracted hospitalization, poor housing conditions or the severe illness of one of her children.

Luckily, this combination of circumstances prevails often enough to deserve being regarded as the average, ordinary mental state of a mother at the onset of pregnancy. If it exists, her medical guides may look forward with a feeling of relief to the likelihood of freedom from untoward psychological complications. There is ground for the same sense of relief as that which obtains when, at the end of a thorough physical examination, the findings warrant a favorable prediction of the course of the biologic process.

However, departures from these healthy preliminary conditions are not at all uncommon. They can and should be studied, diagnosed and treated with the same care, knowledge and interest as are the major and the minor deviations from bodily health and comfort. The principal directions of an unwholesome maternal attitude toward pregnancy present themselves to the knowing observer in the form of two disturbing psychological complexes: (1) fear of the delivery and of the fate of the child to be delivered; and (2) rejection of the child to be delivered.

Fear

Helene Deutsch, whose work on the psychology of women has received great acclaim, wrote in the volume devoted to motherhood: "That great power in human psychic life, *fear*, whatever its nature, certainly has a considerable influence on the emotional course of pregnancy."

A pregnant woman may be beset by two types of fearful anticipations, which often run concurrently: (1) fear for herself; and (2) fear for the baby.

The Mother's Fear for Herself. Every expectant mother knows that there will be pain, hospitalization or at least confinement in bed, perhaps the administration of an anesthetic, and a revolutionary physical change at the end of the pregnancy road. The whole procedure of childbirth, however normal it may turn out to be, must impress her as a sort of surgical intervention to which she will have to submit, and from which there is no possible escape. There is hardly a human being who is entirely devoid of fear of an operation. The astounding progress of medicine and preventive hygiene has greatly reduced the actual dangers; also it has reduced, but not entirely eliminated, the dread. Statistics have shown a marked decline in maternal mortality, but this fact does not remove from the individual woman the anxiously perplexing question: What if it gets *me?* In the not too distant past many more women have lost their lives in pregnancy, labor and soon after giving birth than it is pleasant to contemplate. Even though conditions have improved tremendously, and there is good reason for the expectation of further improvement, the public still is held in awe by the experiences gathered in centuries. Pregnant women's fear of death is therefore understandable and not at all unusual. It has been emphasized by every author who has ever written about the mental hygiene of pregnancy.

There are many possible reactions to fear; some of them are flight, shrinking, avoidance of danger, stupefied inactivity, panic and bravery. No soldier, not even the most courageous, has ever gone into battle without being afraid; when we speak of "fearlessness" on such occasions, we do not refer to absence of fear but the conquest of fear. The conquest is successful if it is prompted and aided by a consistent motive. A pregnant woman is not unlike a soldier with regard to her attitude toward anticipated dangers. When there is an eager desire for a child, when security has been built up by the same kind of confidence in the people important to the mother which brave soldiers have in their commanders and buddies, then the motive is strong enough to conquer fear to the point that it is not even realized. The more the motive has been weakened by anxiety, insecurity and unhappiness, the less strength will the mother have to subdue her fear of childbirth, and the more will the manifestations of her dread come to the fore.

The Mother's Fear for the Child. Pregnancy is in many respects a journey into the unknown. There are justified uncertainties about the expected baby's gender, appearance and general endowment. Uncertainty is a breeder of fear, particularly if previous experiences and orientations have tended to select some special areas of apprehension. Nobody can prophesy the future destiny of a human embryo even with approximate definiteness. But a mother to whom life has been good, who is thrilled by the prospect of having a child, who has fortified herself with a reasonable degree of optimism in all other respects, does not go around imagining all or any of the possible misfortunes which may befall her child. If, however, there is a background of anxiety, then the memory of dire happenings, pseudoscientific notions and folk beliefs may contrive to introduce torturing visions of impending disaster. There are three types of maternal fears for the baby which occur with special frequency.

1. Fear of losing the baby is apt to arise if the pregnancy has been preceded by spontaneous abortions, miscarriages or stillbirths; if previous pregnancies have been, or the present gestation is, accompanied by pathologic complications; or if these things have happened to relatives or close friends.

2. Fear of heredity is based on the layman's vague and frequently distorted interpretations of the results of scientific research. No real scholar ever has claimed that a child's personality development is merely an inherited repetition of some progenitor's antics, that traits are handed down as trinkets are, or that statistics can be applied to individuals. But this is exactly what "heredity" means to many people. As a result, anxious parents consult their respective genealogic trees and, finding an uncongenial ancestor hanging from one of the branches, worry themselves sick in the expectation of similar propensities in the baby-to-come. It can be said with considerable assurance that fear of heredity has caused at least as much mental anguish as heredity itself ever did.

3. Superstitious fears are found not only among the lowly and ignorant; they sometimes seem to be too powerful to be squelched even by a college diploma. The idea of mysterious prenatal influences which are said to "mark the baby" is still prevalent in many quarters. The notion is still abroad that a mother's ex-

periences during her pregnancy will in some fashion shape the baby's fate. If she looks wistfully at a handsome child, the beauty will communicate itself to the embryo in her womb. She must be careful to keep her glances off ugliness and misshapen features, or her baby may grow up to be ugly and misshapen.

Klein, Potter and Dyk collected many samples of such misconceptions. A few quotations may serve as illustrations. One mother thought that if one craved expensive out-of-season food, the baby might have a birthmark, but if the same food were in season, the baby would not be marked. Another believed that if she had a permanent wave during her pregnancy, she might be electrocuted. One young woman, convinced that her own small hemangioma was caused by the fact that her mother had eaten strawberries while carrying her, feared that her child might be "marked by a mouse seen on a stove."

Rejection

Not all children arrive in this world because they have been wanted by their parents. The number of unplanned and unwanted pregnancies in our civilization is truly appalling. Statistics cannot possibly reach the annual total of illegally induced abortions, because every effort is made by the participants to keep them under the cover of secrecy. The unquestionably high figure is augmented by numerous unskillful attempts which do not succeed in destroying the child, who therefore comes into existence as an "unsuccessful abortion." This is a tragic state of affairs, both because of the interference with human life and because of the circumstances and the mental attitudes leading to the interference.

However, rejection of the pregnancy does not always end in the drastic ejection of the embryo from the uterus and from life. It often expresses itself more or less subtly in the parental attitude toward the unwanted pregnancy. It is not too unusual to hear rejecting mothers speak of the conception as an "accident" and describe their feelings at the time of the discovery as a "shock."

Therefore, maternal rejection results in one of three clearly circumscribed reactions: (1) illegal abortion, (2) unsuccessful attempt at abortion, (3) a nonaccepting attitude toward the pregnancy.

It is not easy for the average healthy person to comprehend the fact of a woman's repudiation of her own offspring. Maternal rejection is indeed a very complex phenomenon anchored deeply in the mother's personality and relationships formed over a long period of time. What seems to be solely a matter of her feelings limited to *bearing and borne* has its origins in her own childhood and adolescence, her sexual orientation, her way of facing and adjusting to life in general. Of course, nurses cannot be expected to undertake the specifically psychiatric task of delving into the details or even the essentials of every pregnant woman's life history and its meaning to her. Nevertheless, there are several typical situations, ascertainable without too much difficulty, which play a prominent part in the immediate etiology of maternal rejection.

Socially unsanctioned, "illegitimate" conception is one of the most easily recognized sources of maternal resentment. The child so borne may unfortunately learn that he will be a permanent reminder of his mother's misstep, will either precipitate a "forced marriage" or be a hindrance in the consideration of future matrimonial aspirations, will raise the difficult problem of support, may estrange her from her relatives and friends and may thoroughly alter her status in society. All this naturally makes for an unhappy state of mind. Nevertheless, illegitimate pregnancy is not always synonymous with rejection. In certain ethnic groups —segments of our Negro population, for instance, in which some circles have a tolerant attitude toward babies born out of wedlock— such pregnancies often are accepted by the mothers with far greater ease than is generally the case.

Unplanned, "accidental" pregnancies are often resented because of economic distress. There already are too many mouths to be fed out of a meager budget. The mother already has her hands full, cooking, cleaning, laundering and taking care of her older children. Under such circumstances the newcomer may be viewed chiefly as an added expense and burden. The husband's displeasure with the addition to the family may further aggravate the resentment.

The mother's feelings about her husband and her marital happiness determine to a considerable extent the degree of her acceptance or rejection of her pregnancy. If dissensions and incompatibilities have led to disillusionment and raised the specter of eventual dissolution of the marriage, it is extremely difficult to look forward to the birth of a child with unmixed pleasure and equanimity. This is equally true of pregnancies which, though planned and premeditated, have been entered into with ulterior motives, in which the genuine desire for a child figures much less than the purpose which his existence is intended to serve. Children sometimes are conceived as part of a scheme to keep the husband (or the wife), to appeal to the marital partner's sense of responsibility, to satisfy the family's clamor for an heir to the name. If the mother finds that the disclosure of her pregnancy has not reduced her husband's alcoholism, gallivanting, lack of ambition or indifference toward her, then the child's coming has failed to accomplish the major purpose for which it was designed and therefore is resented as a bad investment.

Our culture has departed healthily and progressively from the idea that childbearing is a woman's only function and fulfillment. Women have embarked fruitfully on many occupations which were not open to them previously. Many women come to matrimony and motherhood from the ranks of stenographers, salesgirls, nurses, teachers, factory workers, entertainers and waitresses. Some continue working while married until some time during the first pregnancy. Few people realize that the transition from a busy vocational life, from participation in group activities (office, store, hospital, school, factory, restaurant, etc.), and from a variety of interests and associations to quiet domesticity, change and narrowing of duties, and limitation of contacts with people calls for major adjustments of routine and attitudes. Stable mothers, happily married, have gained a great deal from their jobs, which gave them an opportunity for personal enrichment, the satisfaction of having had a fling at life before their domestication and practice in dealing with human beings. The new experience of pregnancy is enjoyed, because the mother obtains a richer biologic and psychological gratification from motherhood than she ever obtained from her job, because she wants a child or children from the man whom she loves.

However, if the marriage turns out to be emotionally and economically disappointing,

often there is a compensatory toying with the idea of returning to the former occupation and associates. Then comes the first pregnancy, which is either "accidental" or desired as a means of cementing a brittle husband-wife relationship and giving to the mother a new content in life. With it, however, comes a realization of finality. The child's expected arrival is looked upon with mixed feelings as a trap and a promise of something more precious than a job. This constant swaying between acceptance and rejection creates many quandaries which complicate the mother's attitude toward her pregnancy. I have heard a sizable number of mothers report how, under such conditions, they had felt "trapped," "hemmed in," "confined" or "cooped up" during pregnancy and how, in their night dreams and daydreams, they were not pregnant and were happily back at their jobs.

Though matrimonial unhappiness is one of the outstanding immediate factors in the etiology of maternal rejection, there are many other elements which color the picture in individual instances. A few specific examples may suffice.

Mrs. A. conceived immediately after marriage. A vivacious friend of hers, whose defiance of local bigotry had caused the neighbors' tongues to click for years, had given premature birth to a child 7 months after her wedding; the whole community had raised suspicious eyebrows and cast aspersions. Mrs. A., who was pathetically dependent on the opinions of other people, lived throughout her pregnancy in dread that her child might come prematurely and arouse similar suspicions. She began to resent her pregnancy as coming "too soon." The combination of fear and rejection created an urgent psychiatric problem, caused her to attempt an abortion and almost wrecked the marriage.

Mrs. B. avowedly did not want children. Her husband likewise did not wish to be "bothered." They got along well for 10 years. Their relatives and friends did not approve of their childlessness. They pointed out that, being people of wealth and standing, it was their "duty" to have children. They finally yielded when Mrs. B. decided that, having reached her thirties, she should "hurry up" if she was to have any children at all. But, once pregnant, she felt very bad and hated the child from the moment that she discovered her pregnancy. She hated her advisers and blamed her husband for submitting to their dictates.

Mrs. C. was kept despotically under the thumb of her domineering mother, who consented to her marriage at 19 years on the condition that, being "too young," she promise not to have any children for several years. Mrs. C. was in love with her husband, who was anxious to become a father before his anticipated departure for the Pacific combat zone. When Mrs. C.'s mother learned about the pregnancy, she reproached her daughter, kept reminding her of the broken pledge, and finally refused to speak to her for several weeks. Matters were aggravated by the fact that, after the husband's departure, Mrs. C. was enticed by her mother to live in her house. Worried about her husband, made to feel guilty by her mother, who ascribed recurrent headaches to her daughter's "disobedience," Mrs. C. was driven to despair. She came to accept her mother's endlessly repeated verdict that she should not have become pregnant so soon and looked on her pregnancy as an irreparable mistake destined to be a permanent reminder of her filial disloyalty.

Effect of Fear and Rejection

Fear and rejection, the principal obstacles in the path of good mental health in pregnancy, may be damaging in a variety of ways. An attitude of dread of the things to come and a revulsion against that which has become inevitable are obviously not conducive to comfort and composure.

However, it should be pointed out from the start that mild fear and resentment which are not too deeply rooted in the mother's personality often can be handled by her satisfactorily without too much interference with her equanimity. She is ready to seek and accept from her physician or nurse enlightenment with regard to her apprehensive puzzlements. She is able to overcome the first "shock" of the discovery of her pregnancy and to adjust to, or at least compromise with, the new situation.

A different picture obtains when strong emotional conflicts are at play, when the mother is the victim of powerful unconscious crosscurrents, and when the pregnancy is complicated by fundamental personality difficulties.

It is well known that psychological distress has marked effects on one's ordinary physiologic functions. Everybody is familiar with headache, stomachache and backache which obtrude themselves as "body protests" against emotional conflicts, even though no organic pathology can be demonstrated in the head, the stomach or the back.

Pregnancy is accompanied by a number of physical discomforts on a biologic basis. Nausea and vomiting are among the most frequent and most disturbing. Certainly enough momentous changes are taking place in the mother's somatic condition to explain nausea as a physiologic by-product of the pregnancy. Nevertheless, there are several features which have convinced obstetricians that emotional influences play a significant part in the picture.

1. Nausea, with or with vomiting, is not universal. It has been estimated that in about one third of all pregnancies it is either absent or so mild and fleeting that it constitutes no problem. This has rightly raised the question why identical bodily processes cause severe vomiting in one woman and barely a trace of nausea in another. The search for an answer to this question has led to the observation that the mother's personality and attitudes could be correlated with the degree of severity of the vomiting.

2. This assumption was strengthened by the fact that emotional factors were found to alleviate or aggravate the nausea. There were many instances during the war in which the husband's furlough put a stop to an expectant woman's nausea. A young, "accidentally" impregnated primipara became nauseated as soon as she had discovered the fact. Her husband had a poorly paid job at the time. Her nausea was very disturbing for several weeks but ceased abruptly when her husband was offered a well-paying position.

3. The milder forms of nausea usually are restricted to the early part of pregnancy. This indicates that nausea has a tendency to fade away when there has been a psychological as well as somatic adjustment to the condition.

4. Excessive or pernicious vomiting seems to respond to psychotherapeutic measures at least as well as to other efforts.

Aside from nausea and vomiting, pregnancy is by its very nature associated with other discomforts, which stable mothers taken in their stride. Fear-ridden and rejecting mothers tend to be disturbed by them to a much greater extent. When the pregnancy as such is resented, the necessary changes of routine, the temporary limitation of social activities or the disruption of employment are equally unwelcome. This attitude often results in poor cooperation with the regimen which has been mapped out by the physician and the nurse. Individual behavior differs in accordance with personalities.

One woman will not only follow recommendations anxiously but also be exasperating in her demands for the constant and undivided attention of the nurse, her husband, her relatives and everybody else. Her self-spoiling, forever-complaining and dissatisfied demeanor will calculate to surround her with people expected to cater to her hypochondriac whining or nagging. It is possible, though not certain, that some pregnant women's peculiar appetite for strange and not easily obtainable food items may have an unconscious basis in this type of self-indulgence.

Other women may go out of their way to disregard recommendations. They may continue scrubbing floors, rushing up and down the stairs or—in socially different settings—riding on horseback beyond the time when such strenuous activities are permissible. Their poor mental hygiene may cause them to neglect the essentials of physical hygiene. This devil-may-care or leave-me-alone attitude sometimes poses major problems to the obstetric nurse.

THE MOTHER'S ATTITUDE TOWARD LABOR

Dershimer has called attention to the great facility of childbirth among primitive peoples. Many ethnologists were amazed at the easy labor in civilizations less complex than our own. Deutsch wrote: "In some tribes, the whole confinement period is a matter of minutes. The young mother immediately bathes herself and the newborn infant in the nearest river and returns to her interrupted work as though nothing had happened. If a woman is suddenly seized with labor pains while traveling on land or by water, she resumes her journey immediately after delivery and continues on her way until she reaches her destination."

From this one might—a little too hastily, perhaps—infer that such bliss can be bought for the price of ignorance only. For it is true that primitive woman has not had the day of delivery calculated and marked for her on the calendar; she has not been enlightened about the process of parturition; and she has utter faith in the protective magic of her amulets. But this is not the whole story by far. There are many other primitive tribes, equally untutored, in which there is considerable agitation, kindled by all sorts of rituals, in connection with childbirth. Furthermore, precipitate deliveries occur in our culture as well as in any other. The psychology of labor and delivery is not too well known as yet to afford satisfactory explanations for differences in duration, intensity of pain and psychosomatic relationships in different cultures.

We are on safer ground when we consider differences among individual women in our own midst. We can understand that a stable, well-adjusted mother accepts the confinement as a hoped-for climax, at the end of which comes the coveted reward—the baby. The pain is felt as strongly by her as by any other woman in labor but is tolerated with a determination which keeps the goal in mind. It is recognized as a transition, demanded by Nature, to something that has been eagerly desired. There may be fear similar to that which is felt immediately before a surgical operation. But a stable person, though afraid, submits to the operation because she keeps in mind the goal of relief from the illness which has necessitated the surgeon's intervention. To a woman in good mental health, labor represents not only a first step toward the full restoration of her usual physical adequacy but also the welcome realization of imminent fulfillment.

But long-term anxiety, reinforced by rejection, makes labor appear as something like the painful signing of a contract into which a person has been pushed against her will. Or, if the analogy of an operation may again be resumed, delivery under those circumstances may be compared with a major surgical procedure from which the patient, instead of looking forward to relief, expects lifelong suffering and unpleasantness. Such an attitude rarely appears in undisguised form. No mother can afford to admit even to herself that she does not want her child. The closer the baby's arrival is at hand, the less can the mother's conscience allow her to wish the baby out of the way. There is no such thing as a "maternal instinct," but there is definitely a need for protection against the "unnatural" feelings of rejection. This protection is supplied by an unconscious mechanism called *ambivalence*.

Ambivalence is a fundamental human trait which makes it possible to love and hate the same person simultaneously, to want and not to want a child at the same time. When love and desire predominate, as they do in emotionally healthy mothers, any coexisting negative feelings are weak and negligible and hardly ever come to the surface. But when resentment and rejection are present, the mother has the face-saving need for strenthening and emphasizing whatever positive feelings she has for the baby. The matrimonially unhappy mother discovers that the child, conceived against her wishes, will, after all, be everything that is left to her to live for. She begins to feel guilty about ever having felt an aversion toward the pregnancy and is determined to make up for this when the child arrives.

All these sentiments and attitudes, some of which are intricately embedded in the mother's unconscious, are a significant part of her mental status during labor. It has been said that they may even influence the vigor of uterine contractions, but this, though quite possible, still remains to be demonstrated.

Some obstetricians, realizing the role of fear in labor, have tried to devise methods intended to alleviate the fear. In England, Read, convinced that much of the labor pain is attributable to tension produced by fear, worked out an obstetric regimen intended to keep the mother free from fear and pain by appropriate instruction, preparation and assistance. He described his method in a book entitled *Childbirth Without Fear*. Though in individual cases this may prove to be a helpful contribution to obstetric technic, Read did not pay sufficient attention to the basic mechanisms of the emotional conflicts which are at the bottom of a mother's tensions and fears.

THE MOTHER'S ATTITUDE TOWARD THE NEWBORN

People differ in their attitudes even toward inanimate possessions. One woman will treat her new set of furniture casually. Another will keep dusting and polishing it almost incessantly. A third will have spots and scratches on it in no time. Casualness, obsessiveness and negligence are expressions of personality and, when present, are applied to all phases of living.

A new baby certainly means much more than a new set of furniture. A woman's whole biography, the sum total of her philosophy of life, the background of her attitudes and relationships, her past and her vision of the future are reflected in her mode of adjustment to motherhood and to the newborn. Furthermore, a baby is, unlike a set of furniture, sensitive to the manner in which he is treated. The realization of an infant's responsiveness to affection or lack of affection has been one of the most significant discoveries made by students of human development. Many people are still skeptical when they are confronted with evidences of this discovery. Are not proper nutrition and physical hygiene all that a baby needs? What can he possibly know of his mother's worries or satisfactions? Indeed, he "knows" nothing about them. But he "senses" and responds to a tense or relaxed attitude, a personal or impersonal approach, genuine acceptance or dutiful subjection to regulations.

A series of studies in the past decade brought clinical proof of these observations. Babies reared for the first 2 or 3 years in orphanages under ideal hygienic and nutritional conditions, but without attention to their emotional needs, were found to be severely damaged psychologically. The emotional deprivations had lasting results which showed themselves in behavior deviations, character defects and intellectual deficit. By contrast, control groups reared in foster homes during early infancy achieved a much more satisfactory life adjustment and did far better in intelligence and personality tests.

An infant's need for maternal affection is now recognized as an undisputed scientific fact, as is the need for food and shelter. A loved child is a happy and secure child. An unloved child is unhappy, insecure and riddled with anxieties.

Rejected children are unloved children. A rejecting attitude is apt to push the mother into one of several sets of practices which are harmful to the child's mental hygiene as well as her own. There are, in our civilization, three principal types of maternal behavior in response to the rejection of her baby: open hostilty and neglect, perfectionism and overprotection.

Open Hostility and Neglect

Abandonment and desertion are the extreme forms of such behavior. They are, in a sense, postpartal "abortions"; the baby is tossed out of its mother's existence. But the tossing is sometimes done in a much subtler and more refined form which, though sanctioned by convention, still deprives the baby of a mother. There is no fondling and cuddling. The bottle takes the place of the breast. The mother returns as soon as possible to her work or social functions and leaves the care of her child to relatives or governesses. I have known working mothers who went to see their boarded babies once a week, mainly in order to pay for the board. I have known socialite mothers who had their babies brought to them for a few minutes' inspection "by appointment."

Perfectionism

Ambivalence plays an important part after childbirth, as it has played during pregnancy and labor. The inability to accept a child is coupled with a desire for the ability to accept him. The rejecting mother, justifying her feelings on the basis of the child's imperfections (no "perfect" human has ever existed), goes out of her way to assure the child's acceptability by trying to make him perfect. These are usually mothers who have long had a tendency to obsessive perfectionism, who scrub (or have the maid scrub) the floor until it sparkles, who live by the clock and make a fetish of orderliness and regularity. The baby must be made to fit into this scheme. All sorts of books on child rearing and child psychology are consulted and all but memorized. The advice of doctors and nurses is taken and carried out far too literally. If the baby does not comply with the desired ideal of perfection, the impatient mother resorts to coercion. Psychiatrists have learned that many difficulties of personality development have their origin in forced feeding and coercive bowel training in early infancy. Force and restraint lead to meek submission,

listless withdrawal or rebellious negativism. All of these reactions are signs of frustration of a child who, being human, cannot live up to the demanded standards of perfection.

Overprotection

Some mothers cannot stand the thought that they have resented the pregnancy and the baby's coming. The mother's unsolved conflicts over her own unhappy childhood, matrimonial disillusionment or disrupted career are, after all, not the poor baby's fault. There is a feeling of remorse about the rejection. This feeling is compensated and overcompensated by a determination to sacrifice everything to the baby, to center on him all attention and energy every moment of the day. The child is wrapped in a heavy blanket of overprotection and oversolicitude.

Overprotection is not always the result of rejection. A woman who has lost one or more children through miscarriage, stillbirth or illness, a mother of an only child incapable of having more children because of hysterectomy, a woman whose child has come to her after a long period of childlessness may come to feel that she must be perpetually on guard lest something disastrous befall the child. Her overprotection of the baby is not an expiation for a rejecting attitude but an overdose of mothering and, figuratively speaking, the constant pulling at an uncut umbilical cord.

Regardless of the psychological origin of maternal overprotection, the result is unmerciful "spoiling" of the child. While the neglected or coerced child lives in an emotional refrigerator, the overprotected child lives in a heated oven in which mother love becomes smother love. Maturation and gradual emancipation are made impossible; whenever the child attempts to make use of his newly acquired abilities, he is pushed back into the oven. The mother is alarmed if he cries or if he does not cry, if he wants more food or less food than she believes that he should have, if his stools are softer or harder than she thinks they should be.

Neglect, perfectionism and overprotection are poor substitutes for genuine, natural maternal affection. They indicate emotional difficulties in the mother and create profound emotional difficulties in the infant. A sustained atmosphere of warmth, equally removed from refrigerator and oven, is a sign of the good mental health of the parent and the safest guarantee of an infant's wholesome personality development.

THE PSYCHOSES OF PREGNANCY

In rare instances the mother's emotional conflicts have been so deeply intrenched that they cannot be solved by neurotic mechanisms. The ordinary psychopathologic escapes and defenses, such as neglect, perfectionism and overprotection, are insufficient to keep the mother's personality functioning, even though the function is inadequate. The unconscious conflicts then become so overwhelmingly powerful that a major psychosis results. Estimates about the frequency of psychoses of pregnancy vary widely; they range from 1 in 400 pregnancies to 1 in 1,000 pregnancies.

Puerperal psychoses, with very few exceptions, have their onset after the birth of the child, usually between the 1st and the 14th days following the delivery. Apparently, even though there may have been symptoms of emotional discomfort during the period of gestation, the psychotic break does not come until the process of childbirth has been completed. It is then that the need for new adaptations which confront the mother finds her pathetically unprepared. Psychoses occur in primiparae and multiparae with almost the same frequency. Acute psychotic episodes have been known to repeat themselves in subsequent pregnancies.

There is no specific puerperal psychosis. Its general nature and symptoms may vary considerably. It usually takes the form of one of the two principal types: schizophrenia or manic-depressive psychosis. Recent studies have made it certain beyond question that neither mode of mental collapse is brought about by the pregnancy as such. Childbirth is a strong precipitating factor rather than the actual cause. It is mainly the agent which, shortly after the baby's arrival, tends to disintegrate a personality structure which has long been held together rather loosely and falls apart under the impact of the incisive psychobiologic experience of parturition. Toxic and infectious elements undoubtedly contribute to and hasten the process of disorganization.

The onset is characterized by a noticeable change of general demeanor. Sleeplessness, irritability, anxiety, excessive sadness or excitement, talkativeness, suspiciousness, preoccupation with trivialities and tense agitation should make one very cautious and mindful of psychotic developments. Once the clinical features have established themselves, their recogtion presents no difficulty even to a lay person. Regardless of the type of the psychotic condition, antagonism toward the husband, hostility to the baby and concern over sexual matters are encountered with great frequency. The pathologic attitude toward the child may express itself in a variety of ways. The mother develops an amnesia about the birth of her child; she refuses to believe that the baby is her own; she has the delusional conviction that the baby is dead; she shrinks from contact with the baby because of the tormenting apprehension that she may harm him; she even may actually attempt to kill the baby.

Whenever there is the slightest suspicion of psychotic development, the nurse should immediately inform the physician in charge of the patient. He, in turn, will make immediate provisions for psychiatric care.

THE NURSE'S CONTRIBUTION TO THE MENTAL HYGIENE OF PREGNANCY

Psychiatry has gained important insights into the psychology and the psychopathology of pregnant women. In the great majority of instances psychiatrists are not, and need not be, consulted. This does not mean, however, that in our day and age every pregnant woman should not receive the benefits of existing knowledge. All branches of medicine are now making use of the modern achievements of psychiatry and mental hygiene. Obstetricians, dealing as they do with women who are pregnant, guiding them for a period of almost a whole year, perceiving the great variety of marital and parent-child relationships, have been especially alert in this respect. If proof of this were necessary, one could point to Menninger's questionnaire, the answers to which bespeak great interest and understanding, and to Baker's work, which was carried out at the invitation and under the auspices of the Obstetrical Clinic of the Johns Hopkins Hospital.

The psychiatrically oriented and informed obstetrician and the maternity nurse are the ideal mental hygienists of pregnancy. The nurse, without being a psychiatrist, can contribute a lion's share to the emotional well-being of the mother and to the baby's wholesome start in life. For this purpose, she needs three major attributes: (1) the ability to understand; (2) the ability to listen; and (3) the ability to guide.

The Ability to Understand

Adequate information is one of the first prerequisites. As everywhere else in science, there are a few basic facts which must be learned before any sort of understanding can be reached. Furthermore, a nurse needs this knowledge not only for the sake of her own enlightenment but also to be able to impart it to her patients. Hall and Mohr recorded the types of questions which expectant mothers ask of their mentors in the course of pregnancy. The most frequently recurring questions were about physical care during pregnancy, the initial needs of the child, heredity and "marking." Some of these questions indicate in themselves the presence of quandaries and apprehensions and a desire for clarification.

The Ability to Listen

Patient, empathic listening is one of the greatest assets of anyone who tries to help human beings. People who have problems appreciate nothing more than an opportunity to pour out their troubles. The very act of verbalizing one's perplexities, of trying to hold them before oneself, of setting them forth before someone else, often affords great relief and helps the complainant to gain a better perspective regarding her complaints. There is nothing more frustrating than the experience of a patient who is anxious to talk herself out and is shut off with a remark, however well meant, such as: "Oh, forget it," "Now, don't let that worry you," or "This is just your imagination." It is far more helpful to encourage the speaker by asking interestedly: "What makes you feel that way?" or "Why does this bother you?"

The Ability to Guide

There is a great difference between guidance and direction. Inexperienced, insecure or tactless people often have a tendency to parade their authority and their better knowledge. Advice is given in terms of: "Do as I tell you," and "Take it or leave it." Such an approach does not invite willing cooperation. Patients want to be guided, not bullied. Guidance includes readiness to explain one's directions and to make them acceptable. The aim is voluntary compliance through insight, not blind obedience through intimidation.

Understanding, listening and guidance are the cornerstones of the nurse's positive contribution to the mental hygiene of pregnancy. Without them, mothers will shy away from an otherwise most efficient nurse. They will, and should, shrink back if, having reached out for psychological help, they find that their plea is not recognized or is handled clumsily.

The first contact between the expectant mother and the maternity nurse should be made an occasion for the establishment of a cordial mutual reationship. In this first interview, the pregnant woman should be helped to feel that she has acquired a sympathetic friend to whom she can talk about herself without hesitation. If there is economic distress, the nurse ought to be sufficiently familiar with the communal resources to be able to advise the family about possibilities of applying for and obtaining the necessary financial assistance.

The expectant mother's fears about herself and the baby-to-come should not be dismissed lightly with some indifferent phrase. When the mother has been allowed to reveal the nature and, as far as she can, the sources of her apprehension, she can be reassured by the nurse's explanations based on her better knowledge of the facts. Superstitious fears can thus be dispelled; erroneous notions about heredity and antepartal influences can thus be corrected. There will always be a greater or lesser degree of anxiety about the delivery, especially in primiparae and in mothers whose earlier pregnancy or pregnancies have been aggravated by unpleasant complications. In such instances no amount of reasoning or disputing will succeed in removing the residual fear, but the mother can be helped to accept and adjust to the fear, much as a brave soldier accepts and adjusts to the fear of impending battle. She will be helped particularly by being allowed to live a normal and active life as long as this is possible. Activity is the best prophylaxis against brooding. Though a reasonable amount of rest is needed and highly desirable, modern obstetricians are rightly not in favor of inactivity and inertia during pregnancy. Eastman, discussing "the abuse of rest in obstetrics," wrote: "In whatever class of society, unoccupied life is not conducive to the health of the expectant mother." In view of the experiences with employed pregnant women in both world wars in this country and in England, Eastman felt that "it seems to have been clearly established that it is just as safe, with certain reservations, for pregnant women to work in industrial plants as it is for them to work at home."

The nurse often has an opportunity to contribute to the mental hygiene of the expected baby's older sibling. Profound jealousies among brothers and sisters are created sometimes by the improper preparation of a child for the arrival of a new baby. The existing child, who has had all the attention of his parents, suddenly and unexpectedly finds that an unannounced intruder is occupying his place and, by the very nature of things, seems to be monopolizing his mother's time. Prudishness or ignorance of the possible effects keeps many parents from introducing the new situation to the child gradually and in a manner which would help him to welcome, instead of jealously resenting, the new baby. The nurse can enlighten the family about the best means to prepare the child and bring home to them an understanding of his emotional needs for continued attention and show of affection.

There is little that a nurse can do about the fundamental mechanisms of maternal rejection. Rejection, as we have seen, involves deep-rooted unconscious conflicts which cannot be solved on a conscious level. Nevertheless, even then it helps the mother if she can voice her feelings in the presence of an understanding listener who, by her sympathetic attitude, can at least relieve her of some of her guilty feeling and anxiety. Besides, as Menninger stated, many "prospective parents can accept consciously an unwanted pregnancy with few, if any, manifestations of rejection," especially if they have a chance to discuss their feelings with someone who has insight into their emotional attitudes.

Even though the basic background of rejection is beyond the nurse's scope, she can do much to alleviate some of its most disturbing effects, namely, those of perfectionistic coerciveness and overprotection. In fact, she can be a key figure in the task of parent education.

We have emerged but recently from an era in which physicians and psychologists alike not only sanctioned parental perfectionism but also imposed on mothers rigid rules and regulations which invited obsessiveness. Even then, the average mother, using common sense, did not allow herself to become a mechanized robot to whom the rules were more important than the baby. But insecure mothers, unable to rely on their own resources, inclined to punctiliousness, binding themselves to thou-shalts and thou-shalt-nots, developed a habit of rearing their children "by the book." The psychological school of behaviorism preached the gospel of impersonal "conditioning." Earlier pediatrics tried to cultivate addiction to the clock, a prescribed number of ounces, standard weight charts and calculation of calories. She was considered a good mother who never departed an iota from all these commandments. The sooner and the more persistently she started with toilet training, the higher was her efficiency rating in the eyes of her environment.

The past two decades witnessed a wholesome rebellion against this enthrallment of mother and child. The discovery—or rediscovery—of the character-shaping value of maternal warmth, affection, naturalness and personal handling of the baby initiated a trend toward recognition of "the rights of infants." A baby is no longer regarded as something like a machine to be oiled, cleaned, purged of refuse and immobilized by the clock. He is looked upon as a human being on the way to form relationships with other human beings, relationships which depend on the attitudes of the people closest to him as much as the health of his body depends on proper nutrition, shelter and cleanliness.

This by no means indicates an abandonment of principles and rules based on such principles, but it does indicate an abandonment of obsessive enslavement to rules. It introduces the emphasis on *enjoyment* of the baby, whose care is made a pleasure rather than a succession of chores. It was found that, unless there are physical obstacles, breast feeding makes for a happier contact between mother and child than bottle feeding. It was learned that patient and not too precocious bowel training is far better for the mental hygiene of the child than coercive bowel training. It has been established that occasional picking up and fondling, far from resulting in the dreaded "spoiling," builds in the child a sense of security and of being accepted and loved.

A mother who had reared two children well found herself "accidentally" pregnant again. The discovery was a "shock" to her. Remembering that her two children occasionally refused their spinach and sometimes did not obey her promptly, she made up her mind to rear her third child "scientifically." She lived up to every rule. The child was kept in her crib, was never picked up except to have the diapers changed. Nutrition, ventilation and everything else pertaining to physical welfare were perfect. Yet the baby, who was well endowed, failed to relate herself to her environment. She lived "in a world of her own." When I saw her at the age of 5 years, she was completely withdrawn and, in her schizophrenic aloneness, gave the impression of an idiotic child. This girl, who had been reared "perfectly," became a tragic victim of this type of perfection.

A maternity nurse could have saved this child by helping the mother to recognize the grave hazards of impersonal perfectionism. Pregnancy and puerperium are the best time for implanting healthy methods of child rearing. It cannot be emphasized strongly enough that the maternity nurse, in conjunction with the obstetrician, can do more than any other professional person to engender wholesome attitudes in parents toward their children. The work then can be taken up by pediatricians. Psychiatrists are not called into play until something has gone wrong. It is their job to study the causes of the damage and to communicate these causes to the natural mental hygienists of childhood—obstetricians, pediatricians and professional nurses.

SUMMARY

The mental hygiene of pregnancy, extending over a period of almost a year, is concerned with the emotional health of the expectant mother, the baby-to-come and sometimes the children already present. The mother's fear for herself and the baby and a rejecting attitude toward pregnancy and the child are the most powerful obstacles to emotional well-being. Rejection can manifest itself through neglect, perfectionistic coercion or overprotection. The public health nurse can do much to prevent mental difficulties by her understanding, ability to listen and tactful guidance, by dispelling pseudoscientific and superstitious fears and, above all, by helping the mother to institute adequate methods of child rearing. Such an orientation places the nurse in the front line of mental hygiene.

SUGGESTED READING

Ackerman, Nathan: The Psychodynamics of Family Life, New York, Basic, 1961.

Bowlby, John: Maternal Care and Mental Health, Geneva, World Health Organization, 1952.

———: Child Care and the Growth of Love, Baltimore, Penguin, 1961.

Caplan, Gerald: Preparation for healthy parenthood, Children 1:171, 1954.

———: Concepts of Mental Health and Consultation—Their Application in Public Health Social Work, Publication No. 373, Washington, D. C., U. S. Children's Bureau, 1959.

———: Practical steps for the family physician in the prevention of emotional disorder, J.A.M.A. 170:1497-1506, 1959.

———: An Approach to Community Mental Health, New York, Grune & Stratton, 1961.

Chivers, Norman: Practical approaches to emotional factors in pregnancy, Bull. Maternal and Infant Health 8, No. 1:21-23, 1961.

Deutsch, H.: Psychology of Women, vol. 2, Motherhood, New York, Grune & Stratton, 1945.

Kaplan, D. M., and Mason, E. A.: Maternal reactions to premature birth viewed as an acute emotional disorder, Am. J. Orthopsychiat. 30, No. 3:539-542, July, 1960.

Kartchner, F. D.: A study of the emotional reactions during labor, Am. J. Obstet. Gynec. 60: 19, 1950.

Klein, H. R., Potter, H. W., and Dyk, R. B.: Anxiety in Pregnancy and Childbirth, New York, Hoeber, 1950.

Newton, Niles: Maternal Emotions, New York, Hoeber, 1955.

Newton, Niles, and Newton, Michael: Mothers' reactions to their newborn babies, J.A.M.A. 181:206-210, July 21, 1962.

Peplau, Hildegarde: Anxiety in the mother-infant relationship, Nurs. World. 60:1133-1134, 1960.

Pheshette, Norman, *et al.*: A study of anxieties during pregnancy, labor, the early and late puerperium, Bull. N. Y. Acad. Med. 32:436, 1956.

Selye, Hans: The stress syndrome, Am. J. Nurs. 65, No. 3:97-99, March, 1965.

Straus, Barbara: Mental hygiene in pregnancy, Am. J. Nurs. 56:314, 1956.

CONFERENCE MATERIAL

1. What opportunities are available for teaching in the antepartal clinic while the patients are waiting their "turn" for examination?

2. How would you assist the mother with arrangements for the care of her children during the time that she is in the hospital? What organizations provide such care in your community?

3. For the antepartal patient who never has had any hospital experience, how would you introduce her to the antepartal clinic and prepare her for the complete physical examination?

4. How would you include the father and the other children in helping with the preparations for the new baby and the care of both the mother and the baby after delivery?

5. In discussing antepartal care with parents, how would you explain the relationship of the mother's diet to the baby's development from the time of conception until his birth?

6. In regard to the danger signals of pregnancy, how could you present these to an apprehensive patient without creating undue alarm?

7. What are the reasons for stressing the importance of completing the preparations for delivery by the 7th month of pregnancy?

8. What sources would you consult to find out which states in the United States require premarital and antepartal examinations for the detection of syphilis?

9. What type of referral system is used in your community when it is necessary for the patient to consult other community agencies for health or social services?

Study Questions

UNIT TWO: NURSING IN PREGNANCY

Read through the entire question and place your answer on the line to the right.

1. Below are some signs, symptoms and conditions commonly associated with pregnancy. Those which the patient might notice and describe in the first trimester of pregnancy are:
A. Amenorrhea
B. Enlargement and tenderness of breasts
C. Enlargement of uterus
D. Frequent micturition
E. Goodell's sign
Select the number corresponding to the correct letters.
   1. A and C
   2. A, B and D
   3. B, D and E
   4. All of them   **2**

2. A. In pregnancy, morning sickness is most common during which of the following periods?
   1. First month
   2. First 6 weeks
   3. Sixth to 12th week
   4. First 4 months
   5. Eighth to 16th week   **3**
B. A patient complains of morning sickness. Which of the following measures should the nurse suggest as a possible means of overcoming this discomfort?
   1. Keep the stomach empty when nausea is present.
   2. Drink plenty of water upon arising.
   3. Eat 6 small meals instead of 3 per day.
   4. Increase daily intake of whole milk.   **3**

3. A pregnant woman seen for the first time in the antepartal clinic has a hemoglobin of 70 per cent. The nurse should understand that this condition is:
A. A true anemia
B. Caused by increased blood volume
C. Dangerous to baby's development
D. Predisposing to postpartal hemorrhage   **B**

4. The nurse in the obstetrician's office should instruct the patient regarding the collection of the specimen for the Aschheim-Zondek test by telling the patient to:
A. Save the first voided specimen in the morning.
B. Withhold fluid intake during the night and collect the first voided specimen in the morning.
C. Report to the laboratory in the morning for a blood specimen.
D. Take a warm voided specimen to the laboratory.   **B**

5. Though the pregnant woman is usually advised to include a quart of milk in her diet daily, which of the following, if any, would justify the omission of milk?
A. Milk makes her constipated.
B. She is gaining weight too rapidly.
C. She is not gaining fast enough and needs more concentrated foods.
D. Milk causes a feeling of fullness, decreasing her appetite for other foods.
E. Milk causes heartburn.
F. None of the above; milk should not be omitted.   **F**

6. The most essential foods in a 2,300-calorie diet for a pregnant woman are:
A. High in carbohydrate, low in protein
B. High in protein, low in carbohydrate

C. High in protein, low in fat
D. High in fat, low in protein   ___C___

7. The nurse in the antepartal clinic will encourage the pregnant woman to see her dentist at the earliest convenience because:
A. Each baby causes the mother to lose one tooth.
B. Bone development of the baby requires calcium.
C. Foci of infection should be removed early in pregnancy.
D. The increased carbohydrate needed in pregnancy is detrimental to sound teeth.   ___C___

8. What instruction should the clinic patient be given concerning the care of her breasts during pregnancy?
A. A brassière should:
 1. Not be worn
 2. Be worn snugly enough to support and lift up the breasts
 3. Be worn snugly enough to press the breasts flat against the chest wall
 4. Be worn snugly enough to apply constant firm pressure toward the midline   ___2___
B. Special care of the nipples should begin:
 1. As early as pregnancy is confirmed
 2. Between the 3rd and 4th months
 3. Between the 6th and 7th months
 4. At the beginning of the 9th month   ___3___

9. Psychophysical preparation for childbearing is a term applied to a program in antepartal education.
A. The program includes certain "exercises" as one aspect of preparation. Which of the following are these "exercises" intended to accomplish?
 1. Promote control of muscle tension for coordination and economy of effort in all the mother's activities
 2. Develop intra-abdominal space for uterine enlargement
 3. Obviate the need for pharmaceutical analgesics   ___1___
B. The program prepares the pregnant patient for some of the experiences of labor. In addition to neuromuscular control, which of the following measures will be most helpful to her during labor?
 1. Sympathetic care
 2. Moderately heavy sedation
 3. Understanding the progress of labor   ___3___
C. Which of the following best explains the purpose of conscious control of respiration during the first stage of labor?
 1. Gives mechanical relief of pressure by depression of the diaphragm to expand the abdominal wall
 2. Limits the downward movement of the diaphragm through restriction of breathing to the upper chest
 3. Gives the patient a calming rhythmic activity upon which to concentrate   ___3___

10. A. If the pregnant woman complained of painful, swollen veins in the legs, the nurse would understand that the condition would be likely to be due to:
 1. Infection of the blood-vessel wall
 2. Toxins accumulating in the blood
 3. Pressure against the veins in the pelvis
 4. Pressure directly against the walls of the arteries
 5. Force of gravity   ___3___
B. To remedy this condition, the nurse would expect that the patient would be advised that she should:
 1. Refrain from wearing restricting clothing around the legs or the abdomen
 2. Refrain from wearing a corset
 3. Lie down each day for an hour's rest
 4. Apply an Ace bandage, starting above the source of obstruction   ___1___

11. The nurse teaching parents' classes should stress the importance of which one of the following?
A. Husbands doing the housework for their wives during the period of pregnancy

B. The idea of sharing responsibility in parenthood
C. The causes of invalidism during pregnancy
D. The moral responsibility of being parents

B

12. If a woman 6 months pregnant asked if she should or should not wear a corset, in your opinion the patient should be advised:
A. To avoid wearing any corset
B. To adjust her regular corset loosely
C. To wear a corset that will keep the uterus from rising too high in the abdomen
D. To wear a corset that will firmly support the lower portion of the abdomen and the back
E. To wear a corset that will not disclose her condition

D

13. The reason that pregnant women are warned against wearing high-heeled shoes from the 7th to the 9th months is:
A. To avoid additional backstrain
B. To increase venous pressure in the legs
C. To allow freer movement in taking daily exercises
D. To dress themselves according to current styles

A

14. The expectant mother who is employed as a stenographer should be advised that:
A. Rest periods are unnecessary if the job requires only "desk work."
B. Part-time employment should be requested after the 4th month of pregnancy.
C. A position which requires moderate manual labor would be more advantageous because it affords physical exercise.
D. Employment should be discontinued if the work causes moderate fatigue.

D

15. The clinic nurse would expect the pregnant patient to be advised to get in touch with her doctor *immediately* as soon as she observed which of the following?
A. Abdominal pain
B. Bleeding with bright blood
C. Blood-streaked mucus
D. Chills and fever
E. Constipation
Select the number corresponding to the correct letters.
    1. A, B and D
    2. B, C and E
    3. C, D and E
    4. All of them

1

16. In teaching the pregnant woman how to take a vaginal douche prescribed by the physician, the following should be emphasized:
A. A hand-bulb syringe is satisfactory if the mother is accustomed to using it.
B. The medicated solution must be prepared according to the physician's instructions.
C. The external genitalia should be cleansed with soap and water before taking a douche.
D. The douche may be taken while sitting on the toilet if the douche bag is placed no higher than 2 feet above the level of the hips.
E. The douche nozzle should be inserted gently into the vagina as far as it will go.
Select the number corresponding to the correct letters.
    1. A and B
    2. B and C
    3. B, D and E
    4. All of them

2

17. During her first visit to the clinic the mother confides to the nurse that she is afraid to have a baby. The most appropriate response of the nurse might be:
A. "Modern obstetrics makes having a baby so safe that you have absolutely nothing to fear."
B. "Perhaps if you discussed this with a psychiatrist he would help you to overcome this feeling."
C. "Many women feel this way, so I wouldn't be concerned about it if I were you."
D. "I can understand that you might feel this way. What is it in particular that you are worried about?"

D

Note: The key to the correct answers to these questions is given on page 597.

UNIT THREE

Nursing During Labor and Delivery

Phenomena of Labor
Analgesia and Anesthesia for Labor
Conduct of Normal Labor

Premonitory Signs of Labor • Cause of Onset of Labor • Uterine
Contractions • Duration of Labor • The Three Stages of Labor

Chapter 10

Phenomena of Labor

Labor is an event which follows pregnancy and is, in fact, the climax of the entire maternity cycle. During the 9 months of gestation certain physiologic and psychological adaptations gradually have taken place in the gravid woman, and simultaneously the growth and the development of the fetus have progressed toward maturity in preparation for the transition from intra-uterine to extra-uterine life.

Labor refers to the series of processes by which the products of conception are expelled from the mother's body (Fig. 10-1). The terms "childbirth," "travail," "accouchement" and "confinement" have all been used at one time or another to refer to labor. The word "delivery" refers, as a rule, to the actual delivery of the baby.

PREMONITORY SIGNS OF LABOR

During the last few weeks of pregnancy a number of changes indicate that the time of labor is approaching. Particularly in primigravidas, "lightening" occurs about 10 to 14 days before delivery. This alteration is brought about by a settling of the fetal head into the brim of the pelvis, often to such a degree that the lowest part of the occiput is at the level of the ischial spines (Fig. 10-2). This may occur at any time during the last 4 weeks, but occasionally does not eventuate until labor actually has begun. Lightening may take place

suddenly, so that the expectant mother arises one morning entirely relieved of the abdominal tightness and diaphragmatic pressure that she had experienced previously (Fig. 6-7). But the relief in one direction often is followed by signs of greater pressure below, such as shooting pains down the legs, an increase in the amount of vaginal discharge and greater frequency of urination due to pressure on the bladder. In mothers who have had previous children, lightening is more likely to occur after labor begins.

For a varying period before the establishment of true labor, the patients often will suffer from so-called "false labor," and the nurse should be able to distinguish between this and effective uterine contractions. True labor contractions will produce a demonstrable degree of dilatation of the cervix in the course of a few hours. On the other hand, false labor contractions are painful but do not affect the cervix. The crux of the matter, then, between true and false labor is whether or not the uterine contractions effect cervical effacement and dilatation.

False contractions may begin as early as 3 or 4 weeks before the termination of pregnancy. They are merely an exaggeration of the intermittent uterine contractions which have occurred throughout the entire period of gestation but are now accompanied by discomfort. They occur at decidedly irregular intervals, are confined chiefly to the lower part

211

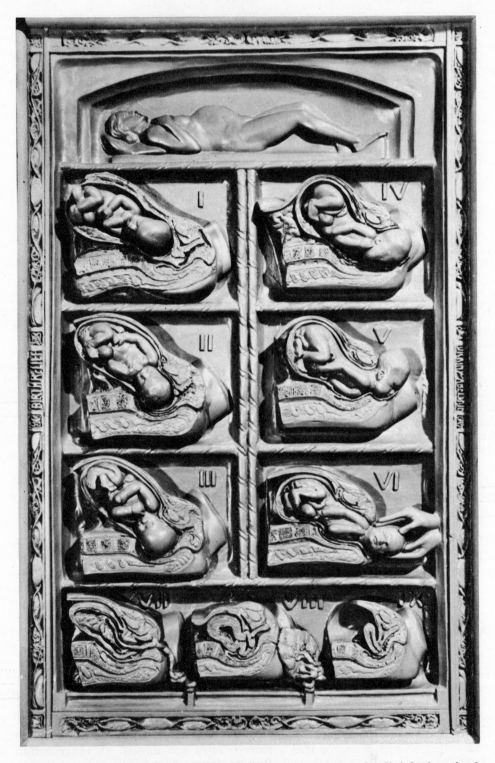

Fig. 10-1. "The Birth Relief." This distinguished sculptured relief depicts the 9 stages of birth with vertex presentation from before labor through the delivery of the placenta. (Dickinson-Belskie models, Cleveland Health Museum, Cleveland)

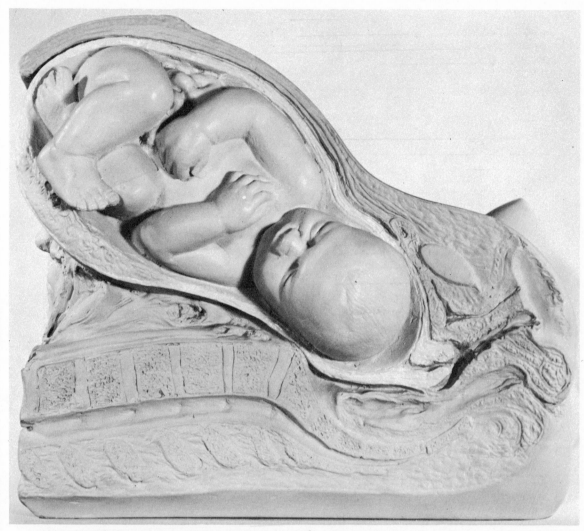

FIG. 10-2. Before labor, showing the uterus relaxed with the cervix closed and thick pelvic floor. (Dickinson-Belskie models, Cleveland Health Museum, Cleveland)

of the abdomen and the groin and do not increase in intensity, frequency and duration. The discomfort rarely is intensified if the mother walks about and may even be relieved if she is on her feet. Examination by the physician will reveal no changes in the cervix. The signs that accompany true labor contractions present a contrasting picture. True labor contractions usually are felt in the lower back and extend in girdlelike fashion from the back to the front of the abdomen. These contractions have a definite rhythm and gradually increase in frequency, intensity and duration. In the course of a few hours of true labor contractions a progressive effacement and dilatation of the cervix would be apparent.

Another sign of impending labor is pink "show." After the discharge of the mucous plug that has filled the cervical canal during pregnancy, the pressure of the descending presenting part of the fetus causes the minute capillaries in the mucous membrane of the cervix to rupture. This blood is mixed with mucus and therefore has the pink tinge. The nurse should understand that pink show is simply the appearance of a small amount of blood-tinged

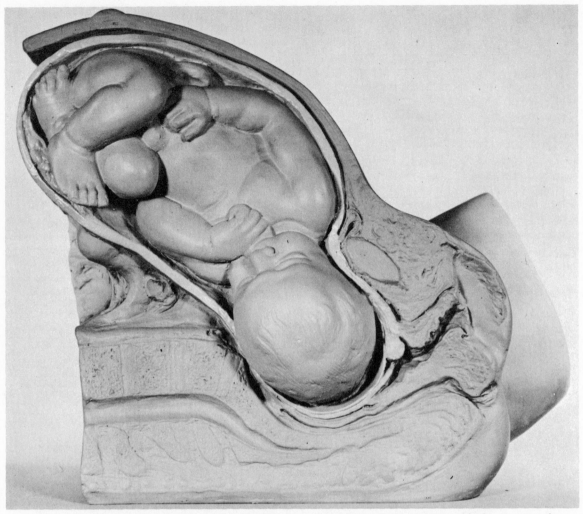

FIG. 10-3. First stage of labor. The rhythmic contractions of the uterus aid the progressive effacement and dilatation of the cervix, as well as the descent of the infant. (Dickinson-Belskie models, Cleveland Health Museum, Cleveland)

mucus, and that any substantial discharge of blood should be reported to the physician.

Occasionally, rupture of the membranes is the first indication of approaching labor. It used to be thought that this was a grave sign, heralding a long and difficult labor, but present-day statistics show that this is not true, and that rupture of the membranes often is followed by labors which are even shorter than the average. Nevertheless, the physician should be notified at once; under these circumstances, he usually will advise the patient to enter the hospital immediately. After the rupture of the membranes there is always the possibility of a prolapsed cord if the presenting part does not adequately fill the pelvic inlet. This might occur if the infant presents as a footling breech, or by the shoulder, or in the vertex presentation when the fetal head has not descended far enough into the true pelvis prior to the rupture of the membranes (see Fig. 19-8).

CAUSE OF ONSET OF LABOR

Regardless of species, whether the fetus weighs 2 Gm. at the end of a 21-day pregnancy, as in the mouse, or whether it weighs 200 pounds at the end of a 640-day pregnancy, as in the elephant, labor regularly begins at the right time for that particular species, namely, when the fetus is mature enough to cope with extra-uterine conditions but not yet large enough to cause mechanical difficulties in labor. The process responsible for this beautifully synchronized and salutary achievement is obscure. Nevertheless, countless theories have been advanced to explain the phenomenon. Among them may be mentioned increased irritability of the uterus as the result of greater distention, growing distention of the lower uterine structures with pressure on the surrounding nerves and the influences of hormones.

UTERINE CONTRACTIONS

In all languages the word for the uterine contractions of labor has been interpreted the same, namely, "pain." Alone among normal physiologic muscular contractions, moreover, those of labor can be painful. The duration of these contractions ranges from 45 seconds to 1 minute and a quarter, averaging about 1 minute. Each contraction presents 3 phases: a period during which the intensity of the contraction increases (increment), a period during which the contraction is at its height (acme), and a peroid of diminishing intensity (decrement). The increment, or crescendo phase, is longer than the other two combined. The contractions of the uterus during labor are intermittent, with periods of relaxation between, resembling in this respect the systole and the diastole of the heart. The interval between contractions diminishes gradually from about 10 minutes early in labor to about 2 or 3 minutes in the second stage. These periods of relaxation not only provide rest for the uterine muscles and for the mother but also are essen-

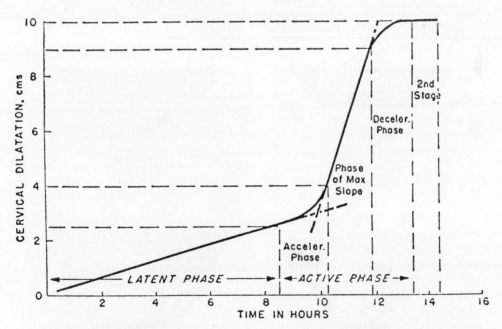

MEAN LABOR CURVE

FIG. 10-4. Graphic appraisal of the time factor in labor. The *latent phase* includes that portion of the first stage between the onset of labor contractions and acceleration in the rate of cervical dilatation. The upswing in the curve denotes the onset of the *active phase* of the first stage of labor, which includes the accelerated phase, the phase of maximum slope and the deceleration phase. (Friedman, E. A.: Graphic appraisal of labor. A study of 500 primigravidas, Bull. Sloane Hosp. Wom. 1:42, 1955)

tial for the welfare of the fetus, since unremitting contractions may so interfere with placental functions that the resulting lack of oxygen produces fetal distress. Another characteristic of labor contractions is that they are quite involuntary, their action being not only independent of the mother's will but also of extra-uterine nervous control. In other words, uterine action in labor, like that of the heart, is under control of nerves located within the organ itself.

DURATION OF LABOR

Although there is usually some degree of variation in all labors, an estimate of the average length of labor can be based on studies of records of some several thousand primigravidas and multiparas (see Suggested Reading). The average duration of first labors is about 14 hours, approximately 12½ hours in the first stage, 1 hour and 20 minutes in the second stage, and 10 minutes in the third stage. The average duration of multiparous labors is approximately 6 hours shorter than for first labors; for example, 7 hours and 20 minutes in the first stage, a half hour in the second stage, and 10 minutes in third stage.

During the first stage of labor full dilatation of the cervix (10 cm.) is accomplished, but for the greater part of this time little cervical dilatation is accomplished. This has been clearly demonstrated in Friedman's study of 500 labors of primigravidous women (Fig. 10-4). From his study labor is divided into the latent phase and the active phase. The *latent phase*, from the onset of uterine contractions, takes many hours and accomplishes little cervical dilatation. But with the beginning of the *active phase*, cervical dilatation proceeds at an accelerated rate and then reaches a deceleration phase shortly before the second stage of labor.

THE THREE STAGES OF LABOR

The process of labor is divided, for convenience of description, into 3 distinct stages.

The first stage of labor, *or the dilating stage, begins with the first true labor contraction and ends with the complete dilatation of the cervix.*

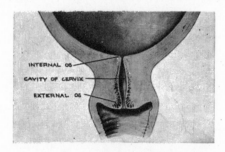
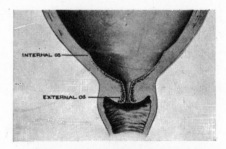
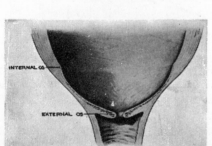
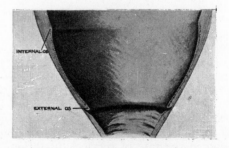

FIG. 10-5. Cervix in primigravida. (*Top, left*) At beginning of labor; no effacement or dilatation. (*Top, right*) About one half effaced, but no dilatation. (*Bottom, left*) Completely effaced, but no dilatation. (*Bottom, right*) Complete dilatation. (Bumm)

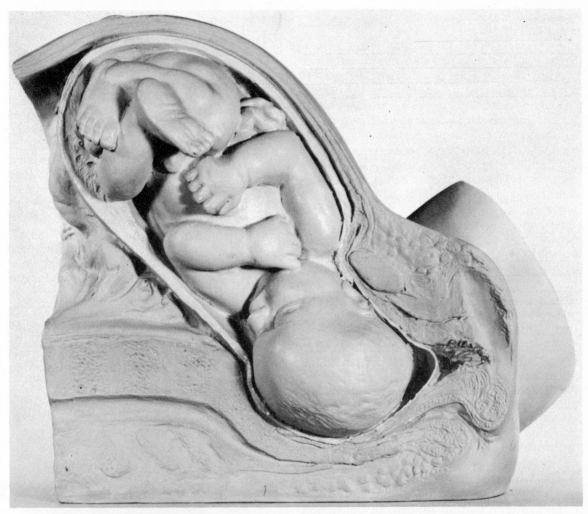

Fig. 10-6. Full dilatation: cervix high, head deep in birth canal, membranes intact. (Dickinson-Belskie models, Cleveland Health Museum, Cleveland)

The second stage of labor, *or the stage of expulsion, begins with the complete dilatation of the cervix and ends with the delivery of the baby.*

The third stage of labor, *or the placental stage, begins with the delivery of the baby and terminates with the birth of the placenta.*

The First Stage of Labor

In the beginning of the first stage the contractions are short, slight, or 10 or 15 minutes or more apart and may not cause the patient any particular discomfort. She may be walking about and between contractions is generally quite comfortable. Early in the first stage the discomfort usually is located in the small of the back, but, as time goes on, it sweeps around, girdlelike, to the anterior part of the abdomen. The contractions recur at shortening intervals, every 3 to 5 minutes, and become stronger and last longer. Indeed, the contractions which precede and accompany full dilatation are often of excruciating severity. At this time, furthermore, there is usually a marked increase in the amount of show due to rupture of capillary vessels in the cervix and the lower uterine segment.

As the result of the uterine contractions, two all-important changes are wrought in the cervix during the first stage of labor—*efface-ment* and *dilatation* (Fig. 10-3).

Effacement is the shortening of the cervical canal from a structure 1 or 2 cm. in length to one in which no canal at all exists, but merely a circular orifice with almost paper-thin edges. As may be seen in Figure 10-5, the edges of the internal os are drawn several centimeters upward, so that the former cervical mucosa becomes part of the lower uterine segment and lies parallel with and contiguous to the chorion membrane. Effacement may be compared with a funneling process in which the whole length of a moldable tube (the cervical canal) is converted into a very large, flaring funnel, with only a small circular orifice for an outlet. In primigravidas, effacement is usually complete before dilatation begins, but in multiparas it is rarely complete, dilatation proceeding, as a rule, with rather thick cervical edges. Synonymous with effacement are the terms "obliteration" and "taking up" of the cervix.

Dilatation of the Cervix. By this is meant the enlargement of the external os from an orifice a few millimeters in size to an aperture large enough to permit the passage of the fetus—that is, to one with a diameter of about 10 cm. When dilatation has reached this figure, it is said to be complete. Although the forces concerned in dilatation are not well understood, several factors appear to be involved. In the first place, the muscle fibers about the cervix are so arranged that they pull upon its edges and tend to draw it open. In the second place, the uterine contractions make pressure on the bag of waters and this, in turn, burrows into the cervix in pouchlike fashion, exerting a dilating action (Fig. 10-6). This is usually called the hydrostatic pressure of the bag of waters. In the absence of the bag of waters, the pressure of the presenting part against the cervix and the lower uterine segment has a similar effect.

It should be noted that the dilatation of the cervix in the first stage of labor is solely the result of uterine contractions which are involuntary. In other words, there is nothing that the mother can do, such as bearing down, which will help the slightest in expediting this period of labor. Indeed, bearing-down efforts at this stage serve only to exhaust the mother and cause the cervix to become edematous.

The Second Stage of Labor

The contractions are now severe and long, lasting 50 to 70 seconds and occurring at intervals of 2 or 3 minutes. Rupture of the membranes usually occurs during the early part of this stage of labor by a gush of amniotic fluid from the vagina. Sometimes, however, membranes rupture during the first stage and occasionally, as already indicated, before labor begins. In rare instances the membranes fail to rupture, and the baby is born with the intact amniotic sac surrounding it. Obviously, in such cases the membranes must be artificially ruptured at once, for otherwise the infant will drown. In some rare cases the baby is born in a "caul," which is a piece of the amnion that sometimes envelops the baby's head. Superstitious parents consider this to be a good omen.

During this stage, as if by reflex action, the muscles of the abdomen are brought into play; and when the contractions are in progress the patient will strain, or "bear down," with all her strength so that her face becomes flushed, and the large vessels in her neck are distended. As a result of this exertion she may perspire profusely. During this stage the mother directs all her energy toward expelling the contents of the uterus.

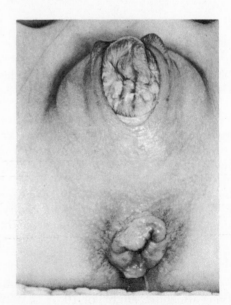

FIG. 10-7. Extreme bulging of perineum showing patulous and everted anus.

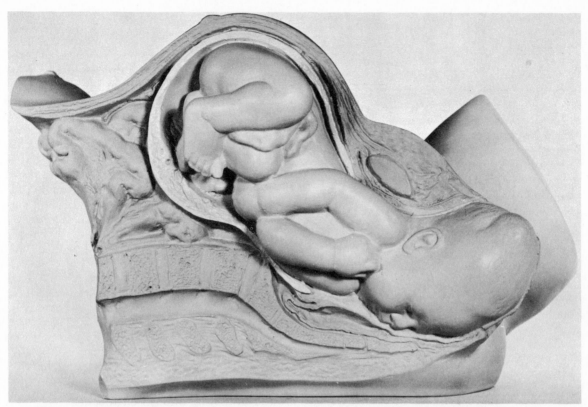

FIG. 10-8. Second stage of labor. "Caput," or top of infant's head, begins to appear through the vulvar opening. (Dickinson-Belskie models, Cleveland Health Museum, Cleveland)

Toward the end of the second stage, when the head is well down in the vagina, its pressure causes the anus to become patulous and everted (Fig. 10-7), and often small particles of fecal material may be expelled from the rectum at the occurrence of each contraction. This condition must receive careful attention to avoid contamination. As the head descends still further, the perineal region begins to bulge, and the skin over it becomes tense and glistening. At this time the scalp of the fetus may be detected through a slitlike vulvar opening (Fig. 10-8). With each subsequent contraction the perineum bulges more and more, and the vulva becomes more dilated and distended by the head, so that the opening is gradually converted into an ovoid and at last into a circle. With the cessation of each contraction the opening becomes smaller, and the head recedes from it until it advances again with the next contraction.

The contractions now occur very rapidly, with scarcely any interval between. As the head becomes increasingly visible, the vulva is stretched further and finally encircles the largest diameter of the baby's head. This encirclement of the largest diameter of the baby's head by the vulvar ring is known as "crowning." The physician now supports the tissues surrounding the perineum and delivers the head between contractions. One or two more contractions are normally enough to effect the birth of the baby.

Whereas in the first stage of labor the forces are limited to uterine action, during the second stage two forces are essential, namely, uterine contractions and intra-abdominal pressure, the latter being brought about by the bearing-down efforts of the mother. (The force exerted by the mother's bearing down can be likened to that used in forcing an evacuation of the bowels.) Both forces are essential to the successful spontaneous outcome of the second stage of labor, for uterine contractions without

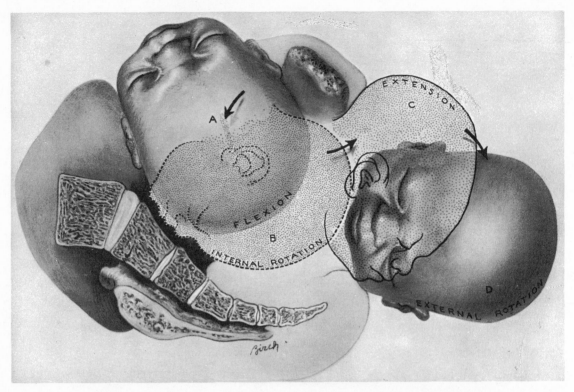

Fig. 10-9. L.O.A. Positional changes of head in passing through birth canal.

bearing-down efforts are of little avail in expelling the infant, while, conversely, bearing-down efforts in the absence of uterine contractions are futile. As explained in Chapter 12, Conduct of Normal Labor, these facts have most important practical implications.

In its passage through the birth canal, the presenting part of the fetus undergoes certain positional changes which constitute the mechanism of labor. These movements are designed to present the smallest possible diameters of the presenting part to the irregular shape of the pelvic canal, so that it will encounter as little resistance as possible. The mechanism of labor consists of a combination of movements, several of which may be going on at the same time. As they occur, the uterine contractions bring about important modifications in the attitude or habitus of the fetus, especially after the head has descended into the pelvis. This adaptation of the baby to the birth canal, as descent takes place, involves the four processes called flexion, internal rotation, extension and external rotation (Fig. 10-9).

For purposes of instruction, the various movements will be described as if they occurred independently of one another.

As previously stated, in the primigravida, engagement usually occurs during the last weeks of pregnancy, but in the multipara it ordinarily does not take place until after labor has begun. When the biparietal diameter of the infant's head is within the pelvic inlet, engagement is said to have occurred.

Descent. The first requisite for the birth of the infant is descent. In primigravidas, because engagement is frequently deep at the onset of labor, further descent does not necessarily begin until the second stage of labor sets in. In multiparas, on the other hand, descent begins with engagement. In either event, once having been inaugurated, descent is inevitably associated with the various movements of the mechanism of labor.

Flexion. Very early in the process of descent the head becomes so flexed that the chin is in contact with the sternum, and, as a consequence, the very smallest anteroposterior

Fig. 10-10. Successive stages of extrusion of placenta: (*left*) by Schultze's mechanism; (*right*) by Duncan's mechanism.

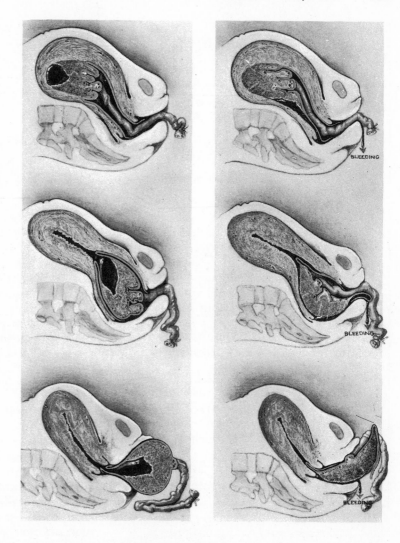

diameter (the suboccipitobregmatic plane) is presented to the pelvis.

Internal Rotation. As seen in Chapter 2, the head enters the pelvis in the transverse or diagonal position. When it reaches the pelvic floor, the occiput is rotated and comes to lie beneath the symphysis pubis. In other words, the sagittal suture is now in the anteroposterior diameter of the outlet (Fig. 2-7). Although the occiput usually rotates to the front, on occasion it may turn toward the hollow of the sacrum. If anterior rotation does not take place at all, the occiput usually rotates to the direct occiput posterior position, a condition known as persistent occiput posterior. Since this represents a deviation from the normal mechanism of labor, it will be considered in

Chapter 19, under Abnormal Fetal Positions.

Extension. After the occiput emerges from the pelvis, the nape of the neck becomes arrested beneath the pubic arch and acts as a pivotal point for the rest of the head. Extension of the head now ensues, and with it the frontal portion of the head, the face and the chin are born (Fig. 10-11).

External Rotation. After the birth of the head, it remains in the anteroposterior position only a very short time and shortly will be seen to turn to one or another side of its own accord—*restitution.* When the occiput originally has been directed toward the left of the mother's pelvis, it then rotates toward the left tuberischii, and in the opposite direction when it originally has been toward the right. This is

---

**SUMMARY OF MECHANISM
OF LABOR**

First Stage—Dilating Stage

Definition. **Period from first true labor contraction to complete dilatation of cervix.**

What Is Accomplished? **Effacement and dilatation of cervix.**

Forces Involved. **Uterine contractions.**

Second Stage—Expulsive Stage

Definition. **Period from complete dilatation of cervix to birth of baby.**

What Is Accomplished? **Expulsion of baby from birth canal—facilitated by certain positional changes of fetus: descent, flexion, internal rotation, extension, external rotation and expulsion.**

Forces Involved. **Uterine contractions plus intra-abdominal pressure.**

Third Stage—Placental Stage

Definition. **Period from birth of baby through birth of placenta.**

What Is Accomplished? **(A) Separation of placenta; (B) expulsion of placenta.**

Forces Involved. **(A) Uterine contractions; (B) intra-abdominal pressure.**

---

known as external rotation and is due to the fact that the shoulders of the baby, having entered the pelvis in the transverse position, undergo internal rotation to the anteroposterior position, as did the head; this brings about a corresponding rotation of the head, which is now on the outside. The shoulders are born in a manner somewhat similar to that of the head. Almost immediately after the occurrence of external rotation, the anterior shoulder appears under the symphysis pubis and becomes arrested temporarily beneath the pubic arch, to act as a pivotal point for the other shoulder (Fig. 10-12). As the anterior margin of the perineum becomes distended, the posterior shoulder is born, assisted by an upward lateral flexion of the infant's body. Once the shoulders are delivered, the infant's body is quickly ex-

truded (expulsion) because of its relative size.

The average duration of the second stage of labor in primigravidas is an hour and a quarter, and in multiparas about 30 minutes or less. Sometimes 2 or 3 contractions suffice for the completion of the period of expulsion.

The Third Stage of Labor

The third stage of labor is made up of two phases, namely, *the phase of placental separation* and *the phase of placenta expulsion.*

Immediately following the birth of the infant, the remainder of the amniotic fluid escapes, after which there is usually a slight flow of blood. The uterus can be felt as a firm globular mass just below the level of the umbilicus. Shortly thereafter, the uterus relaxes and assumes a discoid shape. With each subsequent contraction or relaxation the uterus changes from globular to discoid shape until the placenta has separated, after which time the globular shape persists.

Placental Separation. As the uterus contracts down at regular intervals on its diminishing content, the area of placental attachment is greatly reduced. The great disproportion between the reduced size of the placental site and that of the placenta brings about a folding or festooning of the maternal surface of the placenta (Fig. 10-13); with this process separation takes place. Meanwhile, bleeding takes place within these placental folds, and this expedites separation of the organ. The placenta now sinks into the lower uterine segment or upper vagina as an unattached body.

The signs which suggest that the placenta has separated are: (1) the uterus becomes globular in shape and, as a rule, firmer; (2) it rises upward in the abdomen; (3) the umbilical cord descends 3 or more inches farther out of the vagina; and (4) a sudden gush of blood often occurs. These signs usually occur within 5 minutes after the delivery of the infant.

Placental Expulsion. Actual expulsion of the placenta may be brought about by bearing-down efforts on the part of the mother if she is not anesthetized. If this cannot be accomplished, it is usually effected through gentle pressure on the uterine fundus by the physician after he has first made certain that the uterus is hard. This never should be attempted when the uterus is relaxed, because the organ

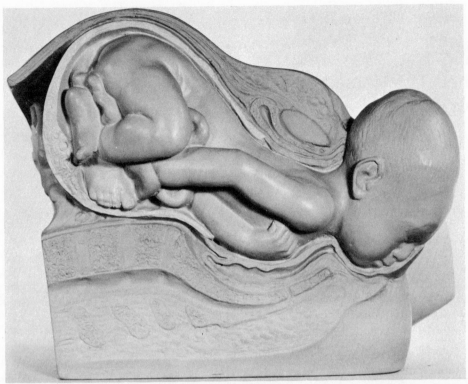

FIG. 10-11. Head extends upward; pelvic floor retreats. (Dickinson-Belskie models, Cleveland Health Museum, Cleveland)

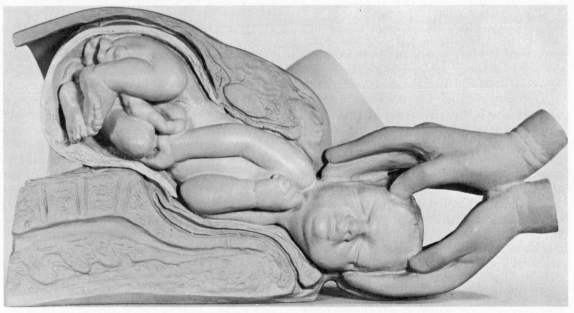

FIG. 10-12. Birth of shoulders: rotating to accommodate to birth passage. (Dickinson-Belskie models, Cleveland Health Museum, Cleveland)

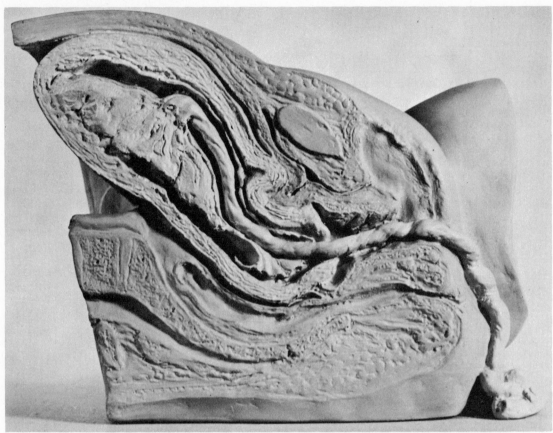

FIG. 10-13. Separation of placenta. (Dickinson-Belskie models, Cleveland Health Museum, Cleveland)

may turn inside-out and result in one of the gravest complications of obstetrics, so-called "inversion" of the uterus (see Chap. 19).

The extrusion of the placenta may take place by one of two mechanisms. First, it may become turned inside-out within the vagina and be born like an inverted umbrella with the glistening fetal surfaces presenting. This is known as Schultze's mechanism and occurs in about 80 per cent of cases. Second, it may become somewhat rolled up in the vagina, with the maternal surface outermost, and be born edgewise. The latter is known as Duncan's mechanism and is seen in about 20 per cent of deliveries (Fig. 10-10). It is believed that the Schultze's mechanism signifies that the placenta has become detached first at its center, and usually a collection of blood and clots is found in the sac of membranes. The Duncan mechanism, on the other hand, suggests that

the placenta has separated first at its edges, and it is in this type that bleeding usually occurs at the time of separation.

The contraction of the uterus following delivery serves not only to produce placental separation but also to control uterine hemorrhage. As the result of this contraction of the uterine muscle fibers, the countless blood vessels within their interstices are clamped shut. Even then, a certain amount of blood loss in the third stage is unavoidable, the average being about 250 to 300 cc. It is one of the aims of the conduct of labor to reduce this bleeding to a very minimum.

SUGGESTED READING

Borell, U. L. F., *et al.*: Effect of uterine contractions on the human uteroplacental blood circulation, Am. J. Obstet. Gynec. 89:881-890, August 1, 1964.

Brady, J. P., and James, L. S.: Heart rate changes in fetus and newborn infant during labor, delivery and the immediate neonatal period, Am. J. Obstet. Gynec. 84:1-13, July, 1962.

Brundin, J., and Engstom, L.: Studies of diuresis during spontaneous and oxytocin induced labor, Obstet. Gynec. 16:577-580, November, 1960.

Burnhill, M. S., et al.: Uterine contractility during labor studied by intra-amniotic fluid pressure recordings, Am. J. Obstet. Gynec. 83: 561-571, March 1, 1962.

Busby, Trent: The duration of labor: mean, median, and mode, Am. J. Obstet. Gynec. 55: 846-851, May, 1948.

Caldwell, W. E., Moloy, H. C., and D'Esopo, D. A.: A roentgenologic study of the mechanism of the engagement of the fetal head, Am. J. Obstet. Gynec. 28:824, 1934.

Cibils, L. A., and Hendricks, C. H.: Normal labor in vertex presentation, Am. J. Obstet. Gynec. 91:385-395, February 1, 1965.

Eastman, N. J.: Williams' Obstetrics, ed. 13, New York, Appleton, 1966.

Fitzhugh, M. L., and Newton, Michael: Muscle action during childbirth, Phys. Ther. Rev. 36: 805-809, December, 1956.

Friedman, E. A.: Graphic appraisal of labor. A study of 500 primigravidas, Bull. Sloane Hosp. Wom. 1:42, 1955.

————: Relation of maternal age to the course of labor, Am. J. Obstet. Gynec. 91:915-924, April 1, 1965.

Friedman, E. A., et al.: The effect of uterine overdistention on labor, Obstet. Gynec. 23:164-172, February, 1964.

Greenhill, J. P.: Obstetrics, ed. 13, Philadelphia, Saunders, 1965.

Guyton, A. C.: Textbook of Medical Physiology, ed. 2, Philadelphia, Saunders, 1961.

Hendricks, C. H., et al.: Pressure relationships between the intervillous space and the amniotic fluid in human term pregnancy, Am. J. Obstet. Gynec. 77:1028-1037, May, 1959.

Hon, E. H.: Electronic evaluation of fetal heart rates, Am. J. Obstet. Gynec. 83:333-338, February 1, 1962.

Hunter, C. A., Jr.: Uterine motility studies during labor, observation on bilateral sympathetic nerve block in the normal and abnormal first stage labor, Am. J. Obstet. Gynec. 85:681-686, March 1, 1963.

Kastell, B.: The facilitation of labour by abdominal compression, Physiotherapy 47:161-162, June 10, 1961.

Kelly, J. V.: Effect of fear upon uterine motility, Am. J. Obstet. Gynec. 83, No. 5:576, 581, March 1, 1962.

Osofosky, H. J., et al.: Changes in blood volume during parturition and the early postpartum period, Am. J. Obstet. Gynec. 88:396-398, February 1, 1964.

Quilligan, E. J., et al.: Correlation of fetal heart rate patterns and blood gas values. II. Bradycardia, Am. J. Obstet. Gynec. 91:1123-1132, April 15, 1965.

Redman, T. F.: Descent of presenting part in pregnancy and labor, Am. J. Obstet. Gynec. 66: 607, 1953.

Taubert, H. D., and Haskins, A. L.: The effect of isoxsuprine hydrochloride upon the contractility of the human uterus in labor, Maryland Med. J. 10:346-348, July, 1961.

Wajdowicz, E. K.: Abdominal decompression during labor, Am. J. Nurs. 64:87-89, December, 1964.

Chapter 11

Analgesia and Anesthesia for Labor

From the time of early civilizations the pains and the tortures endured by women in childbirth have been related in the historical records. It was not until the middle of the 19th century that medical science introduced anesthesia to relieve this pain. Two important pioneers who made important contributions in the use of anesthesia in obstetrics were Sir James Y. Simpson, of Edinburgh, and his contemporary in this country, Dr. Walter Channing, of Boston. A knowledge of the historical development of pain relief used in obstetrics will assist the nurse to gain an increased understanding of modern practices utilized in this approach to providing the mother with more comfort during labor. In addition, she will find that this study provides fascinating reading material. Space will not permit an adequate discussion here; thus the student is advised to pursue it in appropriate texts. (See Suggested Reading and Chapter 24, History of Obstetrics.)

TYPES OF PAIN RELIEF

Pain relief in labor may be of two main types: (1) *obstetric analgesia* and (2) *obstetric anesthesia.*

By *obstetric analgesia* is meant the administration of certain drugs during the first and the second stages of labor, prior to the actual birth of the baby, for the purpose of relieving the discomfort caused by labor contractions.

By *obstetric anesthesia* is meant the administration of certain drugs for the total obliteration of pain and sensation during the procedure of delivery of the infant, the placenta and perineal repair, if required.

In modern obstetric practice various technics may be utilized for pain relief in labor. No one method should be employed universally for all women. In this country, Demerol or one of the other synthetic narcotics, in combination with scopolamine and/or one of the drugs such as Phenergan, is most commonly used to achieve systematic analgesia and amnesia. Systemic anesthesia is produced by the inhalation of anesthetic gases (nitrous oxide, cyclopropane, ethylene) or volatile anesthetics (ether, chloroform) or by the intravenous infusion of thiopental sodium (Pentothal Sodium). Regional anesthesia may be produced by spinal or caudal anesthesia, or by local infiltration of the tissues concerned with an anesthetic solution such as procaine. Certain technics, such as continuous caudal, may be used for both obstetric analgesia and anesthesia. When regional anesthetics are used, the patient is awake, but painful sensation is abolished in the areas concerned. Inhalation or intravenous anesthetics, of course, produce unconsciousness.

GENERAL PRINCIPLES

The proper psychological preparation of the

226

Fig. 11-1. This patient chipped off her right front tooth and bruised her chin when she was under analgesic and amnesic drugs, as the result of throwing herself against a radiator near the bed. Patients receiving such medications during labor must never be left unattended, even for a moment.

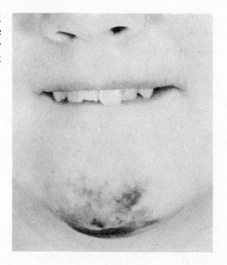

expectant mother in the care she receives throughout her pregnancy and labor is an indispensable basic sedative. A woman who is contented, unafraid and possessed of complete confidence in her obstetrician and nurses usually enjoys a relatively comfortable first stage of labor and requires a minimum of medication. This wholesome attitude toward parturition must be assiduously fostered at all times as an essential phase of pain relief.

When any form of pain relief is administered in labor, the safety of two patients, the mother and her infant, is the most important consideration. When prescribing analgesic medication, the physician's judgment is influenced by many factors, such as the length of gestation; the mother's emotional behavior; her response to pain; her previous obstetric and anesthetic experiences; and, of course, the frequency, intensity and duration of uterine contractions and the general character of the labor. Analgesia should not be initiated too soon. One rule should be absolute: such medication never should be started until positive proof exists that the cervix is showing progressive effacement and dilatation. In general, primigravidas should not be given analgesic medication until the contractions are strong and regular, and the cervix is 3 to 5 cm. dilated; in multiparas the cervix should be 4 to 6 cm. dilated. If the medication is administered before good labor is established, the drugs may appreciably retard the progress of labor or even stop it. On the other hand, when medication is started somewhat later than the optimal time, the efficacy of the analgesia is diminished as a rule, especially in rapid multiparous labors. These drugs also may affect the infant's respirations at birth if sufficient time has not elapsed for their metabolism and excretion prior to the birth of the baby. It is important that the drugs exert little effect on the uterine contractions; otherwise, not only will the progress of labor be impeded but also, after the delivery, if the uterine contractions are suppressed, postpartal hemorrhage may occur.

Any mother in labor should be in a single room if possible, but particularly when drugs are administered to promote obstetric analgesia. When the drugs administered will produce systemic analgesia, the environment should be conducive to rest, that is, free from such forms of external stimuli as bright lights and noises, even conversation. The room should be quiet and dimly lighted, though light enough to permit the nurse in attendance to observe the signs of progress of labor, as well as the mother's general condition.

Before administering the drugs, the nurse should give the patient certain explanations about the therapy so that she understands what is happening and particularly that the darkened quiet environment will enhance the effect of the medication. At this time the patient should be encouraged to empty her bladder. This not only contributes to her immediate comfort but also often avoids the necessity of catheterization if she is not able to void later on in labor. In addition, this is a preventive measure to avoid postpartal urinary retention. The fetal heart tones are taken now, and again after the medication is administered. In the latter instance, only sufficient time should elapse to permit absorption of the medication, which, of course, would be dependent on the route of administration utilized. Most physicians advocate that patients receive nothing by mouth after analgesia is started.

Patients under any form of analgesia require constant and meticulous attention. The nurse must be alert to the signs which indicate progress of labor even more carefully now that the mother is sedated, particularly those signs which herald the second stage of labor. Also, if left alone, a patient may throw herself against the wall or out of bed, or may vomit and aspirate the gastric contents. Numerous injuries and a few deaths are on record as a result of such negligence. Figure 11-1 illustrates the results of an accident which occurred when the patient was under sedation. Similarly, conduction anesthesia demands meticulous attention to the blood pressure and anesthetic levels if safety is to be achieved.

Before any agent is administered to produce general anesthesia, false teeth, chewing gum or any other foreign object must be removed from the mouth, because these may be swallowed or aspirated when the patient loses consciousness. Because vomiting is likely to occur during the induction of anesthesia and during the emergence from the anesthetic state, an emesis basin and towels must be within easy reach. During the entire period of unconsciousness after returning from the delivery room, the patient should lie on her right side, with or without a slight degree of Trendelenburg position, with the neck extended. This position augments drainage of vomitus if emesis should occur and at the same time helps to prevent obstruction of respiration due to relaxation of the tongue. To prevent further interference with respiration until the patient awakens, and until the danger of the tongue slipping back is eliminated, the lower jaw should be supported by pressure against the mandible.

OBSTETRIC ANALGESIA

"Twilight Sleep." The first medication used to produce amnesia in labor was a combination of morphine and scopolamine. Introduced in Germany during the early years of this century, this method of producing "a state of clouded consciousness" met with widespread public interest in the United States about 1918, under the name of "Twilight Sleep." Although it is now seldom employed, it is of great historical interest because the delicate balance between amnesic and depressive drugs that it utilized forms the basis of many modern technics.

Morphine and other opium derivatives are less frequently used in labor today because of the marked depression that these narcotics cause on the maternal and fetal respiratory centers and on uterine contractions. Since these drugs readily cross the placenta, an infant born before the drugs are metabolized and excreted suffers the effects of respiratory depression and at birth may be slow to breathe. However, morphine is a most valuable drug and in specific instances may be the drug of choice, as in the case of uterine dysfunction. Here it affords a means of giving the patient a much needed rest, the so-called "morphine rest." (See Chap. 19, Complications of Labor.)

Narcotic Amnesia

The most commonly employed method of obstetric analgesia used in this country today is a combination of drugs to produce narcotic amnesia of everything which occurred throughout labor. Scopolamine, a drug which produces amnesia, is used in combination with an analgesic agent, such as Demerol, or a hypnotic, such as a barbiturate.

Scopolamine, an alkaloid of belladonna, is a parasympathetic depressant drug with a diversant action on the central nervous system. The action of this drug provides several advantages for the mother in labor (such as its ability to counteract respiratory depression). However, the real aim in using such a drug as scopolamine is to produce forgetfulness or amnesia (Greek for "without memory"), thus obliterating the memory of whatever events occurred under its influence, and not to provide actual pain relief. If the patient is without pain, as in the periods between contractions, the drug acts as a depressant and causes fatigue, drowsiness and sleep. However, prior to sedation, the drug may produce restlessness, excitement, hallucinations and delirium; and these manifestations are most likely to occur in the presence of pain. For this reason an analgesic drug is given with scopolamine to forestall this kind of stimulation during the period of uterine contractions. A woman thus medicated may shriek, make grimaces and show other evidences of pain, but on awakening from the effects of the drug will remember nothing about her labor and will vow that she has experienced no discomfort whatsoever. Unfortunately, this will not be the case if the person in attendance refreshes the mother's memory with an account of the events that have taken place.

The average adult dose of scopolamine is 0.4 mg. ($\frac{1}{150}$ gr.) to 0.6 mg. ($\frac{1}{100}$ gr.), the initial dose usually ordered being 0.4 to 0.45 mg. Subsequent doses in decreasing amounts, i.e., 0.3 mg., 0.2 mg., may be prescribed to follow at 30-minute to 2-hour intervals. When an analgesic drug, such as Demerol, is given in conjunction with this, it may be given with the initial dose of scopolamine and repeated in 4 hours, if necessary, in a somewhat lesser dose. The dosage schedule for sedation must always be individualized according to the progress of labor and the individual patient's needs. However, the total amount of scopolamine given within a 24-hour period should be limited to 1.5 mg.

Meperidine hydrochloride (Demerol) is a synthetic compound which resembles morphine in its analgesic properties and atropine in its antispasmodiclike effects. Hence, in labor it not only relieves pain but is believed to exert also a relaxing effect on the cervix and so expedite dilatation. It is usually administered intramuscularly in dosages of 50 to 100 mg., with repetition of the dosage in a few hours if necessary. The total dose in any 8-hour period should not exceed 200 mg. A moderate sedative effect is produced, the patient usually sleeping between contractions but awakening when spoken to. Demerol, used alone, does not cause excitement or disorientation, but rather a mental state of well-being. The effect of Demerol on the respiratory center is decidedly less depressing than that of morphine. However, many authorities feel that it crosses the placental barrier and has more effect on the fetus than previously thought.

Demerol alone produces analgesia but not amnesia. If amnesia also is desired, scopolamine may be used in conjunction with it. Like morphine, Demerol is included under the Harrison Act, and its distribution and sale are governed by the regulations of the Federal Bureau of Narcotics.

Barbiturates. Since about 1934, derivatives of barbituric acid, usually in combination with scopolamine, have become increasingly popular for obstetric analgesia. Barbiturates are hypnotics and produce relaxation from tension and absence of fear but are not in themselves analgesic. Some of the more commonly employed are Nembutal (pentobarbital sodium), Amytal Sodium and Seconal Sodium. These three drugs are very similar in their action, but Amytal Sodium is likely to be the choice of the doctor when labor gives prospects of being prolonged, because its effect is more enduring than the other two. As an example of the technic employed in barbiturate analgesia, the following program is one which might be carried out when this form of pain relief is desired.

If the patient complains of discomfort and the cervix is effaced and 3 to 4 cm. dilated:

Amytal Sodium or   } 0.3 Gm. (5 grains)
Nembutal or Seconal   }   by mouth
In 20 minutes:
Scopolamine 0.3 or 0.4 mg. ($\frac{1}{200}$ to $\frac{1}{150}$ grain) by hypodermic
One hour after initial dose:
Scopolamine 0.1 or 0.2 mg. ($\frac{1}{600}$ to $\frac{1}{300}$ grain), depending on condition of patient
Repeat scopolamine 0.1 mg. ($\frac{1}{600}$ grain) hourly if necessary, but maximum dosage should not exceed 1.0 mg. ($\frac{1}{60}$ grain).
Barbiturate may be repeated every 4 hours in 0.1 Gm. doses.

Patients with kidney diseases should not be given barbiturates, since the confused state produced may persist for many hours thereafter due to delayed elimination.

Paraldehyde. This pungent-smelling liquid is favored by a few obstetricians as an analgesic and amnesic agent. It may be administered by mouth or by rectum. The average dose of paraldehyde is from 10 to 15 cc., depending on the weight of the patient, and may be repeated in about 6 hours or supplemented by other drugs. When paraldehyde is given orally, it must be prepared in a way that will disguise the objectionable taste, for example, with sugar and chipped ice or with port wine and a little water. For rectal administration it should be mixed with 25 or 30 cc. of olive oil. The effect is similar to that produced by the barbiturate-scopolamine program described above.

Inhalation Analgesia

The intermittent, brief inhalation of *nitrous oxide, ether, trichloroethylene* or *chloroform* ("analgesia à la reine") may also be administered with contractions for analgesia. (See Obstetric Anesthesia, p. 236.)

It is usually the nurse's responsibility to administer oral, subcutaneous or intramuscular medications in providing nursing care for the patient receiving obstetric analgesia. Unless the nurse has had special training in a school of anesthesia, it is highly undesirable to have her master technics for administration of anesthesia, and she should not be expected to assume responsibility for administering obstetric inhalation analgesia or anesthesia. Knowledge of anesthetic drugs and their desired and untoward effects is necessary in order for her to perform her professional role as a maternity nurse. *Only in an emergency, however, and under the direction of a physician, may she administer anesthetic agents.* In such a situation the physician assumes full responsibility for the anesthesia.

Paracervical Block Analgesia

By this term is meant the injection of an anesthetic solution into the region around the cervix to allay the pains caused by cervical dilatation. It is usually followed by pudendal block anesthesia for delivery. Paracervical block anesthesia is being used in a considerable

number of hospitals with eminent success, but some obstetricians believe that it sometimes exerts a depressing effect on the infant. Therefore, its place in obstetrics is not completely established.

OBSTETRIC ANESTHESIA

The most commonly employed methods of obstetric anesthesia are inhalation of narcotic gases or volatile anesthetics, intravenous anesthesia with a soluble barbiturate, and regional anesthesia, such as local infiltration, spinal or caudal. The continuous caudal technic provides both analgesia in the first and the second stages of labor and anesthesia for delivery.

Regional Anesthesia

Local Infiltration. The injection of local anesthetic agents such as procaine, Metycaine and the like may be employed to desensitize the area of the perineum for a spontaneous delivery, or, in the event of an operative delivery, to block the pudendal nerves in order to produce more profound anesthesia of the area supplied by these nerves. This technic is usually of no value for analgesia during labor and is not begun until the delivery is imminent,

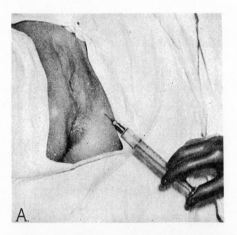 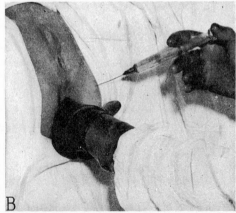

A.   B.

Fig. 11-2. Local infiltration anesthesia for episiotomy. (A) Intradermal wheals raised over ischial tuberosities. (B) Index finger in rectum for palpation of ischial spines and infiltration of internal pudic nerves. Infiltration of perineal fibers of the ilioinguinal nerves and posterior cutaneous femoris nerves completes the procedure. (Eastman: Williams' Obstetrics, ed. 11, New York, Appleton)

when it can be administered by the obstetrician. After the mother is prepared and draped for delivery, the injection is made first to the right and then to the left of the fourchet, using the needle in a fan-shaped manner and following the lower border of the vulva on each side (see Fig. 11-2).

When the *pudendal block* is to be accomplished, a No. 20 spinal needle 10 cm. long, attached to a 10- or 20-cc. Luer syringe, is passed first just below and beyond the ischial spine. Solution then is injected to anesthetize the internal pudendal nerve. The needle is partially withdrawn, then inserted laterally toward the tuberosity of the ischium, where more solution is injected. The needle is again withdrawn in the same manner and inserted to infiltrate the labia. The entire procedure is repeated on the opposite side. In a few minutes, perineal muscles are relaxed, and the skin of the perineum becomes anesthetized.

When one considers an anesthetic agent from the standpoint of safety for both mother and her infant, local infiltration of the tissues has manifold advantages. First of all, there is practically no anesthetic mortality. Since the uterine contractions are not impaired, the progress of the mother's labor is not retarded, and after the delivery the effect of the anesthetic agent will not cause uterine relaxation and thus excessive bleeding. And since there is no direct effect of the anesthetic on the infant, it is protected from asphyxia.

Continuous Caudal. This is a form of analgesia and anesthesia achieved by "blocking" the nerves in the peridural space. The anesthetic agent is introduced into the peridural space via the sacral hiatus (see Fig. 10). It is

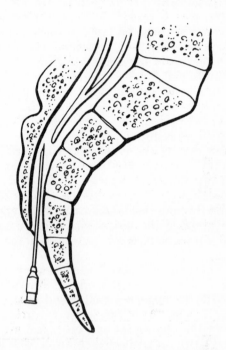

FIG. 11-3. Sagittal section of sacral canal, with caudal needle properly placed in the caudal space.

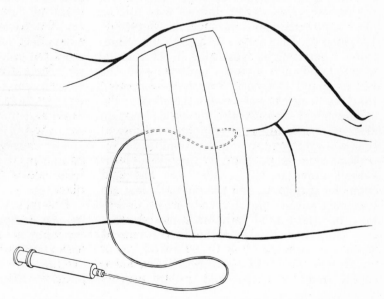

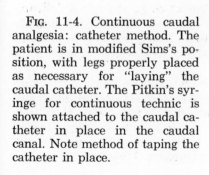

FIG. 11-4. Continuous caudal analgesia: catheter method. The patient is in modified Sims's position, with legs properly placed as necessary for "laying" the caudal catheter. The Pitkin's syringe for continuous technic is shown attached to the caudal catheter in place in the caudal canal. Note method of taping the catheter in place.

screened by a thin layer of fibrous tissue. This opening is called the sacral hiatus and leads to a space within the sacrum known as the caudal canal or the caudal space (Fig. 11-3). This space is really the lowermost extent of the bony spinal canal. Through it a rich network of sacral nerves passes downward after they have emerged from the dural sac a few inches above. The dural sac separates the caudal canal below from the spinal cord and its surrounding spinal fluid.

By filling the caudal canal with a suitable anesthetic solution, pain sense in the sacral nerves is abolished, and anesthesia of the pelvic region is produced.

When the patient is in good labor and the cervix is 5 cm. dilated in the multipara (preferably 7 to 8 cm. in primipara), caudal analgesia may be started. By the addition of anesthetic solution through the caudal catheter at appropriate intervals, the desired effect can be maintained throughout labor (anesthesia for delivery).

To insert the catheter, the obstetric patient is placed on her side in a modified Sims's position, with the upper leg well flexed at the hip and knee joints and the lower leg extended (Fig. 11-4). The sacral and coccygeal area is cleansed with an antiseptic solution. The area is surrounded with sterile towels or a sterile drape. The physician, of course, wears sterile gloves for the procedure, since it requires surgical aseptic technic. After the pliable needle or fine plastic catheter has been inserted into the caudal space, a test dose of 8 cc. of the local anesthetic solution, such as Metycaine 1.5 per cent, Pontocaine 0.15 per cent, Xylocaine 1 per cent or Nesacaine 3 per cent, is injected. When 5 minutes have elapsed, the test for spinal anesthesia is made to be assured that the drug has not been injected into the subarachnoid space. At this time the physician also will check the anal sphincter for loss of tone and examine the lower extremities for increasing skin temperature. If these two observations prove to be positive, i.e., the anal sphincter is relaxed, and the patient's feet are becoming warmer and dry, they are an indication that the caudal catheter is placed properly. Only after this is certain is the patient given the obstetric dose of 20 to 30 cc. of medication which will block the afferent nerve supply from the uterus and usually provide

anesthesia to the 10th thoracic dermatome.

At first the patient experiences a sense of fullness along the distribution of the sciatic nerve in one or both legs, which may cause temporary discomfort. About 15 minutes after the injection, relief is obtained from the abdominal discomfort of uterine contractions, and in about 20 minutes the analgesia should be complete. One observes the lower extremities for pronounced vasodilatation and cessation of sweating as one of the first effective signs. The great toe and the ball of the foot are the first parts to develop vasomotor block; thus this area is the first to become pink, warm and dry. The heel will be the last to show these signs. The effect may be unilateral at first, and some minutes may elapse before it affects the other side, or the physician may have the patient lie on the unaffected side to encourage diffusion of the anesthetic agent. The nurse should remember that the physician should be consulted before changing the patient's position to one side or the other during this early stage of analgesia. After anesthesia has been will established, there is usually no contraindication to changing the patient's position so long as the pliable needle or plastic catheter is protected. If the procedure is successful, the patient experiences no pain whatsoever in labor and is not conscious of either uterine contractions or of perineal distention, except for some minor degree of pressure.

Provided that the maternal systolic blood pressure does not fall below 100 mm. Hg, with resulting fetal hypoxia, a continuous caudal has the advantage of exerting the least possible effect on the infant, because it does not cross the placental barrier in significant pharmacologic doses. This factor is an advantage to the premature infant particularly, as well as the fact that caudal analgesia tends to retard rapid and forceful labor and enables the physician to perform an easy, controlled delivery. It also lessens the strain of labor for mothers handicapped with heart disease, pulmonary tuberculosis, acute respiratory infections or diabetes.

POSSIBLE COMPLICATIONS. One of the commonest complications of conduction analgesia for labor is *maternal hypotension*; thus it is important for the nurse or the physician in attendance to keep a constant check on the patient's blood pressure. Hypotension can be controlled by alertness and prompt action on the part of the attendant. One of the first clues that may alert the nurse that the patient's blood pressure has dropped abruptly is a sudden episode of rather severe nausea, accompanied promptly by the other signs of sudden hypotension. When the mother in labor becomes hypotensive, immediate action should be taken to restore the blood volume to the central circulation. The most expedient measure in this instance is to elevate the patient's legs, either by raising the foot of the bed or merely elevating her legs. The latter measure is easily accomplished by standing at the foot of the bed, grasping the patient's ankles and raising both legs simultaneously to almost a 90-degree angle. This author (E. F.) has been present on numerous occasions when Dr. Robert Hingson has done this successfully—what he refers to as a "bloodless phlebotomy." The patient may require oxygen at this time. If her blood pressure does not return to normal, she should be turned on her left side (with the foot of the bed elevated) and continue to breathe oxygen. Lying on the left side relieves the uterine pressure exerted on iliac veins and the inferior vena cava, and thus facilitates venous return from the lower extremities. If the fall in the patient's blood pressure is severe, the physician may prescribe an intravenous infusion of 5 per cent dextrose in water. Often merely the temporary elevation of the patient's legs, or turning her on her left side, will restore the blood pressure to normal. If the above measures are not successful, the physician may administer small divided doses of a vasopressor drug. It must be remembered that when the patient has been given a vasopressor, she should *not* be given the oxytocic ergonovine or its derivatives (see Chap. 12, Conduct of Normal Labor). This alkaloid of ergot has a synergistic action with vasopressors; the combination of these drugs has been reported to result in very severe headache and cerebrovascular accident(see Suggested Reading).

In addition to its tendency to produce hypotension, *other disadvantages* of continuous caudal are (1) it increases the rate of forceps deliveries, (2) it may prolong labor, and (3) if the anesthetic level reaches above T-10, there is a marked increase in uterine atony. It would be contraindicated in the case of shock or hemorrhage because of its vasodilator tendencies and, for the same reason, should be used cautiously in toxemia. Any infection of the skin over the sacral area, in particular, would likewise be a contraindication for its use.

This type of anesthesia requires hospital facilities and is more demanding on the time and the skill of the medical staff, so that in many smaller hospitals it is not feasible to employ it.

Continuous caudal analgesia was introduced in the autumn of 1942 by Dr. Robert A. Hingson and Dr. Waldo B. Edwards, of Staten Island, N. Y. It was received with wide acclaim and at the present writing is employed in many hospitals.

Spinal Anesthesia. Spinal anesthesia, as used in obstetrics, falls into two major divisions. The first is a semiterminal type of anesthesia which is employed for the latter part of labor and delivery and is provided by low dosage of a hyperbaric solution. The second is a terminal type and is administered either by the single-dosage method or the continuous technic; its largest field of employment is in cesarean section. Although minute doses of spinal anesthesia can be given to provide pain relief throughout labor, this technic is difficult and, by and large, unsatisfactory. Too often labor is stopped by spinal anesthesia.

Low-Dosage Hyperbaric Spinal (Saddle Block). This form of anesthesia is one of the most popular in the United States today. Nearly all the local anesthesia agents have been used in saddle-block anesthesia. By the addition of glucose to the solution of Pontocaine or other anesthetic agent, localization and concentration of the drug in the conus of the dural sac are facilitated. Inasmuch as this anesthetic is of short duration, it is necessary to time its administration properly, and delivery should be anticipated within an hour or so following the onset of anesthesia.

Inhalation Anesthesia

Volatile Anesthetics

Ether, chloroform and *trichloroethylene* are volatile anesthetic agents which are used for obstetric analgesia and anesthesia. These substances cross the placenta readily and are capable of producing narcosis in the fetus.

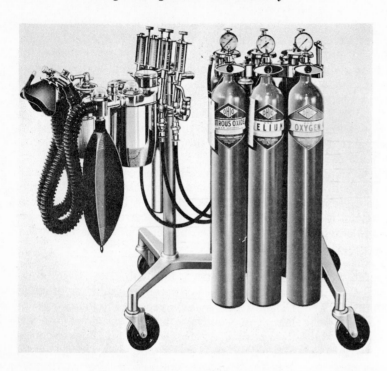

Fig. 11-5. Circle filter anesthesia apparatus. With this type of machine any combination or mixture of gases can be administered to the patient. (Heidbrink Division, Ohio Chemical & Surgical Equipment Co., Madison, Wis.)

From the standpoint of the mother, ether and chloroform inhibit uterine contractions and thus increase the possibility of excessive bleeding both during and following the delivery. These two compounds are better suited to anesthesia for delivery and do not lend themselves to obstetric analgesia. On the other hand, trichloroethylene should *not* be used for anesthesia.

The inhalation of the volatile anesthetics is contraindicated when upper respiratory infection or pulmonary disease exists and, of course, after the patient has had a full meal. This type of anesthesia also is contraindicated in the presence of prematurity or when, for other reasons, one expects possible fetal hypoxia.

Ether. Because of the slowness of its action, the margin of safety is greater with ether than with any other inhalation anesthetic, and with careful administration it is relatively safe even in the presence of severe cardiac or hypertensive disease.

ADMINISTRATION. At the present time, when modern apparatus is employed, ether is administered by the closed circuit or semiclosed circuit technic, so that it is possible to administer an adequate amount of oxygen simultaneously and to complement or to supplement nitrous oxide or ethylene anesthesia when deeper anesthesia is needed or desired (Fig. 11-5).

Ether also may be administered by the open-drop method, using a wire mask covered with gauze and a can of ether (Fig. 11-6). A bent safety pin is put through the cap of the ether can to make a dropper; or a small V-shaped incision is made lengthwise in the cork which comes with the ether can, and after a 1-inch wick of gauze is inserted into this crevice, it is inserted into the can. When the can is tilted, ether will drop off the gauze wick. Some anesthetists prefer to administer ether from a small glass bottle, prepared with the cork and wick, to permit visualization of the amount of ether in the container. When ether is dropped on a mask placed over the patient's nose and mouth, care must be taken to permit an adequate mixture of air to maintain oxygen requirements and prevent any hypoxia. The hypoxia can be averted if oxygen flowing at 4 liters is administered simultaneously through a small rubber catheter placed under the mask. The use of an improvised cone made from newspaper covered with cloth is not advised. Even with the wire mask there is an additional "dead space" of 60 cc., i.e., space filled with

Fig. 11-6. Equipment for administration of ether by the open-drop method. (A) Bottom view of wire mask, showing metal retaining-ring which holds the gauze on the mask and prevents the gauze from touching the skin. (B) Can of ether. (C) Top view of wire mask covered with a few layers of gauze. (D) Nasopharyngeal airway. (E) Glass bottle for dispensing "drop" ether, demonstrating one method of utilizing an incised cork and gauze wick in a bottle. (F) Oropharyngeal airway. (These airways should be available for immediate use when any form of general anesthesia is administered.)

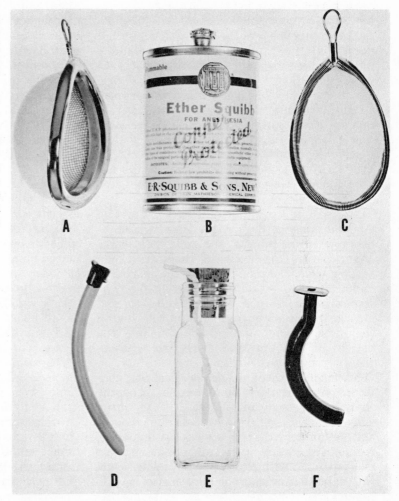

the exhaled air and carbon dioxide. When the paper cone is used, the air exchange is hindered, and the volume of this "dead space" is increased to about 200 cc. Since there is an inadequate supply of fresh air to supply oxygen demands, the patient rebreathes carbon dioxide.

In order to avoid irritation from open-drop ether, care should be exerted that none of the liquid ether touches the skin or the conjunctiva. The face should be anointed with petrolatum and the eyes protected with petrolatum gauze or a towel. When the eyes are covered with a towel, it must be ascertained that the lids completely cover the eyes at all times during anesthesia; otherwise, a corneal abrasion will result from the irritation of the towel. After this preparation, the mask is held

slightly above the patient's nose and mouth, and a few drops of ether are poured onto the mask. This will acclimate the patient to the pungent odor of ether and will help to prevent a coughing attack due to the irritating effect of ether on the laryngeal mucous membrane. Then the mask is lowered to the patient's face, covering her nose and mouth, and, as the patient tolerates the increasing concentration of the ether vapor, the rate of flow of the drops of ether is slowly increased. The increased flow of the drops of ether should never reach a point where it becomes a steady flow of the liquid. In addition, care must be exercised to distribute the flow of ether drops evenly about the mask so that it does not concentrate in one spot. This diffuse saturation of the mask will hasten vaporization of the liquid ether and will cause a steady, even increase in the concentration of ether vapor under the mask. If the patient does not tolerate the rate of flow of ether during this stage of induction of anesthesia, the anesthetist should reduce the rate. At times it is proper to remove the mask and permit the patient to have a few breaths of fresh air until she breathes normally. When respiration is again normal, the anesthetist may slowly reapply the mask to the face and then slowly start to drop ether again.

STAGES OF ANESTHESIA. As long as the patient remains conscious, she is in Stage 1, the analgesia stage of anesthesia.

About 5 to 10 minutes after the start of ether anesthesia, the patient loses consciousness and enters Stage 2, the excitement stage of anesthesia. During Stage 2 the patient may become violent, cry out, pull at the restraints and attempt to get off the delivery table. The respiration is irregular in depth and rate, and muscle tonicity is increased. For this reason the nurse should refrain from touching the patient at this time and await the anesthetist's signal before doing so.

Meanwhile, the anesthetist carefully continues with the rapid flow of ether to hasten the patient's entry into Stage 3, the surgical stage of anesthesia. However, during periodic episodes of apnea, which may occur due to irregular respiration, the mask should not be oversaturated with ether. Such oversaturation with ether will inhibit the vaporization of the liquid ether (by preventing an adequate exchange of air through the wet mask) and will also cause some retention of carbon dioxide by the patient.

When the respiration again regains its regular rate and rhythm, the patient is in Stage 3. At this point one must be careful not to permit the patient to "lighten" in depth of anesthesia and slip back into Stage 2. If this should occur, it will be noticed that the patient starts swallowing, and unless the anesthesia is deepened immediately, the swallowing will be followed by vomiting. If the patient should unavoidably vomit, her head should be turned to the side and the table put into slight Trendelenburg position. In addition, the vomitus should be sucked out of the patient's mouth by adequate suction via either the oral or the nasal route. The finesse with which the anesthetist carries the patient through the first two stages of anesthesia into the surgical stage of

anesthesia is very important. Frequently, this determines the "smoothness" of the anesthesia and influences the occurrence of complications both during and after anesthesia.

It should be remembered that in the period following the delivery the mother often is unconscious. During ether narcosis, her face should be slightly flushed, but never pale or cyanotic; her respiration should be deep, possibly stertorous, but never irregular; and her pulse should be full, of good quality, fairly rapid, but never intermittent. At this time, excessive uterine bleeding may occur due to the direct effect that ether has on the uterine musculature.

Chloroform. In 1847, Sir James Y. Simpson's famous experiment with chloroform convinced him that this anesthetic was far stronger and better than ether and a means to afford painless delivery. But Simpson's discovery was met with tremendous opposition on all sides. The clergy rebelled against his work and defamed him as a heretic and blasphemer for his attempt to ease the suffering which women had experienced since time immemorial. Their attacks were based on the Bible, with such verses as "In sorrow thou shalt bring forth children" (Gen. 3:16). But Dr. Simpson, also a student of the Bible, was able to refute their charges with such quotations from the Scriptures as "And the Lord God caused a deep sleep to fall upon Adam, and he slept; and he took one of his ribs, and closed up the flesh instead thereof" (Gen. 2:21).

ANALGESIA À LA REINE. In 1853, when Queen Victoria's eighth child was born, she was given momentary inhalations of chloroform with each labor contraction. It proved to be a highly efficacious means of pain relief, and since that time the method has been known as "Queen's anesthesia" or anesthesia *à la reine*. Actually, the procedure does not produce complete anesthesia but simply diminishes the intensity of the discomfort and may be best regarded as a form of analgesia.

ADMINISTRATION. Chloroform is now considered to be too toxic a drug for common use and is rejected by most of the large American hospitals. Nevertheless, it is still used in some rural areas when the mother is a normal healthy parturient. This agent must be preserved in tight, light-resistant containers; otherwise decomposition will occur, forming toxic phosgene gas. Since in the liquid state chloroform will produce severe irritation and burns of the skin and the conjunctiva, care must be exercised to ensure that none of the liquid—or objects moistened with the liquid chloroform—touches the skin or the conjunctiva. Before administering chloroform, the patient's face should be anointed with petrolatum and her eyes protected by the instillation of a drop of castor oil, in addition to being shielded with a towel, as previously described for protection during administration of open-drop ether. The chloroform is administered 10 to 15 drops per minute by the open-drop method. The mask should be supported at least 2 or 3 fingerbreadths from the face. At no time should the mask encircle the nose and the mouth tightly, because chloroform must be given with high concentrations of oxygen or fresh air. Under no circumstances should towels be placed around the mask when giving chloroform.

Chloroform is pleasant to take, rapid in action and in recovery, and rarely gives rise to nausea.

POSSIBLE DANGERS. For the mother, on the other hand, it may be dangerous unless handled with care. It must never be "pushed"—that is, anesthetic action must never be hastened by pouring the chloroform on rapidly or by lowering the mask to the face. Nor should it be continued to the point of complete anesthesia, since the prolonged administration of chloroform anesthesia (for the repair of laceration, for instance) may give rise to myocardial damage. For the latter reason, chloroform is used less frequently than formerly. In giving chloroform the following danger signals should be watched for: pallor; shallow, jerky respiration; weak pulse; cyanosis, and deep, stertorous respiration (the last a sign that complete anesthesia has been produced). Should breath-holding occur, the mask should be removed instantly; otherwise the patient may suffer from cardiac arrest due to the massive concentration of the drug inhaled with the next respiration.

Epinephrine and oxytocin *never* should be used in conjunction with chloroform anesthesia because ventricular fibrillation may result. If any of these signs develop, the anesthetic should be discontinued at once.

Trichloroethylene (Trilene). Trilene is a chemical substance which resembles chloroform in many of its properties. In obstetrics it occasionally is employed at the time of each contraction as a self-administered analgesic agent (Trilene à la reine). A suitable inhaler containing Trilene is strapped to the parturient's wrist, and she inhales the Trilene vapor as soon as a contraction begins. If consciousness is benumbed to the point of unconsciousness, the inhaler automatically drops from the patient's face, thus preventing an excessive degree of anesthesia. Although this method has been employed extensively in Great Britain, its use in the United States has been limited.

Gas Anesthetics

Nitrous oxide and *cyclopropane* are two anestheic gases widely used in current obstetric practice. They should always be administered by a physician or a specially trained nurse anesthetist and restricted to use where adequate apparatus is available. Although these anesthetic agents are safe in the hands of the skilled practitioner, in the hands of the inexperienced they may suddenly become dangerous to both mother and her infant.

Nitrous oxide in combination with oxygen is used for pain relief in labor when deep relaxation is not required. The concentration is of extreme importance. For the purposes of analgesia and anesthesia, nitrous oxide should never exceed 80 per cent concentration (frequently referred to as 80-20, meaning 80 per cent nitrous oxide and 20 per cent oxygen), a concentration which has little effect on the uterine activity. Too low a concentration of oxygen will cause asphyxia neonatorum in the fetus, and such asphyxia may cause irreparable damage to the higher centers of the infant's brain.

Once the cervix becomes fully dilated, nitrous oxide may be administered intermittently for pain relief during contractions. When the patient indicates that a uterine contraction has begun, the mask is placed over her nose and mouth, and she is encouraged to take 3 deep breaths of a high flow 80-20 mixture of nitrous oxide and oxygen, or 1 breath with lower concentration of nitrous oxide and a higher concentration of oxygen if it will suffice. As soon as the contraction is over, the mask is removed until the next one begins. The mother should not lose consciousness but will be relieved of the discomfort of the contraction. This method of intermittent pain relief may be continued until the head crowns, when the anesthetic may be deepened to facilitate the control of the infant's head, and for the performance of episiotomy, if it is necessary. When the infant's head is born, the nitrous oxide is shut off temporarily, and the mother is given oxygen until the cord has been clamped.

One cannot overemphasize the importance of keeping an almost constant check on the fetal heart tones when nitrous oxide is administered to the mother in labor. It is not only the nurse's responsibility to listen to the fetal heart tones almost constantly but also to inform both the obstetrician and the anesthetist of her findings.

Cyclopropane. This highly explosive substance is the most potent of the anesthetic gases and is particularly advantageous in cases in which rapid induction with good relaxation is desired because of tumultuous labor. Cyclopropane may be administered with a higher concentration of oxygen than the other anesthetic gases, which one would assume to be of benefit to the unborn infant. However, if the mother's respiratory center is depressed, the oxygen saturation in the maternal arterial blood will be diminished because of her diminished respiration, and thus the oxygen concentration in the infant's arterial blood also will be decreased. In addition, if cyclopropane is administered to the mother for a prolonged period of time, the fetal respiratory center will be depressed.

Uterine contractions are not decreased when the concentration of cyclopropane given is maintained at a low level, but they are rapidly abolished as this level is increased. For this reason, when cyclopropane is given for a prolonged period, excessive uterine bleeding may occur.

Cardiac irregularities in the mother may occur when oxytocin or certain vasopressors are given during the administration of cyclopropane anesthesia. As in the case when either Trilene or chloroform is given to the mother, such drugs as oxytocin, epinephrine and those drugs which have a sympatheticlike action or mimic sympathetic nervous system response (sympathomimeticamines) should not be used in conjunction with cyclopropane. The nurse should be familiar with this principle, since she may be given a verbal order to administer the oxytocic drug at the time of delivery.

Because of the explosion hazard, every protection should be used to protect the mother as well as the hospital personnel. Cyclopropane is usually administered with the closed system machine and with continuous flow of the gas.

Intravenous Anesthesia

Thiopental Sodium (Pentothal Sodium). Intravenous Pentothal, one of the soluble barbiturates, may be used to produce anesthesia for rapid spontaneous deliveries, for uncomplicated outlet forceps deliveries or to induce anesthesia for the extraction of an infant by cesarean section. It may also be indicated in some cases of toxemia, when convulsive seizures are anticipated; in certain neurologic diseases, such as epilepsy; or in neuropsychiatric problems, when the patient is psychotic. This technic requires the skills of a competent physician anesthesiologist and, therefore, cannot be employed by the inexperienced or "occasional" anesthetist.

Recent studies have shown that within 5 minutes after the introduction of Pentothal Sodium into the mother's circulation there is an equalization of barbiturate in the mother's and the infant's blood. Therefore, when the use of the drug is elective, the anesthesia should not be started until the patient has been fully prepared and draped and the obstetrician is ready to start the delivery immediately after induction of anesthesia. Experience has shown that with the limitation of the amount of drug (a maximum dosage of 200 mg. of 2 or 2½ per cent Pentothal) used for induction and to aid expediency on the part of the operating obstetrician, there are very few, if any, deleterious effects on either mother or infant. Anytime a mother receives a soluble barbiturate, such as Pentothal Sodium, for anesthesia she should also be given continuous oxygen. If the anesthesia becomes prolonged, then the anesthetist will supplement it with another agent, such as nitrous oxide or cyclopropane, and repeat doses of the intravenous barbiturate will not be given until after the infant is delivered.

THE MAJOR DISADVANTAGES of intravenous Pentothal anesthesia for delivery are (1) the possibility of *fetal narcosis* due to overdosage of the drug, delay in delivery or synergistic action with the analgesic drugs given during the first and second stages of labor; (2) *fetal hypoxia* due to hypotension in the mother, which may occur as a result of the intravenous Pentothal; and (3) *maternal laryngospasm.* The latter hazard is very serious and is due to the fact that Pentothal is not a true anesthetic, but rather a hypnotic. It does not depress the laryngeal reflex, which remains active, so that any foreign object such as saliva or mucus can cause a severe episode of laryngospasm. Another factor to consider is that there is also a rectal reflex which, when stimulated, will cause laryngospasm. In this instance, the passage of the head through the birth canal is apparently adequate stimulus to initiate this reflex.

SUGGESTED READING

Apgar, V., *et al.*: Comparison of regional and general anesthesia in obstetrics, J.A.M.A. 165: 2155, 1957.

Black, M. E.: Psychorelaxation management for labor and delivery, Clin. Obstet. Gynec. 4:108-116, March, 1961.

Buxton, C. L.: A Study of Psychophysical Methods for Relief of Childbirth Pain, Philadelphia, Saunders, 1962.

Casady, G. U., *et al.*: Postpartum hypertension after use of vasoconstrictor and oxytocic drugs: etiology, incidence, complications and treatment, J.A.M.A. 172:1011-1015, 1960.

Council on Drugs, American Medical Association: New and Nonofficial Drugs, 1964, Philadelphia, Lippincott, 1964.

Dosser, Clarissa, and O'Connor, John: Continuous epidural block for obstetric anesthesia, Am. J. Nurs. 60, No. 9:1296-1299, September, 1960.

Duncan, C., Hindman, J., and Mayberger, H.: Chloroform as an obstetrical anesthesia, Am. J. Obstet. Gynec. 72:1004, 1956.

Eastman, N. J.: Williams Obstetrics, ed. 13, New York, Appleton, 1966.

———: Editorial comment on abstract of article by Herbert Thoms and Robert Wyatt: A natural childbirth program (*in* Obstet. Gynec. Survey 6:163, 1951), Obstet. Gynec. Survey 20, No. 3:484-486, June, 1965.

Ellison, G., Philpott, N., and Simpson, G.: Obstetrical anesthesia, Am. J. Obstet. Gynec. 74: 283, 1957.

Flowers, C. E., Jr.: Increasing the safety of obstetrical anesthesia, Bull. Maternal Welfare 2:9, 1955.

———: Trilene, an adjunct to obstetrical anesthesia and analgesia, Am. J. Obstet. Gynec. 65: 1027, 1953.

Frohman, I. P.: Demerol, Am. J. Nurs. 53:567, 1953.

Griffin, N. L.: Preventing fires and explosions in the operating room, Am. J. Nurs. 53:809, 1953.

Grollman, Arthur: Diurectics, Am. J. Nurs. 65, No. 1:84-89, January, 1965.

Gross, H. N., and Posner, N. A.: An evaluation of hypnosis for obstetric delivery, Am. J. Obstet. Gynec. 87:912-920, December 1, 1963.

Hingson, R., and Hellman, L.: Anesthesia for Obstetrics, Philadelphia, Lippincott, 1956.

Hingson, R. A., and Cull, W. A.: Conduction anesthesia and analgesia for obstetrics, Clin. Obstet. Gynec., 4, No. 1:87-107, March, 1961.

Krug, E. M.: Pharmacology in Nursing, ed. 9, St. Louis, Mosby, 1963.

Lock, F. R., and Greiss, F. C., Jr.: The anesthetic hazards in obstetrics, Am. J. Obstet. Gynec. 70: 861, 1955.

Maternity Center Association: Psychophysical Preparation for Childbirth: Guidelines for Teaching, ed. 2, New York, Maternity Center Association, 1965.

National Fire Protection Association: Recommended Safe Practice for Hospital Operating Room, Bulletin No. 56, National Fire Protection Association, 60 Battery–March St., Boston 10, Mass.

Nicholson, M. J.: Case history: postpartum hypertension after use of vasoconstrictor and oxytocic drugs, Anesth. Analg. 39:382-383, July-August, 1960.

Nyirjesy, I., *et al.*: Hazards of the use of paracervical block anesthesia in obstetrics, Am. J. Obstet. Gynec. 87:231-235, September 15, 1963.

Ulin, P. R.: The exhilarating moment of birth, Am. J. Nurs. 63, No. 6:60-67, June, 1963.

Vellay, Pierre: Childbirth without pain, New York, Dutton, 1960.

Dimensions of Effective Nursing Care • Prelude to Labor • The Onset of Labor • Admission to the Hospital • Establishment of the Nurse-Patient Relationship • Continuing Care • Examinations in Labor • Conduct of the First Stage • Conduct of the Second Stage • Conduct of the Third Stage • Immediate Care of the Infant • Emergency Delivery by the Nurse • Lacerations of the Birth Canal • Episiotomy and Repair

Chapter 12

Conduct of Normal Labor

DIMENSIONS OF EFFECTIVE NURSING CARE

Perhaps at no other time during the maternity cycle is the nurse in such an advantageous position to give nursing care as she is during the time of parturition. It is a unique and humbling experience, this miracle of giving birth, not only for the mother and the father, the main participants, but also for the physician and the nurse who share this experience, and upon whom so much depends. From the parents' point of view, labor looms as a critical period in the process of childbearing; often it is considered by them, and especially by the mother, as the end of a long-drawn-out process rather than the beginning of new life. Hence they attribute enormous significance to events and people who are necessary and helpful to them at this time. They indicate repeatedly that they consider the nurse in particular to be one of those necessary, helpful people. Indeed, she can be if she utilizes the opportunity.

Effective nursing care during labor provides for maximum well-being and comfort for both mother and infant and at the same time allows the father to participate in the process, in so far as he is able, and to derive a sense of satisfaction from that participation. The nursing intervention is purposeful but flexible, based always on the needs of each individual patient, infant and husband. To execute such care, the nurse must have knowledge and understanding of the course of normal labor, ability to recognize deviations from the normal, and judgment and ability to cope with stressful and emergency conditions. In addition, she should have a mastery of certain skills, both technical and communicative, which she can apply appropriately to meet the exigencies of the situation. The importance of teamwork between doctor and nurse should not be overlooked, and especially it is important to keep the physician informed through accurate reporting and recording of the progress of the mother in labor.

However, knowledge and technical ability are not sufficient in themselves, for the nurse must be able also to convey warmth and empathy if she is to be really effective. The empathic nurse is able to enter into the feelings of her patient and at the same time to retain her separateness. Thus, objectivity is maintained, which contributes to more effective care.[1] Yet the worth and the individuality of each mother always are recognized. In addition, the nurse should be accepting and nonjudgmental regarding the behavior of the mother or the father, realizing that this is a stressful period, and that their usual behavior may be drastically different. She strives to sustain her patient and to reinforce her confidence whenever necessary, thus helping the mother to attain the greatest amount of comfort and

[1] See article by C. Aring in Suggested Reading for differentiation between empathy and sympathy.

241

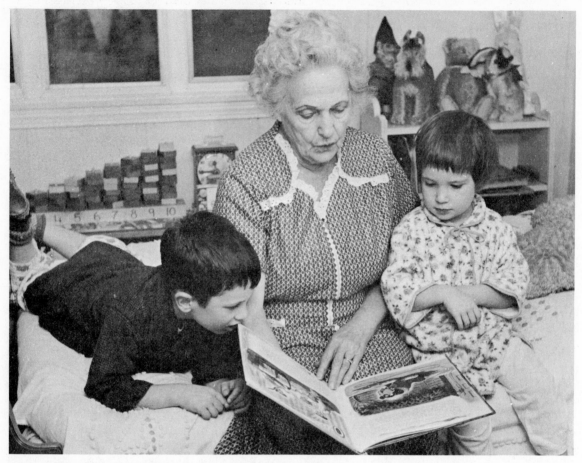

FIG. 12-1. Grandmother comes to care for Flip and Kathy when mother goes to the hospital.

satisfaction from the labor experience. By assisting the patient and her husband to mobilize their resources and strengths, she is able to work with them in a positive way and to reinforce their concept of themselves as adequate people.

The mind and body of the nurse boggle a bit when she is faced with this considerable responsibility; certainly the young student has some trepidation when she is called upon to assume these duties. Yet with competent guidance and instruction she learns to function efficiently in this role. In order to help the student and/or young graduate prepare for her responsibility, the authors in this chapter have focused on both the patient and the nurse as they move through the successive stages of labor. Although it is the mother who truly delivers her infant, the other important people

in this event—the husband, the doctor and ancillary personnel—are not to be forgotten, for they also play important roles.

PRELUDE TO LABOR

The prodromal signs heralding the onset of labor begin several weeks before true labor commences (see Chap. 10). Lightening may occur any time during the last 4 weeks of pregnancy; in primigravidas it usually occurs about 10 days to 2 weeks prior to labor. This phenomenon causes a sensation of decreased abdominal distention produced by the descent of the presenting part of the baby into the pelvis. In multigravida this may not occur until the labor has begun. The painless Braxton Hicks contractions which have occurred intermittently throughout the latter part of pregnancy may increase so much that they become annoying. They may cause the mother many restless or sleepless nights that contribute to her gradually increasing tension and fatigue. Since the rise in the anxiety level contributes to heightened awareness, the mother becomes more sensitive to various stimuli: if the baby is generally less active, she may worry; if he moves more than usual, she may worry. She wonders about the 2- to 3-lb. weight loss that may occur 3 to 4 days before the onset of labor; ordinarily this would be an occasion of great rejoicing, but now it may give her some concern. Even the increased vaginal mucous discharge may have an ominous significance for her. The spurt of energy that may occur 1 to 2 days before labor begins often leads her into activities that are overfatiguing, and she will need anticipatory guidance from the nurse and the physician to help her to set limits on activity.

This is the time to finish packing her suitcase and to simplify her housekeeping duties. She may want to complete meal preparations for the family's use when she is in the hospital; if this is done daily little by little, then it should not become bothersome. Last-minute details for the care of the other children or the functioning of the household can be taken care of at this time. Short walks in the fresh air are a good way to release extra tension without overfatigue. The mother should be encouraged to achieve a happy balance between activity and rest.

During the latter part of pregnancy the mother will have been instructed about what she should do when she thinks labor has begun. As term approaches, it is wise for the nurse to explore with the mother her preparations for coming to the hospital. The patient and her husband should know approximately how long it will take them to reach the hospital and what alternate means of transportation are available if the husband may not be able to take his wife. What entrance to the hospital they should use and what admission procedures they must go through also are important. A tour of the ward for the parents should be arranged during the antepartal period so that they can become more familiar with the surroundings.

THE ONSET OF LABOR

Most physicians instruct their patients to notify them if the labor contractions become rhythmic and regular and/or the bag of water breaks. To prepare the patient adequately for what to expect, and to instruct her on an appropriate course of action, it is necessary that the nurse have an understanding of the physiology of labor as well as other factors (p. 247). Since the nurse will be with the patient more constantly than the doctor after the patient is admitted to the hospital, the nurse will be expected also to report on the general character of the labor contractions as well as the other symptoms of labor. First, it must be determined whether the patient is actually in labor. Although this is occasionally a difficult problem to settle, usually a decision can be reached on the basis of the differential points between true and false labor (Table 8). It is important that the patient be aware of the difference, too, since it will save herself and the doctor innumerable telephone calls and concern if she does not think every contraction is indicative of true labor.

TABLE 8. DIFFERENTIAL FACTORS IN TRUE AND FALSE LABOR

TRUE LABOR	FALSE LABOR
Contractions:	*Contractions:*
Occur at regular intervals	Occur at irregular intervals
Intervals gradually shorten.	Intervals remain long.
Intensity gradually increases.	Intensity remains the same.
Located chiefly in back	Located chiefly in abdomen
Intensified by walking	Walking has no effect; often gives relief
Show:	*Show:*
Usually present	None
Cervix:	*Cervix:*
Becomes effaced and dilated (this can be determined by digital examination)	Usually uneffaced and closed

TABLE 9. GUIDELINES TO MOTHER'S PARTICIPATION IN LABOR*

WHAT IS HAPPENING	HELPING YOURSELF	BREATHING PATTERN IN CONTRACTION	OTHER HELPS
PRELUDE TO LABOR Lightening (2-4 weeks before 1st baby comes) Braxton-Hicks contractions may increase Increased vaginal mucous discharge Weight loss of 2-3 lbs. (3-4 days before labor) Baby less active Spurt of energy (1-2 days before labor)	Have hospital suitcase packed. Simplify housekeeping. Conserve energy.		
ONSET OF LABOR You may notice any one or a combination of: Regular contractions (felt as backache, pelvic pressure, gas, menstrual cramp, etc.) Show Rupture of membranes	Check signs; time contractions. Call doctor and report. If daytime, continue usual light activity. If night, rest.		Husband or other chosen companion offers diversion and relieves possible tension-producing situations in home.
EARLY FIRST STAGE Cervix effacing, dilatation beginning Contractions become strong enough so that you feel need to do something Dilatation continuing; contractions becoming somewhat closer and stronger If contractions are causing backache	When contractions start, breathe out and relax. Continue slow deep breathing through contraction. Try sitting positions (3, 4). In between contractions rest, read, watch TV, etc. Go to hospital as doctor directs. Relax as much as possible in sitting or lying positions during travel and admitting procedures. Lie on side: breathe deeply and slowly while rocking pelvis very gently through-out contraction (8a, 8b).		Admitting procedures, including questions, examinations, checking baby's heart, perineal shave, enema: medication as indicated. Firm pressure against lower back or slow deep massage during contractions.

WHAT IS HAPPENING	HELPING YOURSELF	BREATHING PATTERN IN CONTRACTION	OTHER HELPS
LATE FIRST STAGE Dilatation continuing, contractions becoming markedly closer, stronger, and of longer duration.	Try lying on back (1a1). Breathe regularly but more shallowly during contraction. When further need felt, change to accelerated breathing, shallow at height of contraction. Relax during contraction.		Direction in control of relaxation and of breathing rhythm and depth. Face sponged with cool cloth: lips moistened. No distracting conversation. Medication as indicated.
TRANSITION: 10 to 20 strong, long contractions, close together but may be somewhat irregular. These contractions complete dilatation. Rectal pressure may cause desire to bear down. There may be tremors, nausea, perspiration, hiccups.	During contractions continue to try to relax. Concentrate on breathing control. As contraction starts, begin breathing fairly deeply; blow out occasionally if there is urge to push (see fig. 33). Don't hold breath. Don't push.		Reassurance about normality of sensations and probable limitation of their duration. Understanding acceptance of possible expressions of irritability.
SECOND STAGE Baby moves gradually through birth canal. Contractions change in character, remaining very strong but slightly farther apart. Continuing strong contractions pushing baby down against pelvic floor and causing stretching, perhaps burning sensation. Baby's head seen at vaginal opening. As doctor slowly delivers head, there may be strong desire to push. Shoulders are born one at a time. Relief is experienced as birth of baby is completed.	During contractions use position fig. 34. Push toward vaginal opening as directed, relaxing pelvic floor and steadily reinforcing work of uterus. (see fig. 35) Between contractions relax completely. While being moved to delivery room, pant deeply through contractions. When settled on delivery table, push as directed through contractions, remembering to relax pelvic floor and thighs. Rest completely between contractions. Pant deeply to control pushing urge; relax thighs. (see figs. 36, 37) If requested to push, push very gently.		Pillows arranged to support mother in comfortable position for pushing. Direction of pushing effort and encouragement of complete relaxation between contractions. Transfer to delivery room. Anesthesia as indicated. Episiotomy as indicated. Direction for controlled pushing and panting.
THIRD STAGE Rhythmical contractions, less intense Abdomen sensitive Placenta delivered	Push as directed. Lie back and enjoy baby!		

* Psychophysical Preparation for Childbearing: Guidelines for Teaching, ed. 2, pp. 44, 45, New York, Maternity Center Association, 1965.

Certain Figures in this quoted table correspond to Figures in our text, as follows: 8a, 8b to Fig. 8-17; Fig. 33 to Fig. 8-27; Fig. 34 to Fig. 8-28; Fig. 35 to Fig. 8-29.

ADMISSION TO THE HOSPITAL

As previously stated, the mother who has been given adequate antepartal care will have received instruction from the physician or the nurse on what to anticipate when she comes to the hospital to have her baby. If this is the mother's first hospital experience, it will be much easier for her if she has been told about the necessary preliminary procedures, such as vulvar and perineal preparation, the methods of examination employed to ascertain the progress of labor, and the usual routines exercised for her care in the course of labor. The mother should understand that she should come to the hospital at the onset of labor, for as labor progresses, these activities are more difficult to carry out and are much more distressing to the patient. The preparation for delivery will of necessity vary in different hospitals, since every hospital has its own admission procedure. The nurse should be aware that many details may be accomplished in a number of ways. Very few institutions employ precisely the same technic in preparing a mother for delivery. Actually, the differences are in details only, for the principles are the same everywhere—namely, asepsis and antisepsis, together with careful observation of the mother for any deviations from the normal.

ESTABLISHMENT OF THE NURSE-PATIENT RELATIONSHIP

For many a young mother in labor, admission to the maternity unit may mark her first acquaintance with hospitals as a patient. Her immediate reaction may be one of strangeness, loneliness and homesickness, particularly if the husband is not permitted to stay with her in the labor room. Regardless of the amount of preparation for this event, whether she is happy or unhappy, whether she wants the baby or not, every mother enters labor with a certain amount of normal tension and anxiety (see p. 197). Moreover, not infrequently mothers are thoroughly afraid of the whole process. This may be attributed in part to the fact that the mother's preparation for childbearing has been limited, or she may have been reared in an environment fraught with mysteries of childbirth and old wives' tales. If she has had previous children, she may have had unfortunate and fear-producing experiences. All these factors make her fear understandable.

Encouragement. Accordingly, one of the first responsibilities of the nurse is to recognize that, in addition to the physical manifestations, there are psychosocial factors that influence each mother's pregnancy and have a bearing on her individual needs for care (see Chaps. 8 and 9). Therefore, every mother deserves encouragement that tends to inspire assurance during her labor. Her discomfort never should be minimized, and an effort should be made to help her to keep in control when her labor is painful. Attention should be directed to the fact that progress is being made, and that her efforts to work cooperatively with her labor are helpful and necessary.

Awareness of Physical and Behavioral Signs. In addition, the nurse must be constantly alert to the physical and behavioral signs associated with the progress of normal labor. She can be extremely helpful by giving the couple anticipatory guidance in this repect so that they will know what to expect during this experience. At the same time, she must watch vigilantly for any sign that may point to abnormal developments. For instance, an increase in pulse rate, a rise in temperature, excessive bleeding, changes in the character of uterine contractions, passage of meconium with a vertex presentation, or alterations in the fetal heart sounds are changes which may have profound implications for the mother's welfare.

Rapport. The nurse who is cordial, empathic and interested in the welfare of her patients establishes good rapport with relative ease and, with astute interviewing, secures the necessary information that will enable her to gain greater insight into the mother's nursing needs. The establishing of rapport is essential in giving effective supportive care. Rapport may be thought of as a relationship consisting of interrelated thoughts and feelings that include empathy, compassion, sympathy, interest and respect for each individual as a unique human being. The concept involves positive communication that contributes to mutual understanding and acceptance. The nurse who establishes rapport with her patient demonstrates understanding and acceptance of the mother. The mother, in turn, is able to trust the nurse, and an effective nurse-patient relationship is facilitated.[2]

First Impressions. The kind of greeting that the patient receives as she enters the delivery suite is extremely important and sets the tone for future interaction with the health team. Some institutions permit the father to accompany his wife to the area, to visit a while and then to depart temporarily, leaving the mother to be admitted and prepared. Others prefer to admit the mother first and then let the husband and the wife remain together; still others do not allow the husband to be with his wife at all during labor. If the husband is present, the nurse should be mindful that he is to be considered and welcomed in an appropriate way, as is his wife.

The mother should be made to feel welcome, expected and necessary (remember that it is she who delivers the baby). Thus she and her husband, if he is present, should be called by name and shown personally by the nurse to the labor room that the mother will occupy. Once there, the patient can be helped, if necessary, to undress and to get into bed.

Orientation. The mother and the father will need to know some of what will be expected of them, and what they in turn can expect as participants in this new situation. Hence, the nurse can begin an orientation to the process of labor as well as to the general environment. It is to be remembered that there is no set form or content for this orientation and no set time for the introduction and the continuation of this process; rather the nurse must first explore what the parents do know about the environment and the labor process, so that she can judge what needs to be introduced, reinforced, etc., and when the most appropriate time to do this would be. An easy conversational manner may be employed rather than a rapid-fire explanation of dos and don'ts.

The rationale for any procedures and/or restrictions always should be given. The patient should not be overloaded with too much stimuli at one time and should be allowed to absorb any new information and explanation before additional material is presented. The nurse can

structure the situation to allow the patient to "feedback" information, so that the nurse knows how much the mother really understands.

Generally, the mother and her husband will need to know what procedures and activities will be performed and the reason for them. In addition, the couple should know the limits of the mother's activity, and what restrictions of food and fluids there will be. What the patient and her husband can expect regarding the progress of labor should be included also, i.e., what will be happening physically, how the mother will be feeling, and how she and her husband can participate in the labor experience. (See Table 9, Guidelines to Mother's Participation in Labor, and Chap. 10.) The father, if present, should be included in any explanations, etc., since he may be participating in the care of his wife. As implied, this orientation will continue throughout the entire course of labor and possibly delivery. The nurse will determine when and how each phase will be instituted, according to the cues given by the mother and the husband.

CONTINUING CARE

After making the mother comfortable in the labor room, the nurse will need to find out some rather specific information regarding the mother's general condition, i.e., the frequency, the duration and the intensity of her contractions, the amount and the character of show, and whether the membranes have ruptured or are intact. At this point it is expedient to learn when the first signs of labor became apparent to the mother and the nature and timing of the uterine contractions from that time. Since the mother's emotional status often has bearing on her physical labor, it is wise to be continuously alert to her behavior—whether she seems *unduly* apprehensive, or whether she is relatively relaxed or calm. Restlessness, excessive conversation, rapid, darting eye movements, arm and body rigidity, and plucking at the bedclothes are all signs of the former. The nurse should report all findings to the physician as soon as possible.

Although the nurse should avoid any outward display of rush or hurry, she should proceed with the admission as quickly as pos-

---

[2] A more thorough discussion of the various concepts involved in rapport and their implementation has been described in the writings of Travelbee, Aring, Kachelski, and Jourard (see Suggested Reading).

sible. It must be remembered that the mother's labor usually will become progressively stronger; hence the more procedures, orientation, etc., that can be accomplished early in labor, while she is able to be more responsive with relative ease, will enhance the patient's comfort and well-being. Also, there generally will be several other people who will be concerned with the care of the mother—the doctor, intern, laboratory technician, etc.—and they often cannot carry out their activities until the patient is fully admitted. Finally, an expeditious completion of the admission procedures leaves more time for the mother and her husband to be together before the actual delivery.

Prior to the physician's examination the nurse will take the mother's temperature, pulse, respiration and blood pressure and listen to the fetal heart tones. A voided urine specimen should be obtained for the admission specimen and to facilitate the physician's vaginal examination. If the patient is allowed to use the bathroom, a receptacle should be placed under the toilet seat since the physician should have available for examination whatever material may be passed per vagina, as well as the urine specimen. If the patient is in labor, the doctor probably will order such procedures as shaving and cleansing of the vulva.

Enema. Unless labor is progressing too rapidly, a cleansing enema may be ordered. The nurse will use the same principles in giving the enema as for any other patient; however, she may find it more difficult to insert the tube because of the pressure of the presenting part of the fetus or of hemorrhoids that the mother may have. Hemorrhoids and/or the strength of the contractions may make the enema discomforting for the patient. It is essential that the nurse let the mother know that she is aware of the possible discomfort, and that she will do all she can to give the enema carefully and comfortably. Giving a step-by-step explanation of the procedure as well as telling the mother specifically what she can do to help to allay the discomfort will go far to alleviate the discomfort. Helpful remarks are: "Let me know when you're having a contraction, and I'll clamp the tubing. Relax your buttocks when you begin to feel the tube being inserted. I'll give this very slowly, so as not to increase cramping. Let me know if it's too uncomfortable, and I can stop the flow for a little while."

An admission bath is rarely a routine procedure. Most patients have sufficient warning at the onset of labor to enable them to bathe prior to coming to the hospital. When a bath is deemed desirable, the type used will depend to some extent on the facilities of the hospital. The types usually given are the shower and the sponge bath. The hand spray may be used as an improvised shower when the shower stall is not available.

Vulvar and Perineal Preparation. The aim in shaving and washing the vulva should be to cleanse and disinfect the immediate area about the vagina and to prevent anything contaminated from entering the birth canal. During labor, pathogenic bacteria ascend the birth canal more readily, and every effort should be made to protect the mother from intrapartal infection. In some hospitals a sterile gauze sponge or a folded towel is placed against the introitus to prevent contaminated matter, such as hair or soapy fluid, from entering the vagina during the preparation procedure. In addition, the nurse should be aware that infection from the nasopharynx is possible, and she should avoid unnecessary coughing or talking which might contaminate the vulva from this source.

In most hospitals the pubic and the vulvar hair are lathered prior to shaving to facilitate the procedure and make it more comfortable for the patient. An ordinary safety razor is used, and, beginning at the mons veneris, with the direction of the stroke being from above downward, the area of the vulva and the perineal body is shaved. The nurse should stretch the skin above each downward stroke and permit the razor to move smoothly over the skin without undue pressure. When the entire area anterior to an imaginary line drawn through the base of the perineal body has been shaved, the patient can be turned to her side to enable the nurse to complete the shaving of the anal area. With the upper leg well flexed, the anal area is lathered and shaved, again with a front-to-back stroke. It must always be remembered that anything which has passed over the anal region must not be returned near the vulvar orifice.

The solutions as well as the technics used in cleansing the genitals will vary in different hospitals, but warm water with soap is probably the most commonly employed. More re-

Fɪɢ. 12-2. Rectal examination, showing flexion of thumb of the gloved hand to prevent contamination of the vulva.

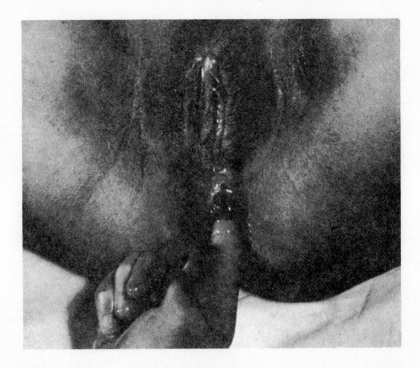

cently, pHisoHex has come into popular usage. A little of this antibacterial liquid cream, used with water and applied to the area with friction, creates a lather and cleanses the skin. On repeated use it develops cumulative bacteriocidal and bacteriostatic properties. Some patients do get a local mucosal reaction manifested by edema and tenderness when pHiso-Hex is used full-strength. In these cases the pHisoHex should be discontinued and a non-irritating soap substituted. The reaction disappears spontaneously in several hours, and no specific treatment is required other than to remove the solution thoroughly with water.

In washing the genitals, the nurse should cleanse thoroughly first the surrounding areas, using sterile sponges or disposable washcloths for each area and gradually working in toward the vestibule. The strokes must be from above downward and away from the introitus. Special attention should be paid to separating the vulvar folds in order to remove the smegma which may have accumulated in the folds of the labia minora and/or at the base of the clitoris. Finally, the region around the anus is cleansed. It should be emphasized here again that a sponge which has passed over the anal area must not be returned near the vulvar orifice but should be discarded immediately. The patient is instructed not to touch the genitals lest she infect herself.

EXAMINATIONS IN LABOR

General. The pulse, respiration and temperature are taken, as previously stated, and are repeated every 4 hours. In cases in which there is fever, or in which labor has lasted more than 24 hours, it is desirable to repeat these observations every 2 hours. The blood pressure is recorded by either the physician or the nurse and is repeated every hour; in cases of toxemia of pregnancy, this may be done more frequently, according to the physician's instructions. As soon as possible after admission, a complete examination of the heart and the lungs is carried out by the physician to make certain that there are no conditions present which might contraindicate the type of analgesia or anesthesia to be used.

Abdominal. The abdominal examination is similar to that carried out in the antepartal period, comprising estimation of fetal size and position and listening to the fetal heart sounds.

Rectal. The majority of the examinations during labor are abdominal and rectal; vaginal examinations are performed only for special

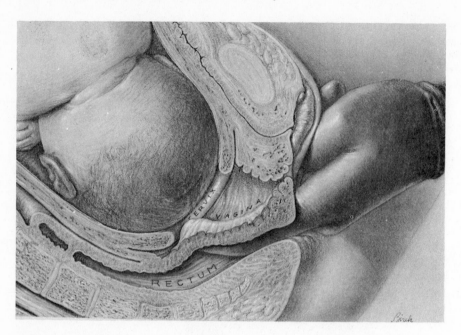

reasons. It was previously thought that rectal examinations were much safer than vaginal examinations, since they reduced the risk of carrying pathogenic bacteria from the introitus and the lower vagina to the region of the cervix and the lower uterine segment. Studies and general experience show that this supposed advantage of rectal examinations over vaginal examinations has been greatly exaggerated. Nevertheless, rectal examinations do have the advantage of not requiring preliminary disinfection on the part of the physician or the patient.

For either rectal or vaginal examination the patient should lie on her back with her knees flexed. The nurse should drape the patient so that she is well protected, but with the perineal region exposed. In making a rectal examination the index finger is used, the hand being covered by a clean but not necessarily sterile rubber glove. As shown in Figure 12-2, the thumb should be fixed into the palm of the hand, because otherwise it may enter the vagina and introduce infection. The finger is anointed liberally with a lubricating jelly and introduced slowly into the rectum. The cervical opening usually can be felt as a depression surrounded by a circular ridge (Fig. 12-3). The degree of dilatation and the amount of effacement are noted. Very often the membranes can

be felt bulging into the cervix, particularly during a contraction. The level of the fetal head is now ascertained and correlated with the level of the ischial spines as being a certain number of centimeters above or below the ischial spines. After the completion of the examination the patient's perineum is wiped, and the examiner's hands are washed. The rectal glove is cleansed and sterilized if it is to be reused; otherwise, it should be discarded.

The frequency with which rectal examinations are required during labor depends on the individual case; often one or two such examinations are sufficient, while in some instances more are required. The nurse who stays with the mother constantly will find that she becomes increasingly skillful in her ability to follow the progress of labor to a great extent by careful evaluation of subjective and objective symptoms of the mother, i.e., the character of the uterine contractions and the show, the progressive descent of the area on the abdomen where fetal heart sounds are heard, the mother's over-all response to her physical labor, etc.

Vaginal. If the mother is to have a vaginal examination, she may be prepared by cleansing the vulvar and the perineal region in a manner similar to that used in preparation for delivery. The physician scrubs his hands as for an operation and dons sterile gloves. Before introducing his fingers into the vagina, he takes care to separate the labia widely in order to minimize possible contamination of his examining fingers if they should come in contact with the inner surfaces of the labia and the margins of the hymen. Then the index and the second fingers of the examining hand are gently introduced into the vagina (Fig. 12-4). Vaginal examination is more reliable than rectal, since the cervix, the fontanels, etc., can be palpated directly with no intervening rectovaginal septum to interfere with the tactile sense. Some authorities feel that the danger of introducing infection into the birth canal is increased with repeated vaginal examinations and thus attempt to limit the number of times the examination is repeated, using it only as necessary.

CONDUCT OF THE FIRST STAGE

The first stage of labor (dilating stage) begins with the first symptoms of true labor and ends with the complete dilatation of the cervix. The physician examines the patient early in labor and sees her from time to time throughout the first stage but may not be in constant attendance at this time. In normal labor his examinations (fetal heart, rectal, etc.) will show that the baby is in good condition and that steady progress is being made. Furthermore, the rate of progress often will give some indication as to when delivery is to be expected. Since the physician is usually unable to be with the mother constantly during this stage, he must rely on the nurse not only to safeguard the welfare of mother and fetus but also to notify him concerning the progress of labor.

Support During Labor

As already emphasized, it is as important for the nurse to have an empathic supportive attitude toward the mother as to have the ability to interpret the progress of labor and to perform certain technical procedures skillfully. It should be pointed out that "supportive care" includes not only aspects of emotional support but also aspects of physical care which in the total context of care contribute to the well-being and the comfort of the mother and hence

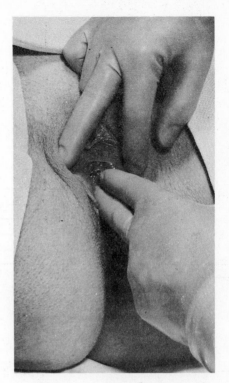

Fig. 12-4. Vaginal examination.

to her emotional equilibrium. Thus, a sponge bath, oral hygiene, a backrub, an explanation before a procedure, etc., all enhance her comfort and help the mother to feel that she is a special, worthwhile person. Many of the physical care activities that nurses perform consist, in part at least, of "laying on of hands," which is known to be necessary and helpful to patients in maintaining or reachieving good health. These activities, then, can be valuable entrées in establishing and maintaining rapport and hence an effective relationship. Even the intrusive procedures which are so often painful or distasteful, if done with gentleness and skill, show the patient that her dignity and integrity are respected.

Related to this "laying on of hands" aspect is the effectiveness of the use of touch. Although this has not been explored to any great degree scientifically, its importance was recognized as far back as the mid-19th century.[3]

[3] Mauriceau, A. M.: The Married Women's Private Medical Companion, New York [publisher unknown], 1859.

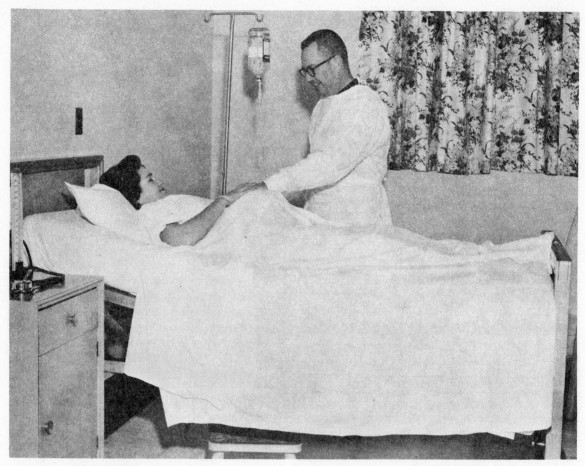

Fig. 12-5. Expectant parents share experience of labor together. (MacDonald House, University Hospitals of Cleveland)

More recently, authors have found that the patient's ability to work effectively with her labor contractions increased when extensive physical contact was introduced and then decreased when physical contact was withdrawn (see Suggested Reading). This contact can take the form of a backrub, allowing the patient to grasp the nurse's hand, stroking the patient's brow, etc. However, touch should not be used indiscriminately, as excessive and/or inappropriate touching is offensive to many people. The need will vary from patient to patient, and the mother will indicate which type of touch is helpful and who will be the most appropriate person to give it. The nurse must use her professional judgment regarding its use, and her rapport with the patient will help her to make a correct decision. This type of communication can be a way of demonstrating the nurse's concern and empathy, especially when verbal communication is difficult or impossible. It is also an effective means of incorporating the husband into the care and the support of his wife.

The more cheerful, flexible environment of the modern labor room undoubtedly is conducive to putting the patient and her husband more at ease, but this in itself is not enough. Once labor is well established, the mother should not be left alone. The morale of women in labor is sometimes hopelessly shattered, regardless of whether or not they have been prepared for labor during pregnancy, when they are left by themselves over long periods of time. During labor the mother is more sensitive to the behavior of those about her, particularly in relation to her perception of how much concern there is on the part of the personnel about her safety and well-being. As labor progresses, there is a normal narrowing of the phenomenal field, an "inward turning," which results in easy distortion of stimuli and perception. For instance, careless remarks dropped in conversation often are misinterpreted as indicative of negligence or unfeelingness. It is well to remember that comments and laughter overheard in the corridor outside the patient's room may contribute to her uneasiness. Therefore, the nurse must be on guard against unfortunate happenings of this kind.

The nurse should be aware that her own anxieties in the situation may be communicated to the patient. The process of labor and the forthcoming delivery will produce normal anxieties which are no more than a healthy anticipation of the events to come (in both patient and nurse). Thus, most patients tolerate their labor much better if they are told the kind of progress that is being made and assured that they are doing a good job working with their contractions. This is part and parcel of the continuing orientation to the labor process that was mentioned earlier (see p. 247).

Another point that is apropos here is the usefulness and the effectiveness of suggestion for the mother in labor. It has been shown that the pregnant woman is extremely passive and vulnerable; this increases her sensitivity and makes her receptive to both positive and negative suggestion from virtually total strangers. The nurse can utilize this suggestibility to great advantage in her supportive care, since the mother responds very readily to suggestions, especially in early labor. The groundwork can be laid at this time for the more complicated instructions that may be necessary later in labor concerning relaxation, breathing technics and the management of pain.

The mother who has attended antepartal classes that have included exercise and relaxation technics is usually better prepared for labor, but nevertheless she needs to be coached in utilizing the technics which will enable her to cooperate with the natural forces of labor. During early labor the patient usually prefers to move about the room and frequently is more at ease sitting in a comfortable chair. She should be permitted and encouraged to do this and whatever else seems to be most relaxing and pleasant to her. If hospital policy permits the husband to be in the labor room, his presence can be a valuable asset because of the support that it gives his wife. Several studies have documented the presence of the husband during labor as a major source of support for the mother (see Suggested Reading). This not only benefits the mother but also helps the father to feel that he has a more vital role in participating with his wife in the birth of their child (Fig. 12-5).

Progression of Active Phase of Labor. When the mother begins to mind her labor, she may need help to get into a comfortable position and to relax. During the contractions she should be coached as necessary in the application of the slow deep-breathing technic described in Chapter 8. Regardless of how diligently the mother has practiced the various breathing and relaxing technics during pregnancy, or the level of her understanding about the physiology of labor, the situation is changed somewhat for her by active labor. Each mother may react in a slightly different way, for each is an individual. Some analgesic medication may be required for the mother's comfort after good labor is established (see p. 228). The nurse may observe in time that as the active phase progresses, i.e., the 7- to 10-cm. dilation, slow deep breathing becomes difficult for the patient. The mother herself is aware that "her diaphragm won't cooperate." Encouraging her to change to rapid, shallow breathing (accelerated breathing) with the contractions is usually easier and more effective.

Uterine Contractions

The term "pains" has been associated with uterine contractions of childbirth since time immemorial. One finds this term of reference still in common usage, so that even today many young women approach childbirth with fear of pain. It is no easy task to dispel this age-old fear, but throughout the childbirth experience a conscious effort must be made to instill a wholesome point of view in the mother. The nurse should avoid the use of the word "pain" whenever possible because of the very connotation of the word, and it is hoped that

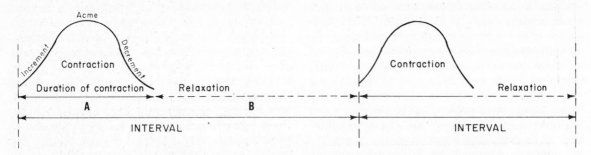

FIG. 12-6. The interval and the duration of uterine contractions. The frequency of contractions is the interval timed from the beginning of one contraction to the beginning of the next contraction. The interval consists of two parts: (A) the duration of the contraction and (B) the period of relaxation. The broken line indicates an indeterminate period, since this time (B) is usually of longer duration than the actual contraction (A).

she will not use it in reference to uterine contractions. It is important to remember, however, that as labor progresses, the contractions often become painful. This is not just a figment of the patient's imagination. Therefore, it is the nurse's responsibility to help the mother to distinguish bétween the *fear and anticipation* of pain and the *actual* pain she may be experiencing, and to help her to cope effectively.

Studies of pain have demonstrated that the anticipation of pain raises the anxiety level significantly to cause the pain reaction threshold to lower. Thus, the patient reacts sooner to even minimal pain stimuli. The pain is subjectively intensified and even a slight amount of pain seems to be much greater. Furthermore, other sensations are misinterpreted as pain, e.g., pressure, stretching, etc., which explains why the digital examinations and even the pressure of the nurse's fingers on the abdomen as she times contractions "hurts." Therefore, "everything" is painful, and the heightening of the anticipation of pain in turn increases the response to pain, and soon a vicious cycle is established. The nurse can help to break this cycle or to prevent it from becoming established by intervening at the anticipation-anxiety junction. She does this by reminding the patient when a contraction is over (and the pain is gone), that another contraction is not expected for several minutes: thus, this is the time for the mother to rest and to relax. The anxiety related to the anticipation of pain then is lowered or eliminated (the mother

knows now she is free from pain for several minutes and can rest), and the subjective intensification is diminished. It is obvious that the nurse or some other reliable person must be in continuous attendance in order to do this.

The frequency, the duration and the intensity of the contractions should be watched closely and recorded. The frequency of contractions is timed from the beginning of one contraction until the beginning of the next contraction. The duration of a contraction is timed from the moment the uterus first begins to tighten until it relaxes again (Fig. 12-6). The intensity of a contraction may be mild, moderate or strong at its acme. Since this is a relative factor, it is difficult to interpret unless one is at the mother's bedside. For the sake of description, one might say that during a mild contraction the uterine muscle becomes somewhat tense, during a moderate contraction the uterus becomes moderately firm, and during a strong contraction the uterus becomes so firm that it has the feel of woody hardness, and at the height of the contraction the uterus cannot be indented by pressure of the examiner's fingers.

When the mother first becomes aware of the contractions, they may be 15 to 20 minutes apart and lasting perhaps 20 to 25 seconds. Since these are of mild intensity, she usually can continue with whatever she is doing, except that she is alert to time the subsequent contractions to have specific information to give the physician when she calls him. If this is her first pregnancy, he may advise her to wait until the contractions are 5 to 10 minutes apart before coming to the hospital (depending on the other signs of labor). However, if she is a multipara, she will more than likely be told to come to the hospital as soon as a regular pattern of contractions is established (again, depending on other criteria).

As labor progresses, the character of the contractions will change (see Chap. 10). They will become stronger in intensity, last longer (a duration of 45 to 60 seconds) and come closer together (at a frequency of every 2 to 3 minutes). The only effective method the nurse can employ to time contractions is to keep her fingers lightly on the fundus. The fingers are recommended because they usually are more sensitive than the more calloused palm. However, for some people the whole hand is helpful.

It should be emphasized that enough of the fingers should be used to ensure adequate contact with the abdomen; too slight a contact does not enable the nurse to ascertain the contractions accurately.

As the nurse times in this manner, she is able to detect the contraction, as it begins, by the gradual tensing and rising forward of the fundus, and to feel the contraction through its 3 phases until the uterus relaxes again. The inexperienced nurse can get some idea of how a contraction will feel under her fingertips if she feels her own biceps contract. First, the forearm should be extended and the fingertips of the hand on the opposite side placed on the biceps. Then, the arm is gradually flexed until the muscle becomes very hard, held a few seconds, and gradually extended. This should

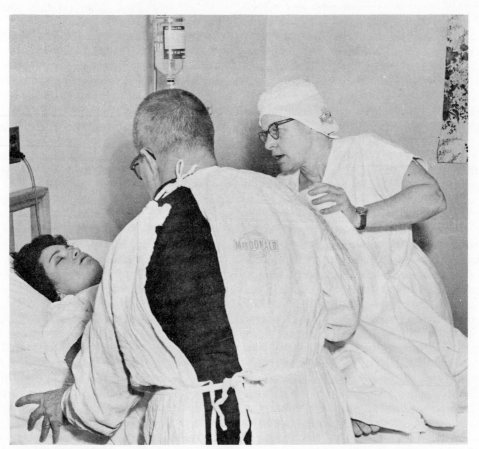

FIG. 12-7. Mother in active first-stage labor (cervix 8 cm. dilated) being assisted by husband and nurse to accomplish conscious relaxation. (MacDonald House, University Hospitals of Cleveland)

take about 30 seconds to simulate a uterine contraction. It is not reliable to ask the mother to let you know when contractions begin, because often she is unaware of it for perhaps 5 or 10 seconds, sometimes even until the contraction reaches its acme. It is important for the nurse to observe the rhythm of the contractions and to be assured that the uterine muscle relaxes completely after each contraction. As the labor approaches the transition, the contractions will be very strong, last for about 60 seconds and occur at 2- to 3-minute intervals. If any contraction lasts longer than 70 seconds and is not followed by a rest interval with complete relaxation of the uterine muscle, this should be reported to the physician immediately because of its implications for both the mother and her infant (see Chap. 19, Complications of Labor).

Particularly during the late active phase the need for human contact—someone to hold on to—during the severe contractions will be seen. The mother responds less well to other physical contact, stroking, sponging, etc.; she may even say, "Leave me alone," meaning, of course, "Don't disturb me." It is helpful for her, however, to have someone's hand to hold, and she should be allowed to do this if she indicates the need.

Since during the first stage of labor the uterine contractions are involuntary and uncontrolled by the patient, it is futile for her to "bear down" with her abdominal muscles, because this only leads to exhaustion. The mother who has been prepared for "natural childbirth" has been schooled in breathing technics, such as diaphragmatic breathing or rapid shallow costal breathing, and with coaching from her husband or her nurse is usually able to accomplish conscious relaxation.

With the "unprepared" mother a different situation exists. These mothers best can be helped to relax by encouraging and coaching them to keep breathing slowly and evenly during the early contractions and then more rapidly and shallowly during the late active phase. They should be reminded not to hold their breath during the contractions. One should not expect perfection in the breathing technics with these patients; however, this activity gives the inexperienced mother a point of concentration, and her feeling that she is actually participating and "controlling" her labor to some degree is helpful to her. Most mothers in labor, whether they are "prepared" or not, want to cooperate, and the calm, kind, firm guidance of an interested nurse can do much to help the mother utilize her contractions effectively.

Show

This mucoid discharge from the cervix is present after the discharge of the mucous plug. As progressive effacement and dilatation of the cervix occur, the show becomes blood-tinged due to the rupture of superficial capillaries. The presence of an increased amount of bloody show (blood-stained mucus, not actual bleeding!) suggests that rather rapid progress may be taking place and should be reported immediately, particularly if associated with frequent severe contractions.

A perineal pad should not be worn during labor because of the nature of the vaginal discharge. The tenacious mucoid discharge frequently comes in contact with the anus and could easily be smeared about the external genitalia and vaginal orifice when the patient moves about the bed or adjusts the pads. A quilted pad placed under the mother's buttocks serves very well to absorb material discharged from the vagina. This pad should be changed frequently and the perineum cleansed as necessary to keep the mother clean and dry.

Fetal Heart Tones

The behavior of the fetal heart beat in labor is of great importance. When taking the fetal heart sounds, one should listen and count for 1 full minute in order that any irregularity or slowing may be detected. As already explained, the fetal heart rate normally is between 120 to 160 beats per minute, except during and immediately after a uterine contraction, when it may fall to as low as 70 to 110. Hon[4] found that in multigravidas the fetal heart rate might fall from 140 to 110-120 beats per minute at the acme of a contraction. In primigravidas the drop is greater, at times reaching 60 to 70 beats per minute (Fig. 12-8). This physiologic bradycardia begins after the onset of a con-

[4] Hon, E. H.: Electronic evaluation of fetal heart rates, Am. J. Obstet. Gynec. 83:333-358, February 1, 1962.

traction and ends 10 to 15 seconds prior to its end. It is believed to result from compression of the fetal skull by the partially dilated cervix rather than from fetal hypoxia. It appears to occur most commonly between 4 and 8 cm. of cervical dilatation.

It may be difficult to hear the sounds during a contraction, because the uterine wall is tense, and, in addition, it is more difficult for the mother to lie still during this period. But it is particularly important to listen at this time, since these observations inform the listener how the fetus reacts to the contraction. From a clinical standpoint any prolonged slowing should be reported to the obstetrician. Should the slowing be below 100 beats per minute, and should it last more than 30 seconds after the termination of a contraction, then it is no longer considered to be physiologic and is taken as a sign of fetal distress. Occasionally, this prolonged slow rate is accompanied by the passage of meconium, another sign indicative of fetal distress if it occurs in a vertex presentation. It must be remembered that unless the membranes have ruptured, the meconium will not be apparent. Any unusual observations must be reported to the physician promptly so that measures can be instituted before permanent damage is done to the infant.

Repeated auscultation of the fetal heart sounds constitutes one of the most important responsibilities in the conduct of the first and the second stages of labor (see Chap. 6, Normal Pregnancy). During the early period of the first stage of labor the nurse should record the fetal heart rate every hour, and once good labor is established, every half hour, or even more often if indicated. During the second stage of labor it should be done every 5 minutes and recorded.

The fetal heart tones should be checked immediately following the rupture of membranes, regardless of whether they rupture spontaneously or are artificially ruptured by the physician. With the gush of water that ensues, there is a possibility that the cord may be prolapsed, and any indication of fetal distress from pressure on the umbilical cord can thereby be detected.

Other Aspects of Care

Temperature, Pulse and Respiration. The pulse in normal labor is usually in the 70's or the 80's and rarely exceeds 100. Sometimes the pulse rate on admission is slightly increased because of the excitement of coming to the hospital, but this returns to normal shortly thereafter. A persistent pulse rate over 100 suggests exhaustion or dehydration. The temperature and respiration should also be normal. If there is an elevation of temperature

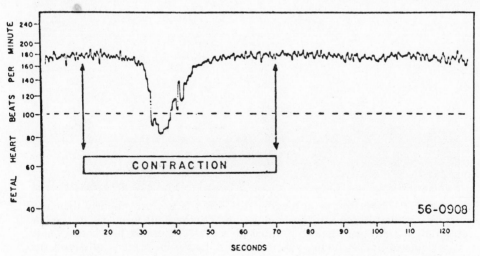

FIG. 12-8. Electronic evaluation of fetal heart rates, showing normal slowing of the fetal heart rate during uterine contraction. (Hon, E. H.: Observations on "pathologic" fetal bradycardia, Am. J. Obstet. Gynec. 77:1084, 1959)

over 37.2° C. or 99° F. (orally), or the pulse and respiration become rapid, the physician should be notified. The temperature should be recorded every 4 hours, or more frequently if indicated. On the other hand, the pulse and respiration should be taken every hour.

Blood Pressure. The blood pressure should be recorded every hour during labor. During the first stage of labor there is little change in blood pressure between contractions, but during contractions an average increase of 5 to 10 mm. Hg may be expected. For this reason the blood pressure readings should be taken between the contractions. Any unusual recordings of either systolic or diastolic pressure should be reported immediately.

Fluid and Food Intake. The practice here varies greatly among different physicians and in different institutions. Therefore, the wishes of the physician in charge should be ascertained before proceeding. In general, it is customary to urge the mother to take water or clear fluids, such as tea with sugar, during the early phase of the first stage of labor, but she should not be given solid or liquid foods because their digestion is delayed during labor. Evidence that the powers of digestion are impaired at this time is demonstrated by the fact that it is not unusual for nausea and/or vomiting to occur near the end of the first stage of labor. It may be necessary to administer a general anesthetic for the delivery, so that if the patient takes fluid or food shortly before delivery, vomiting and consequent aspiration may occur. On the other hand, in a prolonged labor, it is most important to maintain adequate fluid and caloric intake in order to forestall dehydration and exhaustion, in which case the physician may find it desirable to administer intravenous glucose solutions.

Bladder. The patient should be asked to void at least every 3 or 4 hours. The mother in labor often attributes all of her discomfort to the intensity of uterine contractions and therefore is unaware that it is the pressure of a full bladder which has increased her discomfort. In addition to causing unnecessary discomfort, a full bladder may be a serious im-

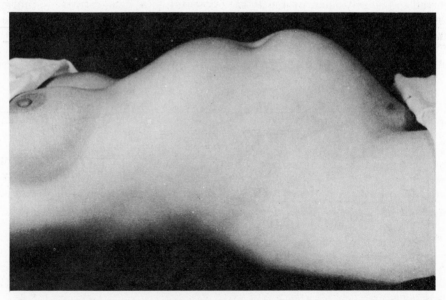

FIG. 12-9. Dystocia due to bladder distention. The tremendously distended bladder is plainly seen in the photograph. This patient was sent to the hospital after 3 days of ineffectual labor at home. The cervix had been dilated, it is believed, for 24 hours, yet no progress had been made. Catheterization of the greatly distended bladder yielded 1,000 cc. of urine. Following this, the infant's head descended at once, and delivery was easy. (Eastman: Williams' Obstetrics, ed. 11, New York, Appleton)

Fig. 12-10. Technic of catheterization, showing use of 6-inch sterile tissue forceps to insert catheter.

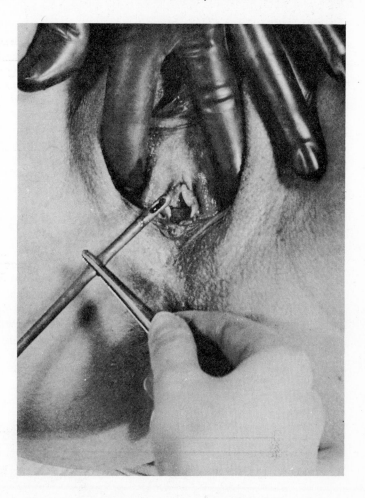

pediment to labor (Fig. 12-9) or the cause of urinary retention in the puerperium. If the distended bladder can be palpated above the symphysis pubis, and the patient is unable to void, the physician should be so informed. Not infrequently he will order catheterization in such cases. Various technics are used, all designed at maintaining strict asepsis. One technic, illustrating the use of sterile tissue forceps to hold the catheter, is shown in Figure 12-10.

Analgesia. (See Chap. 11, Analgesia and Anesthesia.) Before administering the medication prescribed to promote analgesia, the nurse should inform the mother that she is going to give her medication which will make her more comfortable and help her in labor. She should encourage the mother to try to rest and assure her that she will not be left alone. It is wise to tell her also that you will remain quietly at the bedside and keep conversation at the very

minimum in order for her to get the maximum benefit from the medication. Her bladder should be emptied prior to administering the drugs, and the fetal heart tones and the mother's vital signs should be recorded before and after such medication is given. Once analgesic therapy has been instituted, the mother should not receive fluids or food by mouth and should remain in bed. The environment should be conducive to rest, the room quiet and darkened but with sufficient light to permit accurate observation of the patient. Many institutions require that side rails be applied when the patient is medicated, even though there is someone in attendance. The necessity of this should be explained to both the patient and her husband, so that any undue fears or misinterpretations are avoided. The father, especially, should be alerted to the importance of keeping the rails up if he is attending to any of his wife's needs, since he is not used to their presence and is apt to forget to reapply them if he steps away from the bedside for a time. This can be a difficult experience for the husband. Thus, if he is showing the strain at this time, he may welcome the suggestion of having a cup of coffee and a change of scene for a while. If the mother has received scopolamine or other drugs in dosage sufficient to cause her to be heavily sedated, she *never* should be left unattended.

Signs of Second Stage. There are certain signs and symptoms, both behavioral and physical, which herald the onset of the second stage of labor. These signs and symptoms should be watched for carefully. They are as follows: (1) The patient begins to bear down of her own accord; this is caused by a reflex when the head begins to press on the perineal floor. (2) Her mood of increasing apprehension, which has been building since the contractions became well established, deepens; she becomes more serious and may appear bewildered by the force of the contractions. (3)

There is usually a sudden increase in show that is more blood-tinged. (4) The patient becomes increasingly irritable and unwilling to be touched; she may cry if disturbed. (5) The mother thinks that she needs to defecate. This symptom is due to pressure of the head on the perineal floor and consequently against the rectum. (6) Although she has been "working" successfully with her contractions during most of her labor, the uncertainty that she has been experiencing (since 4- to 8-cm. cervical dilatation) as to her ability to cope with the contractions becomes overwhelming; she is frustrated and feels unable to manage if left alone. (7) The membranes may rupture, with discharge of amniotic fluid. This, of course, may take place any time but occurs most frequently at the beginning of the second stage. (8) The mother may be eager to be "put to sleep"; or if she is given appropriate help, she may narrow her concentration to trying to cope with the contractions and/or pushing according to instructions. It is important to remember that the mother's consciousness is somewhat altered

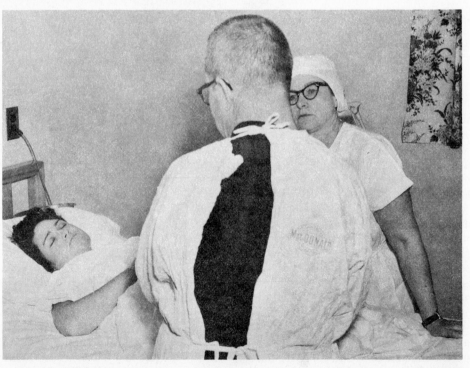

FIG. 12-11. Mother is encouraged to relax and sleep between contractions (cervix 10 cm. dilated but fetal head needs to descend further). (MacDonald House, University Hospitals of Cleveland)

because of the pain, her enforced concentration and possibly medication; therefore, any coaching should be short and explicit and may need to be repeated with each contraction. The nurse also must be firm but gentle in setting limits with the mother, so that she can conserve her energy for the second stage. Thrashing about and continued crying only lead to exhaustion, and the mother needs the firm guidance of a skillful person to help her to maintain control. (9) The perineum begins to bulge and the anal orifice to dilate. This is a late sign, but if signs numbered 1, 3, 5, and 7 occur, it should be watched for with every contraction. Only rectal or vaginal examination (or the appearance of the head) can definitely confirm the suspicion. Emesis at this time is not unusual.

In order to spare the mother a hurried trip to the delivery room and permit adequate time to cleanse and drape her properly for the delivery without unnecessary rush, the nurse should report promptly any or all of these symptoms which she observes. If these signs are overlooked, a precipitate delivery may occur without benefit of medical attention. In general, primigravidas should be taken to the delivery room when the cervix is fully dilated, and multiparas when it is 7 or 8 cm. dilated.

CONDUCT OF THE SECOND STAGE

The second stage of labor (expulsion stage) begins with the complete dilatation of the cervix and ends with delivery of the baby. The complete dilatation of the cervix can be confirmed definitely only by rectal or vaginal examination. However, the nurse often is able to make a nursing diagnosis on the basis of her observations of the progress of labor, particularly if she correlates these findings with knowledge of the mother's parity, the speed of any previous labors, the pelvic measurements, etc., noted in the antepartal record. Although the general rule regarding the optimal time for taking a mother to the delivery room has been stated, it must be remembered that, in addition, the physician will be guided in his decision to give such an order by such factors as the station of the presenting part and the speed with which labor is progressing. If on

examination of a primigravida, the physician finds the cervix to be fully dilated but the presenting part of the fetus only descended to the level of the ischial spines (midpelvis), he undoubtedly will want the mother to remain in the labor room to permit the forces of labor to bring about further descent of the fetus before taking the mother to the delivery room. During this period he may want the patient to exert her abdominal forces and "bear down." In most cases bearing-down efforts are reflex and spontaneous in the second stage of labor, but, occasionally, the mother does not employ her expulsive forces to good advantage, particularly if she has had caudal analgesia. The nurse will be asked to coach and encourage the mother in this procedure. The thighs should be flexed on the abdomen, with hands grasped just below the knees when a contraction begins. Instructions should be given to take a deep breath as soon as the contraction begins and, with her breath held, to exert downward pressure exactly as if she were straining at stool. Pulling on the knees at this time, as well as flexing the chin on the chest, is a helpful adjunct to maintain downward pressure of the diaphragm and to stabilize the chest and the abdominal musculature. In addition, maintaining the legs flexed as for the "push" position deters the mother from pushing her feet against the table. Avoiding such pressure on the feet is important, because it discourages tensing of the gluteal muscles and thus contributes to further relaxation of the pelvic floor. The "bearing down" effort should be as long and sustained as possible, since short "grunty" endeavors are of little avail. If at this time the mother is in the delivery room, but her legs as yet have not been put up in stirrups or leg holders, she can be coached in the same manner. In most hospitals the delivery tables have firmly attached hand grips which can be adjusted in position so that the mother can reach them comfortably to pull against, if she wishes. However, in doing so her hands are not free to pull up on her knees with the contraction, so that the nurse or other person in attendance needs to assist her. This can be accomplished by assisting the mother to bring her legs up into position and exerting proper pressure against her knees as she bears down with the contraction. Care should be

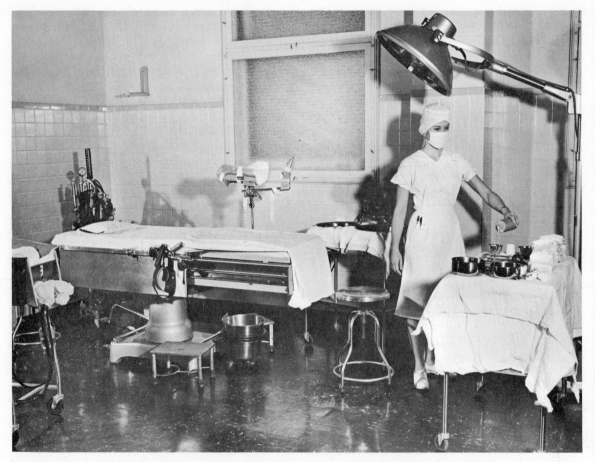

Fig. 12-12. The delivery room. Nurse is preparing instrument table.

exercised to grasp the mother's knees from above, since doing so under the knees could exert undesirable pressure on the popliteal veins. At the end of each contraction the mother is assisted to put her legs down and encouraged to rest until the next contraction begins. Usually, these bearing-down efforts are rewarded by increased bulging of the perineum, that is, by further descent of the head. The patient should be informed of such progress, for encouragement is all-important. In certain instances it may be undesirable for the mother to bear down; thus the nurse should not encourage the mother to do so without the physician's request. In these cases, if the mother has an urge to bear down, she can be instructed to pant during each contraction; this will obviate her bearing down since it is impossible to push while panting.

When the mother is ready to be transferred to the delivery room, it is more helpful if the same nurse who has been attending her in labor accompanies her to the delivery room. This transfer will mean a new environment for the patient to cope with under very stressful circumstances. There may be great physical and mental exertion called for with little preparation or practice. To the mother in labor who is unfamiliar with such surroundings, the "sterile" atmosphere of the delivery room can be strange, cold and uninviting, what with its obstetric furnishings and supplies that become even more foreboding as they reflect the glittering lights of the room. Under such circumstances the sight and the sound of familiar faces and voices, even though partially concealed and muffled by the surgical caps, masks and gowns, do give the patient some sense of

FIG. 12-13. Bassinet infant Kreiselman resuscitator. An explosion-proof bassinet for the immediate care of the newborn infant. (Ohio Chemical and Surgical Equipment Co., Madison, Wisconsin)

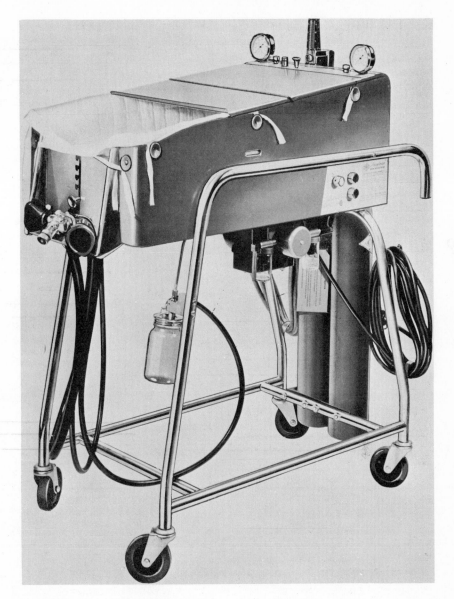

continuity and security. Furthermore, by this time the nurse and the patient should have established a communication pattern, each able to pick up the other's more covert cues. Thus, the coaching, guidance and follow-through necessary in the second stage of labor will be expedited if the same person continues with the care.

The nurse will notice that the mother has become increasingly involved in the whole birth process. The seemingly panicky frustration of the late active phase subsides a bit (with appropriate coaching and reassurance), and the patient may experience a sense of relief that the expulsive stage has begun. The desire to push and to bear down is very strong now—uncontrollable, in fact—and the patient generally gets enormous satisfaction with each push. Some patients, however (e.g., those with a highly charged emotional labor), experience acute pain and need all available help and encouragement to continue bearing down. The nurse will note that in most instances there is complete exhaustion after each expulsive effort, and the mother often drops off to sleep, only to be roused by the next contraction. Since consciousness is still altered, it may be difficult for the mother to follow directions readily even though she may want to. Again, repeated, short, explicit directions are required to encourage her to rest or to work but more especially to prepare the mother for the expulsive effort if she is sleeping between contractions and awakens abruptly.

Muscular cramps in the legs are common in the second stage because of pressure exerted by the baby's head on certain nerves in the pelvis. To relieve these cramps, the leg should be straightened and the ankle dorsiflexed by exerting pressure upward against the ball of the foot until the cramp subsides (see Fig. 8-16). Meanwhile, the knee should be stabilized with the other hand. These cramps cause excruciating pain and must never be ignored.

Good obstetric care during the second stage of labor demands the closest teamwork among physician, nurse and anesthetist. By previous understanding, or more often by established hospital routine, each has his or her own responsibilities in the delivery room, and, if the best interests of the mother and her infant are to be fulfilled, the responsibilities of each must be carried out smoothly and efficiently.

Up to now, the primary focus for the nurse has been on direct patient care. Now she must enlarge her focus to include the obstetrician and other allied professionals; that is, there will be more activities which will require the actual assistance of these persons than was necessary during the first stage of labor. Thus, the nurse must be sensitive not only to the cues sent by the mother but also to those relayed by the other personnel.

Preparation for Delivery

Preparation of the Delivery Room. There are no two hospitals in which the set-up of a

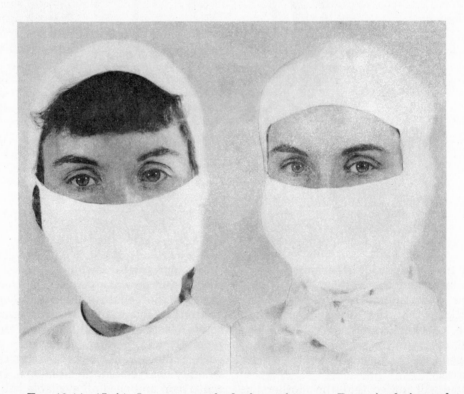

Fig. 12-14. (*Left*) *Incorrect* method of wearing cap. Bacteria, hairs and other infectious particles can readily fall from exposed hair and contaminate sterile fields. (*Right*) *Correct* method of adjusting cap so that *all* hair is covered.

delivery room or the procedure for delivery is precisely the same, and this is one phase of the nurse's work which she must learn wholly from actual observation and experience in her own institution. Nevertheless, she can obtain a general idea of the main equipment used from Figure 12-12.

The delivery table is designed so that its surface is actually composed of two adjoining sections, each covered with its own mattress. This permits the patient to lie in the supine position until it is desired to put her legs up into stirrups, that is, put her in the lithotomy position. At this time the table is "broken" by a mechanical device. The retractable or lower end of the table drops and is rolled under the main section of the table. Thus ready access is given to the perineal region. Or, if it is desired to deliver the patient in the dorsal recumbent position, the lower portion of the table can be allowed to remain in place.

The instrument table opposite the foot of the delivery table contains the principal sterile supplies and instruments needed for normal delivery, including, among other articles, towels, sponges, catheter, solutions, basins and the "cord set." The cord set is a group of instruments used for clamping and cutting the umbilical cord, namely, 2 hemostats, a pair of scissors and a cord tie or clamp. Other instruments often are included, because it may be necessary for the physician to perform an episiotomy or to repair lacerations (p. 286). Other instruments frequently included are 2 hemostats, 2 Allis clamps, 1 mouse-tooth tissue forceps, 2 sponge sticks, 1 vaginal retractor, 2 tenaculae, 1 needle holder, assorted needles and a pair of obstetric forceps.

A double-bowl solution stand or basin rack generally is used to hold the basins, one for wet sponges and the other to receive the placenta. Emergency instruments, a crib and a resuscitator, such as the Kreiselman (Fig. 12-13), which provides heat in addition to mechanical suction and oxygen equipment, are part of standard delivery room equipment. Even if the infant does not require resuscitation, the resuscitator affords him a warm, protected environment, and it is a convenient place in which to give him care. To facilitate the delivery, all equipment should be in readiness at all times.

Asepsis and Antisepsis. Persons who have a communicable disease or persons who have been in contact with a communicable disease should be excluded from maternity service until examined by a physician. The examining physician should certify that the employee is free from infections before he or she is allowed to return to duty. Personnel with evidence of upper respiratory infections or open skin lesions, diarrhea or any other infectious disease also should be excluded. Furthermore, all persons working in the maternity area should have a pre-employment physical examination and thereafter an annual physical examination and such interim exminations as may be required by the hospital.[5]

Of prime importance in the conduct of the second stage are strict asepsis and antisepsis throughout. To this end everyone in the delivery room must wear a clean cotton uniform, cap and mask, and those actually participating in the delivery are in sterile attire. Masking must include both nose and mouth. Caps should be so adjusted as to keep *all* hair covered (Fig. 12-14). If the nurse scrubs to assist the doctor, the strictest aseptic technic must be observed. The hands should be disinfected as carefully as for a major surgical operation. Scrubbing the hands should be started sufficiently early so that full time may be allotted, as well as to don gown and gloves.

Transfer of the Mother to the Delivery Room. When the physician deems the birth to be imminent, he will ask that the mother be transferred to the delivery room and prepared for delivery. If the mother is awake, she should be told what is happening and be informed in advance about any procedure. If the husband will not be accompanying his wife to the delivery room, then time should be allowed, if possible, for them to bid each other a temporary goodbye. This kind of planning not only is supportive but also enables both to cooperate more fully. Care should be taken to have only one person instruct or coach the mother at any one time. When delivery is imminent, her attention will be limited necessarily, as already illustrated, and the sound of several voices at one time is confusing. If the physician, for example, is coaching, it is well for nurse not to

[5] Recommendations from the Manual of Standards in Obstetric-Gynecologic Practice, p. 11, Chicago, The American College of Obstetricians and Gynecologists, 1963.

participate verbally; however, she should remain alert and ready to step into the role
whenever it is appropriate.

Prior to the actual transfer to the delivery
room the nurse should find out what type of
anesthesia the physician is planning to use.
Since the immediate positioning of the patient
in the delivery room will depend on the type
of anesthesia used, this preplanning will expedite activities during delivery and promote
smoother functioning of the team.

Delivery

If spinal anesthesia is to be administered,
the patient is turned on her side for the administration. If she is given a saddle block, she
may be placed on her side or assisted to a
sitting position on the side of the delivery
table, with her feet supported on a stool and
her body leaning forward against the nurse.
Her back should be toward the operator and
bowed (the position requires flexion of the
neck and the lumbar spine). This principle of
cervical and lumbar flexion is used also in the
side lying position (see Chap. 11).

Although the positioning and the administration of the anesthesia take only a few minutes, the mother undoubtedly will be extremely
uncomfortable due to the severity of the contractions at this time; she should be assured
that this discomfort is only temporary, and
soon she will be pain-free. The fetal heart tones
and the maternal blood pressure should be
checked frequently—every 5 minutes or so. In
addition, the mother should have her head
elevated with two small pillows to help to prevent the anesthetic level from rising beyond
the desired height. So that the anesthetic level
may stabilize, the nurse should wait for instructions from the anesthetist before putting
the mother's legs in stirrups or performing any
other manipulations. If the mother is to receive general anesthesia, she lies supine on the
table. Local or pudendal anesthesia are administered with the mother in the lithotomy
position (see Chap. 11).

As has been previously stated, anesthesia
should be administered only by a qualified
physician or a nurse anesthetist. This entire
subject is discussed in more detail in Chap-

ter 11, Analgesia and Anesthesia for Labor.

During the time that the anesthesia is being
administered, the circulating nurse can un-
cover the sterile tables, check the resuscitator
and attach a sterile suction catheter and oxygen mask, and perform other duties for which
she is responsible. Once the anesthesia has
been administered, the nurse should resume
checking the fetal heart tones every 5 minutes.

Before elevating the mother's legs into the
stirrups, cotton flannel boots which cover the
entire leg should be put on. In putting the legs
of the patient up into stirrups or leg holders,
care should be used not to separate the legs
too widely or to have one leg higher than the
other. Both legs should be raised or lowered at
the same time, with a nurse supporting each
one if the mother is unable to help in the positioning. Failure to observe these instructions
may result in straining the ligaments of the
pelvis, with consequent discomfort in the puerperium. Care should be taken to avoid pressure
on the popliteal space, and to angle the stirrups
so that the feet are not dependent. The mother
also is given handles to grip and pull on, which
aid her in her bearing-down efforts. Wrist
straps usually are attached to these, which are
secured about the wrist and allow some limited
movement but prevent her from reaching up
to touch the sterile drapes. The purpose of the
handles and the cuffs should be explained to
the mother, since many patients often complain about being "strapped down."

With the patient in the lithotomy position,
the nurse carries out the procedure for cleansing the vulva and the surrounding area. If the
delivery is to be conducted with the mother in
the recumbent position, this may be carried
out with the knees drawn up slightly and the
legs separated. Then, the physician, who meanwhile has scrubbed his hands and donned sterile gown and gloves, drapes the patient with
towels and sheets appropriate for the purpose
(Fig. 12-15).

After the patient has been prepared for delivery, catheterization, if done, is carried out
by the physician. Sometimes it is difficult to
catheterize a patient in the second stage of
labor, since the infant's head may compress
the urethra. If the catheter does not pass
easily, force never should be employed. Whenever it is possible and appropriate, all

procedures, of course, should be explained to the mother as they occur.

As the infant descends the birth canal, pressure against the rectum may cause fecal material to be expelled. The physician will employ sponges (as a rule soaked with saline solution) to remove any fecal material which may escape from the rectum.

Fundal pressure should not be used to accomplish spontaneous delivery or to bring the head deeper into the birth canal. Severe fundal pressure may cause uterine damage or rupture of the uterus.

As soon as the head distends the perineum to a diameter of 6 or 8 cm., the physician often will place a towel over the rectum and exert forward pressure on the chin of the baby's head while the other hand exerts downward pressure on the occiput (Figs. 12-16 to 20).

This is called Ritgen's maneuver, and allows the physician to control the egress of the head; it also favors extension so that the head is born with the smallest diameter presenting. The head usually is delivered between contractions and as slowly as possible (Fig. 12-21). At this time the mother may complain about a "splitting" sensation due to the extreme vaginal stretching as the head is born. All these measures (control of head by Ritgen's maneuver, extension and slow delivery between contractions) help to prevent lacerations. If a tear seems to be inevitable, an incision which is called an episiotomy may be made in the perineum. This will not only prevent lacerations but also will facilitate the delivery (see p. 286). Immediately after the birth of the infant's head the physician passes his finger along the occiput to the infant's neck in order

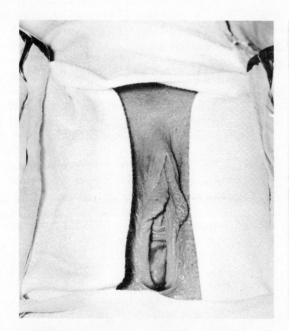
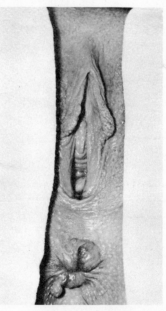

FIG. 12-15. Proper draping for delivery showing appropriate placement of sterile towels, one of which covers the anus. (The Johns Hopkins Hospital, Baltimore, Md.)

FIG. 12-16. Scalp of the infant detected through a slitlike vulvar opening as the perineal region begins to bulge and the skin over it becomes tense and glistening. Pressure of the descending head causes the anus to become patulous and everted. For purposes of showing changes which take place in the anus the lower towel has been removed from this photograph and the succeeding ones of this series, but this is for illustrative purposes only. (The Johns Hopkins Hospital, Baltimore, Md.)

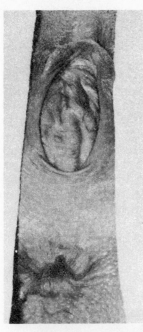

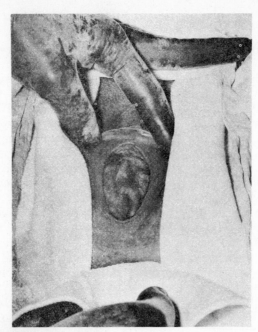

Fig. 12-17. (*Left*) Appearance of the infant's head with subsequent contractions. The vulva becomes more dilated and distended by the infant's head so that the opening is gradually converted into an ovoid. (The Johns Hopkins Hospital, Baltimore, Md.)

Fig. 12-18. (*Right*) Control of the progress of the head to preserve the perineum from tearing. (The Johns Hopkins Hospital, Baltimore, Md.)

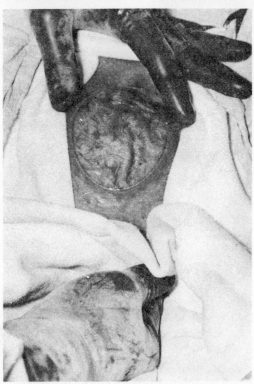

Fig. 12-19. Farther advanced extension of the head. The left hand is used to prevent sudden expulsion of the head as it crowns, while pressure on the infant's chin through the perineum by the right hand expedites extension and delivery. This is Ritgen's maneuver. (The Johns Hopkins Hospital, Baltimore, Md.)

to feel whether a loop or more of umbilical cord encircles it. If such a coil is felt, it should be gently drawn down and, if loose enough, slipped over the infant's head. This is done to prevent interference with the infant's oxygen supply, which could result from pressure of his shoulder on the umbilical cord. If the cord is too tightly coiled to permit this procedure, it must be clamped and cut before the shoulders are delivered; then the infant must be extracted immediately before asphyxiation results. As shown in Figure 12-22, the anterior shoulder usually is brought under the symphysis pubis first and then the posterior shoulder is delivered, after which the remainder of the body follows without particular mechanism (Figs. 12-23 and 24). The exact time of the baby's birth should be noted. The infant usually cries immediately, and the lungs become expanded; about this time the pulsations in the umbilical cord begin to diminish. The physician usually will defer clamping the cord until this occurs, or for a minute or so if practicable, because of the marked benefit of the additional blood to the infant. Using sterile instruments, he cuts the cord between the 2 Kelly clamps, which have been placed a few inches from the umbilicus, then the umbilical clamp or tie is applied. The tie, a sterilized linen tape ligature, is usually applied about an inch from the abdomen, with care to secure it

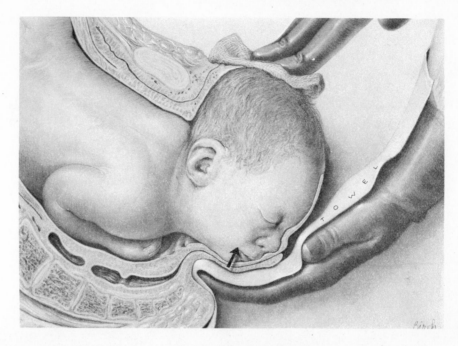

FIG. 12-20. Ritgen's maneuver, as it appears in median section. Arrow shows direction of pressure.

tight enough to prevent bleeding without its cutting into the cord (Figs. 12-25, 28). A second ligature may be applied for further protection if it is desired, or if it is necessary because of any bleeding. There are several types of umbilical clamps, such as the Kane, the Zeigler and the Hesseltine, which are used extensively in many institutions (Fig. 12-27). With these the possibility of hemorrhage is minimized.

The first 15 minutes after the infant's birth is the most hazardous period of life, when more infants succumb than during any subsequent time. The responsibility for much of the care during this period is delegated to the nurse, so that the physician may devote his attention to the mother during the third stage of labor (see p. 277 and Chap. 15).

CONDUCT OF THE THIRD STAGE

Delivery of the Placenta

The third stage of labor (placental stage) begins after the delivery of the baby and ter-

minates with the birth of the placenta. Immediately after delivery of the infant the height of the uterine fundus and its consistency are ascertained. The physician may do this by palpating the uterus through a sterile towel placed on the lower abdomen, but it is a duty which often is delegated to the nurse, at least while the physician is engaged in clamping and

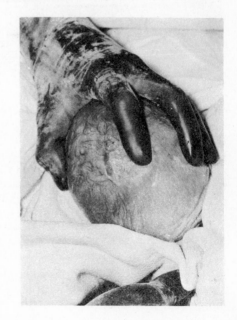

FIG. 12-21. Birth of the head. The full hand is used to control the progress with emergence of the forehead and face. (The Johns Hopkins Hospital, Baltimore, Md.)

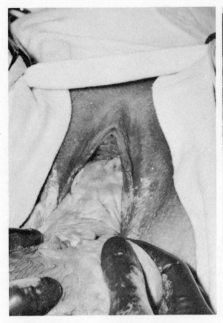
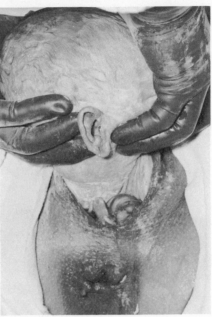

FIG. 12-22. Delivery of the shoulders. (*Left*) The anterior shoulder is brought under the symphysis pubis. (*Right*) Delivery of the posterior shoulder. (The Johns Hopkins Hospital, Baltimore, Md.)

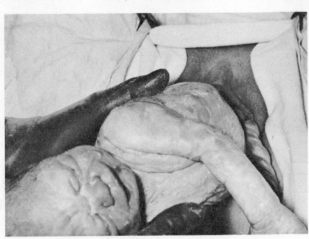

FIG. 12-23. Delivery of the infant's body. (The Johns Hopkins Hospital, Baltimore, Md.)

cutting the umbilical cord. The nurse may do so by placing her hand on the abdomen *under* the sterile drape. The uterus should be held very gently with the fingers behind the fundus and the thumb in front. So long as the uterus remains hard, and there is no bleeding, the policy is ordinarily one of watchful waiting until the placenta is separated; no massage is practiced, the hand simply resting on the fundus to make certain that the organ does not balloon out with blood. Since attempts to deliver the placenta prior to its separation from the uterine wall are not only futile but may be dangerous, it is most important that the signs of placental separation be well understood. If the responsibility of "guarding" the fundus is delegated to the nurse, she should watch for signs of placental separation and report such to the physician. The signs which suggest that the placenta has separated are as follows:

1. The uterus rises upward in the abdomen; this is due to the fact that the placenta, having been separated, passes downward into the lower uterine segment and the vagina, where its bulk pushes the uterus upward.

2. The umbilical cord protrudes 3 or more inches farther out of the vagina, indicating that the placenta also has descended.

Fig. 12-24. (*Left*) Upon delivery the infant is held in the head-down position to promote drainage of secretions from the respiratory passage. Mucus is gently wiped from the infant's face, then suctioned from the nostrils and the mouth with an ear bulb syringe or other suction device. Note that there is no traction on the cord, which is still attached to the placenta. (The Johns Hopkins Hospital, Baltimore, Md.)

Fig. 12-25. (*Right*) The cord is cut between the two Kelly clamps, which have been placed a few inches from the umbilicus. (The Johns Hopkins Hospital, Baltimore)

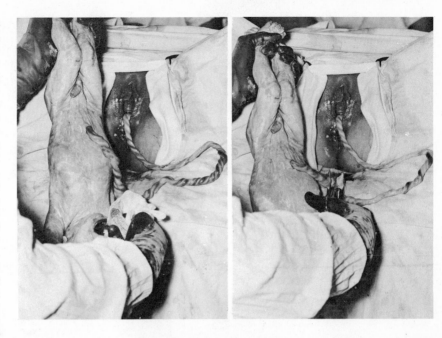

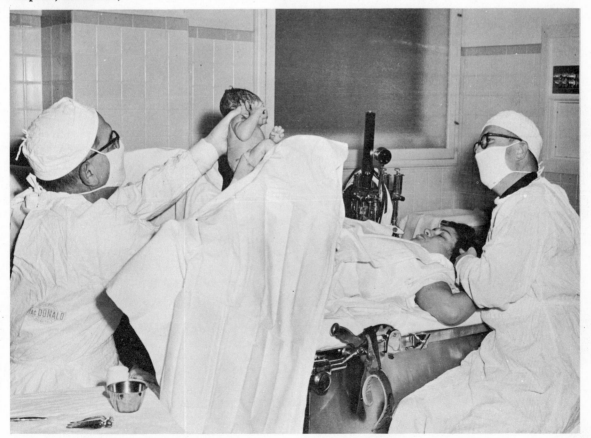

Fig. 12-26. Doctor lifts baby for parents to see immediately upon delivery.

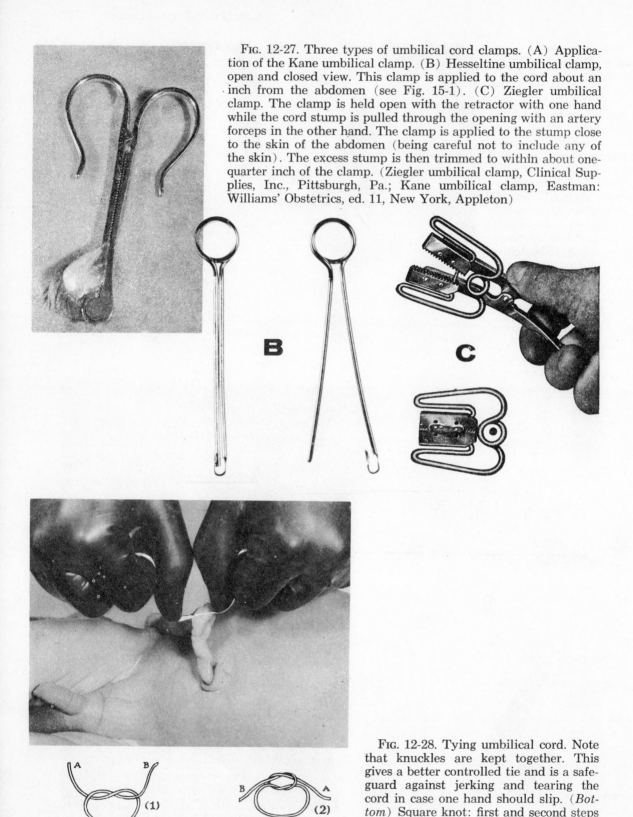

FIG. 12-27. Three types of umbilical cord clamps. (A) Application of the Kane umbilical clamp. (B) Hesseltine umbilical clamp, open and closed view. This clamp is applied to the cord about an inch from the abdomen (see Fig. 15-1). (C) Ziegler umbilical clamp. The clamp is held open with the retractor with one hand while the cord stump is pulled through the opening with an artery forceps in the other hand. The clamp is applied to the stump close to the skin of the abdomen (being careful not to include any of the skin). The excess stump is then trimmed to within about one-quarter inch of the clamp. (Ziegler umbilical clamp, Clinical Supplies, Inc., Pittsburgh, Pa.; Kane umbilical clamp, Eastman: Williams' Obstetrics, ed. 11, New York, Appleton)

B

C

FIG. 12-28. Tying umbilical cord. Note that knuckles are kept together. This gives a better controlled tie and is a safeguard against jerking and tearing the cord in case one hand should slip. (*Bottom*) Square knot: first and second steps in tying.

FIG. 12-29. Waiting for the separation of the placenta.

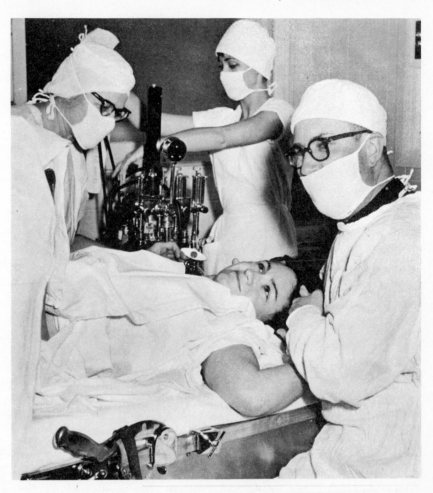

3. The uterus changes from a discoid to a globular shape and becomes, as a rule, more firm.

4. A sudden trickle or spurt of blood often occurs.

These signs are apparent sometimes within a minute or so after delivery of the infant and usually within 5 minutes. When the placenta has certainly separated, the physician first ascertains that the uterus is firmly contracted. He then may ask the patient, if not anesthetized, to "bear down," and the intra-abdominal pressure so produced may be adequate to expel the placenta (Fig. 12-31). If this fails, or if it is not practicable because of anesthesia, the physician, again having made certain that the uterus is hard, exerts gentle pressure downward with his hand on the fundus and, employing the placenta as a piston, simply moves the

placenta out of the vagina. This procedure, known as placental "expression," must be done gently and without squeezing (Fig. 12-30). It never should be attempted unless the uterus is hard; otherwise the organ may be turned inside out. This is one of the gravest complications of obstetrics and is known as "inversion" of the uterus (p. 498). The physician carries out a careful inspection of the placenta to make sure that it is intact (Fig. 12-32); if a piece is left in the uterus, it may cause subsequent hemorrhage.

Oxytocin and/or ergonovine, or their derivatives, may be administered at the physician's request to increase uterine contractions and thereby to minimize bleeding. These agents are employed widely in the conduct of the normal third stage of labor, but the timing of their administration differs greatly in various hos-

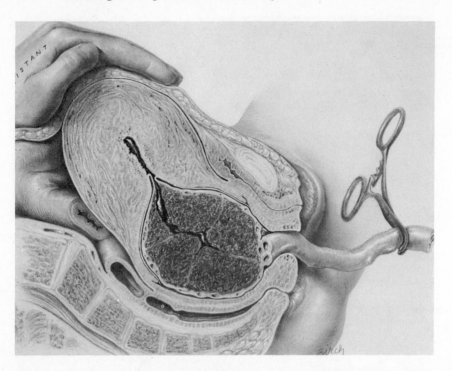

FIG. 12-30. Expression of placenta is usually done by the physician, if necessary, but *on his instructions* may be done by an assistant. The *uterus must be hard* if this is attempted. Note that the uterus is not squeezed.

pitals. These oxytocics are not necessary in most cases, but their use is considered ideal from the viewpoint of minimizing blood loss and the general safety of the mother.

The Oxytocics. Ergonovine is an alkaloid of ergot. It is a powerful oxytocic; i.e., it stimulates uterine contractions and exerts an effect which may persist for several hours. When administered intravenously, the uterine response is almost immediate, and within a few minutes after intramuscular or oral administration. This response is sustained in character with no tendency toward relaxation and so is ideal for the prevention and the control of postpartal hemorrhage. This drug will cause an elevation of blood pressure. More recently a semisynthetic derivative of ergonovine, methylergonovine tartrate, has been widely employed

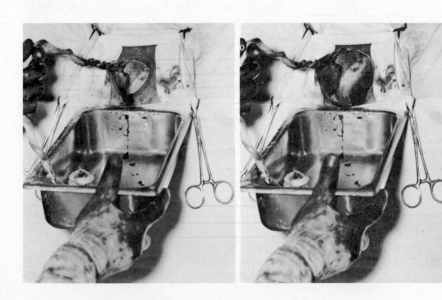

FIG. 12-31. Third stage of labor. The delivery of the placenta. (The Johns Hopkins Hospital, Baltimore, Md.)

FIG. 12-32. Inspecting the placenta: (A) the fetal side, (B) the maternal side. (The Johns Hopkins Hospital, Baltimore, Md.)

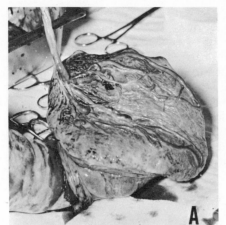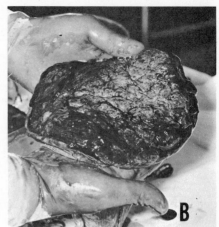

because it possesses several advantages over the parent drug. Usually called by its trade name, Methergine, it has the ability to produce stronger and longer contractions and is less likely to cause elevation of the blood pressure. Both drugs when given intravenously may cause transient headache and, to a lesser extent, temporary chest pain, palpitation and dyspnea. These side-effects are less likely to occur with intramuscular administration of the drugs.

Oxytocin is another agent which, like ergonovine, causes a marked contraction of the uterus. However, the response of the uterus to oxytocin resembles the response to ergonovine for only the first 5 or 10 minutes; then normal rhythmic contractions of amplified degree return, with intermittent periods of relaxation. The oxytocic fraction separated from posterior pituitary extract is referred to by the name oxytocin; it is widely used because it does not possess the strong vasopressor and antidiuretic effects of Pituitrin, which was used more extensively in former years. Recently, a synthetic oxytocin injection has been developed and marketed under the brand name of Syntocinon. Its action, dosage and indications are similar to those of oxytocin. Another drug which re-

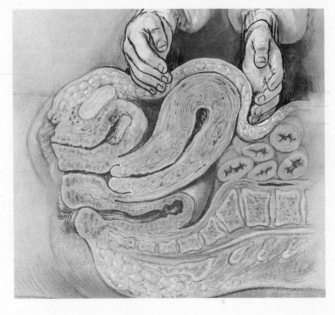

FIG. 12-33. Proper method of palpating fundus of uterus during first hour after delivery to guard against relaxation and hemorrhage. The right hand is placed just above the symphysis pubis to act as a guard; meanwhile the other hand is cupped around the fundus of the uterus.

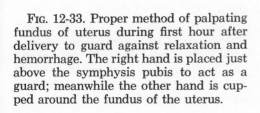

cently has been developed is sparteine sulfate (Tocosamine). It is used primarily in dysfunctional types of labor and for induction of labor. When used as recommended, it produces a gradual onset of regular uterine contractions similar to that encountered in normal labor.

On the obstetrician's order the nurse administers the oxytocic intramuscularly, the intravenous medications being administered by a physician. The average doses of the drugs are as follows: oxytocin, 10 units (1 cc.) intramuscularly or intravenously; Syntocinon, 10 units (1 cc.) intramuscularly or intravenously; Tocosamine, 150 mg. (1 cc.) intramuscularly administered at $1\frac{1}{2}$- to 2-hour intervals to maintain satisfactory uterine stimulation until a total of 4 doses (600 mg.) has been given; ergonovine, 0.2 mg. ($\frac{1}{320}$ gr.) or 1 cc. intramuscularly or intravenously; and Methergine, 0.2 mg. ($\frac{1}{320}$ gr.) or 1 cc. intramuscularly or intravenously. Various institutions use the drugs separately or in conjunction as is necessary to produce the desired results. The choice of the oxytoxic usually will depend on the anesthetic agent administered. Oxytocin is contraindicated for use with drugs that have a sympathomimetic action.

Immediate Postpartal Care

Physical and Psychological Care. Constant massage of the uterus during the period after the delivery of the placenta is unnecessary and undesirable. However, if the organ shows any tendency to relax, it must be massaged immediately with firm but gentle circular strokes until it contracts effectively, in order to prevent blood loss.

After the delivery has been completed, the drapes and the soiled linen under the mother's buttocks are removed, and the lower end of the delivery table is replaced. The mother's legs are lowered from the stirrups simultaneously, and after a sterile perineal pad is applied, she should be covered with a blanket to avoid chilling. She is now ready to be transferred to her own bed. Many delivery suites have a designated postpartum recovery area or adjacent recovery room where the mother remains for an hour or so or until she has recovered from the anesthesia, her vital signs have stabilized, and there is no unusual bleeding from the birth canal.

If the mother is awake at this time, she will be eager to have a closer look at her baby and hold it, if this is possible. One should remember that although she is quite exhausted, she is usually elated, proud of her accomplishment of giving birth, and eager to share this with her husband. Whenever possible, all efforts should be made to allow the father, the mother and the infant to share this momentous time together. At one hospital the baby is placed in the mother's arms as soon as she is transferred to her bed, and the husband is permitted to remain at her bedside while she is in the recovery area. This arrangement provides an excellent opportunity to let both mother and father have a close, thorough look at their baby and to let them begin the necessary process of incorporating him into their family unit. Since all three are under the watchful (but unobtrusive) eye of the nurse, there is little danger to the infant from undue exposure, choking on mucus, smothering, etc.

Immediately after delivery, or perhaps later, the parents, particularly the mother, may relieve tension by giving way to some emotional displays, i.e., laughing, crying, incessant chatter, anger (if all has not gone well or as expected, etc.). These emotions often are quite unexpected and shock and embarrass those involved. A calm, accepting, nonjudgmental attitude on the part of the nurse is very effective in allaying any embarrassment and in helping the patient to gain control.

The nurse must remember that the patient is beginning a period that is enormously important; she is, in fact, now a "mother" with all its concomitant responsibilities; glimmerings of this already are reaching the consciousness. This is not the "end" but only the beginning of a whole new role! In addition, she is physically and emotionally exhausted from the great effort she has put forth; thus, there may be a temporary emotional upheaval.

Several comfort measures can be employed to restore calm and to help the mother to relax enough to get some much needed rest and sleep. A soothing backrub, change of gown and linen, a quiet conversation with the nurse and/or the husband in which the patient is allowed to ventilate her feelings, an environment conducive to rest, all are helpful. In addition, a warm beverage can be offered to help to allay undue excitement; since the mother is apt to be extremely hungry and thirsty, this is welcome nourishment as well as a therapeutic soporific.

Many mothers, of course, do not have an emotional outburst per se, although the majority do experience some degree of excitement and elation when the delivery is accomplished. Any of the above nursing activities are suitable also for them. Some patients experience a great need for sleep and drop off as soon as they ascertain that the baby is "all right." If the patient is sleeping continuously or intermittently, she should be allowed to do so, being disturbed only for those nursing observations that are necessary. When she indicates readiness (after the first hour after delivery), her baby should be presented, and she should be allowed to examine and to explore to her heart's content.

The mothers who have not been conscious during the delivery have rather different reactions than those patients who have participated in the birth process. Often they do not seem to believe that delivery has taken place, or that the baby shown them "is really mine." They will question again and again: "Is it really all over?" "What is it again?" (This refers to the sex of the child.) "Did I have the baby?" The apparent alteration in awareness seems to be related to the anesthesia and the unconsciousness. These patients need more firm reassurance and contact with their infants to help them realize that they have had a baby. Even though the repeated questioning may become annoying, the nurse should recognize that this is necessary for the mother so that she can begin the important process of disengagement from the symbiotic relationship that she had with her infant during pregnancy. She must now establish the baby as a real entity outside her body rather than inside. All mothers have this task to perform, but it is harder for the mother who has been delivered under heavy anesthesia, for as far as she is concerned, she was not "there" when it all happened.

Maternal feelings, as we know, do not spring unbound at the time of delivery. Rather they are developed, often slowly, as is the case in any other developmental process (see Chap. 15). The early encounters and care that the mother receives in the delivery area help to pave the way for later responses in the postpartal period.

The first hour following the delivery is a most critical one for the mother. It is at this time that postpartal hemorrhage is most likely to occur as the result of uterine relaxation. Thus, it is mandatory that the uterus be watched constantly throughout this period by a competent nurse who keeps her hand more or less constantly on the fundus and at the slightest sign of diminishing contraction massages it, to make sure that it does not relapse and balloon with blood (Figs. 190, 202). It is important for the nurse to be constantly alert not only to the condition of the mother's uterus but also to any abnormal symptoms related to her general condition. Checking of the maternal vital signs is usually included in the nursing observations. These signs are checked as often as necessary until they become stable, as previously stated.

IMMEDIATE CARE OF THE INFANT

As soon as the infant is born, measures should be taken to promote a clear air passage before the onset of respiration. Often, as the head is delivered, it is necessary to wipe the mucus and fluid from the infant's nose and mouth before he has a chance to gasp and aspirate with this first breath. From the moment of delivery the infant should be kept in the head-down position until his upper respiratory passage is cleared of mucus, amniotic fluid, etc. A small rubber bulb syringe, or a soft rubber suction catheter attached to a mechanical suction or mouth aspirator, should be used promptly to suction the oropharynx and to remove fluids which may be obstructing the airway. If there seems to be much mucus present, the physician will hold the infant up by his ankles to encourage more mucus to drain from the throat. The mucosal surfaces of the palate and the posterior pharynx should not be wiped with gauze, since its rough texture can lead to abrasions and thus provide a portal of entry for pathogenic organisms.

The baby may not "cry" at once, but he usually gasps or cries after the mucus has been removed, as he now needs oxygen by way of the lungs, since the accustomed supply was

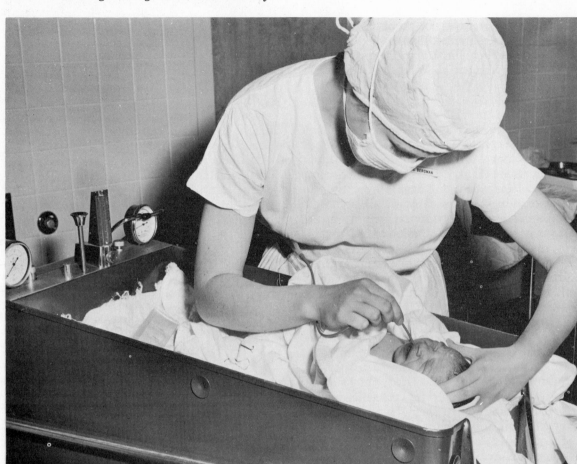

Fig. 12-34. Suctioning the newborn in the delivery room.

cut off when the placental circulation stopped. If crying has to be stimulated, it must be done with extreme care. As the infant is being held in the head-down position to promote the drainage of mucus from the respiratory passages, gentle rubbing of the infant's back is usually sufficient stimulus to initiate crying. And, in the act of crying, mucus is forced from the nose and the throat, thus enabling the infant to be better able to breathe. Vigorous, external irritants are *unnecessary* and *dangerous* and should not be employed. These include spanking the soles of the feet and/or buttocks, forcible rubbing of the skin along the spine, alternate hot and cold tubbing of the infant, and dilatation of the anal sphincter. These procedures are obsolete and shocking to the infant.

A sterile receiver should be available for the physician to wrap around the infant until it can be placed in a warm crib. It must be remembered that any room is much cooler than the mother's body, and the infant never should be exposed to chilling. As soon as the physician has clamped and cut the cord, he usually places the infant in a heated crib or resuscitator (previously draped with a sterile receiver to avoid contaminating his gloves) so that he may devote his attention to the mother during the third stage of labor. As mentioned previously, even for the infant who requires no resuscitation, the resuscitator affords a warm protected environment for the infant and, in addition, a convenient place for the nurse now to proceed with the infant's care. If a circulating nurse is responsible for the infant's care in the delivery room, she will have cleansed her hands thoroughly with some agent such as pHisoHex or surgical soap in preparation, preferably while the physician is delivering the infant's head.

Appraisal of the Newborn Infant

Once the physician has placed the infant in the heated crib (or incubator or resuscitator) in the delivery room, the responsibility for the infant's care usually is delegated to the professional nurse. It is imperative that the infant's condition be evaluated accurately immediately after birth, and that close observation be continued by the nurse. As she makes her observations, her interpretation of the baby's responses will result in a nursing diagnosis and consequent plan for nursing intervention.

Suctioning. Since it is important to maintain a clear airway for the infant, it may be necessary to suction further mucus from the oropharynx. It is important *not to oversuction* at any time, because this merely deprives the infant of oxygen and irritates the mucous membrane. If further suctioning is necessary, the nurse may use the suction apparatus on the electric infant resuscitator, a bulb syringe, or a soft rubber catheter attached to a De Lee glass trap, which was designed especially for aspirating mucus in the treatment of newborn infants (Fig. 12-34). Care should be taken not to traumatize the tissues of the oropharynx with the tip of the catheter or with forceful suction. When the nasopharynx is obstructed by mucus which must be removed via the nostrils, the nurse may safely pass a small French catheter into the nostril if she avoids using force. The catheter must *not* be inserted far back. If the catheter is directed horizontally, as if passing over the roof of the mouth, instead of directing it upward as for the adult patient, it usually slips into the tiny infant nostril with more ease. If a bulb syringe is used, it should be collapsed before it is inserted in the baby's mouth; otherwise the material in the oropharynx will be forced into the bronchi and lungs when the bulb is collapsed.

The Apgar Scoring System. The Apgar score provides a valuable index for evaluating the newborn infant's condition at birth. Every nurse who is responsible for the care of new-

TABLE 10. THE APGAR SCORING CHART*

SIGN	0	1	2
Heart rate	Absent	Slow (less than 100)	Over 100
Respiratory effort	Absent	Slow, irregular	Good, crying
Muscle tone	Flaccid	Some flexion of extremities	Active motion
Reflex irritability	No response	Cry	Vigorous cry
Color	Blue, pale	Body pink, extremities blue	Completely pink

* Special Committee on Infant Mortality of the Medical Society of the County of New York: Resuscitation of the Newborn, Philadelphia, Smith, Kline & French Laboratories, 1963.

born infants, not merely those in the delivery room, should be familiar with the principles set forth by Apgar for infant evaluation because they provide a simple, accurate and safe means of quickly appraising the infant's condition. The Apgar scoring system is based on the following five signs (ranked in order of importance). In general, they are made at 1 minute of life and repeated again in 5 minutes. Each sign is evaluated according to the degree to which it is present and is given a score of 0, 1, or 2. (See Table 10.) The scores of each of the signs then are added together to give a total score (10 is maximum).

HEART RATE. This sign is the most important and the last to be absent when the infant's condition is grave. It may be evaluated by palpating the pulsation of the cord or by observing the pulsation where the cord joins the abdomen. Listening to the heartbeat with a stethoscope is surely the most accurate method of ascertaining the beat. The beat may range from 150 to 180 beats per minute during the first few minutes of life; later, within the hour, it usually slows to between 130 and 140 beats per minute. Crying or increased activity will increase the number of beats. If the rate is 100 per minute or under, asphyxia is present, and resuscitation is indicated.

RESPIRATORY EFFORT. A baby who is responding well cries vigorously and has no difficulty in breathing. "Regular" respiration usually is established in a minute or so. Depressed, irregular respiration or apnea indicates that respiratory difficulty is present, and these signs should be reported immediately so that prompt treatment may be instituted (see p. 528).

MUSCLE TONE. An infant who has excellent tonus will keep his extremities flexed and resist efforts to extend them. A baby who does not keep his extremities flexed consistently usually has only moderate tonus; one who is flaccid is in extremely poor condition.

REFLEX IRRITABILITY. Although there are several ways to test this sign, the one most frequently used is a slap on the sole of the infant's foot. This sign can be observed when a vigorous infant is suctioned for mucus by the way in which he resists the catheter. A baby who is in excellent condition will respond with a vigorous cry. He is judged to have a poor response if he cries weakly or merely makes a grimace. If there is a good deal of central nervous system depression, the infant will not respond at all.

COLOR. Cyanosis is seen in all infants at the moment of birth. As the infant's circulation makes the change from fetal to extra-uterine existence, and he begins to breathe, the body of a healthy infant usually will become pink within 3 minutes (see Chap. 4). Since acrocyanosis usually is present for a short while, even in infants who are in excellent condition, those who have scored 2 for each of the other signs may receive only a score of 1 for this part of the evaluation. This will, of course, influence his total score.

INTERPRETATION. An Apgar score of 7 to 10 indicates that the infant's condition is good. If he breathes and cries (or coughs) seconds after delivery, there are usually no special procedures necessary other than those of routine close observation, maintaining a clear airway, and supplying warmth as necessary. A score of 4 to 6 means that the baby is in fair condition. There may be moderate central nervous system depression, some muscle flaccidity, cyanosis, and respiration will not establish readily. *These infants must have their air passages cleared and be given oxygen promptly.* Administration of oxygen can best be done by mask, and the flow should not exceed 4 liters. Gentle patting and rubbing with the receiving blanket to dry the infant's body usually acts as an additional stimulus. A score of 0 to 3 denotes an extremely poor condition. Resuscitation is needed immediately (see Chap. 21).

Other Aspects of Care

Care of the Cord. In many hospitals no dressing is applied after the cord has been clamped or ligated and cut; in others a sterile plain gauze dressing is applied around the cord stump and secured with a binder, which is removed at appropriate times. Regardless of the technic employed, it is imperative that frequent inspection be done to note any signs of bleeding and that strict aseptic precautions be utilized in caring for the cord stump. The method of leaving the cord stump exposed has proved to be very satisfactory. If it is left free, it apparently dries and separates more quickly than when it is kept covered. There is also

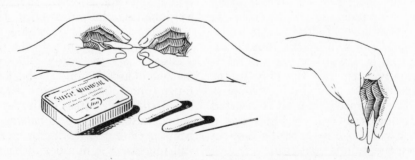

FIG. 12-35. (*Left*) Silver nitrate 1 per cent solution for the care of the eyes of newborn babies; needle puncture of wax ampule. (*Right*) Showing how to manipulate the ampule in administering the drug. (Eli Lilly and Company)

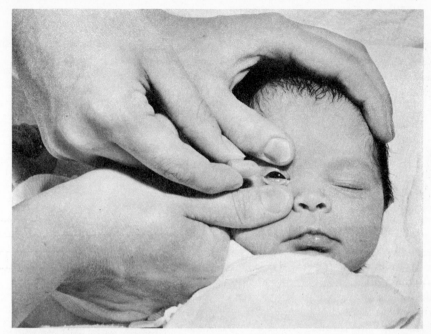

FIG. 12-36. Silver nitrate prophylaxis. (*Top*) Instillation of 2 drops of silver nitrate 1 per cent solution from a wax ampule into the conjunctival sac of each eye. (*Bottom*) After the medication has diffused over the entire conjunctiva (2 minutes), the conjunctival sac of each eye is gently flushed with sterile distilled water or normal saline solution to remove the excess silver nitrate.

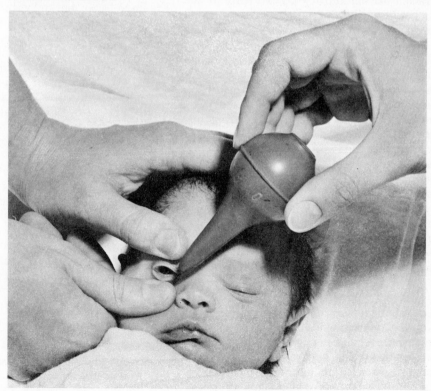

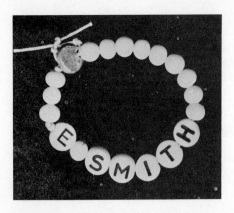

Fig. 12-37. Identification method, using strand of beads. If surname is at all common, use initial of mother's first name also, as shown above. The beads must be sealed around baby's wrist or ankle before he leaves the delivery room.

less irritation of the abdomen and the back, which sometimes results from a moist binder. Some pediatricians think that the abdominal muscles become stronger by not being bound.

Care of the Eyes. As soon as the cord is cared for and the infant's respiration is well established, the eyes should receive prophylactic treatment for protection against ophthalmia neonatorum (see Chap. 21, Disorders of the Newborn). This treatment is so important that at the present time the use of a silver preparation is mandatory by statute in all states. It is supplied in wax ampules containing silver nitrate 1 per cent solution, especially prepared for eye instillation (Fig. 12-35).

Instilling drops in the infant's eyes is more easily accomplished if the nurse shades the eyes from the light while putting the drops first in one eye, allowing time for the baby to recover from the shock and the smarting before she puts the drops in the other eye. One of the best methods is to draw down the lower lid gently and carefully instill 2 drops of the solution in the conjunctival sac, using great care not to drop it on the cornea. After 2 minutes, when it will have diffused itself over the entire conjunctiva, the lids should again be held apart and the conjunctival sac of each eye flushed gently with normal saline solution or sterile distilled water (Fig. 12-36). The prompt irrigation of the eyes following instillation of silver nitrate drops is said to reduce the incidence of chemical conjunctivitis without affecting the prophylactic efficacy. The nurse must take especial precautions against allowing any contamination of the eyes and against dropping any silver solution upon the face. Silver nitrate prophylaxis may cause signs of irritation, such as redness, edema or discharge, but

these manifestations are transient and in no way cause permanent damage if the silver nitrate solution used is in correct concentration.

Hypoprothrombinemia Prophylaxis. Many physicans prescribe that a single dose of phytonadione solution (Aquamephyton) 1.0 mg. (0.5 cc.) be administered intramuscularly during the course of the immediate care of the newborn after delivery. This water-soluble form of vitamin K_1 acts as a preventative measure against neonatal hemorrhagic disease. Amounts of the medication in excess of 1.0 mg. may predispose to the development of hyperbilirubinemia and should be avoided.

Identification Methods. Some method of identification of the newborn is applied before the cord is cut or before the baby is removed from the delivery room. There are several satisfactory methods in use. Some hospitals use the linen tapes marked with the mother's name and hospital number, fastening one to the baby's arm or ankle and the other to the mother's wrist. The identification beads are made up with the mother's surname and initials and sealed with a lead bead. This bracelet or anklet is applied before the baby leaves the delivery room (Fig. 12-37). The pliable plastic bracelet or anklet has space for the mother's name and initials as well as a permanent lock which has to be cut to be removed.

The palmprint and footprint method of identification consists of a stainless procedure made on chemically treated sensitized paper. It is designed to take the palmprints or footprints of the baby and the thumbprint of the mother at the time of delivery and may be repeated at the time of discharge from the hospital. It is a simple, quick and permanent method.

The following editorial comment presents the recommendations of the American Hospital Association.

Mix-ups involving two or more babies are quite rare in hospital nurseries, but they still can happen. In one state alone in a period of 18 months eight mix-ups or alleged mix-ups occurred. When such a mix-up, alleged or actual, does occur, a torrent of unfavorable publicity is unloosed and the parents concerned may be haunted by a lifetime of doubt about their child. The confusion sometimes arises because two mothers in a hospital at the same time have the same surname; it sometimes arises because a single identification becomes detached from the baby; or it may even arise because parents get to wondering after they leave the hospital how the attendants maintained the identity of the babies. Sometimes the confusion is easily straightened out, and sometimes it leads to giving the wrong baby a harmless prescription; only rarely does it lead to an actual exchange of babies. The American Hospital Association has long been aware of this problem, and, because it has been found that photographs, footprints, handprints, and fingerprints are adjuncts but cannot yet be considered reliable as the sole means of identifying the newborn infant, the Association has urged the adoption of a standard operating procedure that if applied would reduce mix-ups to the vanishing point.

The main features of this procedure are as follows: (1) Each baby should be marked in the delivery room with two items of identification. (2) The identification items should show the mother's full name, date and time of birth, and some correlation with the mother, such as her fingerprint or number. (3) Each time the baby comes to the mother, the mother should be informed that it is her responsibility to identify her baby by the marking. (4) When the baby and mother are discharged, one of the bands should be removed, preferably by the mother, and, after the mother has properly identified her baby, the removed identification should then be pasted to the baby's chart. The mother should acknowledge in writing that this is how her baby was marked, and that she identified it as hers. The leaflet that gives the full procedure in detail has been available since December, 1949. Once established as a routine, this procedure, far from being a burden, would prevent a type of mistake that would otherwise be easy to make but is nonetheless inexcusable.[6]

Current practice emphasizes that the newborn should be discharged without removing the identification band. Several states now have laws making it mandatory not to remove the identification bands on hospital premises. The mother should be taught how to remove the band as part of the discharge instructions.

As already discussed in Chapter 1, the reg-

istration of the infant's birth is a legal responsibility. It is mandatory that a birth certificate, such as that shown in Figure 1-4, be filled out on every birth and submitted promptly to the local registrar.

After the Delivery. After caring for the infant, the nurse will continue to assist the physician with the care of the mother and her infant. If the mother is awake, she may be anxious to have her baby brought near so that she may see it at close range. If she is drowsy, it may be better to wait until she is more alert. The nurse will be governed by each mother's response at this time. Some mothers want to touch their babies; others are eager to hold their babies at this time, and if this is sanctioned by the physician, there is no reason that it should not be permitted for a brief period. In this instance the nurse should be careful to keep her hand under the infant for support and added protection, should this be necessary, because of the mother's excitement in her first contact with her newborn.

If the infant is well wrapped and warm, he may be kept in a crib at the mother's side until the mother leaves the delivery room. He should be kept in a modified Trendelenburg position (at an angle of 30°) to promote drainage of mucus, and on his side to avoid aspiration of this mucus. Care should be taken to avoid placing the infant in an exaggerated Trendelenburg position (almost directly downward), since the relatively large amount of abdominal contents will press against the diaphragm and the partially expanded lungs and may impede the infant's respiratory efforts.

The nurse should observe the infant at frequent intervals to make sure that he is breathing properly, that the mouth and the nose are free from mucus, and that there is no bleeding from the cord. Because this period may be a critical one for the infant, many hospitals have facilities, such as a receiving nursery on the labor and delivery division, where the infant is transferred at this time. This not only provides closer supervision and care for the infant but also permits the nurse in the delivery room to devote her undivided attention to the mother.

Baptism of Infant. If there is any probability that the infant is in imminent danger and may not live, the question of baptism should be considered in cases in which the religion of the family is Roman Catholic; this also applies

[6] Editorial Comment: Identification of the newborn infant, J.A.M.A. 162:44, 1956.

to some of the other denominations of the Christian church. This is an essential duty and means a great deal to the families concerned, and thoughtfulness in this matter will never be forgotten by them. (It is to be understood that such baptism would be reported to the family.)

The following simple instructions were given by the late Rev. Paul L. Blakely, S.J., Ph.D.

The Catholic Church teaches that in case of emergency, any one may and should baptize. What is necessary is to make the intention of doing what the Church wishes to do and then to pour the water on the child (the head by preference) saying at the same time, "I baptize thee in the name of the Father and of the Son and of the Holy Ghost." The water may be warmed if necessary but it must be pure water and care should be taken to make it flow. If there is any doubt whether the child is alive or dead, it should be baptized, but conditionally; i.e., "If thou art alive, I baptize thee," etc.

On page 281 of the Book of Common Prayer of the Protestant Episcopal Church, it is stated: "In cases of extreme sickness, or any imminent peril, if a Minister cannot be procured, then any baptized person present may administer holy Baptism, using the foregoing form" (i.e., the form given above).

EMERGENCY DELIVERY BY THE NURSE

In the course of labor one occasionally encounters the so-called *precipitate delivery,* a rapid spontaneous delivery in which the infant is born without adequate preparations on the part of the physician or the nurse, sometimes even without benefit of their immediate care. This may occur in certain multiparous women, particularly if the soft parts of the pelvis offer little resistance, if the contractions are unusually strong and forceful, or if the mother does not experience painful sensations during labor and thus has inadequate warning that the delivery is approaching. The mother, of course, may suffer lacerations of the tissues as the result of tumultuous labor. The infant is endangered because, in its rapid progress through the birth canal, it may suffer cerebral trauma; or the umbilical cord may be torn in the process of the delivery. In addition, if the

mother is unattended, the infant may be in jeopardy from lack of care during the first few minutes of life.

Whether the nurse is caring for a mother in the hospital labor room, making a home visit, or involved in some emergency situation, it is well for her to be prepared for a precipitate delivery. It seldom happens that the nurse is alone with her patient in the hospital when the delivery is imminent; but knowing what to do in such a situation, in the event that the physician is not present, is advantageous for all concerned. In the excitement which may ensue, the nurse's concern for the immediate safety of the mother and the baby usually demands all of her attention.

However, it should be stressed that the nurse's composure and her ability to convey this is one of the cornerstones in a successful delivery. Whenever possible, the nurse should let the mother know what to anticipate and instruct her as best she can in what she can do to cooperate effectively. Here teamwork with the mother is essential and can be accomplished if the nurse instills confidence by demonstrating her competence in both the physical and the emotional aspects of care. If the father is present, he can be utilized in the care of his wife in whatever capacity seems most appropriate and in accord with his ability. He might help best by taking care of the other children or by calling the physician, or he might be involved directly in some aspect of the delivery. If it seems more desirable that he be away from the immediate vicinity, then the reasons for his leaving should be given. He should not be dismissed summarily from the situation.

The nurse who is consistently conscientious about applying principles of asepsis and antisepsis will automatically apply them in this instance, to the best of her ability. Usually, there is inadequate time for proper cleansing of the vulva, or scrubbing her own hands and donning sterile gloves, or draping the mother, all of which would be ideal. However, a clean delivery area should be maintained, and, if time and facilities permit, the nurse's hands should be cleansed.

Delivery of the Head. As the head distends the perineum at the acme of a contraction, gentle pressure is exerted against the head to control its progress and thereby to prevent undue stretching of the perineum. This kind

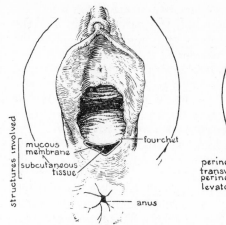
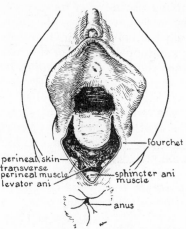
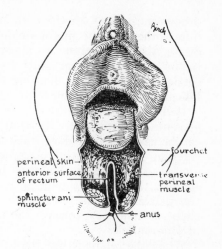

FIG. 12-38 A. First-degree tear. FIG. 12-38 B. Second-degree tear. FIG. 12-38 C. Third-degree tear.

of *control* applied to the descending head during each contraction will prevent its sudden expulsion through the vulva, reducing the possibility of consequent complications. *The head must never be held back.* The mother should be encouraged to pant during the contraction to deter bearing down efforts on her part, particularly as the head, which will be supported by the nurse, is being delivered. Whenever possible, the infant's head should be delivered between contractions.

Rupture of the Membranes. If the membranes have not ruptured previously, they may remain intact until they appear as a smooth, glistening object at the vulva. If they protrude, they may rupture with the next contraction. But if the membranes have not ruptured before the head is delivered, they must be broken and removed immediately (by nipping them at the nape of the infant's neck) to prevent aspiration of fluid when the infant takes its first breath.

Precautions Concerning the Cord. As soon as the head is delivered, the nurse should feel for a loop or loops of cord around the neck and, if any is found, gently slip it over the baby's head, if this can be done easily. But, as stated on page 268, if the cord is coiled too tightly to permit this, it must be doubly clamped and cut (between the clamps) before delivery of the rest of the body. One or more loops of cord around the fetal neck occur in about a quarter of all deliveries.

Delivery of the Infant's Body. After external rotation of the head, which is usually spontaneous, there is no occasion for haste in the delivery of the body. Gentle downward pressure with the hands on either side of the head may be exerted to direct the anterior shoulder under the symphysis pubis, then reversed upward in order to deliver the posterior shoulder over the perineum. The infant's body now will follow easily and quickly and should be supported as it is born.

Immediate Care of the Infant. As soon as the face appears, mucus and fluids should be wiped from the nose and the mouth. Then, after the infant is born, if he does not cry spontaneously, or if there seems to be mucus in the respiratory passages, the infant should be held up by his ankles to encourage the mucus to drain from his nose and mouth. In doing this, care must be exercised to avoid any traction on the umbilical cord and, at the same time, to prevent the infant's head from pressing down against the bed. Drainage of mucus is stimulated when the infant cries but can be encouraged by "milking the trachea," i.e., with the forefinger, stroking the neck from its base toward the chin. Further stimulation by gentle rubbing of the back may stimulate breathing.

Care of the Cord. There is *no* hurry to cut the cord, so this should be delayed until proper equipment is available. It is a good plan to clamp the cord after pulsations cease (but not imperative at the moment) and to wait for the physician to cut the cord after he arrives. One must always bear in mind that sterile conditions must exist for the cord-cutting procedure; otherwise the infant's safety is jeopardized. Also, the technic for applying the cord tie or umbilical clamp must be assiduously carried out to prevent bleeding from the umbilical stump (see p. 268).

Delivery of the Placenta. When signs of placental separation are apparent, the mother can be asked to bear down with the next contraction to deliver the placenta. Since the danger of hemorrhage is always to be guarded against, the fundus should be massaged after the delivery of the placenta if there is the slightest tendency toward relaxation of the uterine muscles.

When the infant is breathing satisfactorily, he can be placed on his side across his mother's abdomen (with his head kept low to promote postural drainage and his body covered to prevent chilling). This accomplishes several things: the mother is given her baby, she can touch him and is usually enthralled by the close physical contact with him; the warmth of the mother's body prevents the infant from being chilled; and the pressure exerted on the uterus by the weight of the infant helps it to contract.

One must remember to proceed slowly and carefully throughout the delivery. As stated earlier, the nurse's reaction to the situation undoubtedly will be transferred to the mother; if the nurse remains poised and unfaltering, the mother and other people involved are more likely to do so.

LACERATIONS OF THE BIRTH CANAL

During the process of a normal delivery lacerations of the perineum and the vagina may be caused by rapid and sudden expulsion of the head (particularly when it "pops" out), the excessive size of the infant and very friable maternal tissues. In other circumstances they may be caused by difficult forceps deliveries, breech extractions or contraction of the pelvic outlet in which the head is forced posteriorly. Some tears are unavoidable, even in the most skilled hands.

Perineal lacerations usually are classified in 3 degrees, according to the extent of the tear.

First-degree lacerations are those which involve the fourchet, the perineal skin and the vaginal mucous membrane without involving any of the muscles (Fig. 12-38 A).

Second-degree lacerations are those which involve (in addition to skin and mucous membrane) the muscles of the perineal body but not the rectal sphincter. These tears usually extend upward on one or both sides of the vagina, making a triangular injury (Fig. 12-38 B).

Third-degree lacerations are those which extend completely through the skin, the mucous membrane, the perineal body and the rectal sphincter (Fig. 12-38 C). This type is often referred to as a complete tear. Not infrequently these third-degree lacerations extend a certain distance up the anterior wall of the rectum.

First- and second-degree lacerations are extremely common in primigravidas; their high incidence is one of the reasons that episiotomy is widely employed. Fortunately, third-degree lacerations are far less common. All 3 types of lacerations are repaired by the physician immediately after the delivery to ensure that the perineal structures are returned approximately to their former condition. The technic employed for the repair of a laceration is virtually the same as that used for episiotomy incisions (see p. 287), although the former is more difficult to do because of the irregular lines of tissue which must be approximated.

EPISIOTOMY AND REPAIR

An episiotomy is an incision of the perineum made to facilitate delivery. The incision is made with blunt-pointed straight scissors about the time that the head distends the vulva and is visible to a diameter of several centimeters. The incision may be made in the midline of the perineum—a median episiotomy. Or it may be begun in the midline and directed downward and laterally away from the rectum —a mediolateral episiotomy (Fig. 12-39). In the latter instance the incision may be directed to either the right or to the left side of the mother's pelvis.

As the infant's head distends the vulva, if a laceration seems to be inevitable, the physician undoubtedly will choose to incise the

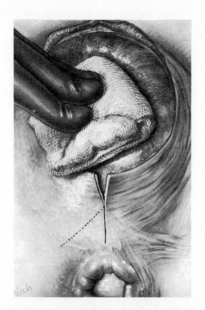

FIG. 12-39. Episiotomy. Showing lines of incision for median and mediolateral episiotomy.

(Technic employed at the Johns Hopkins Hospital. Many other methods are equally satisfactory.)

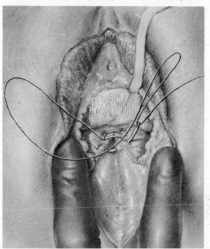

FIG. 12-40. Episiotomy. "Tail-sponge" in vagina to occlude bleeding, continuous suture in vaginal mucosa.

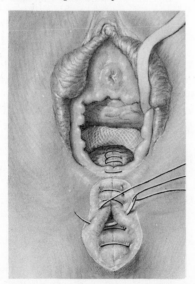

FIG. 12-41. Episiotomy. After the levator ani muscle has been united by two or more sutures (shown tied and cut), the fascia covering the muscle is sutured. Note the "tail-sponge."

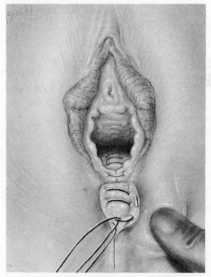

FIG. 12-42. Episiotomy. After suturing to the lowermost angle of the fascia, the round needle is replaced by cutting needle and the running suture continued upward in subcuticular fascia.

perineum rather than allow that structure to sustain a traumatic tear. This operation serves several purposes:

1. It substitutes a straight, clean-cut surgical incision for the ragged, contused laceration which otherwise is likely to ensue; such an incision is easier to repair and heals better than a tear.

2. The direction of the episiotomy can be controlled, whereas a tear may extend in any direction, sometimes involving the anal sphincter and the rectum.

3. It spares the baby's head the necessity of serving as a "battering ram" against perineal obstruction; if prolonged, this "pounding" of the infant's head against the perineum may cause brain injury.

4. The operation shortens the duration of the second stage of labor.

In view of these several advantages of episiotomy, many physicians employ it routinely in the delivery of the primigravida.

There are many equally satisfactory methods utilized by different physicians for episiotomy repair. The suture material ordinarily used is a fine chromic catgut, either 00 or 000. The technic employed at the Johns Hopkins Hospital is shown in Figures 12-40 through 42. A round needle and continuous suture is used to close the vaginal mucosa and fourchet, and then laid aside while several interrupted sutures are placed in the levator ani muscle and the fascia. Then the continuous suture is again picked up and used to unite the subcutaneous fascia. Finally, the round needle is replaced by a large, straight cutting needle, and the running suture is continued upward as a subcuticular stitch.

SUGGESTED READING

Allen, S.: Nurse attendance during labor, Am. J. Nurs. 64:70-74, July, 1964.

Anderson, B.: Training course for obstetric technicians, Pediatric Nursing Currents, Ross Laboratories, 12:1-2, May, 1965.

Aring, C.: Sympathy and empathy, J.A.M.A. 16: 448-452, May, 1958.

Berrien, C.: Evaluating the newborn, Nurs. Outlook 9:93-96, February, 1961.

Black, M.: Psychorelaxation management for labor and delivery, Clin. Obstet. Gynec. 4:108-116, March, 1961.

Bonica, J. J.: An atlas on the mechanisms and pathways of pain in labor, What's New, No. 217:16-26, Spring, 1960.

Bradley, R. A.: Fathers' presence in delivery rooms, Psychosomatics 111:474-479, November-December, 1962.

Brady, J. P., and James, L. S.: Heart rate changes in the fetus and newborn infant during labor, delivery and the immediate neonatal period, Am. J. Obstet. Gynec. 84:1-13, July, 1962.

Buxton, C. L.: A Study of Psychophysical Methods for Relief of Childbirth Pain, Philadelphia, Saunders, 1962.

Carbary, L. J.: The fetal heart monitor, Nurs. Outlook 11:835, November, 1963.

Carter, E. W.: Support: a lay concept in nursing *in* Burd, S., and Marshall, M.: Some Clinical Approaches to Psychiatric Nursing, New York, Macmillan, 1963.

Chambers, W.: Nursing Diagnosis, Am. J. Nurs. 62:102-104, November, 1962.

Christian, J. R.: Comparison of ocular reactions with the use of silver nitrate and erythromycin ointment in opthalmia neonatorum prophylaxis, J. Pediat. 57:55-60, July, 1960.

Cibils, L. A., and Hendricks, C. H.: Normal labor in vertex presentations, Am. J. Obstet. Gynec. 91:385-395, February 1, 1965.

Cummins, H., and Midlo, C.: Fingerprints, Palms and Soles, New York, Dover, 1961.

De Agustina, J., *et al.*: Ward study: The meaning of touch in intrapersonal communication *in* Burd, S., and Marshall, M.: Some Clinical Approaches to Psychiatric Nursing, New York, Macmillan, 1963.

Eastman, N. J., and Hellman, L. M.: Williams Obstetrics, ed. 13, New York, Appleton, 1966.

Fitzhugh, M. L., and Newton, M.: Muscle action during childbirth, Phys. Ther. Rev. 36:805-809, December, 1956.

Goodman, R. R.: Psychological support in labor, a supervisor's view, Hosp. Topics 42:99-100, August, 1964.

Hardy, F. M.: Management of labor, Nurs. Times 58:598-600, May, 1962.

Hellman, L. M., *et al.*: Some factors affecting the fetal heart rate, Am. J. Obstet. Gynec. 82:1055-1063, November, 1961.

Hendricks, C. H., *et al.*: Pressure relationships between the intervillous space and the amniotic fluid in human term pergnancy, Am. J. Obstet. Gynec. 77:1028-1037, May, 1959.

Hendricks, C. H., and Pose, S. V.: Intranasal oxytocin in obstetrics, J.A.M.A. 175:384-387, February 4, 1961.

Herschelmann, R. F., and Partridge, A.: Deladumone for breast discomfort, Am. J. Nurs. 59: 1252-1254, September, 1959.

Hon, E. H.: Electronic evaluation of fetal heart

rates, Am. J. Obstet. 83:333-338, February 1, 1962.

Ioris, J.: Effective support during labor and delivery, R.N. 25:70-78, 88, February, 1962.

Johnson, B. S.: Meaning of touch in nursing, Nurs. Outlook 65:59-60, February, 1965.

Jourard, S.: The bedside manner, Am. J. Nurs. 60:63-66, January, 1960.

Kachelski, A.: The nurse-patient relationship, Am. J. Nurs. 61:76-81, May, 1961.

Karmel, M.: Thank You, Dr. Lamaze, Philadelphia, Lippincott, 1959.

Kelly, J. V.: Effect of fear on uterine motility, Am. J. Obstet. Gynec. 83:576-581, March 1, 1962.

————: Effect of hypnotically induced anxiety on uterine muscle, Am. J. Obstet. Gynec. 83:582-587, March 1, 1962.

Kendall, B., and Farell, D. M.: Use of fetal electro-cardiography, Am. J. Nurs. 64:75-79, July, 1964.

LeFever, J.: View from the side of the table, Am. J. Nurs. 63:67-69, June, 1963.

Lesser, Marion, and Keane, Vera: Nurse-Patient Relationships in a Hospital Maternity Service, St. Louis, Mosby, 1956.

Manning, R. E.: To do or not to do—a critical review of vaginal examination during labor, Am. J. Obstet. Gynec. 82:1356-1358, December, 1961.

Montgomery, T. L.: Immediate care of the newborn, Clin. Obstet. Gynec. 5:30-43, March, 1962.

Naeye, R. L.: The fetal and neonatal development of twins, Pediatrics 33:546-553, April, 1954.

Newton, N., and Newton, M.: Mothers' reactions to their newborn babies, J.A.M.A. 181:206-210, July 21, 1962.

Novack, J.: Psychological support and labor—a nursing educator's views, Hosp. Topics 42:97-98, August, 1964.

Peplau, H.: Anxiety in the mother-infant relationship 60:1133-1134, May, 1960.

Pettit, R.: Palliation of common obstetrical discomfort, Am. J. Obstet. 85:125, January, 1963.

Psychophysical Preparation for Childbearing: Guidelines for Teaching, ed. 2, New York, Maternity Center Association, ed. 2, 1965.

Read, G. D.: Childbirth Without Fear, rev. ed., New York, Harper, 1953.

Reardon, H. S., et al.: Chemical stimuli of respiration in early neonatal period, J. Pediatrics 57:151-170, August, 1960.

Riker, A. P.: How it feels to be a maternity patient, R.N. 26:47-50, October, 1963.

Rosengren, W. R.: Some psychological aspects of delivery room difficulties, J. Nerv. Ment. Dis. 132:515-521, June, 1961.

Saltenis, I. J.: Physical Touch and Nursing Support in Labor, unpublished master's thesis, Yale University, New Haven, Conn., 1962.

Schafer, G.: Induction of labor, Am. J. Nurs. 61:89-92, September, 1961.

Stanley, J. L.: The effect of pain relief for labor and delivery on the fetus and newborn, Anesthesiology 21:405-430, July-August, 1960.

Taylor, P. M., et al.: Venous hypertension in the newborn associated with delayed clamping of the umbilical cord, Acta Pediat. 50:149-159, March, 1961.

Thoms, H., and Billings, W.: A consideration of childbirth programs, New Eng. J. Med. 552:860, 1956.

Travelbee, J.: What do we mean by rapport?, Am. J. Nurs. 63:70-72, February, 1963.

Tryon, P. A., and Leonard, R. C.: The effect of the patient's participation on the outcome of a nursing procedure, Nurs. Forum 3, No. 2:79-89, 1964.

Ulin, P. R.: The exhilarating moment of birth, Am. J. Nurs. 63:60-67, June, 1963.

Wiedenbach, E.: Family-Centered Maternity Nursing, New York, Putnam, 1958.

Willson, J. R.: Management of Obstetric Difficulties, ed. 6, St. Louis, Mosby, 1961.

CONFERENCE MATERIAL

1. A mother who is contemplating the delivery of her first child is worried for fear that she may not get her own baby if another infant is born at the same time she is delivered. How would you reassure this mother concerning the identification methods for newborn infants?

2. An 18-year-old mother having her first baby is admitted to the hospital in early labor. It is obvious from her behavior that she has had no preparation for this experience and is frightened and apprehensive. What specific measures would you include in your nursing plan for her care?

3. An unwed mother goes into labor, having made no arrangements for the care of her 2-year-old girl and her 12-year-old boy. What resources could you suggest in this situation? What is the responsibility of hospital and community agencies in this case?

4. How do the public health organizations and hospitals in your community help the patient and her family to prepare for the delivery?

5. Why is prophylaxis for the eyes of the

newborn required by law in all states? How would you go about securing the desired information concerning such legislation in the various states of the United States?

6. You are caring for a mother having her fourth child, who is in very active labor. Suddenly, the membranes rupture, and she begins to bear down. As you observe the perineum, you see the infant's head crowning. Since you are alone with this mother at the time, what will you do?

7. A 21-year-old mother at term, who has attended "natural childbirth" classes for a previous pregnancy, comes to the hospital on her physician's instructions because her membranes have ruptured. She is apologetic because her contractions are only 10 to 12 minutes apart, of mild intensity, lasting about 35 seconds and "not really good enough yet to come to the hospital." On examination, her cervix is found to be 2 cm. dilated and 10 per cent effaced. Discuss the nursing care you would plan for this mother if she were assigned to your care.

Study Questions

UNIT THREE: NURSING DURING LABOR AND DELIVERY

Read through the entire question and place your answer on the line to the right.

1. Give the term or the phrase which best fits each of the following statements:
A. Enlargement of the external os to 10 cm. in diameter   *full dilitation*
B. Maximum shortening of the cervical canal   *effacement*
C. A type of drug used in obstetrics which blots out memory of whatever occurs under its influence   *amnesia*
D. A condition caused by failure of the uterine muscle to stay contracted after delivery   *uterine atony*
E. A surgical incision of the perineum during second-stage labor   *episiotomy*
F. Settling of the baby's head into the brim of the pelvis   *lightening*

2. The character and the frequency of uterine contractions and the location of the discomfort experienced by the mother during labor often provide pertinent information regarding the labor.
Situation No. 1: In the case of a multipara who is having discomfort but is not in real labor, which of these symptoms would most probably serve to identify false labor contractions?
    A. Discomfort may begin as early as 3 or 4 weeks before the onset of true labor.
    B. Discomfort occurs 3 or 4 days before the onset of true labor.
    C. Contractions occur at regular intervals.
    D. Contractions occur at irregular intervals.
    E. Discomfort is confined to the lower abdomen and the groin.
    F. Discomfort is felt in the upper abdomen and the back.
Select the number corresponding to the correct letter or letters.
    1. A only
    2. A and C
    3. A, D and E
    4. All of them   **3**
Situation No. 2: In the case of a primigravida in the beginning of the first stage of labor, which of the following symptoms would most probably describe her labor contractions?
    A. Contractions occur at regular intervals.
    B. Contractions occur at irregular intervals.
    C. Discomfort is confined to the lower abdomen and the groin.
    D. Discomfort is located in the lower back and the abdomen.
    E. Contractions occur at intervals of from 2 to 3 minutes.
    F. Contractions occur at intervals of from 10 to 15 minutes.
Select the number corresponding to the correct letters.
    1. A and C
    2. A, D and F
    3. B, C and E
    4. All of them   **2**
Situation No. 3: In the case of a primigravida approaching the end of the first stage of labor, which of the following symptoms would most probably give an accurate description of her labor?
    A. Contractions occur at regular intervals.
    B. Contractions occur at irregular intervals.
    C. Contractions occur at intervals of every 1 to 1½ minutes.
    D. Contractions occur at intervals of from 2 to 3 minutes.
    E. Duration of contraction is from 45 to 60 seconds.
    F. Duration of contractions is from 50 to 70 seconds.

Select the number corresponding to the correct letters.
1. A, C and E
2. A, D and F
3. B, D and E
4. All of them   2

3. Labor is divided into the first, the second and the third stages.
A. When is the first stage of labor considered to be terminated?
   1. When contractions occur at 10- to 15-minute intervals
   2. When the cervix is completely dilated
   3. When the baby is delivered   2
B. When is the second stage of labor considered to be terminated?
   1. When the cervix is completely dilated
   2. When contractions occur at 2- to 3-minute intervals
   3. When the baby is delivered   3
C. When is the third stage of labor considered to be terminated?
   1. When the baby is delivered
   2. When the placenta is delivered
   3. After the uterus has remained firm for 1 hour   2

4. The nurse is caring for a mother during the first stage of labor. Which of the following observations would she report promptly to the physician?
A. Small amounts of bright blood in the vaginal discharge
B. Plugs of blood-streaked mucus in the vaginal discharge
C. Sudden gush of amniotic fluid from the vagina
D. Mother has a frequent desire to urinate.
E. Fetal heart rate slows during uterine contractions but returns to its usual rate 10 to 15 seconds following the contractions.
Select the number corresponding to the correct letters.
1. A and C
2. A, C and E
3. B, D and E
4. All of them   1

5. On admission of the mother to the labor suite, which of the following procedures are usually carried out routinely?
A. Check mother's temperature, pulse, respirations and blood pressure.
B. Take the mother to the bathroom and have her void.
C. Cleanse and shave the vulvar and perineal area.
D. Listen to the fetal heart sounds.
E. Prepare the mother for vaginal examination.
Select the number corresponding to the correct letter or letters.
1. A only
2. A and E
3. A, C and D
4. All of them   3

6. Why is an enema frequently given to a mother during the early part of the first stage of labor?
A. To obtain a stool specimen
B. To avoid straining as the mother bears down with contractions
C. To cleanse the lower bowel and/or stimulate labor contractions   C

7. After the cervix is dilated, and particularly if the membranes have ruptured, what facilities would provide the mother with the greatest degree of comfort and safety to expel an enema?
A. Use of toilet facilities in bathroom
B. Remain in bed and use the bedpan
C. Use the bedpan on a chair close to the bed   B

8. Often it is the nurse's responsibility to decide when the mother is ready to be moved from the labor room to the delivery room. Which of the following signs would signify to the nurse that the time of delivery is near?
A. Mother has a desire to defecate.
B. Increase in frequency, duration and intensity of uterine contractions
C. Mother begins to bear down spontaneously with uterine contractions.
D. Bulging of the perineum
E. Increase in amount of blood-stained mucus from the vagina
Select the number corresponding to the correct letter or letters.
   1. D only
   2. A, C and E
   3. B, D and E
   4. All of them

4

9. A physician was busy draining mucus from the mouth of the baby immediately after its birth and asked the nurse to let him know as soon as the placenta seemed to be separated. Which of the following would indicate that it was separated?
A. Gradual descent of the uterus farther into the pelvis
B. Protrusion of several more inches of umbilical cord
C. Uterus becomes more firm and rounded
D. A sudden gush of blood from the vagina
E. Large clots of blood slip out of the vagina
Select the number corresponding to the correct letters.
   1. A and C
   2. B, C and D
   3. B, C and E
   4. All of them

2

10. As soon as the physician had clamped and cut the umbilical cord, he handed the infant over to the nurse to care for. Which of the following acts would the nurse perform in the immediate care of the infant?
A. Place the infant so that he lies in a modified Trendelenburg position in a heated crib or resuscitator.
B. Wipe the mucus out of the infant's mouth with sterile gauze.
C. Slap the infant's back and soles of the feet sharply to stimulate crying.
D. Gently remove all vernix caseosa and blood in drying the infant's body with the receiving blanket.
E. "Label" infant with required item of identification as soon as he is transferred to the nursery.
Select the number corresponding to the correct letter or letters.
   1. A only
   2. A and C
   3. B, D and E
   4. All of them

1

11. After the delivery the infant is cared for by a nurse in the receiving nursery. The nurse who is caring for the mother during the first hour after the delivery of the placenta would include which of the following in her nursing care plan?
A. Keep the mother warm and out of drafts.
B. Express blood clots if they should accumulate in the uterus.
C. Massage the fundus continuously.
D. Administer ergotrate 0.2 mg. intramuscularly.
E. Check the mother's vital signs at frequent intervals.
Select the number corresponding to the correct letter or letters.
   1. B only
   2. A and C
   3. A, B and E
   4. All of them

3

12. Possibly the most dangerous stage of labor for the mother is the third stage because of the possibility of postpartal hemorrhage and shock.

A. Because there is a certain amount of blood loss, hemorrhage is said to take place when the loss exceeds what amount of blood?
1. 100 cc.
2. 300 cc.
3. 500 cc.   *3*

B. The most common cause of postpartal hemorrhage is atony of the uterus. What is the first thing to do as a preventive measure if the uterus appears to be atonic?
1. Take a firm grasp on the uterus.
2. Massage the uterus firmly.
3. Administer an oxytocic drug.   *2*

13. The physician told the nurse to watch a mother during labor for evidence of a prolapsed cord which he feared might occur.

A. When would the nurse consider that a prolapsed cord would be most likely to occur?
1. During the second stage of labor
2. In breech presentation
3. If the presenting part was not engaged in the pelvic brim
4. If the amniotic sac were intact
5. If the mother were particularly fatigued   *3*

B. If the nurse did suspect the cord to be prolapsed, what position should she put the mother in, with the hope of relieving the pressure on the cord?
1. Knee-chest position
2. Fowler's position
3. Sims' position
4. A prone position   *1*

C. In addition to changing the mother's position to relieve pressure on the cord, what other measures may the nurse employ if she observes the umbilical cord prolapsed out of the vagina?
1. Immediately wash the cord with warm antiseptic solution and replace in vagina.
2. Cover the cord with a wet sponge.
3. Apply a clamp to the exposed cord and cover with a sterile towel.
4. Keep the cord warm and moist by continuous applications of sterile saline compresses. *4*

D. What are the chief objectives of the emergency care given when prolapsed cord occurs?
1. To prevent cold air from prematurely stimulating respiration
2. To prevent drying of the cord while it is still pulsating
3. To stimulate and restore circulation in the cord by vasodilation
4. To prevent or relieve pressure on the cord   *4*

Note: The key to the correct answers to these questions is given on page 597.

UNIT FOUR

Nursing in the Normal Puerperium

The Physiology of the Puerperium
Nursing Care During the Puerperium

Chapter 13

The Physiology of the Puerperium

INTRODUCTION

This chapter deals with the study of the anatomic and the physiologic changes that normally occur during the puerperium. Knowledge and understanding of the reproductive process concerning pregnancy and labor will serve as a basis for understanding how the generative organs and the various systems of the human body adapt following the delivery.

The term puerperium (from *puer*, a child; and *parere*, to bring forth) refers to the 6-week period elapsing between the termination of labor and the return of the reproductive organs to their normal condition. This includes both the *progressive changes* in the breasts for lactation and *involution* of the internal reproductive organs. Although the changes brought about by involution are considered to be normal physiologic processes, they border closely between a condition of health and disease, for under no other circumstances does such marked and rapid involution of tissues occur without a departure from a state of health. For this reason, the quality of the mother's care at this time is essential to ensure her immediate as well as her future health.

ANATOMIC CHANGES

Uterus

Involution of the Uterus. Immediately following the delivery of the placenta the uterus becomes an almost solid mass of tissue, about the size of a grapefruit. Its thick anterior and posterior walls lie in close opposition, so that the center cavity is flattened. The uterus remains about the same size for the first 2 days after delivery but then rapidly decreases in size by an atrophic process called involution. This is effected partly by the contraction of the uterus and partly by autolytic processes in which some of the protein material of the uterine wall is broken down into simpler components which then are absorbed and eventually cast off through the urine.

THE PROCESS OF INVOLUTION. The separation of the placenta and the membranes from the uterine wall takes place in the outer portion of the spongy layer of the decidua, and, therefore, a remnant of this layer remains in the uterus to be cast off in part in the lochia. Within 2 or 3 days after labor this remaining portion of decidua becomes differentiated into 2 layers, leaving the deeper or unaltered layer attached to the muscular wall from which the new endometrial lining is generated. The layer adjoining the uterine cavity becomes necrotic and is cast off in the lochia. The process is very like the healing of any surface; there is oozing of blood from the small vessels on this surface. The bleeding from the larger vessels is controlled by compression of the retracted uterine muscle fibers. The process of regeneration is rapid, except at the site of former placental attachment, which requires 6 or 7 weeks to

297

heal completely. Elsewhere, the free surface of the endometrium is restored in half that time.

THE PROGRESS OF INVOLUTION. The normal process of involution requires 5 or 6 weeks, and at the end of that time the uterus regains its normal size, although it never returns exactly to its virgin state. One can realize more fully the rapidity of this process by comparing the changes which occur in the weight of this organ. Immediately following the delivery the uterus weighs approximately 2 pounds; at the end of the first week, about 1 pound; at the end of the second week, about 12 ounces; and by the time that involution is complete, it should weigh only about 2 ounces. By observing the height of the fundus, which may be felt through the abdominal wall, the nurse is able to appreciate more fully these remarkable changes. Immediately after the birth of the placenta the uterus sinks into the pelvis, and the fundus is felt midway between the umbilicus and the symphysis, but it soon rises to the level of the umbilicus (5 or 5½ inches above the pubes); and 12 hours later it probably will be found a little higher. Day-by-day careful measurements will show that it is diminishing in size, so that at the end of 10 days or so it cannot be detected by abdominal palpation. The approximate rate of decrease in the height of the fundus is a little over half an inch or one fingerbreadth a day. Observation of this rate of involution is very important; the physician will want to be informed about any marked delay, especially if accompanied by suppression of the lochia or retention of clots. In measuring the height of the uterus, care should be taken that the observations are made after the bladder is emptied, as a full bladder will raise the height of the fundus.

Apparent indications that involution is not occurring satisfactorily are: the uterus fails to decrease progressively in size, it remains "flabby" and causes the mother much discomfort (see Subinvolution in Chap. 20, Complications of the Puerperium).

Changes in the Cervix. After the delivery the cervix is a soft, flabby structure but, because it is retracting, by the end of the 1st week it becomes so narrow that it would be difficult to introduce anything the size of a finger. Unlike the process of involution which is now occurring in the body of the uterus, a very considerable new formation of muscle cells is taking place in the cervix and, simultaneously, any lacerations are healing. Once a mother has delivered a child vaginally, the cervix does not assume its pregravid appearance, but the external os remains open in varying degrees, although the internal os is closed. This is one of the characteristics of the uterus of a multiparous woman.

The Lochia. A knowledge of the healing process by which the lining of the uterus becomes regenerated is a valuable adjunct to the nurse in understanding and interpreting the lochial discharge. At first the discharge consists almost entirely of blood with a small amount of mucus, particles of decidua and cellular debris which escape from the placental site. It should not contain large clots or membrane or be excessive in amount. This discharge lasts about 3 days and is called *lochia rubra*. As the oozing of blood from the healing surface diminshes, the discharge becomes more serous or watery and gradually changes to a pinkish color, the so-called *lochia serosa*. Toward the 10th day the lochia is thinner, greatly decreased in amount and almost colorless, the so-called *lochia alba*. By the end of the 3rd week the discharge usually disappears, though a brownish mucoid discharge may persist a little longer. Lochia possesses a peculiar animal emanation which is quite characteristic and should never, at any time, have an offensive odor.

The quantity of lochia varies with individuals, but, generally speaking, it is more profuse in multiparas. It is to be expected that when a mother is out of bed for the first time there may be a definite increase in the amount of discharge. Nevertheless, the recurrence of fresh bleeding after the discharge has become dark and diminished in amount, or the persistence of bright blood in the lochia or the suppression of the discharge (which may be caused by cold, fright, grief or other emotion) should be reported to the obstetrician. The daily observation of the amount and the character of the lochia is of the greatest importance as an index of the progress of healing of the endometrial surface.

The Pelvis

The vaginal walls, the vulva and all other tissues which have become hypertrophied during pregnancy also undergo a process of involution in their return to normal. The *vagina* requires some time to recover from the distention brought about by the delivery. This capacious passage gradually diminishes in size, although rarely returns to its nulliparous condition. The *labia majora* and the *labia minora* become flabby and atrophic as compared with their condition before childbearing. Any abrasions and lacerations of the genital canal caused by the passage of the fetus should heal completely during the puerperium. The *ligaments* that support the uterus, the ovaries and the tubes, which have also undergone great tension and stretching, are now relaxed and will take considerable time to return almost to their normal size and position. This is one of the reasons that the mother must be given intelligent interpretation of early ambulation.

Abdominal Wall

The abdominal wall recovers partially from the overstretching but remains soft and flabby for some time. The striae, due to the rupture of the elastic fibers of the cutis, usually remain but become less conspicuous because of their silvery appearance. The process of involution in the abdominal structures requires at least 6 weeks. Provided that the abdominal walls have retained their muscle tone, they gradually return to their original condition. However, if these muscles are relaxed because they have lost their tone, there may be a marked separation or *diastasis of the recti muscles*, so that the abdominal organs are not properly supported. Rest, diet, prescribed exercises, good body mechanics and good posture may do much to restore the tonicity of these muscles.

The Breasts

During pregnancy progressive changes occur in the breasts in preparation for lactation (see Chap. 6). It is believed that the circulating levels of estrogen and progesterone during pregnancy inhibit the activity of the anterior pituitary hormone *luteotrophin* (sometimes referred to as LTH, prolactin, the lactogenic hormone or the mammogenic hormone). With the delivery of the placenta, however, this inhibition is removed, and luteotrophin is then free to initiate lactation.

After the delivery the breasts continue much the same for about 2 days. The breasts secrete a small amount of *colostrum*, which appears as a thin yellowish fluid. It will be remembered that colostrum is formed at the end of pregnancy, and women who carry out special breast care preparation during the last weeks of pregnancy often are able manually to express small amounts of it before the birth of the baby. The nutritive value of colostrum is low in comparison with that of normal breast milk. Colostrum contains more protein (lactalbumin) and inorganic salts but less fat and carbohydrate than human breast milk. During these first days after the delivery breast feeding is advantageous for both mother and infant. The infant's sucking at the breast helps to stimulate lactation, and, in addition, it stimulates the uterus to contract. These early breast feeding experiences simultaneously fulfill the infant's need for sucking.

On the 3rd or the 4th day postpartum the breast milk usually "comes in." There is an obvious change in the color of the secretion from the nipples; it becomes bluish white, the usual color of normal breast milk. At this time the breasts suddenly become larger, firmer and more tender as the lacteal secretion is established, causing the mother to experience throbbing pains in the breasts, extending into the axillae. This congestion, which usually subsides in 1 or 2 days, is caused in part by the pressure from the increased amount of milk in the lobes and the ducts but even more by the increased circulation of blood and lymph in the mammary gland, producing tension on the very sensitive surrounding tissues. This is sometimes referred to as *primary engorgement*.

Breast milk varies markedly in its quality and quantity, not only in different individuals, but also in the same individual at various times. In general, the amount of breast milk increases as the infant's need for it increases. Nature seems to have coordinated carefully the mother's need for rest and the infant's need for food during the first 2 days, when only colostrum is secreted. But during this time lactation is definitely stimulated by the infant's sucking, and although the secretion of breast milk would occur naturally, without this stimulation and the complete emptying of the breasts the secretion of breast milk would not continue for more than a few days. If the infant is put to breast consistently, by the end of the first week a healthy mother usually has about 6 to 10 ounces of breast milk a day. By the end of 4 weeks this amount about doubles, so that she produces about 20 ounces a day. Breast milk is produced on the basis of "supply and demand"; i.e., the amount secreted gradually adjusts in relation to what the baby takes at an average feeding. In time, as the baby grows, the mother may have about 30 ounces of breast milk a day.

The supply of breast milk is dependent on several factors, such as the mother's diet, the amount of exercise and rest she gets, and her level of contentment. An adequate diet for lactation requires increased amounts of protein, calcium, iron and vitamins as well as an ample fluid intake (see p. 333). The mother who is breast-feeding needs a good night's sleep, a rest period in the middle of the day and normal exercise. Worry, emotional tension and too much activity (overexertion and fatigue) have an adverse effect on lactation (see Chaps. 8 and 15). In relation to lactation, the actual size of the breast is not as important as the amount of glandular tissue, since the secreting tissues of the mammary gland produce the breast milk and not the fat. It has been verified that certain drugs, if administered to the lactating mother, are excreted in the breast milk, for example, large doses of salicylates, certain cathartics, iodides, bromides, quinine, atropine, opium, etc.

CLINICAL ASPECTS

Temperature

Slight rises in temperature may occur without apparent cause following the delivery, but, in general, the mother's temperature should remain within normal limits during the puerperium, that is, below 38° C. (100.4° F.) when taken by mouth. Any mother whose temperature exceeds this limit in any two consecutive 24-hour periods of the puerperium (excluding the first 24 hours postpartum) is considered to be febrile.

It was formerly believed that an elevation of temperature naturally occurred with the establishment of lactation on the 3rd or the 4th day after the delivery, and the so-called *milk-fever* was considered to be a normal accompaniment of this process. At the present time this is considered to be a fallacy. On rare occasions a sharp peak of fever for several hours may be caused by extreme vascular and lymphatic engorgement of the breasts, but this does not last longer than 12 hours at the most.

In judging the significance of a rise in temperature, the pulse rate provides a helpful guide, for in a puerperal patient with a slow pulse, a slightly elevated temperature is not likely to signify a complication. Nevertheless, any rise of temperature in the puerperium should excite the suspicion of endometritis (see Chap. 20, Complications of the Puerperium).

Pulse

In the early puerperium a pulse rate which is somewhat slower than that at other times is a favorable symptom. The rate usually averages between 60 and 70 but may even become a little slower than this in 1 or 2 days after the delivery. This is merely a transient phenomenon, so that by the end of the 1st week or 10 days the pulse returns to its normal rate. On the other hand, a rapid pulse after labor, unless the mother has cardiac disease, may be an indication of shock or hemorrhage.

Blood

Most of the blood and metabolic alterations characteristic of normal pregnancy disappear within the first 2 weeks of the puerperium.

After-pains

Normally, after the delivery of the first child, the uterine muscle tends to remain in a state of tonic contraction and retraction. But if the uterus has been subjected to any marked distention, or if tissue or blood clots have been retained in the cavity, then active contractions occur in an effort to expel them, and these contractions may be painful. In multiparas a certain amount of the initial tonicity of the uterine muscle has been lost, and these contractions and retractions cannot be sustained. Consequently, the muscle contracts and relaxes at intervals, and these contractions give rise to the sensation of pain, the so-called "after-pains." These after-pains are more noticeable after a pregnancy in which the uterus has been greatly distended, as with multiple births or hydramnios. They are particularly noticeable in the breast-feeding mother, when the infant is put to breast (because sucking stimulates the uterus to contract), and they may last for days, although ordinarily they become quite bearable in about 48 hours after delivery. Often after-pains become so sharp that the administration of a sedative is necessary. Any time that they are severe enough to disturb the mother's rest and peace of mind, the physician should be notified.

Digestion

Although the mother's appetite may be diminished the first few days after labor, the digestive tract functions normally in the puerperium. Her thirst is considerably increased at this time due to the marked diaphoresis and loss of fluids associated with the puerperium. Moreover, the fact that the mother has probably gone without fluids for some hours in labor undoubtedly increases her thirst.

Loss of Weight

In addition to the 10- or 11-pound loss of weight which results at delivery, there is generally a still further loss of about 5 pounds of body weight during the puerperium due to the marked increase in excretions.

Kidneys

The amount of urine excreted by the kidneys in the puerperium is of particular significance. As previously stated, during pregnancy there is an increased tendency of the body to retain water, so that now the tremendous output of urine represents the body's effort to return its water metabolism to normal. Diuresis regularly occurs between the 2nd and the 5th days after delivery, sometimes reaching a daily output of 3,000 cc. After the delivery, in particular, the bladder may distend without any awareness on the part of the mother, especially if she has received any form of analgesia. Therefore, it becomes a major responsibility of the nurse to be alert to signs of a full bladder and thus to prevent distention from occurring.

During the first few days after labor there may be a marked increase in the amount of acetone and nitrogen in the urine. The acetone

is due to an excessive breakdown of carbohydrate resulting from the increased muscular activity in labor, while, on the other hand, the nitrogen excretion is due to the breakdown of protein material of the uterine wall in the process of involution, as previously mentioned. Occasionally, during the first weeks of the puerperium the urine contains substantial amounts of sugar which has no relationship to diabetes but is due to the presence of lactose, milk sugar, which is absorbed from the mammary glands.

Intestinal Elimination

The mother is nearly always constipated during the first few days of the puerperium. This is due to the relaxed condition of the intestinal and the abdominal muscles, in particular, and to the inability of the abdominal wall to aid in the evacuation of the intestinal contents. In addition, if hemorrhoids are present, the mother often is afraid to have a stool because of the discomfort these varicosities cause during elimination.

Skin

It is to be expected that elimination of waste products via the skin is accelerated in the early puerperium, often to such a degree that the mother is drenched with perspiration. These episodes of profuse sweating, which frequently occur in the night, gradually subside and do not require any specific treatment aside from protecting the mother from chilling at such times as they occur.

Menstruation

If the mother does not breast-feed her infant, the menstrual flow probably will return within 8 weeks after delivery. Ordinarily, menstruation does not occur so long as the mother is breast-feeding, but this is not a certainty. During lactation the first menstrual period may occur as early as the 2nd month but usually occurs about the 4th month following the delivery. It has been known not to reappear until as late as the 18th month. Studies have shown that failure to menstruate during lactation is due to suppression of ovulation, but, since some mothers have been known to become pregnant in the course of breast-feeding an infant, we know that this is not always the case.

POSTPARTAL EXAMINATIONS

The condition of the mother is confirmed before she is discharged from the hospital to make sure that her progress has been satisfactory during the early puerperium. In addition to verifying her vital signs and present weight, observations are made to determine the condition of her breasts, the progress of involution and the healing of the perineal wound. A pelvic examination is deferred, since findings made by palpation of the uterus and inspection of the lochia will give satisfactory evidence as to the progress of involution at this time.

Follow-up Examinations

As has been mentioned previously, the reproductive tract should return to its normal condition by the end of the puerperium. In order to investigate the general physical condition of the mother and determine with what normalcy she has completed her maternity experience, she should return to her physician for examination about 6 weeks postpartum. During the visit the weight and the blood pressure are taken, the urine is examined for albumin, and a blood count may be done. The condition of the abdominal walls is observed, and the breasts are inspected. If the mother is breast-feeding, the condition of the nipples and the degree of lacteal secretion are a significant part of the observation. If the mother is not breast-feeding, the breasts should be observed to see that physiologic readjustments have occurred. A thorough pelvic examination is carried out to investigate the position of the uterus, the healing of perineal wounds, the support of the pelvic floor, and whether involution is complete. In addition, this return examination provides an opportunity for the mother and the obstetrician to discuss any other problems relating to this maternity experience. If abnormalities are found, they may be treated at this time and arrangements made for further examinations and treatments as necessary. Regardless, most physicians in-struct their patients to return in 6 months for a check-up examination. Many encourage the mothers to return for a check-up again at the end of 1 year.

SUGGESTED READING

Bare, W. W., *et al.*: Double-blind evaluation of two androgen-estrogen preparations and a placebo for suppression of lactation, Am. J. Obstet. Gynec. 87:276-279, 1963.

Beicher, S. J., *et al.*: Carbohydrate metabolism in pregnancy. V. The interrelations of glucose, insulin and free fatty acids in late pregnancy and postpartum, New Eng. J. Med. 271:866-872, October 22, 1964.

Bruni, J. R., *et al.*: Controlled double-blind evaluation of three analgesic medications for post-partum discomfort, Obstet. Gynec. 25:76-81, January, 1965.

Dennis, K. J.: Changes in body weight after delivery, J. Obstet. Gynec. Brit. Comm. 72:94-102, February, 1965.

Eastman, N. J., and Hellman, L. H.: Williams Obstetrics, ed. 13, New York, Appleton, 1966.

Fleming, A. R.: Prophylaxis of postpartum urinary retention, Am. J. Obstet. Gynec. 64:134, 1952.

Gioiosa, R.: Incidence of pregnancy during lactation in 500 cases, Am. J. Obstet. Gynec. 70:162, 1955.

Greenhill, J. P.: Obstetrics, ed. 13, Philadelphia, Saunders, 1965.

Guyton, A. C.: Textbook of Medical Physiology, ed. 2, Philadelphia, Saunders, 1961.

Herschelmann, R. F., and Partridge, Ann: Deladumone for breast discomfort, Am. J. Nurs. 59:1252-1254, September, 1959.

Kessler, W. B., *et al.*: Hepatic function during pregnancy and puerperium, Obstet. Gynec. 23:372-380, March, 1964.

Lennon, G. G., *et al.*: The puerperium, Brit. Med. J. 5399:1687-1690, June 27, 1964.

Love, E. J., *et al.*: Evaluation of oral and intravenous glucose tolerance in tests for the diagnosis of prediabetes in the puerperium, Am. J. Obstet. Gynec. 88:283-290, February 1, 1964.

Metcalfe, J.: The maternal heart in postpartum period, Am. J. Cardiol. 12:439-440, October, 1963.

Naish, F. C.: Breast Feeding, ed. 2, London, Lloyd Luke, 1956.

Newton, Michael, and Newton, Niles: The normal course and management of lactation, Clin. Obstet. Gynec. 5:44-63, March, 1962.

Nickerson, K., *et al.*: Oxytocin and milk ejection, Am. J. Obstet. Gynec. 67:1028-1034, 1954.

Pritchard, Jack A., *et al.*: Blood volume changes in pregnancy and the puerperium. II. Red blood cells loss and changes in apparent blood volume during and following vaginal delivery, cesarean section, and cesarean section plus total hysterectomy, Am. J. Obstet. Gynec. 84:1271-1282, November 15, 1962.

Rubin, Reva: Puerperal change, Nurs. Outlook, 9, No. 12:753-755, December, 1961.

Slotnick, I. J., Stelluto, M., and Prystowsky, H.: Microbiology of the female genital tract. III. Comparative investigation of the cervical flora of parturients receiving either rectal or vaginal examinations, Am. J. Obstet. Gynec. 85:519-526, February 15, 1963.

Steiner, G. J.: Late postpartum eclampsia: report of a case, Obstet. Gynec. 24:594-596, October, 1964.

Tuttle, W. W., and Schottelius, B. A.: Textbook of Physiology, ed. 15, St. Louis, Mosby, 1965.

Udesky, I. C.: Ovulation in lactating women, Am. J. Obstet. Gynec. 59:843, 1950.

Womack, William S., *et al.*: A comparison of hormone therapies for suppression of lactation, Southern Med. J., 55, No. 8:816-820, August, 1962.

Chapter 14

Nursing Care During the Puerperium

INTRODUCTION

Changes brought about in the medical management of the puerperium in the last decade have brought about corresponding changes in this phase of nursing care. These changes have redirected the emphasis and given new significance to what heretofore was considered rather routine nursing. The care of the patient during the postpartal period is very important and presents a real challenge to the nurse. The newly delivered mother is a healthy patient who is adjusting physically and emotionally from the experience of pregnancy and labor. In addition, with the arrival of the infant, she must adapt to a new family structure. Her needs for physical care have been greatly modified because of two important developments, namely, the advent of early ambulation following the delivery and the subsequent evolvement of more simplified maternity nursing procedures.

Increased insight into the psychosocial needs of the newly delivered mother has resulted in greater attention to the emotional aspects of care. As has been emphasized before, the mother, the infant, the father and the other children are considered as a unit. In the hospital the nurse may not necessarily have the responsibility of caring for the mother and her new baby at the same time; nevertheless, the infant must be considered in relation to the mother's care, and their care in turn must be related to the total family constellation. The simplification of certain aspects of physical care in no way diminishes the need for professional nursing care, for the astute nurse can use physical care activities as valuable entrées in developing a productive nurse-patient relationship (see Chap. 12). Moreover, she must use her observational and communicative skills continuously. The mother's physiological functioning must be observed accurately, her dependency needs must be met, anticipatory guidance and health teaching must be given according to the mother's readiness to learn, and the developing relationship between the mother and the infant should be appropriately observed and guided.

CHANGES AND REACTIONS DURING THE PUERPERIUM

As stated in Chapter 12, the mother immediately after labor experiences a sense of complete fatigue which is comparable to that which would normally follow the exertion of any strenuous muscular activity. At the same time, if she has been awake during the delivery of her infant, she may be so exhilarated by the experience and the feeling of relief which accompanies it that she is not aware of being exhausted. She is interested in seeing and holding her baby and visiting with her husband. Although this first visit of the family to-

304

gether may be rather brief, it is an experience which is particularly gratifying to the parents. Following this, every effort should be made to help the mother to rest, and with little encouragement she usually passes off into a sound natural sleep. The discomforts and activities which may interfere with sleep, such as soreness of the vulva, hemorrhoids, "after-pains," and frequent postpartal observations, should be expedited and/or mitigated as much as possible.

Many mothers complain of feeling chilled immediately after labor; a few even appear to have a shaking chill. Such chills may be due in part to nervous reaction and exhaustion. There is some disturbance of equilibrium between internal and external temperature caused by excessive perspiration during the muscular exertion of labor. Some authorities believe that the "chill" may be due partly to the sudden release of intra-abdominal pressure which results as the uterus is emptied at delivery. This

reaction may be avoided if the mother is made comfortable in a warm bed and given a warm beverage when possible (see Chap. 12). If her body does begin to quiver, an extra cotton blanket should be placed over her or tucked close around her body for comfort. Many mothers (and their husbands) are frightened or disturbed by the chill; thus, reassurance by the nurse that this is not an unusual occurrence following delivery is extremely helpful.

Physiologic and Psychological Changes

Specific anatomic and physiologic changes already have been discussed in Chapter 13. However, it is well for the nurse to keep in mind that these alterations occur abruptly and are sizable. They involve profound diminution in circulating blood volume, a weight loss, displacement of internal organs, etc. It is truly marvelous that the new parturient copes so

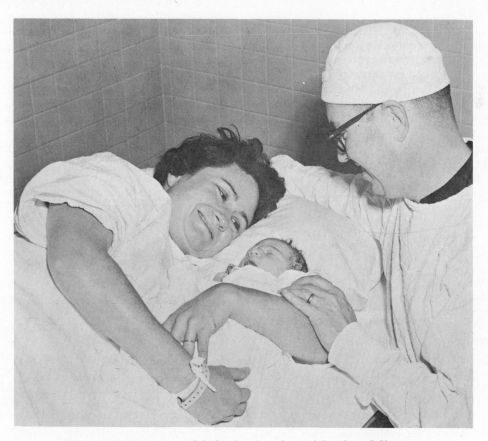

FIG. 14-1. Parents and baby having first visit after delivery.

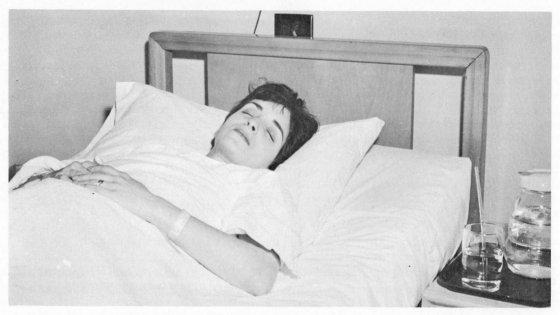

FIG. 14-2. Rest after delivery. (MacDonald House, University Hospitals of Cleveland)

adequately, and that she complains so little (see Suggested Reading).

The normal puerperal course follows a predictable healing and regenerative pattern, one that is not confined to the physical aspects of the patient. A new role must be assumed along with all of its concomitant tasks, new attitudes must be formed, and these adjustments must be undertaken before physical restoration is complete.

As with any regenerative process, energy is involved—energy that is needed to survive and to meet the everyday obligations of the mother's social and individual role. During the time that the mother coped with the increasing demands of labor there was a progressive withdrawal of social energy, i.e., a narrowing of attention and an inward turning (see Chap. 12). During the postpartal period the reverse process occurs: the mother is slowly able to extend the sphere of physical and psychic energy from herself to others in the immediate environment and thence to events and persons outside her immediate environment.

Phases of the Restorative Period of the Puerperium. "TAKING-IN" PHASE. One author[1] has described certain phases that occur during

[1] Rubin, Reva: Puerperal change, Nurs. Outlook 9:753-755, December, 1961.

the restorative period of the puerperium. The first of these seems to be a "taking-in" period (this lasts 2 or 3 days), in which the mother is passive and dependent. She tries to do what she is told, she gratefully accepts what she is given, and she initiates little or no action; rather she awaits the action of others. She seems to be grateful when decisions are made for her, and even simple decision-making as well as slight physical activity seems to fatigue her. It becomes apparent to the nurse that the needs she expresses are more in relation to herself than in relation to her baby. The wise nurse attempts to meet these needs to the mother's satisfaction, thus enabling her to move on to the more complex tasks of mothering her baby.

Sleep and food play an important part during this phase. The mother is far more able to begin the activities required of her if she is allowed to have a well-earned refreshing sleep. If this necessary rest is disrupted, the mother may experience a "sleep-hunger" which may last for several days; this results in irritability, fatigue and general interference with the normal restorative process. Thus, the necessity of appropriate intervention by the nurse to allow the mother to get adequate sleep cannot be stressed enough.

The nurse will note, also, that the mother usually has a good appetite and, in fact, may talk a good deal about food, about either the adequacy or the inadequacy of her meals. In-between nourishment is appreciated and needed (especially by nursing mothers). The concern about food seems to be a part of the mother's general need to be restored. Food, as we know, has tremendous psychological significance in terms of care-asking and care-giving (see Chap. 8). The nurse should be especially cognizant of the mother's need for hearty meals and should expedite extra nourishment whenever possible. Moreover, she should be aware that a poor appetite often is one of the first symptoms that all is not proceeding normally in the puerperal period.

Psychological Adjustment. During the "taking-in" phase the mother begins to relive the delivery experience in order to integrate it fully with reality. She is apt to be very talkative at this time, and she may want to know certain specifics and details so that she can form a total picture of what "really happened" during delivery. As she obtains this information, she is able to realize more fully that the pregnancy and the delivery are truly over, and that her baby now is born and is an individual outside of and separate from herself. This is a considerable task and involves rather profound changes in attitudes and feelings. The symbiotic relationship between mother and

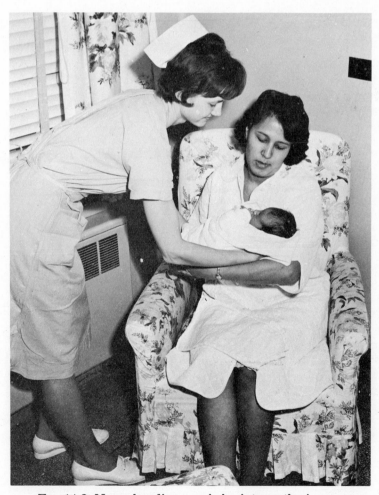

Fig. 14-3. Nurse handing new baby into mother's arms.

infant during pregnancy is at an end, and the mother now must identify her child as a separate individual (see Chap. 15).

TAKING-HOLD PHASE. The second phase in the puerperal period has been described as a "taking-hold" phase; that is, the mother strives for independence and autonomy and finally begins to be the initiator. One of her main concerns at this point seems to be her ability to control her bodily functions; her bowels and bladder must perform well, and she takes an active part in seeing that they do. If she is nursing her infant, she is concerned about producing an acceptable quantity and quality of milk. She often will ask the nurses and the doctors anxiously (referring to the milk), "Has it come in yet?" And later she wants to know: "Do you think I have enough?" She cannot have enough explanation and reassurance that she is "performing" well at this time. She wants to walk, to sit, to move as she did before delivery and is very anxious and impatient if she cannot make her body behave as it once did. It is as though she is thinking, "How can I possibly assume all my responsibilities for others if I cannot control my own body?"

Her first mothering tasks are especially important to her, and "failures" (inability to elicit a bubble from her infant, poor sucking response on the part of the baby, her awkwardness in handling her child), no matter how small and expected (by the staff), can send her to the depths of despair. Even the skillful

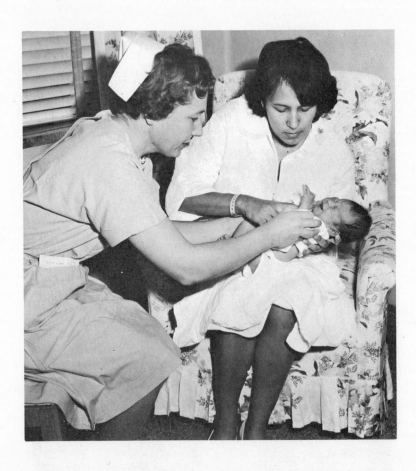

FIG. 14-4. Under guidance from the nurse, the mother learns to change baby's position.

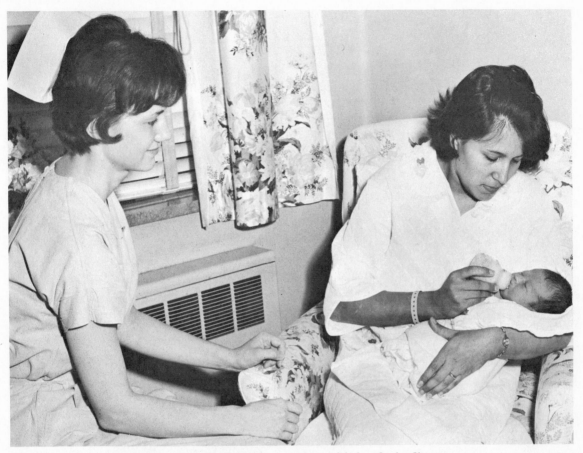

FIG. 14-5. Assisting the mother with bottle feeding.

intervention of the nurse seems only to point up her "inadequacy" as a mother. She often will voice her feelings with an "Oh, I'll never be able to bathe him as easily as you do." Or she says: "He always seems to take his milk better when *you* feed him." Conversely, when she succeeds at a task, her delight and relief are wonderful to behold. It is difficult to imagine (for anyone other than a new mother) how thrilling a hearty bubble from a small infant can be.

Since there is a good deal of anxiety as well as activity in this phase, fatigue and exhaustion may occur if the mother is not helped to set realistic expectations and limits for herself. Since this "taking-hold" phase lasts about 10 days, much of it will take place at home.

The nurse can be invaluable in giving the mother, as she appears able and ready to accept it, anticipatory guidance about what to expect and how to manage. During the hospital stay the mother profits greatly from reassurance and explanation regarding the various processes and hour-by-hour events. She finds guidance and reinforcement of appropriate behavior by the nurse particularly helpful when she attempts to perform her mothering tasks.

When assisting the mother, the nurse must be careful not to impose herself between the mother and her baby (no matter how awkward or maladroit the mother seems). Rather, the nurse should allow the mother to perform the actual task (after necessary demonstration or instruction) and then encourage, reinforce, etc., whatever behavior was appropriate. In this way she demonstrates that she has confidence in the mother's ability to cope with new tasks. In order to gain skill and confidence in her mothering ability, the mother needs the opportunity to make decisions about the

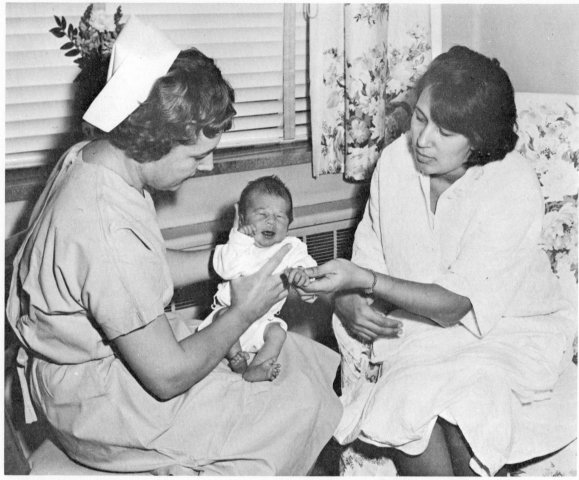

Fig. 14-6. Nurse demonstrates for mother how baby can be safely supported between her hands (as in bubbling).

baby's needs as well as guidance regarding his physical care. When she is allowed to find answers to her questions (again with guidance as necessary) and is reassured that her judgment is correct, she is able to feel confident in her ability to perceive needs accurately and to make decisions. Thus, she is better able to meet problems in the future. (See Suggested Reading for a more thorough discussion of changes and behavior during the puerperium.)

Postpartal Blues. Sometime during the puerperium, for no apparent reason, the mother quite suddenly may experience a "let-down" feeling. She may become irritable and tearful, may even lose her appetite and find it difficult to sleep. These are the usual manifestations of the so-called "postpartal blues";

they usually are very temporary and may occur while the mother is in the hospital or after her discharge home. This temporary depression is <u>thought to be related to the hormonal changes that occur during this time and the ego regression that can accompany the increased dependency needs and responsibilities.</u> Discomfort, fatigue and exhaustion certainly contribute to this condition, if they do not actually precipitate it. The mother may release tension by crying and thus become more comfortable. However, since she usually does not know exactly why she is crying, she may feel guilty about this somewhat unaccustomed emotional display.

The nurse can help the mother most effectively if she is able to recognize and to inter-

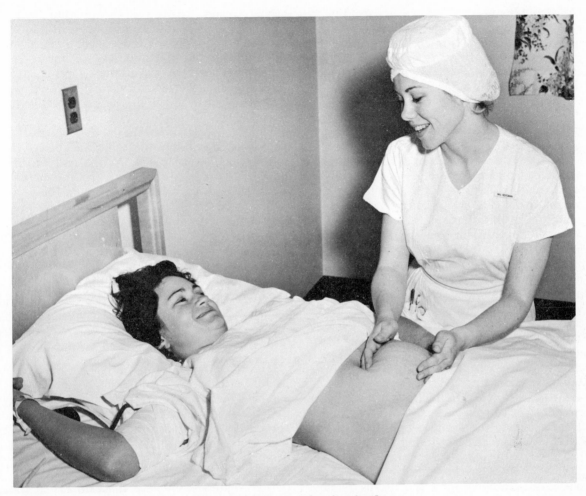

Fig. 14-7. Nurse palpating fundus.

pret the mother's behavior and, in turn, is kind and understanding. If the mother does want to cry, her privacy should be respected, and she should be assured that this behavior is not only acceptable but therapeutic. Accurate reporting and recording of the mother's emotional state is important at all times, since occasionally a more serious and pathologic psychological upheaval occurs, and the prodromal signs may become apparent during the hospital stay (see Chap. 20).

Summary. It is well for the nurse to keep in mind during the early days of the puerperium that although the mother appears to recover with amazing rapidity after the delivery, this very rapid apparent recovery helps to obscure the fact that the mother's entire being still is

going through a period of transition. Therefore, she is more vulnerable to stress at this time. Problems that she otherwise might handle with relative ease may stimulate emotionally charged situations as she faces the increased responsibilities for the nurturing and the care of her new baby, her family and home. At the same time, the mother's own need for affection and attention may bring about feelings of jealousy, guilt, etc., when the major attention more often than not is directed to the infant. Therefore, care should be focused on providing physical rest for the mother as well as an environment that is as free from tension and worry as possible. In addition, the mother should be given as much help as she needs to gain self-confidence in caring for her baby and perceiving his needs. This will mean that the old cliché "routine postpartum care" is not to be taken literally. Nursing care during the puerperium, as during any other period of the childbearing cycle, must be "tailored" to meet the needs of each individual patient.

IMMEDIATE CARE

Intelligent interpretation of the patient's physiologic and behavioral responses is essential to the mother's safety and welfare. Paramount among the physiologic responses is the condition of the uterus. The mother must be observed carefully for bleeding during the first 6 hours after labor and particularly during the 1st hour after delivery (see Chap. 12).

Considerable information can be gained by palpating the fundus through the abdominal wall to be assured that the uterus remains firm, round and well contracted. At the same time it is also important to inspect the perineal pad for obvious signs of bleeding, as well as to take the pulse and the blood pressure. During the first hour these observations should be made at least every 15 minutes, or more often if indicated. In some hospitals it is customary to have a nurse (or a properly prepared nurse's aide) sit at the bedside during this hour, with her hand on the mother's abdomen so that she can feel the fundus constantly. As long as the bleeding is minimal, and the uterus remains firm, well-contracted and does not increase in size, it is neither necessary nor desirable to stimulate it. However, if the uterus becomes soft and boggy because of relaxation, the fundus should be massaged immediately until it becomes contracted again. This can be best accomplished if one hand is placed just above the symphysis pubis to act as a guard, as the other hand is cupped around the fundus and rotated gently. It should be remembered that the uterus is a sensitive organ which, under normal circumstances, responds quickly to tactile stimulation. Care must be taken to avoid overmassage, because, in addition to causing the mother considerable pain, this may stimulate premature uterine contractions and thereby cause undue muscle fatigue. Such a condition would further encourage uterine relaxation and hemorrhage. If the uterus is

atonic, blood which collects in the cavity should be expressed with firm but gentle force in the direction of the outlet, but only after the fundus has been first massaged (Fig. 14-7). Failure to see that the uterus is contracted before pushing downward against it could result in inversion of the uterus, an exceedingly serious complication.

During the 1st hour the mother should be kept clean, dry and comfortable but allowed to rest as much as possible. At the end of this hour it is usually customary to give the mother a partial bath as necessary and take the temperature, in addition to other vital signs, before transferring her to the postpartal division. The nurse must be constantly alert for any changes in the mother's condition, such as her color, character of the pulse, respiration and blood pressure, the status of the fundus and the amount of vaginal bleeding.

GENERAL PHYSICAL CARE

The daily routine procedures for the postpartal patient vary in different hospitals, but the principles of care are essentially the same. Certain observations should be made and recorded daily. These would include such findings as temperature, pulse and respiration; urinary and intestinal elimination; the physical changes which occur normally in the puerperium. One should note the changes in the breasts, the height and consistency of the fundus, the character, the amount and the color of the lochial discharge and the condition of the episiotomy (see Chap. 13). Furthermore, it is equally important for the nurse to be alert to the mother's general comfort and well-being—how she rests and sleeps, her activity, her appetite, her emotional status and, particularly, because of its vast influence, how she is adjusting to her role as a new mother (see Chap. 15).

Temperature, Pulse and Respiration

The temperature should be carefully watched during the first 2 weeks of the puerperium, as fever is usually the first symptom of an infectious process. And, as has been stated previously, the pulse rate provides a helpful guide in determining the significance of a rise in temperature. These observations are usually made and recorded every 4 hours for the first few days after delivery, omitting the 2 A.M. observations, which would disturb the mother's sleep. Thereafter, they are made every night and morning, as long as the mother is progressing normally. If the temperature rises above 37.8° C. (100° F.) or the pulse rate above 100, the physician should be notified immediately. Usually, the blood pressure is not checked regularly unless there has been some abnormality. Then observations and recordings are made every 2 to 4 hours or more frequently, as indicated.

Nutrition

Very shortly following the delivery, after having gone without food or fluids for some hours, the mother may express a desire for something to eat. When food is put before her, however, she may have little appetite. Unless she has received a general anesthetic or is nauseated, there is usually no contraindication to giving her some nourishment. However, it is prudent to give her small amounts of easily digested foods, such as milk or tea and toast, for this first meal. Thereafter, she enjoys a normal diet.

The two factors which the nurse must bear in mind when considering the mother's diet are (1) providing for her general nutrition and (2) providing enough nourishing foods to supply the additional calories and nutrients required during lactation. If these nutritional requirements are provided for, the mother's convalescence will be more rapid, her strength will be recovered more quickly, and the quality and quantity of her milk will be better. She will also be more able to resist infections.

The daily diet of the lactating mother should be like that taken during pregnancy, with the addition of 1,000 calories and amounts of the various nutrients (protein, calcium, iron, vitamin A, thiamine, riboflavin, niacin and ascorbic acid) as recommended by the Food and Nutrition Board of the National Research Council[2] (see Chap. 8, Antepartal

[2] Recommended Dietary Allowances, rev. ed., Publication No. 1146, National Academy of Sciences, National Research Council, Washington, D. C., 1963.

Care). These increased demands in the diet during lactation can be supplied with the addition of a pint of milk, one serving of vegetable and one of citrus fruit, an egg and one large serving of meat. Foods which the mother knows from experience disagree with her should be avoided; but the old belief that certain foods eaten by the mother will cause colic in her infant is now discredited. However, as previously stated in Chapter 13, certain drugs may be excreted in the mother's milk in sufficient quantity to affect the breast-fed infant.

Mothers in general, and particularly mothers who are breast-feeding, usually have good appetites and become hungry between meals. For this reason it is advisable to see that they receive intermediate nourishment consisting of a nourishing beverage or a snack 3 times a day. If the nourishment is in the form of a glass of milk or some milk product, this helps to incorporate the additional milk requirement for the nursing mother.

Rest and Sleep

During the puerperium the mother needs an abundance of rest and should be encouraged to relax and sleep whenever possible. This can best be accomplished if she is comfortable and free from worry and other anxiety-producing situations. The need for rest has even more significance for the mother who is breast-feeding, because worry and fatigue inhibit her milk supply. With the exception of the husband, visitors should be limited during the first week or so because they can be tiring. A mother who is not getting sufficient rest is usually anxious and worries over minor things that otherwise might cause her little concern. Furthermore, many emotional problems often are precipitated by sleeplessness and fatigue.

It becomes the nurse's responsibility to adjust the hospital routine whenever possible to provide the mother with uninterrupted periods of rest. Routine procedures can be delayed or rearranged to meet the mother's needs. A bottle-fed infant may be fed occasionally by the nurse if the mother is sleeping and does not want to be awakened. If the mother is unable to nap during the day (and she may not, due to excitement and fatigue), she can be encouraged to rest as quietly as possible for certain continuous periods. The need for rest and sleep may have to be explained and reiterated to her, especially during the "taking-hold" phase, as she is eager to be up and about and may tend to overdo.

Early Ambulation

Although early ambulation of the so-called "normal" mother had its inception out of necessity during World War II, experience with this aspect of management of the puerperium has shown that it possesses certain intrinsic advantages to the mother, and as a result it is almost generally accepted as routine practice today. The mothers seem to get their strength back more quickly and appear to be stronger on the 5th or 6th day than they used to be at the time of discharge under the old regimen. This is proved by multiparas who were kept on best rest for 7 to 14 days following previous deliveries, who state that they feel better and stronger with early ambulation. With this increase in exercise for the newly delivered mother, her circulation is stimulated, and there are fewer complications of thrombophlebitis. Moreover, bladder and bowel functions are improved, with the result that bladder complications leading to catheterization are greatly reduced. Abdominal distention and constipation occur less frequently. The majority of healthy mothers are allowed out of bed in 8 to 24 hours.

If the patient has had a conduction anesthesia which involves entering the dura, she may be kept in a recumbent position for about the first 8 hours. It is felt by many physicians that keeping the patient flat in bed for this time helps to prevent the occurrence of a postspinal headache, since headache is precipitated and aggravated when the head is elevated. Postspinal headache is thought to be due to a leakage of the spinal fluid through the puncture hole of the dura, with subsequent decrease in cerebrospinal fluid volume and pressure. Therefore, the use of a small gauge needle for making the puncture, a recumbent position while the puncture hole is sealing, and encouraging the patient to force fluids (to hasten fluid replacement) are all measures which may be helpful in the prevention of this condition.

The first time that the mother is out of bed she should "dangle" for a short time before actually getting up. Then usually she can walk a few steps from the bed and sit in a chair for a brief period. On succeeding times up, she can increase her activity gradually. The newly delivered mother needs someone to assist her in and out of bed and to go with her when she walks to the bathroom. The nurse should remain close at hand while the mother is in the bathroom so that she can give immediate assistance if the mother becomes weak or faint.

It is important that the nurse explain the purposes of early ambulation to the mother and help her to learn how she can achieve an effective combination of sitting, walking and lying in bed. All too many mothers feel that once they are out of bed they are "on their own" and expected to take care of themselves entirely. Most of them are afraid of being a nuisance and hesitate to ask for help, whereas others do not realize that help is available. The nurse's attitude is important, for if she acts friendly and interested in the mother, demonstrates a desire to help her and makes her feel comfortable, the mother is more likely to ask for help. New mothers, in particular, are sensitive to the attitudes of those responsible for their care. Many of them are experiencing an enforced dependency for the first time in their adult lives and find this difficult. Others become resentful because they feel that they are being forced toward independence too quickly. It is only as the nurse recognizes each patient as an individual that she is able to gain insight in providing for the mother's total nursing needs.

Although it is customary for mothers to be discharged home on the 5th to the 7th day, and in some instances as early as the 3rd or the 4th, it should be remembered that early ambulation and the duration of hospital stay are two entirely different matters. Regardless of the day of discharge, mothers should be cautioned to proceed slowly at home during the puerperium, resting a large part of the time. If teaching about "getting back to routine gradually" was begun early in the antepartal period, the mother will be better prepared.

Bathing

As previous mentioned, the mother is prone to have marked diaphoresis in the early puerperium, so that she will find the daily bath or shower refreshing and a source of comfort. The first complete bed bath after delivery should be given by the nurse, even if the mother has already been allowed out of bed for a brief period. This not only conserves a considerable amount of the mother's energy but permits the nurse on the postpartal division, who may be caring for the mother for the first time, to have an opportunity to make certain observations. If the mother is not fatigued, this is an opportune time also to include a considerable amount of health teaching. The nurse will be guided in her teaching by the "readiness" of the mother to learn and should remember that she can absorb only so much information at one time. In addition to answering specific questions asked by the mother, the nurse might include information about breast care, perineal hygiene, elimination, general activity and hospital routines.

After the first bath the mother usually is able to shower or, if she is on bed rest, to bathe herself at least partially. Nevertheless, help should be given as necessary. Showers usually are permitted as soon as the patient becomes ambulatory, if such facilities are available. The first time or two that the mother takes a shower, the nurse or the attendant should remain nearby for safety. It is particularly important that a patient who has had a cesearean section be instructed regarding her bathing. Usually, these patients are not allowed to shower even though they are ambulatory, since the incision should be kept dry until it has closed, and/or the sutures have been removed. These patients see other patients enjoying their showers and often assume that this type of bathing would be suitable for them.

Tub baths usually are allowed in 2 weeks, and some physicians permit tub bathing earlier (see Suggested Reading).

Urinary Elimination

The newly delivered mother does not usually express a desire to void, in part because the bladder capacity is now increased as a result of reduced interabdominal pressure. In addition, if the mother has received analgesia or anesthesia during labor, the sensation of a full bladder may be further diminished. The mother should be encouraged to void within the first 6 to 8 hours following the delivery. It is not prudent, however, to adhere to a designated lapse of time to indicate when the mother should empty her bladder, but rather on evidence indicating the degree of bladder distention. It should be kept in mind that there is an increased urinary output during the early puerperium. Moreover, mothers who have received intravenous fluids, or who are having them, are very likely to develop a full bladder. As the bladder fills with urine, it gradually protrudes above the symphysis pubis and can be observed bulging in front of the uterus. If the bladder is markedly distended, the uterus may be pushed upward and to the side and may be somewhat relaxed. When a hand is cupped over the fundus to massage it and to bring the uterus back to its midline position, the bladder will protrude still further. When the hand is removed, the uterus will return to its displaced position. Further evidence of bladder distention can be gained by palpation and percussion of the lower abdomen, which will reveal a difference in consistency between the uterus and the bladder. The latter will be ballotable and filled with liquid in contrast with the uterus, which will have a firm tone. Such observations are of extreme importance and demand immediate attention, first, because a full bladder is considered to be one of the causes of postpartal hemorrhage, and, second, because if the bladder is permitted to become distended, urinary retention will follow inevitably.

Some mothers have difficulty in voiding at first. As a result of the labor itself, the tone of the bladder wall may be temporarily impaired, or the tissues at the base of the bladder and around the urethra may be edematous. Often the patient's inability to void is due to the fact that she is not accustomed to using the bedpan and would have this same difficulty using one any time. If the mother is allowed early bathroom privileges, urinary elimination may present no problem. On the other hand, some efforts may be needed to excite normal urination. First of all, a positive approach, asking the mother, "Will you try . . ." rather than "Do you feel as if you want to . . ." is often helpful to get the mother to void. Also, making her feel at ease by helping her to assume a comfortable position, providing privacy and giving her assurance will help to avoid build-

ing up tensions which might further inhibit
normal urination.

The nurse should offer the mother a bedpan
at intervals of 2 to 3 hours at first and measure
the urine at each voiding during the first few
days until it has been established that the
mother is emptying her bladder completely. A
voiding must measure 100 cc. to be considered
satisfactory. At the first attempt the mother
may void a small amount of urine and obviously not empty her bladder. If the bladder
is not distended, she may be allowed to wait
an hour or so before trying again to empty it,
because then she may do so. But if she continues to void in small amounts at frequent
intervals, one may suspect that she has a residual urine, and thus these voidings are
merely the overflow of a distended bladder.
Every effort should be made to encourage the
mother to void in sufficient amount so that
catheterization will not have to be resorted to,
but any time she is unable to do so, and there
is evidence of bladder distention, she should
be catheterized immediately.

Catheterization. Although the procedure for
catheterization varies to some degree in different hospitals, the principles involved are
essentially the same. Aseptic technic must be
maintained throughout to avoid introducing
bacteria into the bladder or contaminating the
birth canal. If the mother is given routine
perineal care prior to beginning the catheterization procedure, the potential danger of
infection is further reduced.

Because there is a certain amount of soreness of the external genitalia, the nurse should
proceed with extreme gentleness and convey
to the mother the impression that she is aware
of the additional tenderness. As the labia are
separated to expose the vestibule, care should
be exercised to prevent pulling on the perineal
sutures. The nurse will find that the meatus
may be difficult to locate due to the edema and
consequent distortion of the tissues; therefore
a good light is imperative.

The urinary meatus and surrounding area
are cleansed prior to the insertion of the catheter; the nurse should proceed gently, but remember all the while that a certain degree of
friction is necessary for proper cleansing of the
area. None of the cleansing solution should be
permitted to run into the vaginal orifice because of the danger of contaminating the birth

canal. Immediately following the cleansing,
a dry cotton ball should be placed at the introitus to prevent excretions from the vagina,
i.e., blood or lochia, from spreading upward to
the urinary meatus, from whence it can be carried into the bladder when the catheter is
inserted.

Intestinal Elimination

Because the bowel tends to remain relaxed
in the early puerperium (as in pregnancy),
intestinal elimination may be somewhat of a
problem. In view of the sluggishness of the
bowels during this time, constipation can be
anticipated unless certain measures are instituted to prevent it. Although obstetricians'
orders vary, it is common to give a stool
softener each night after delivery and/or a
laxative or mild cathartic on the evening of the
2nd day following delivery. If a bowel evacuation has not occurred by the morning of the
3rd day, a cleansing enema or a suppository
may be prescribed. The latter is very effective
and less traumatic for most patients.

If there has been no elimination for several
days, and especially if the mother has had
more extensive perineal repair done, an oil
retention enema, followed some hours later by
a cleansing enema, sometimes is ordered.

Certain laxatives are excreted in breast
milk and therefore affect the infant. The
mother who is breast-feeding should be advised to follow her physician's prescription if
laxatives should need to be used to encourage
proper elimination after the mother is discharged from the hospital. In addition, the
usual measures employed to encourage good
bowel habits, i.e., adequate fluid intake, roughage foods in the diet, establishing a habit time,
etc., should be included in the health teaching.

SPECIAL PHYSICAL CARE ASPECTS

Throughout the care of the obstetric patient, emphasis has been directed to the prevention of infection by application of principles of antiseptic and aseptic technics. In view
of this, the special procedures employed in the
care of the mother during the puerperium
should be planned so that individual care technic can be maintained whenever possible. Each

mother should have her own equipment for breast care, perineal care, etc., and her equipment should be kept in a designated place separate from her neighbor's. This is facilitated in hospitals where the physical plan of the postpartal unit provides a bathroom adjoining each room, in which separate shelves are provided for each mother's equipment and supplies. Such practices are important in the over-all effort to prevent cross contamination.

Breast Care

The care of the breasts during pregnancy has been discussed in Chapter 8, Antepartal Care. Although some aspects differ after the delivery, depending on whether or not the mother is breast-feeding, the principles of good breast hygiene continue to be of primary importance.

The routine care is directed to maintain cleanliness and adequate breast support necessary for the normal function of the breasts and the comfort of the mother. Precautions should always be exercised to handle the breasts gently, and above all to avoid rough rubbing, massage or pressure on these organs.

The mother who is bottle-feeding her infant should bathe her breasts daily with mild soap and water; this is done most conveniently at the time of the daily shower or bath. No other special care need be given. Recent research[3] has indicated that the mother who is breast-feeding should avoid the use of soap on her nipples, since this substance removes the protective skin oils and leaves the nipple more prone to damage. It is recommended that she wash her breasts daily with plain water at the bath or shower time. No further cleansing before each nursing need be done (see Chap. 15). However, the hands should be washed in soap and water if they are to come in contact with the breast. The nurse has an excellent opportunity for health teaching about postpartal care of the breasts while she is giving the mother her first bath after the delivery.

Some kind of breast support should be worn 24 hours a day after delivery. Various types of binders or brassières may be used as long as they support the entire breast in the natural position. When a breast is well supported, it is not only more comfortable, but also, if it is pendulous, proper support aids in preventing congestion caused by interference with circulation (Fig. 14-8). Following the delivery, the breasts are soft, but by the 3rd or the 4th postpartal day, as milk replaces colostrum in the breasts, they become heavier, firmer and more tender. The mother may experience throbbing

[3] Newton, Michael, and Newton, Niles: The normal course and management of lactation, Clin. Obstet. Gynec. 5:44-63, March, 1962.

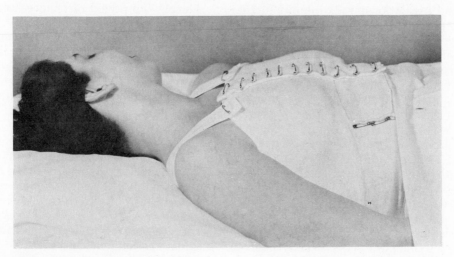

Fig. 14-8. Breast binder made from straight binder, 10 inches wide. Shoulder straps are attached. (MacDonald House, University Hospitals of Cleveland)

pains in her breasts, which extend back into the axillae. During this time, analgesic medication may be required for pain relief until the congestion subsides in 1 or 2 days. Even the mother who is breast-feeding experiences temporary discomfort when the breasts become full.

The mother who is breast-feeding should wear a binder or brassière not only for support of the breasts but also to ensure further cleanliness. Since the milk secretion is likely to leak from the nipples, they should be directly covered with breast squares, such as sterile 4 x 4 gauze dressings. During the mother's hospital stay she may wear a binder which is convenient for breast feeding (such as the bikini), unless her breasts are pendulous. Heavy breasts require the additional support afforded by the more conventional type breast binder (Fig. 14-8). Many mothers prefer to wear a nursing brassière even before the milk comes in. But regardless of which one is used, it should provide uplift support and be well fitted so that it is not too tight and avoids undue pressure on the nipples.

Drying Up the Breasts. The breasts fill with milk initially, unless lactation is suppressed, whether or not the mother nurses her infant. The anterior pituitary gland manufactures and releases the lactogenic hormone after delivery; this hormone stimulates the secretion of milk in the breasts. Tenseness and engorgement result as the milk fills the breasts (see Chap. 15). Since the accumulation of milk inhibits further secretion, engorgement generally subsides in 1 or 2 days; however, until the breasts soften, the mother may experience considerable discomfort. In the event that the mother is not going to breast-feed, the physician will prescribe orders accordingly. The breasts may be dried up either by inhibiting the production of the lactogenic hormone or by not removing the milk from the breasts after it has been secreted.

Many physicians use estrogenic or androgenic hormones, either alone or in combination, to suppress the production of the lactogenic hormone. Diethylstilbestrol, an estrogenic hormone, is one of the more common drugs in use today for this purpose. It usually is given orally in relatively large doses during the early postpartal period and is decreased gradually.

It is felt that when estrogens and androgens are used in combination, they not only suppress the production of the lactogenic hormone but also counteract the undesirable side-effects of each other. Deladumone is an example of such a compound. It is a long-acting drug and is given intramuscularly; one injection is all that is necessary. To achieve maximum effectiveness, the antilactogenic hormones must be given as soon as possible after delivery, since the anterior pituitary begins production of the lactogenic hormone immediately. Lactation is not always effectively suppressed by the administration of hormones, and there may be a mild transient filling or engorgement either a few days after delivery or later, in 1 or 2 weeks. This soon disappears spontaneously. It is important for the nurse to remember that side-effects sometimes accompany the administration of hormones. For instance, the androgens have the potential for retarding the onset of menstruation. Uterine bleeding may follow a prolonged course of estrogen therapy. The nurse will observe that after a course of stilbestrol the lochial discharge is heavier and contains a greater proportion of bright red blood.

If hormones are not used, the breasts usually become engorged 2 to 3 days after delivery, and the tenseness and discomfort last from 24 to 48 hours. Since the breasts are not emptied, the accumulated milk suppresses further secretion of milk. As secretion subsides, engorgement wanes, and the breasts become more comfortable.

During the period of engorgement, discomfort may be considerable, and the mother should receive as much symptomatic relief as possible. A well-fitting uplift brassière or a correctly applied breast binder relieve discomfort from the weight of the breasts. If the latter is ordered, wearing it before the milk "comes in" is helpful. The breast binder should fit snugly but not to the extent that in itself it causes discomfort. The mother can assist by supporting her breasts in the normal position while the binder is being applied. To encourage uplift support, the binder should be pinned from the bottom up. A good principle to remember in providing support for the breasts is that a variety of methods may be adequate as long as they lift the breasts, suspend the weight from the shoulders and do not exert pressure on any area.

The application of ice caps to the breasts also may contribute to the mother's comfort when the breasts are full and tender. Analgesics such as aspirin or a similar compound are helpful in relieving discomfort. The nurse must remember that the milk should not be pumped or expressed from the breasts, since this only stimulates the secretion of more milk. In the past it was thought that the application of very tight binders, restriction of fluids and the administration of diuretics all suppressed lactation; these practices are no longer in general use and have been found to be of little value (see Suggested Reading).

Care of the Perineum

Perineal care is a procedure employed to cleanse the vulva, the perineum and the anal region as a means of preventing infection, promoting healing of the perineum and making the mother comfortable. In addition, it provides an opportunity for the nurse to inspect the area and the lochial discharge. Regardless of whether or not an episiotomy has been performed, perineal care should be done as a routine part of morning care, each time that the mother voids, and after each bowel evacuation. The nurse usually attends to this aspect of care until the mother becomes ambulatory; then, after proper instruction, the mother herself may assume this care. However, it should be emphasized that even though the nurse may not be performing the acutal procedure, she should make a point of inspecting the mother's perineum daily, preferably in the morning, to ascertain whether the stitches are healing properly and to check the character and the amount of lochia. If the mother is allowed to shower, these observations should be made first so that the nurse can observe the lochial discharge more accurately.

There has been much discussion concerning the "best way" for the nurse to give perineal care in the time immediately following delivery. The technic for individual care has simplified the procedure to a large measure, but procedures will vary according to hospital routines. Some hospitals still maintain aseptic technic throughout this procedure, but the majority advocate that this is a "clean" procedure rather than a sterile one, and that the safety of the mother is ensured if antiseptic precautions are adhered to conscientiously.

Disposable washcloths, cotton balls or gauze sponges may be used for cleansing. Although many hospitals continue to use cotton balls for this purpose because they are soft, absorbent and economical, the other materials are preferable. When the pubic hair begins to appear, cotton balls tend to catch on the stubble, and particles of cotton remain unless they are picked off. Another variation found is in relation to the cleansing agent, which might be a mild soap or detergent solution.

In preparation for the procedure, the nurse should wash her hands thoroughly. After preparing the mother, remove the perineal pad, noting the amount, the odor and the appearance of the lochia and discard the pad in a paper bag. Whether removing the perineal pad or in using the sponges or washcloths in the actual cleansing process, always proceed from the front toward the back to avoid contamination of the vestibule from the anal region.

The labia is cleansed first, working from the pubis to the perineum, taking care not to separate the labia with the fingers. The cleansing is done by using a single downward stroke with each sponge, which then is discarded in the paper bag. This cleansing is repeated with as many sponges as necessary. The area then is dried in the same manner.

The cleansing of the anal region can be accomplished most effectively if the mother is turned on her side and the buttocks separated before wiping from the perineum to the anus. If the mother's thighs or buttocks are soiled with profuse lochia, these areas should be bathed with soap and water, for these parts do not have to be cleansed in the same manner as the vulva.

When disposable washcloths are used, the first cloth is soaped and the labia washed down on one side to the perineum and then on the other side. Then the anus is washed last, and the soaped washcloth is discarded. The area is rinsed in the same manner with a second washcloth and dried with a third one. The perineum should be kept clean and dry to promote healing.

The nurse must be mindful of the potential danger of infection if pathogenic organisms ascend the birth canal to the uterus. Care should always be exercised to see that none of the cleansing solution seeps into the vagina because of the possibility of contamination. If the washcloths or moist sponges are used, they should not be dripping wet.

The clean perineal pad should be grasped on

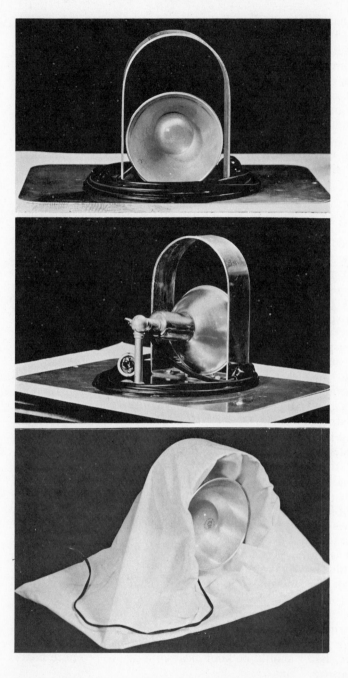

Fig. 14-9. Three views of a lamp designed for "light treatment" of the perineum. This lamp is simple in design and inexpensive. It is equipped with a bracket which acts as a "cradle" over which the bedclothes may be supported. When in use, the frame is completely covered with a pillowcase. The heat provided by such a lamp gives great comfort to patients when perineal stitches are painful. (University Hospitals of Cleveland)

the outside so that the nurse's fingers do not touch the side which will come in contact with the mother's perineum. Then the pad is applied to the vulva (front to back) and secured to the sanitary belt in front before turning the mother to her side to secure the back tab.

Perineal Self-Care. The first time the mother is allowed up to the bathroom, the nurse should take her and show her where her equipment is kept and how to do perineal self-care. The principles of personal hygiene which were stressed when the nurse gave the mother perineal care in bed should be reviewed again. Instruct the mother to wash her hands carefully before and after carying out the procedure. Show her how to assemble the necessary equipment, the paper bag, box of small cleansing tissues and wrapped perineal pad, all of which can be placed on a small stool or table adjacent to the toilet. A box of small cleansing tissues is preferable to a roll of tissue for obvious reasons. Have the mother unfasten the perineal pad she is wearing, and instruct her to grasp it by the tabs and remove it from front to back. This perineal pad is placed in the paper bag, which will be disposed of in a step-on can or other covered waste receptacle. After the mother voids, instruct her to cleanse herself from front to back with tissues, using fresh tissues for each stroke and discarding them in the toilet. The mother should again be instructed how to handle the clean perineal pad so that the inner surface is not contaminated by her fingers and to put it on from front to back. It should be fastened immediately to prevent the pad from moving forward. The toilet should be flushed after the mother assumes a standing position to avoid having any of the flushing water spray the perineum.

Perineal Discomfort. Following a spontaneous vaginal delivery without laceration, mothers usually do not experience perineal discomfort. It is most likely to be present if an episiotomy has been performed, or if lacerations have been repaired, particularly if the perineum is edematous, and there is tension on the perineal sutures. Almost all primigravidas experience some degree of discomfort from an episiotomy, depending largely on the extent of the wound and the amount of suturing done. For the most part during the first few days, local treatment in the form of dry heat, analgesic sprays or ointments is all that is necessary to alleviate the discomfort. But if the pain is more severe in the first day or so, such treatment may not be sufficient, and analgesic medications may have to be administered by mouth or hypodermic injection. Later on, sitz baths may be ordered if the discomfort persists.

Exposure of the perineum to heat from the perineal lamp not only provides a considerable measure of comfort to the mother but also supplies a safe amount of heat to promote local healing of the perineal wound. The physician may prescribe such treatment for 20- to 25-minute periods, 2 or 3 times a day. If a lamp such as the one shown in Figure 14-9 is used,

the mother can recline in bed with the lamp between her knees during the treatment, without spreading the thighs too far apart. This lamp is so constructed that the frame can be completely covered with a pillowcase. The excess cover is brought forward over the arch of the frame and tucked securely between it and the shield which is around the bulb. The heat is provided by an ordinary 25-watt light bulb. When the mother has assumed the dorsal recumbent position, the lamp can be easily slipped between her legs and placed about 10 to 12 inches from the perineum. After the perineum is exposed, the bulb should be adjusted so that the light shines directly on it. The mother can be completely covered during the treatment, because the arch of the lamp frame acts as a cradle to support the top bedclothes.

Mothers who have discomfort from perineal sutures usually will find it uncomfortable to sit for the first few days. Many of them will be observed sitting in a rigid position, bearing their weight on one side of the buttocks or the other, with obvious discomfort to the back as well as the perineum. Therefore, it is important to teach the mother how to sit comfortably with her body erect. In the sitting position, the perineum is suspended at the lowermost level of the ischial tuberosities, which bear the weight of the body. Thus, in order to achieve a greater measure of comfort, the mother must bring her buttocks together to relieve pressure and tension on the perineum, in the same manner as that described in the exercise for contraction and relaxation of pelvic floor muscles (see p. 179). After assuming a sitting position the mother should be instructed to raise her hips very slightly from the chair, only enough to permit her to squeeze her buttocks together and contract the muscles of the pelvic floor, and hold them this way momentarily until after she has let her full weight down again. This exercise will also prove to be helpful to the mother when she is reclining in bed.

Abdominal Support

At the present time there is general agreement that an abdominal binder is unnecessary. It was formerly routine practice to apply one to the newly delivered mother because it was thought that it aided involution and helped to restore the mother's figure. Actually, a binder is of no value for such purposes, and because it inhibits the movements of the abdominal wall, it may actually retard the soft, flabby structures in regaining tone. However, the physician may advise the use of a binder if the mother's abdomen is unusually flabby or pendulous, particularly if the mother believes that she would feel more comfortable with some support. If the mother is ambulatory, the straight abdominal binder may be preferable to the scultetus binder because it is more likely to stay in place when the mother moves about. It must be remembered that the binder is applied from the waist down to avoid pushing the uterus upward.

THE MOTHER WHO IS NURSING

Making the Decision

The type of infant feeding is an important decision for the parents to make. Their ultimate choice will be influenced by a variety of factors, physical and psychological as well as social. Ideally, the subject of the method of infant feeding will be raised during the antepartal period, and the parents will have time and guidance from the doctor and the nurse in making a decision that is most suitable for them.

It is no longer essential that the mother breast-feed her infant to ensure his survival or well-being. The development of modern methods of artificial feeding adequately meet the infant's needs for nutrition and growth (see p. 386). However, breast-feeding has several advantages (see p. 386). Particularly important is the fact that if the mother wants to nurse her infant, this method of feeding can enhance a close relationship between her and her baby.

A variety of factors will influence the couple's decision to breast-feed the infant. The term *couple* is used here deliberately, since the husband's attitudes, feelings and behavior may be as important in terms of decision-making as the mother's. Moreover, they usually have a profound influence on the outcome of the nursing experience. It is wise for the physician and the nurse to explore adequately with the mother (and the father, if necessary) their mutual attitudes, since they are so relevant.

The nurse will note that there seems to be a wide range of commitment to breast-feeding. For instance, some mothers are very eager to nurse their infants; others want to breast-feed but do not feel bad (or "inadequate") if for some reason they cannot. Others try to nurse in spite of the fact that they would prefer to give the baby a bottle; still others flatly refuse to attempt to nurse. Some mothers feel that breast-feeding is too tiring, confining or simply repulsive; many are afraid that it will disfigure their breasts. The mores and pressure of the mother's class and peer group also are important. Bottle-feeding may be the acceptable practice in the community or neighborhood; relatives, friends, etc., may be either very much for or against breast-feeding. Return to employment for the mother may be a very significant factor.

Certain conditions in both the mother and the infant also can have a bearing on the decision and outcome. The mother's physical condition is particularly important. Diseases and infection (i.e., syphilis, tuberculosis, heart and kidney disease, staphylococcal infections, communicable diseases) generally are contraindications for breast-feeding. Similarly, certain infections and anomalies in the infant may make nursing impossible, or at least temporarily impossible (see Chap. 21). Breast infection or painful, cracked or fissured nipples also may require temporary discontinuance of nursing. Pregnancy usually is considered to be an indication for weaning because of the physiologic strain that it places on the mother.

The attitudes of the doctor and nurse influence the couple a good deal, as well as the amount and the kind of help that the mother gets in the hospital when she is first attempting to nurse. The willingness on the part of the staff to impart information and to give assistance helps the parents immensely, especially if they have little information about the process or are actually misinformed about it. However, it is unwise to try to persuade a mother to nurse if she has very negative feelings about breast-feeding. This situation often leads to emotional conflicts in the mother and may impede the adjustment between mother and infant.

Mechanisms in Lactation

The anatomy of the breasts and the physiology of lactation have been discussed in

Chapters 2 and 13, to which the student is referred for a renewal of background understanding of the subject.

Secretion of Milk. Two major mechanisms are involved in lactation. The first of these is the secretion of milk. It is believed, as was previously stated, that the hormone luteotrophin (prolactin, LTH, the lactogenic or mammogenic hormone) is responsible for the initiation of lactation. It is thought that the release of this hormone is enhanced by the sucking of the infant. The milk itself is secreted by the alveoli or acini cells. This secretion commences 3 to 4 days postpartum and continues for as long as the breasts are sufficiently emptied. Frequency of emptying the breasts also is a very important factor, especially when lactation is becoming established. Thus, both the production of milk and the quantity produced are dependent on *frequent* and *complete* emptying of the breasts. The nurse will recall that if the breasts are not entirely emptied, and the back pressure in the alveoli is not relieved, milk secretion decreases and eventually stops (see p. 318).

When lactation is becoming established, milk secretion can be stimulated by having the infant nurse both breasts at each feeding and by increasing the frequency of the feedings. Care should be taken not to tire the mother unduly. Milk production is slow in some mothers, but it can be stimulated by allowing the infant to nurse both breasts every 3 to 4 hours.

Milk-Ejection Reflex. This is the second mechanism involved in lactation. This reflex has been called also expulsion mechanism, the let-down reflex and the draught reflex. It is postulated that the mechanism works in the following way: Impulses from the baby's sucking cause release of oxytocin from the posterior portion of the pituitary. This hormone causes the contractile tissue (myoepithelial cells) around the alveoli to squeeze the milk into the larger ducts and eventually to propel it to the ducts leading to the nipples. The milk then is removed by the compression and suction action of the baby's nursing. It is important to remember that the let-down reflex can be influenced profoundly by psychic factors and the emotions of the mother. For instance, some mothers find that the let-down reflex is elicited (i.e., their breasts begin to drip milk) by an infant's cry or some other sound, sight,

etc., that has become associated with nursing. Often they will say that they can feel their milk "come down" in anticipation of nursing. Fear, worry, pain and tension, all may affect the expulsion mechanism adversely. Thus, it is particularly important for the nurse to help the mother to avoid these emotional disturbances whenever possible. A relaxed atmosphere for nursing, adequate assistance, effective pain relief, and a supportive attitude on the part of the nurse are essential components of effective nursing care for the mother who is breastfeeding. Sometimes oxytocin is given the mother during early lactation to facilitate the milk flow. It may be administered by injection or by a nasal spray (40 U.S.P. units per ml. of solution). This hormone assists the ejection of milk when the let-down reflex is inhibited (as in times of stress) and also is effective in facilitating the milk flow when the breasts are engorged.

Engorgement

When the milk "comes in," the breasts suddenly become larger, firmer and more tender; consequently, many mothers experience varying degrees of discomfort. Some do not seem to be bothered by this transitory condition (and produce a large quantity of milk), but the majority usually have at least a moderate amount of tenderness and pain. A few experience a great deal of discomfort, with throbbing pains in the breast, extending to the axilla. The peak incidence of discomfort seems to occur on the 4th or the 5th day postpartum. It is believed that the engorgement is caused by the pressure from the increased amount of milk in the lobes and ducts as well as from the increased blood and lymph circulation in the breasts.

Symptoms. The engorgement may distend the breasts so much that the skin appears to be shiny. The tissue surrounding the nipple may become taut also to the extent that it actually retracts the nipple, making it extremely difficult for the baby to grasp the nipple and the areola adequately. It used to be thought that fever was a normal consequence of this condition; however, engorgement is *not* an inflammatory process, and if fever occurs, some other cause should be suspected. The breasts may be reddened and feel warm to the touch. They can be very painful, and they become more so when touched or moved.

Although this condition is transitory and usually disappears in 24 to 48 hours, prompt treatment should be instituted, not only for the mother's comfort but also to prevent the condition from progressing. If engorgement is allowed to become marked, then emptying of the breasts (which is the basis of treatment) becomes very difficult because of the occlusion of the ducts by the surrounding congested tissues and the thick and tenacious character of the retained secretions. Secondary lymphatic and venous stasis may occur because the milk cannot be emptied.

Treatment usually consists of removal of the milk, support of the breast, hot packs and/or ice bags and analgesics for the relief of pain. Removal of the milk may be facilitated by the use of oxytocin before the baby nurses to encourage the let-down reflex. Interestingly enough, this drug sometimes is used to relieve discomfort from engorgement in mothers who are *not* nursing. The mechanism of the way in which the drug relieves pain in breasts that are not being emptied is unclear. In addition, manual expression of the milk and pumping (see p. 330), as well as the use of a nipple shield (to help the baby to grasp the nipple), may be recommended. Some mothers find the use of hot packs 15 to 20 minutes before nursing beneficial in improving the flow of milk. Often ice packs between nursing periods are very useful in alleviating discomfort. A good uplift support for the breasts cannot be stressed enough (see p. 159), particularly during the period of engorgement, and a well-fitting brassière should be worn night and day. Analgesics such as aspirin, Darvon or codeine frequently are used for pain relief. These should be given in adequate dosage and with appropriate timing so that the mother can be relatively comfortable during nursing. Since engorgement is transitory, the drugs are needed for a very short time; hence any danger to the infant is minimal.

Initiation of Breast-Feeding

Depending on the condition of both the mother and the infant, nursing usually is started from 8 to 24 hours after delivery. Some physicians prefer to give the baby one or two bottle feedings of water before he begins to breast-feed. It is felt that this helps the infant to regurgitate any mucus or secretions that have been swallowed during delivery. If mucus is a problem with the baby, postponement of nursing is thought by some to be beneficial until the baby can rid himself of it. Usually, the baby is clear of mucus in 24 hours. Many infants indicate their readiness to suck from birth. However, others do not seem to be so eager; these infants need a short period of rest before they demonstrate their readiness. Similarly, the mother may be rested enough a few hours after the baby's birth to commence nursing, or she may need several hours or a day in which to restore herself after delivery. Usually, in 24 hours or so both mother and baby (barring complications) are ready for the nursing experience.

Colostrum will be the chief source of the infant's nourishment until the milk comes in. Putting the infant to breast early is advantageous for both mother and baby, since the sucking stimulates the milk production and helps the uterus to contract; moreover, nursing satisfies the infant's need for sucking. It is important for the nurse to remember that *both* mother and baby must learn how to work as a team in the nursing process. Hence, practice is essential. Even though the mother has breast-fed before, there is a wide range in nursing behavior[4] among infants, and the experience of breast-feeding each infant can be somewhat "new." The mother will need to learn how to handle the infant appropriately, how to interpret his cues of hunger and satiety, and how to help him to grasp the nipple and to withdraw the milk successfully. The infant, in turn, must learn to associate the nipple with food and to coordinate his grasping of the nipple with his sucking and swallowing in such a way as to get his food successfully. No wonder that mother and baby often take a few days to become adept at this process!

When the infant is placed at the breast during the early feedings, the nurse should be present to give any necessary assistance. Preparation of the mother before the actual nursing experience plays a large part in giving effective care. The mother should be instructed

[4] Barnes, G. R., Jr., *et al.*: Management of breast feeding, J.A.M.A. 151:192-199, January 17, 1953.

FIG. 14-10. Both the mother and the baby should be comfortable during the nursing period. The mother should hold the breast so that it does not interfere with the baby's breathing. When he cannot breathe freely, he becomes irritated and may refuse to nurse altogether.

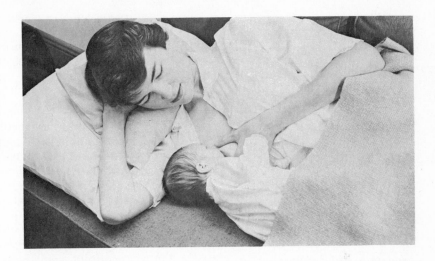

to wash her hands carefully before beginning to nurse. This is a good principle to follow before attempting any infant care. Care of the breasts has been discussed on pages 317 to 318. Whenever it is indicated, the mother should be informed about the feeding reflexes of her infant (see p. 385). During the actual nursing period the nurse can reinforce this information (as necessary) and *show* the mother how to elicit these responses. It is essential that the mother be able to evoke these reflexes herself, since she ultimately must assume total responsibility. All too often the nurse takes over these aspects, and the mother does not get sufficient practice to acquire any skill during these first days in the hospital.

Position. Instructing and assisting the mother to experiment with various positions which are comfortable during nursing is another important facet of care. If the infant is to nurse satisfactorily, he must be held properly by the mother; although some mothers seem to know how to support a baby at the breast, many are awkward, and definite instructions are helpful. Both the mother and the baby must be comfortable and in such a position that the baby can grasp the nipple *and the areola* without any undue effort. If the baby grasps only the nipple, he will not be able to draw out the milk; moreover, the mother's nipples are likely to be damaged. If the mother is lying down (Fig. 14-10), she should be on her side with her arm raised and

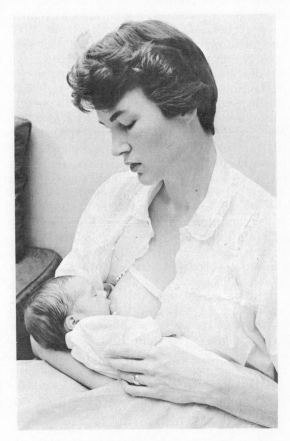

FIG. 14-11. Babies nurse better if the mother is relaxed and both the mother and the baby are comfortable.

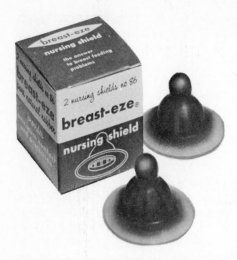

Fig. 14-12. Nursing shield. In the treatment of sore or cracked nipples this soft, natural rubber shield may be used for their protection during the nursing periods. (The Pyramid Rubber Company, Ravenna, Ohio)

her head comfortably supported. The baby should lie on his side, flat on the bed or so supported that he can grasp the breast easily. If the mother prefers to sit up to nurse, she should use a comfortable chair and a stool to support her feet, as necessary. It is often helpful to place a pillow under the arm that is supporting the infant (to reduce the tension on the muscles, Fig. 14-11); or to place a pillow under the baby to raise him to a sufficient height so that he may reach the breast easily. If the stitches of the episiotomy are bothersome, a rubber ring or a pillow under the mother's buttocks may be helpful. The nurse may have to work with the mother a bit to be sure that she is comfortable. Often mothers in their eagerness to get the baby on the breast become very tense and assume quite uncomfortable positions (although they assure the nurse that they are "comfortable"). Patience and gentle reminding on the part of the nurse encourages these mothers to relax more readily.

Orientation of Infant. After the baby is placed beside the mother, he should be allowed a little time to accustom himself to the new environment and to hunt for the nipple himself. He should not be forced to nurse immediately, especially if he is hesitant or shows disinclination. If the rooting reflex is well developed (and as he smells the milk), he will turn toward the nipple or any object that brushes his cheek (see p. 357). Thus, if the mother or the nurse touches his cheek gently with the nipple, he will turn toward it, open his mouth and grasp it. Sucking usually follows closely thereafter. If the infant seems to have some difficulty in finding and grasping the nipple, although he seems to be eager, the mother or nurse can gently cup a hand around the baby's head and guide him to the nipple. Care should be taken, however, not to touch his cheek or to force his head, since he will only turn away and resist the pressure on his head. In addition, he may cry, and a crying baby tends not to grasp a nipple successfully even though he may be hungry.

Sucking Behavior of Infant. Babies will exhibit a wide variety of sucking behavior. Some, after finding the nipple, suck vigorously without stopping until they are satisfied. Others may suck vigorously for a time, appear to sleep or to rest and then resume sucking. Still others mouth the nipple before actually sucking but eventually nurse well. Others seem rather disinterested in the whole thing and dawdle throughout the nursing period. When the milk comes in, however, a change usually is noted, and even these infants begin to nurse more in earnest.

The important point here is that individual differences do exist in infants, apparently from birth; hence care must be taken to allow for these differences. To try to force the infant into a style or speed that is not his will only result in screaming and resistance and refusal; the nursing period should be adapted to the infant and not the infant to the nursing period. Mothers, especially, are appreciative of learning about this; often they think there is "*a* way to nurse" and do not realize the differences in eating behavior that infants have. Giving mothers anticipatory guidance and instruction in this aspect of nursing a baby is a very important component in nursing care.

If the infant is to suck effectively, he must place the nipple well back in his mouth, close his lips tightly around the areola, and squeeze the nipple against his palate with his tongue. He then can compress the lactiferous sinuses behind the areola and draw the milk into his mouth by sucking. He empties the breast through a combination of compression and suction. As he nurses, he moves his jaws up and down to compress and empty the sinuses; his tongue, as it draws the nipple back against the palate, suctions the milk from the nipple. Swallowing occurs when enough milk has been obtained to induce the reflex. This activity is carried on rhythmically, interspaced with periods of rest, until the infant is satisfied.

When the nurse assists the mother, she should be sure that the baby has the nipple on top of his tongue and that enough of the areola is in his mouth to prevent damage to the nipple. If he has a good grasp, his jaws will move up and down regularly, and sucking and swallowing movements can be seen in his cheeks and throat. If his grasp is poor, sucking and swallowing may be infrequent and/or absent, although his jaws may continue to move. If the nurse notes that the breast tissue seems to press against the infant's nose and thus obstructs his breathing, she can instruct the mother to take her forefinger and gently compress the tissue so that it no longer impinges on the infant's nose. Care should be taken not to pull the nipple away from the infant in this maneuver.

Usually, getting the nipple in his mouth and tasting the milk seem to increase the baby's interest and ability to nurse. If the infant does not seem too interested or adept, moistening the nipple by expressing a few drops of colostrum or milk often encourages sucking.

Occasionally, a breast shield (Fig. 14-12) may be used to start the infant nursing if for some reason he cannot grasp the nipple. Continued use of this appliance is unwise, since the breasts cannot be emptied because the lacteal sinuses are not compressed during the nursing. The shield can be useful during the first few minutes of nursing to draw the nipples out if they are flattened by engorgment or inversion. Usually, however, even inverted nipples become prominent if the alveolar area is compressed gently by the fingers before nursing; they generally evert more when the infant sucks. The shield may be used also for a short period if the mother's nipples become sore; some nipple pain is experienced by most women during the first days of nursing, but generally it subsides as milk secretion begins, and the baby becomes satisfied. Mothers often state that the pain disappears when the let-down reflex occurs. The care of sore nipples is discussed on page 328.

Length of Nursing Time. Nursing in the initial feedings usually is limited to between 1 and 5 minutes, so that the nipples will not become irritated. Many authorities do not feel that this amount of time is sufficient (see Suggested Reading) and recommend longer nursing periods (5 to 10 minutes for the initial feedings) to provide sufficient stimulation for milk secretions, time for the let-down reflex to operate and adequate time for the breasts to empty. It is important that the nurse be aware of the physician's wishes in these matters and convey them to the mother with an adequate explanation of the underlying rationale. The length of the first nursing periods can become confusing to the mother if she observes other mothers doing differently, and she has not been given adequate instruction. How the mother tolerates the first nursings is important also; if she does not appear to have much discomfort, and the baby wants to nurse longer, then she may be able to increase her nursing time more quickly. Conversely, if she is experiencing a good deal of pain, then she may not be able to increase her nursing time as fast as her neighbor. This information should be given to the doctor. Usually, nursing time is increased a few minutes each feeding or day until the baby is nursing 15 to 20 minutes at one period.

Opinions differ as to whether the infant should nurse at one breast, or both breasts, each feeding period during the first days. Nursing at one breast, alternating breasts for each feeding, is advantageous until the mother's nipples become accustomed to nursing; thereafter, the infant may be offered both breasts at each feeding. Some authorities feel that nursing both breasts may be done at first to stimulate milk secretion; later, the alternate breast may be used for each feeding. Some mothers continue to use both breasts each feeding even when lactation is well established.

Bubbling. The mother should be instructed in the technic of bubbling her infant (see Chap. 15). This may be done when she changes breasts, or midway and at the end of the feeding period. If the infant has had difficulty in beginning to nurse, it is usually better to bubble him at the end of the feeding. Breast-fed babies tend not to swallow as much air as bottle-fed infants; hence the need for bubbling usually does not present much of a problem.

Giving Support and Supervision. If the infant has taken the nipple without difficulty and has been sucking well for several minutes, the nurse can feel fairly assured that no further assistance is necessary *at this time*. If she leaves the mother and infant, however, she should place the bell cord within reach and instruct the mother to ring if she feels that she needs further help. Moreover, she should make a point of looking in occasionally to observe the progress of the two. Letting the mother have reasonable periods of managing the nursing process by herself will instill confidence in her, but she never should be left without adequate instruction and reassurance. Often, the presence of the nurse is all that is necessary to give the mother the necessary encouragement.

Both the mother and the nurse must realize that many infants do not nurse too well during the first week of life. Unfortunately, the shortened hospital stay only diminishes the time that professional assistance can be given. Therefore, a referral to a public health agency may be indicated, and this possibility should be explored with the mother before she leaves the hospital. If the infant does not seem to respond satisfactorily to the nursing situation during the time that he is in the hospital, he should not be forced. As previously stated, a crying, upset baby will not take a nipple well; rather, he should be cuddled and soothed until he becomes quiet. If the baby still refuses or cannot nurse after about 10 or 15 minutes of effort on the part of the nurse and mother, it is better to stop and to try again when the baby seems to be more ready. If the infant does not appear to be hungry, it is permissable to omit a feeding. If he is evidencing hunger, some physicians advise giving a bottle but still offering the breast at the next feeding. Often, after a few days and with bottle feedings, an infant who has been disinterested and resistant to the breast suddenly takes hold and begins to nurse with vigor. Since the mother can become very discouraged, when her baby is nursing poorly, it is important that the nurse support the mother in her attempts to continue nursing. Patience, reassurance and adequate guidance are key

factors in helping the mother over this initial adjustment.

Care of the Nipples

Too much emphasis cannot be placed on the care of the nipples to facilitate breast-feeding. Cleanliness is a cardinal principle. Thus, keeping the nipples clean and dry is basic to keeping them in good condition (see p. 317).

Sore nipples are a frequent "complaint" during the mother's early breast-feeding experience, and so she should be instructed to report any discomfort in order that corrective measures may be instituted at once.

The nipples are best treated after each nursing period with the application of a bland cream or ointment, such as lanolin or one of the commercially prepared compounds, e.g., Massé Nipple Cream or Vitamin A and D Ointment. Painting the nipples with tincture of benzoin or alcohol has long been used to toughen tender nipples, but this has a tendency to dry the skin; in fact, alcohol has been demonstrated to be destructive to the nipple during lactation. Many hospitals are now advocating the use of a thermalite (therapeutic) lamp for tender or cracked nipples; the affected breast is exposed for 20 to 30 minutes twice a day. The mother should be advised that even the exposure of the breast to fresh air for similar periods is beneficial, because this is a measure she may resort to after she returns home.

When a sore nipple is examined, it may be found to be fissured (cracked) or to have a small erosion (raw area). The primary treatment for either condition is rest, in order to avoid further irritation and to allow time for healing. In the majority of cases a nipple shield (Fig. 14-12) may be used for protection so that the infant may continue to nurse. If there is any bleeding from the fissure or erosion, nursing usually is discontinued. Under such conditions, manual expression should be instituted to empty the breast, not only to continue to stimulate lactation, but also to relieve engorgement. The nurse should make every effort to recognize the early symptoms of "cracked nipples" so that further problems can be avoided. These raw areas afford an easy portal of entry for pathogenic bacteria to gain access to the breast and to cause mastitis. Abscess of the breast is very painful and often disastrous. Not only does it result in the immediate suspension of breast-feeding but it also may prevent the suckling of future babies (see Chap. 20, Complications of the Puerperium).

Length of Nursing Time

The infant will begin nursing, from 1 to 5 minutes, from one or both breasts. Gradually, the time is increased according to the tolerance of the mother's nipples. When lactation is well established, the nursing period is approximately 20 minutes, although there may be a wide variation, depending on the infant's sucking pattern. When the breasts are full, and the milk flow is easily ejected, the breast usually is emptied in the first 5 minues or so of nursing. The baby may continue to suck, or he may fall asleep. If the infant continues to suck for an inordinately long length of time (30 to 45 minutes), this may be an indication that there is not enough milk present, and that he is still hungry, or it may be an indication that he sucks intermittently and therefore takes longer to get the milk. Again, he may wish merely to suck, even though he is not hungry. If secretion of milk is not the problem, it is wiser to let him proceed at his own pace than to attempt to hurry him, so long as nipple irritation does not occur. Sometimes the let-down reflex is so active that the milk literally streams, and the baby not only does not have to suck very hard but may have difficulty in swallowing fast enough to keep up with the stream. Placing the baby in a more upright position is sometimes helpful in preventing choking in these cases. He may have to nurse a bit, stop, and then continue as he learns to cope with the increased stream.

Schedule. A self-regulatory or self-demand schedule is the usual accepted practice today, especially for breast-fed babies; that is, the baby is fed when he indicates hunger by crying and body posture. The infant cries when he is hungry because actual contractions in his stomach cause him pain. If he is fed when he cries and is experiencing pain, he learns to associate food with the relief of pain. Thus food (and mother who supplies it) become pleasant factors in his life. If, on the other hand, he is made to wait until "time" for

feeding, he may not nurse well because he is exhausted from crying or has lost his feeling of hunger. Similarly, if a baby is "sleepy" and not allowed to wake up sufficiently by himself, he also will not nurse well and will soon resent efforts made to wake him up. Slapping the soles of his feet, spanking his bottom and the like generally are not effective. These infants may want to nurse only every 6 to 8 hours for the first few days; later they enjoy more frequent nursing periods.

Most average-sized babies regulate themselves on an *approximate* 4-hour schedule. Smaller infants may prefer 3 hours. However, the nurse and the mother must remember that a wide variation will exist; the interval at times may be from 2 to 6 hours and sometimes as long as 8 hours. Usually, however, there will be 6 to 8 feedings in 24 hours. Each infant also will vary his own schedule. For instance, after a few days the mother may notice that the infant wants to eat every 2 hours or so. She usually can meet the demand, since the more frequent nursing stimulates the milk production. Care must be taken that her nipples do not become sore because of the frequent sucking, or that she does not become fatigued. The nurse will want to be particularly careful in observing mother and baby during this time. If the mother does evidence the above signs, then the nurse, after checking with the doctor, may suggest that a bottle be given for one feeding so that the mother may rest.

Complemental Feedings. This subject has long been controversial. Some physicians (and mothers) feel that giving the infant any artificial feedings diminishes the success of breast-feeding and is extremely detrimental to establishing and maintaining lactation (see Suggested Reading). Others feel that there are legitimate indications for an occasional artificial feeding. A variety of feedings may be used, i.e., plain water, glucose water, dilute formula, full-strength formula. If the mother is to use complemental feedings when she gets home, the nurse will want to be sure that she understands their preparation, the kind and the amount of feedings, and the indications for their use.

Expression of Milk

There are some instances in which the

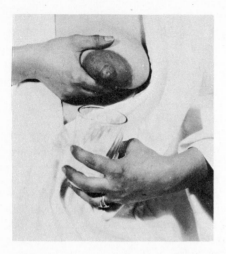

FIG. 14-13. First position in the expression of breast milk from a large, pendent breast, showing the thumb and fingers properly placed and pressing backward.

FIG. 14-14. Second position, showing the thumb and finger pressed deeply into the breast, at the same time compressing the breast well behind the nipple. This deeper pressure is necessary in a round, virginal-shaped breast.

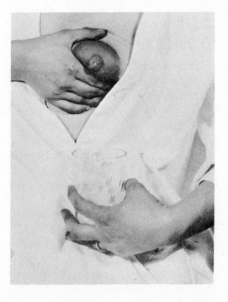

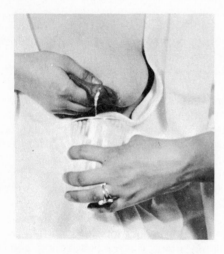

FIG. 14-15. Second position, showing compression of the breast between the thumb and fingers, well behind the nipple, and the milk coming in a stream. Care is exercised to avoid pinching or bruising the breast tissue.

mother is desirous of breast-feeding, but for certain reasons the infant cannot be "put to breast." There are also situations in which the breast-fed infant is not able to empty the breast completely. At such times it becomes necessary to utilize artificial means to empty the breasts of milk; otherwise, if this condition is allowed to persist for several days, lacteal secretion is inhibited, and the future milk supply may be jeopardized.

The hands of the person expressing the milk should be washed thoroughly with warm water and soap and dried on a clean towel. Since the daily care of the breast is designed to maintain cleanliness, the same cleansing ritual required before putting the baby to breast would be utilized here.

Manual Expression. This can be done by nurse, but it is preferable to teach the mother how to carry out this procedure while she is in the hospital. In this way she can have guided practice under the supervision of the hospital nurse, so that when she has to do it after she returns home, her confidence and ability will be increased.

A sterile glass or wide-mouthed container should be in readiness before beginning, and if the milk is to be fed to the infant, a sterile bottle and cap also will be needed. It may be desirable first to massage the breast for a few seconds to stimulate the flow of milk, and in such instance it is helpful to lubricate the hands with a drop of mineral oil. Breast mas-

FIG. 14-16. Illustrating the movements needed to force milk out of the little pockets "P" in which it collects. Place a finger and a thumb on opposite sides of the nipple at "Deep." Press deeply into the breast in the direction of the black arrows. Then compress the breast together in direction of the arrows toward center point "P." This will force the milk out of the ducts in streams. "Deep" and "together" express in two words the motions required. (After U. C. Moore, Nutrition of Mother and Child)

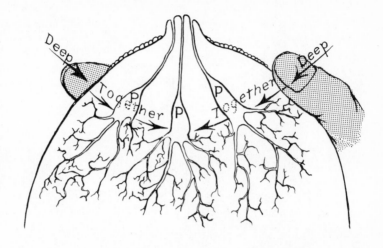

FIG. 14-17. Diagram showing the method of expressing the milk from the breast, as the mother would view it from above, by compressing the milk pockets between the thumb and forefinger. The 3 unused fingers are used to support the breast. This represents the second or "together" motion. (After U. C. Moore, Nutrition of Mother and Child)

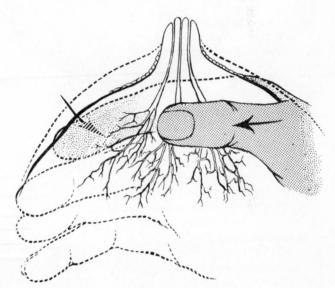

sage should be done with a gliding movement of the hands. The pressure exerted should be firm, even, and, above all, gentle. First, place one hand on top of the other above the breast, then as they are drawn apart turn the fingers downward and encircle the breast. As the hands sweep forward toward the areola, they should cup the breast, drawing it forward and upward, and glide off without ever touching the areola or the nipple. If the breast is pendulous, care should be taken to allow it to fall gently.

One hand is used to support the breast and to express the milk; the other, to hold the container which will receive the milk. Although some authorities advocate that the right hand be used to milk the left breast, the decision as to which hand is used should depend on how the mother can accomplish this with the greatest of ease. The forefinger is placed below and the thumb above the outer edge of the areola. The forefinger should be kept straight so that pressure can be exerted between the middle of this finger and the ball of the thumb. As they are alternately compressed and released, with the area of the collecting sinuses between them, milk is forced out in a stream (Figs. 14-13 to 17). It is of paramount importance here to avoid pinching and possibly bruising the breast tissue. The fingers should not slide forward on the areola or the nipple during the milking

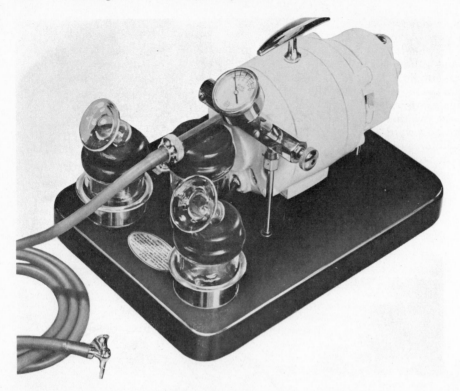

Fig. 14-18. Electric breast-pump. Suction system provides vacuum up to 15″ of mercury. Control allows patient to regulate degree of suction to her requirements and comfort. (Gomco Surgical Manufacturing Corp., Buffalo, N. Y.)

process. However, they must be moved in clockwise fashion around the areola, each time compressing and releasing the fingers on that area, so that all the collecting sinuses may be emptied.

Many obstetricians advocate this method of emptying the breasts rather than using the breast pump, because the action more nearly simulates the action of the infant's jaws as it nurses. Furthermore, since no mechanical equipment is required, it is a method which can be readily used when necessary after discharge from the hospital.

Electric-Pump Expression. Several types of electric breast pumps employing the principle of intermittent negative pressure are used in hospitals (Fig. 14-18). The physician may prescribe their use to empty the breasts of milk, as in some cases to reduce engorgement, or to draw out inverted nipples.

The nurse should be familiar with the instructions pertaining to the particular electric pump that she is using. If she is teaching the mother how to pump her breasts, it is wise to make sure that she understands how to use is, and especially how to control the vacuum.

Low suction will express the milk without discomfort or injury. For whatever purpose the electric breast pump is used, the suction should be increased gradually to prevent irritation to the nipple and needless pain which, in turn, might cause anxiety in the mother and retard the flow of milk. The suction should be intermittent to simulate the sucking of the infant. It takes approximately 5 to 12 minutes to empty a breast completely, depending on the stage of lactation, but pumping should be stopped as soon as milk ceases to flow. If it is used solely to draw out inverted nipples, it should be used only until the nipple becomes erect. A breast should never be pumped longer than 15 minutes at any one time. However, if the mother experiences back or chest pain, and indication the the breast is dry, the pumping should be stopped immediately.

The breast milk obtained should be measured and the amount recorded. When only one breast is pumped at a time, the record should indicate whether it was the right one or the left, so that the next time the other breast can be pumped. If the milk is to be fed to the infant, it should be poured into a sterile nursing bottle, labeled with the infant's name, the time and the date and refrigerated immediately. To ensure further safety in the hospital, milk that is saved for an infant in this way should be sterilized before it is fed to him.

The electric breast-pump machine may be used for more than one mother and thus should be washed with soap or detergent each time that it is used. In addition, certain removable parts, such as the breast-pump bottle and cap, the breast funnel and the rubber connection tubing, must be washed thoroughly, wrapped and autoclaved immediately after use.

Hand-Pump Expression. At times a hand breast-pump may be used. Suction is obtained by alternately collapsing and releasing the rubber bulb. The principles of use and action are the same as those for the electric pump. Since this appliance is used also for more than one mother, it should be washed thoroughly in soap or detergent, rinsed and autoclaved.

Hygiene of the Mother

Rest and Adequate Nutrition. Perhaps these two are the most important considerations for the lactating mother. The detrimental effects of fatigue and worry already have been discussed. In the hospital the nurse is able to act as a buffer between the mother and some of these problems. In addition, the mother is relieved of household responsibilities and is able to have meals served to her. When she leaves the hospital, she no longer has this somewhat protected environment. Thus, it is important that the nurse make sure that the parents understand the importance of rest and adequate nutrition, and that the parents have made adequate plans to provide for them. If it is at all possible, the mother should have help at home. Her main energies then can be directed to the care of the infant and giving attention to her husband and other children. Housekeeping chores will have to be simplified and the mother's activity restricted so that she will get sufficient rest. Since her sleep will be broken at night, naps during the day become particularly *essential*—they should not be considered a luxury. Without adequate rest, the milk supply soon will be reduced to a dribble. If heretofore the woman has been very active, she may need special help to realize the importance of naps and rest periods. It is helpful, also, if visitors (including relatives) are restricted; they can become fatiguing to the mother, and they may be a source of potential infection to the newborn.

Diet. The nutritional requirements of lactating women are high. The total protein, vitamin and mineral intake, as stated in Chapter 13, should be increased over that of the normal requirements for a pregnant woman. The lactating woman needs about 700 calories more than the pregnant woman and 1,000 calories more than the nonpregnant woman (see Table 7, p. 144). This high caloric requirement is necessary, since the lactating mother must meet the caloric needs of her own body, as well as produce the energy needed to convert the food into breast milk. Approximately 39 calories in the diet are required for each ounce of breast milk. Thus, when lactation has reached its maximum, the daily production of about 30 ounces of breast milk would necessitate an additional 1,000 calories in the diet.

The value of a high protein diet to the mother cannot be stressed enough. The mechanism by which food is converted into milk protein is not very efficient; therefore, approximately 2 Gm. of food protein is needed to produce 1 Gm. of milk protein. The greater part of this protein intake (98 Gm. daily) should be in the form of animal protein, since this type supplies all the essential amino acids. The vitamin and mineral intake should be adjusted also to supply the needed amounts for lactation (see p. 144).

A high fluid intake also is necessary for milk production. Between 2,500 and 3,000 cc. is recommended for the mother engaged in usual activity under pleasant environmental conditions. More may be required in hot weather or with physical exertion. This fluid intake should include a good deal of water as well as other beverages. Many mothers find that taking a beverage prior to nursing facilitates the letdown reflex.

If the mother's diet was adequate in pregnancy, then additions rather than changes are all that will be necessary. It is important that the nurse ascertain that the mother is aware of these additions. If she is not, then guidance must be given. Often nursing mothers do not

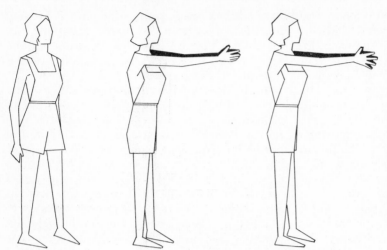

Fig. 14-19. Breast exercise. After breast feeding has been discontinued the breasts seem to be soft and flabby. These simple exercises may help to restore firmness of tissues because they involve the pectoral muscles which lend secondary support to the breasts. Stand with feet apart, toes turned in slightly, abdomen in and up, buttocks tucked under and head held high. Hold fingertips together, with arms at shoulder level. Press fingers together sharply and firmly. Relax and repeat 10 times.

realize that their nutritional needs increase even over the needs of pregnancy, and they try to go back to their prepregnant diet. Increasing the milk intake to at least 1½ quarts daily will meet the additional protein, thiamin, riboflavin, calcium, phosphorus and niacin needs. Supplementing the citrus fruit recommendations in pregnancy with generous servings of other fruits and vegetables will meet the vitamin C requirements. An adequate vitamin D intake can be obtained by supplementing the vitamin-D-rich foods recommended during pregnancy. To further ensure optimum vitamin and mineral intake, many physicians will prescribe that the vitamin supplement capsules taken during pregnancy be continued.

The mother's weight is one of the best criteria in determining adequate caloric intake. It should remain stationary; wide fluctuations will necessitate adjustment of her diet, usually in carbohydrate and fat intake (this statement is based on the assumption that she has an adequate protein intake). The mother may take all foods in moderation as long as they agree with her. The old notion that certain foods (chocolate, the "strong" vegetables such as cabbage, onions, garlic) were excreted through the milk and would upset the baby is no longer universally held.

DEBATABLE ITEMS. Some physicians feel that certain foods, such as berries and chocolate, may produce an allergic reaction in the baby. If the mother has any question regarding these matters, she should consult her physician. Alcohol may be taken in moderation; many mothers find that a glass of sherry or beer before nursing relaxes them considerably and facilitates the let-down reflex. Smoking does not directly influence the lactation process when it is done in moderation, but it should be avoided for the reasons stated in Chapter 8.

Drugs. Many drugs are excreted in the milk, as was explained in Chapter 13, and it is particularly important for the mother to consult her physician before she attempts any self-medication, *even though she has taken the drug before.* Small doses of aspirin, milk of magnesia, mineral oil and some of the bulk-producing laxatives usually may be taken without passing harmful effects to the infant; however, it is well to advise the mother to inform her doctor if she feels she must continue to use any of them.

Weaning

Occasionally, it becomes necessary to wean the baby suddenly. In these cases the physician will follow the regimen for "drying up the breasts" as described on pages 318 to 319. Most often, however, weaning is done gradually. There does not appear to be any "best" time for this procedure. Sometimes, with the introduction of solid foods the infant tends to take the breast less, and the milk supply consequently will diminish. However,

FIG. 14-20. Breast exercise. Lie flat on back with knees and thighs flexed to place spine firmly on the floor. Abdomen is kept flat. Breathe naturally and do exercises slowly. (1) Holding a small book in each hand, stretch arms out level with shoulders. (2) Raise arms forward from body to bring books together, keeping arms straight. Lower arms to outstretched position. (3) Raise arms forward as in No. 2; then carry them, held straight together, to floor behind head. Return arms to outstretched position. Repeat. Stop all exercises before feeling tired.

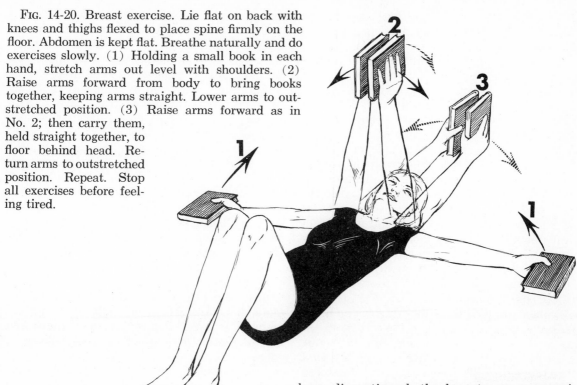

many infants appear to relish solids and still continue to nurse well. It is essential to good health that the baby have solid foods by the age of 6 months at the latest. By this time his iron reserve has been depleted, and foods rich in protein and iron are particularly important. Provided that the baby receives a varied diet that includes meat, eggs, fruits and vegetables, there is no indication for weaning other than the natural inclinations of the mother and the baby. The process can be done gradually, with a cup and/or bottle offered in place of the breast. As the stimulation decreases, so does the milk supply, and lactation gradually ceases. Usually no engorgment ensues; if any should occur, the mother should be instructed to consult her physician.

Breast Exercises

Mothers are sometimes concerned about the temporary increase in the size of the breasts during lactation. When breast-feeding has been discontinued, the breasts soon approximate their previous size and firmness, particularly if needed support has been maintained. There are exercises which, if done regularly, may be helpful. The breast itself is made up of glandular tissue and fat (see Fig. 2-35), and since there is an absence of elastic tissue, exercises cannot directly hasten the return of the breasts to their former state. However, exercises that involve the pectoral muscles may be helpful, because these muscles lend secondary support to the breasts (Figs. 14-19, 20). These exercises may be started when the mother is no longer breast-feeding, should be limited at first and increased only as the mother can tolerate them without fatigue.

PARENTAL GUIDANCE AND INSTRUCTION

A considerable amount of health supervision throughout the mother's pregnancy is devoted to anticipatory guidance, not only to provide for her immediate care, but also to help her plan and prepare for the time when she takes her new infant home from the hospital. A good foundation to facilitate this transition has been laid in this way, but it may lose some of its effectiveness unless certain aspects are reinforced in the immediate puerperium.

Each mother's understanding and ability will vary, depending largely on her background and previous experiences. Undoubtedly, the primipara who has not been accustomed to infants will have much to learn about the care and handling of her new baby. On the other hand, the multipara may feel uncertain about the response of an older child to the new baby and thus require guidance in understanding and dealing with sibling rivalry. Many mothers need to know more about their own care; others need to know how to facilitate certain adjustments within the home or the family group. If the mother knows what she can expect and what to do, she usually can handle simple problems which might otherwise cause fear or apprehension.

Proper care for the mother during the puerperium emphasizes the need for rest, nourishing food and protection from worry. Parents, as a rule, seem to be under the impression that once the delivery is over, normality is restored and they can resume their usual activities immediately. However, it is agreed that it may be weeks before the generative organs have returned to normal size and position, and the emotional and endocrine adjustments may be even more delayed.

Since the nurse is in close and continuous contact with the mother, she should assume the responsibility of giving this anticipatory guidance and/or reinforcing or delegating that part which might be done more suitably by others. One of the most important points to be emphasized is that the mother should proceed *as slowly as possible* in the postpartal period at home. The general feeling of well-being and the excitement of having the baby, together with the emotions aroused in the "taking-hold" phase, all too often provide so great a stimulus that the mother has a tendency to overdo. If there are other children in the household, especially toddlers, the demands on the mother may be considerable.

If it is at all possible, the major responsibilities of housekeeping should be taken over by a "helper," so that the mother can be more relaxed and devote herself primarily to caring for her new infant and spending more time with the immediate family. At this time family rela-

tionships can be strengthened if the mother is not overwhelmed with apprehension and fatigue. The subject of household assistance needs to be explored thoroughly with the mother (and if necessary, the father). The parents may need help in realizing what possibilities and alternatives they have in this matter. Some parents, for instance, manage very nicely when the husband takes some vacationtime and assumes management of the household. However, it must be remembered that not all husbands are able (or willing) to shoulder this considerable task. Other parents can rely on parents, in-laws or relatives for a time. Still others must hire outside help; in these cases the expense and consequent budgeting may have to be discussed. If outside help is employed, then the mother may have some question as to whether a housekeeper or a "nurse" (to take care of the baby) would be more desirable. This, of course, will depend on many factors. Most mothers find that when they are relieved of the heavy housekeeping chores, the "care" of the baby is relatively easy and provides an opportunity to get thoroughly acquainted with the new addition to the household.

The nurse should not "recommend" one type of helper over another. Rather, she should explore the subject with the mother, point out the alternatives that the parents have, and let them make the final decision. This approach would be appropriate for any other aspect of guidance.

By the time that the mother leaves the hospital she should have at least a basic understanding of her own condition and status, and she should know what physical and emotional changes to expect. In addition, she should be familiar with the daily care of her baby and know what to expect of him, together with any other important details related to his care. Parents should know how and where to contact the physician if before the next scheduled visit there should arise any medical problem pertaining to either the mother or the infant.

Since the present-day maternity stay is rather short, some type of follow-up service often is desirable and necessary. Therefore, parents should be offered information about the services of the public health nursing agency in their community, and how they may use these services. In cases of obvious need a re

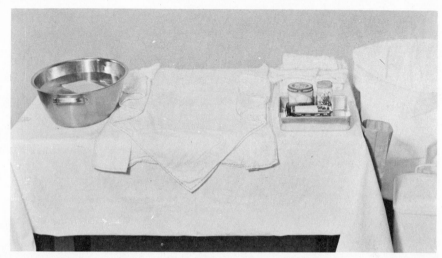

FIG. 14-21. Setup used for baby bath demonstration in the mothers' classroom. Note paper bag for discarded cotton balls, pillowcase for a laundry hamper and step-on can for diaper pail. (MacDonald House, The University Hospitals of Cleveland, Cleveland, Ohio)

ferral to an agency should be instituted before the patient leaves the hospital.

Husbands who have accompanied their wives to parents' classes are usually much more conscious of this period and prepared for it. Often they plan their time at home so that they can help to assume some of the responsibilities. It is not so much physical help that is needed as it is the satisfactions gained by the mutual "sharing" engendered by the partnership. If the mother takes special care to express her appreciation of her husband's awareness and consideration, then this initial readjustment period becomes less tedious and truly gratifying to both.

Group Classes

Many hospitals now provide regularly scheduled mothers' classes in which certain aspects

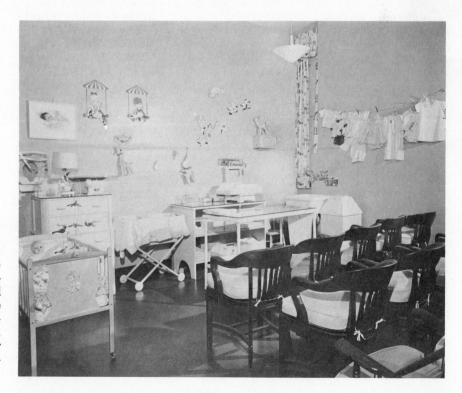

FIG. 14-22. Sloane Babies Alumni Classroom. Well-cushioned chairs add to the mother's comfort during postpartal classes. (Sloane Hospital for Women, Medical Center, New York)

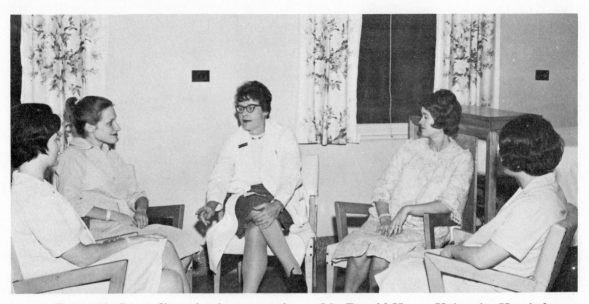

FIG. 14-23. Group discussion for new mothers. (MacDonald House, University Hospitals of Cleveland)

of the care of the infant and the mother at home are demonstrated and/or discussed by a member of the nursing staff. Some of these classes are structured and proceed according to a certain agenda of instruction. A baby bath (Fig. 14-21) and formula preparation demonstration lends itself well to this type of approach. Other classes are less structured; there is no set agenda, and the nurse acts as the discussion leader. All patients may participate, and often members of the group reply to one another's questions. The mother's questions are answered as they arise, and the topics are developed and explained as the comments made by the group are reflected and expanded. This approach enables the group to move at its own speed and to discuss, under the guidance of the nurse, subjects that are of real interest to them. Many classes use a combination of approaches; for instance, the demonstration is structured, and the discussion is unstructured. These classes are particularly valuable, because the new mother is usually most receptive and ready for such learning after her new baby has arrived.

When the mother is permitted to leave her room, she should be encouraged to attend the demonstration and discussion classes in the mothers' classroom. Even mothers who are

breast-feeding benefit from a formula-preparation class, because they learn about the care of nursing bottles used for orange juice or water and how to prepare a supplementary feeding. Some hospitals have special classes for mothers who are breast-feeding. Such classes have the advantage of encouraging the mothers to share, under the guidance of a nurse, experiences and problems related to feeding their infants. More recently, some hospitals have included a pediatrician's class for all mothers, in which the physician discusses the newborn infant—its appearance, behavior, growth, development and, in general, the care of the normal newborn infant.

Individual Teaching

Regardless of the fact that a mother may attend all the group classes offered in the maternity hospital, each mother should be given individual help to learn how to handle and care for her infant while she is in the hospital, particularly if this is her first baby. Many new mothers are timid at first because they do not know what to expect of their infants, or they are afraid of what they will do to them because of their own feelings of inadequacy. A mother who has had no previous experience with infants will need some guided practice in changing diapers, dressing her baby and handling the infant in general (Fig. 14-24). Rooming-in units provide an environment in which the mother can have such an experience over an extended period of time. However, even in situations where the infants are kept in a central nursery, the nurse should plan to spend some time with the mother, in addition to the regular feeding periods, to help her learn to care for her baby. If hospital staffing permits the time, it may be desirable for some mothers to bathe their own infants at the bedside, under the nurse's guidance, before leaving the hospital. There is no reason that such practices should violate the "clean nursery technic" if they have been properly planned. A rooming-in experience is undoubtedly bene-

ficial for mother, father and baby. But when this is not possible because of hospital facilities or policies, a daily extended visiting period can be extremely helpful. In this way the parents and the baby can become better acquainted in the security of the maternity division, where experienced personnel are near at hand to answer the mother's questions and to offer advice.

Postpartal Exercises

Certain exercises are advantageous to the mother during the postpartal period to strengthen the abdominal muscles, to promote involution and a general sense of well-being. Such exercises are *advised and regulated by the physician,* according to the individual

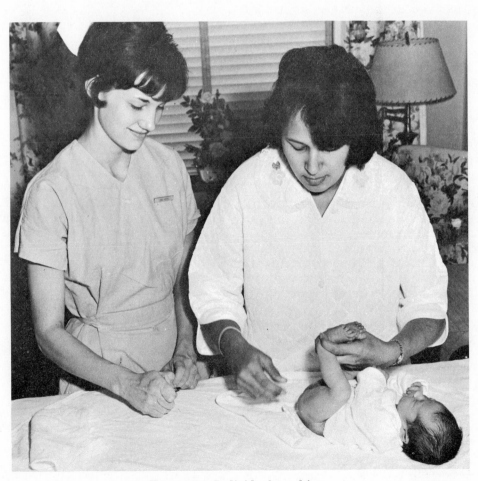

Fig. 14-24. Individual teaching.

Fig. 14-25. Knee-chest position may be advised by the physician if the uterus has not returned to its almost normal position.

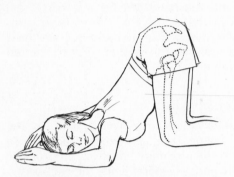

CORRECT—Chest resting on bed, thighs perpendicular to surface.

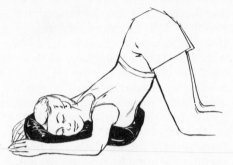

INCORRECT—Chest on pillow, thighs slant away from body.

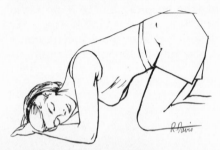

INCORRECT—Resting on elbows, thighs slant inward toward body.

mother's condition. If the mother has had an abnormal delivery or any extensive perineal repair, exercises may not be advisable. Any exercises prescribed for the mother should not be strenuous or tiring when used in moderation. They should be practiced slowly and rhythmically, only a few times at first and gradually increased from day to day (see Chap. 8).

The knee-chest position may be advised by some physicians to encourage the uterus to return to its normal position, particularly if the organ is retroverted. When this exercise is employed, the physician usually instructs the patient to start the exercise about the 3rd postpartal week, beginning with 2-minute periods each morning and evening and gradually increasing the time to 5 minutes twice daily. Patients should never be put in the knee-chest position *without specific orders from the physician.* Because of the anatomic relationship of the bladder to the uterus, the patient should empty her bladder first. The advantage to be gained from this exercise depends on the position of the pelvis. In order to attain the correct attitude of the pelvis, the patient's thighs should remain erect (perpendicular to the floor) while her back is carefully positioned so that it does not sag (Fig. 14-26). Care must be taken to see that the external genitalia are not drawn open to allow air to enter the vagina. The danger of an air embolism occurring in such situations has been reported.

Discharge Instructions

Before the mother is discharged from the hospital, the physician will give her instructions about her care and the rate at which it is prudent for her to resume normal activities in the following weeks at home. She is told to avoid any heavy work and to get as much rest as possible during the next 3 weeks (see p. 313). Her schedule should be planned to include morning and afternoon rest periods and adequate sleep at night. Stair climbing should be limited until the 2nd week at home. If the mother is advised to take exercises to strengthen abdominal and perineal muscles, the physician will specify when they may be started and the frequency with which they are to be done. The hair may be washed at any time, and tub baths or showers are permissible. The mother usually is advised not to have intercourse or to take a vagina douche until after the "6-week check-up" to prevent infection and trauma to the newly healing organs and structures. Instructions concerning eating habits and regulation of the bowels are discussed.

If the medical care of the infant is being supervised by a pediatrician, he may give the mother home-going instructions concerning her baby; otherwise this is taken care of by the obstetrician. The mother should be given specific information about feeding, skin care, clothing, sleep, bowel habits, behavior and the early growth and development of her infant.

Many hospitals provide printed home-going instructions for maternity patients. When these are used, it is the responsibility of the nurse to make sure that the mother understands them before she leaves the hospital.

The maternity programs of most public health agencies include home visits by the nurse. When a referral has not been made by the hospital nurse, the mother should be informed that such services are available in the community and told how to secure them if she should need help with the care of the baby.

The importance of follow-up care for both mother and baby should be stressed. The mother is instructed that it is essential for her to keep the appointment for her "6-week check-up." The infant should be checked in 4 weeks and regularly thereafter by a private physician or in one of the well-baby clinics sponsored by the department of health.

Family Planning

Brutally high death rates approximated so closely the high birth rates for vast aeons that the population of the world remained stationary or almost so. The human female, a relatively slow breeder even among mammals, had to reproduce close to her physiologic maximum if the family, the tribe and the nation were to survive. It took the human population from the beginning of time to about 1850 to reach its first billion. It reached 2 billion in approximately another 80 years. The third billion was added in about 30 years; and at the present rate of growth the prospects are that the next 30 years will add not just 1 billion inhabitants to the globe, but a number that may approximate 3 billion. Dr. Irene Taeuber, one of our most conservative demographers, forecasts another 391 million people for Africa by the end of the century (only 34 years hence), 421 million more for Latin America, and 2 billion, 350 million additional for Asia.

The reasons for these soaring figures are plain enough. As the result of worldwide and highly efficacious public health measures, the death rates, especially in developing countries, have fallen precipitously. But in these very countries the same high birth rates prevail as obtained decades ago. This imbalance between births and deaths leads inevitably to such figures as those just cited. Since it would be unthinkable to suggest any measures to increase death rates, the only solution to the problem, short of the Four Horsemen of the Apocalypse, is reduction in the number of births.

Even at present population levels, the majority of the world's populace subsists on near-starvation diets. Malnutrition is the inevitable forerunner of anemia and increased vulnerability to infectious diseases. Infants and children are the hardest hit. Overcrowding abets the dissemination of infectious diseases and vitiates any attempts at hygienic living. Excessive population is therefore an all-important health problem. For this reason the American Public Health Association, the American Medical Association and other pertinent organizations have long since endorsed family planning as an urgent health need.

The important role that the nurse, both the maternity and the public health nurse, can play in the extensive movement to control excessive fertility is reflected in the numerous articles in nursing journals on this subject, as indicated by the bibliography of this chapter. For example, the Associate Editor of *Nursing Outlook*, Alice M. Robinson, writes in an editorial:

There is no need to advocate any particular concept or belief or method; but it is the nurses' grave and imminent responsibility to give the widest possible help and hope and understanding to the end that guidance in family planning is made unequivocally and universally available to parents, regardless of their socioeconomic status.[5]

She properly points out, moreover, that "*all* major religious groups—Jewish, Catholic and Protestant—agree on the necessity for *responsible, planned* parenthood." It might be added in this connection that at least one method of contraception has the approval of all religions. Certainly, in this modern, changing age it is incumbent on every nurse to be cognizant of

[5] Alice M. Robinson: The principle, not the method, Nurs. Outlook 12, No. 9:27, September, 1964.

the commonly used methods of fertility control, with their advantages and disadvantages, so that she may discuss this important problem with patients in an intelligent manner. Those who are in conscience committed to the moral teachings of the Roman Catholic Church will find that only two of these methods are ethically acceptable to them. For the benefit of our Catholic readers, we have asterisked both. The commonly used methods of contraception are as follows:

Newer Methods

Oral Progestins. Oral contraceptives ("The Pill") have been publicized so extensively in the lay press that their existence is common knowledge. They owe their effect to the suppression of ovulation caused by the administration of certain hormones, and they constitute the most efficacious contraceptive method known. The program involves setting up a "controlled menstrual cycle" by administering one of these pills daily for 20 days, beginning with the 5th day of the menstrual cycle. Because these compounds have estrogenic as well as progestational effects, they provoke endometrial withdrawal bleeding 3 or 4 days after discontinuance. Since it is possible to control the menstrual cycle by these agents, they are used extensively as therapeutic measures in women with menstrual abnormalities. As contraceptive agents, the chief objection that has been raised is the possibility of ovarian damage and various side-effects. Although pregnancy has ensued promptly in many women who have discontinued the method after many years of continued use, these objections have not been completely met.

Intra-uterine Devices (IUCD). This technic (actually an ancient practice but only recently validated scientifically) involves the insertion into the uterine cavity of a small, usually flexible appliance, the length or diameter of which is approximately three quarters of an inch. This foreign object is allowed to remain in the uterus as long as contraception is desired. These devices have been made in various shapes (spirals, loops, rings) and of various materials (plastic tubing, nylon thread, stainless steel). Although the mechanism by which these appliances prevent conception is obscure, they are highly efficacious, ranking second only to oral progestins in the protection that they provide. The advantages of intra-uterine devices are that they are inexpensive and, once inserted, require no further attention, provided that they remain in place. This brings us to the main drawback of these appliances: they frequently are expelled. Moreover, some of the appliances have to be removed because of bleeding or cramps. Spontaneous expulsion or necessary removal by the physician occurs in 15 to 20 per cent of all cases with the devices now being used. With improvement in their size and shape, however, it is expected that the frequency of spontaneous expulsions and necessary removals will be reduced. These devices are being widely used throughout the world, especially in developing countries, where their low cost and lack of any need for continuing motivation constitute particular advantages.

Conventional Methods

The Diaphragm. The diaphragm is a dome-shaped rubber cup, which may range in diameter from 7 to 10 cm. and is inserted digitally into the vagina and over the cervix prior to intercourse and then removed subsequently. A spermicidal jelly usually is applied to the rim of the diaphragm to afford more effective sealing at its rim. The chief objection is the vaginal manipulation necessary to insert it, a procedure which is repugnant to some women. Although its efficacy is good, the diaphragm has lost favor in view of the greater efficacy and acceptability of the oral contraceptives and intra-uterine devices, as discussed in the foregoing paragraphs.

*****The Safe Period or Rhythm.** The rationale of the safe period or rhythm method is as follows: (1) Ovulation *usually* occurs at *approximately* the same date in any given menstrual cycle. (2) The ovum is capable of being fertilized only for a period of 48 hours at the most after ovulation. (3) Spermatozoa are likewise short-lived and are thought to be incapable of fertilizing an ovum for more than 48 hours after ejaculation. Theoretically, therefore, if the date of ovulation could be known with precision *beforehand*, abstinence from sexual intercourse on that day and for the 2 days before and after would forestall conception.

In actual experience, however, ovulation does not occur with clocklike precision. Hence, when the rhythm method is used, only an approximate ovulation date can be estimated in advance, and abstinence must be practiced for several days before and after that date to allow for errors in its estimation. Hence the precision with which the date can be calculated is an all-important factor in the dependability of this method. The calculation of the expected date of ovulation is the responsibility of the attending physician. The accuracy of the estimated day of ovulation can be increased if the woman will take her oral temperature each day during three cycles, record the figures, and submit these to her physician for analysis (see Fig. 3-4 and Chap. 3). Special thermometers are sold at most drug stores for this purpose.

The advantages of this method are that no paraphernalia or spermicidal chemicals are required, no local manipulations are necessary, and it is approved in principle by all religious faiths. The objections are the period of abstinence required and the fact that it is not satisfactory in women with irregular menstrual cycles. When this method is used by intelligent couples eager to postpone the next pregnancy, its efficacy is comparable with that of creams, jellies, foam tablets, and suppositories used for this purpose. Much research now is being directed at pinpointing more precisely the fertile days in order to increase the acceptability of this method.

Douches. Douches taken after intercourse either for cleanliness or contraception are perhaps the least dependable method of contraception, the reported pregnancy rates being very high.

Jellies, Creams and Suppositories. Jellies and creams are inserted into the vagina by means of a special nozzle provided for this purpose, which can be attached to a tube of some spermicidal jelly or cream. The chief objection is messiness, and, as indicated, the efficacy in general is not appreciably better than the rhythm method when the latter program is followed meticulously.

Withdrawal. Withdrawal or *coitus interruptus* is an extensively used method of contraception and appears to be satisfactory to a large proportion of couples. Data on its efficacy are sparse, but the evidence available indicates that it is less dependable than the rhythm method.

*Lactation. As long as lactation is maintained (without supplementary feedings), the likelihood of conception is greatly reduced. This is Nature's way of child spacing. It is well known that ovulation ceases altogether during pregnancy, and in the presence of active lactation, ovulation *usually* is held in abeyance but not to the same degree as in pregnancy. It is not, therefore, a dependable method, but in the majority of cases it may postpone the next conception by several months.

SUGGESTED READING

Adels, M. J., and Rogers, S. F.: Use of a new non-narcotic analgesic for postpartum pain, Am. J. Obstet. Gynec. 84:952-955, October 1, 1962.

American Public Health Association: Policy statement on population, Am. J. Public Health 104:2102, December, 1964.

Beckwith, D. B.: Recent developments in management of the puerperium, Nurs. Mirror 156:29-31, April 12, 1963.

Brodsky, J. D., and Greenstein, C.: Air embolism associated with pregnancy and the puerperium, Illinois Med. J. 112:5, 1957.

Bumgardner, H. D., and Zatach, G. J.: Prevention of episiotomy pain with oral chymotrypsin, Am. J. Obstet. Gynec. 42:514-517, June 15, 1965.

Caplan, G.: The mental hygiene role of the nurse in maternal and child care, Nurs. Outlook 2:14-19, January, 1954.

Chesterman, H.: The public health nurse and family planning, Nurs. Outlook 12:32-34, September, 1964.

Day, G.: Early discharge of maternity patients, Nurs. Outlook 11:825-827, November, 1963.

Gelber, Ida: Family planning in a growing world, Am. J. Nurs. 64:98-103, August, 1964.

Gorden, R. E., and Gorden, K. K.: Social factors in prevention of postpartum emotional problems, Obstet. Gynec. 15:433-438, April, 1960.

Guillot, Ellen: Patterns of help for postpartum mothers, Children 11:147-151, July-August, 1964.

Herschelmann, R. F., and Partridge, A.: Deladumone for breast discomfort, Am. J. Nurs. 59:1252-1254, September, 1959.

Hilliard, M. E.: The evolution of a maternity nurse, Nurs. Forum 4, No. 2:6-29, 1965.

Hornick, G. M., and Howard, E. M.: A hospital postpartum teaching program, Canad. Nurse 59:359-360, April, 1963.

Joint Committee on Family and Child Welfare

and Committee on Health: The Right to Birth Control Information in Family Planning, New York, Community Service Society of New York, June, 1964.

Josselyn, I. M.: Cultural forces—motherliness and fatherliness, Am. J. Orthopsychiat. 26:264-271, April, 1956.

Kallaus, Jane: The mother in the maternity unit, Am. J. Nurs. 65:120-127, April, 1965.

Lesser, M. S., and Keane, V. R.: Nurse-Patient Relationships in a Hospital Maternity Service, St. Louis, Mosby, 1956.

McFarland, M. B., and Reinhart, J. B.: The development of motherliness, Children 6:48-52, March-April, 1959.

Mainwaring, C.: Clean voided specimens for mass screening, Am. J. Nurs. 63:96-97, October, 1963.

Marie Christine, Sister: Postpartum nursing care, Canad. Nurse 61:29-30, January, 1965.

Maternity Center Association: Psychophysical Preparation for Childbearing: Guidelines for Teaching, ed. 2, New York, Maternity Center Association, 1965.

Meir, Gilta: The role of hospital nurses in family planning, Am. J. Nurs. 65:86-91, July, 1965.

Minkler, D.: Public policy in family planning, Nurs. Outlook 12:28-31, September, 1964.

Murray, B. L.: A challenge for nursing in maternal infant care, Bull. Maternal Infant Health 8, No. 1:15-19 ff., 1961.

Murray, B. L., et al.: Implications for learning: Persistent aspects of maternal-child nursing situations, J. Nurs. Ed. 11:5-9 ff., February-March, 1963.

Newton, Niles: Maternal Emotions, New York, Hoeber, 1955.

Newton, N., and Newton, M.: Mother's reactions to their newborn babies, J.A.M.A. 181:206-210, July 21, 1962.

———: The normal course and management of lactation, Clin. Obstet. Gynec. 5:44-63, March, 1962.

Owens, Charlotte: Parents' reactions to defective babies, Am. J. Nurs. 64:83-86, November, 1964.

Poffenbarger, R. S., Jr.: The picture puzzle of the postpartum psychosis, J. Chronic Dis. 13:161-173, February, 1961.

———: Epidemiological aspects of parapartum mental illness, Brit. J. Prev. Soc. Med. 18:189-195, 1964.

Proudfit, F. T., and Robinson, C. H.: Normal and Therapeutic Nutrition, ed. 12, New York, Macmillan, 1961.

Recommended Dietary Allowances, rev. ed., Publication No. 1146, Washington, D. C., National Academy of Sciences, National Research Council, 1963.

Robinson, A. M.: The principle, not the method, Nurs. Outlook 12:27, September, 1964.

Rose, P. A.: Identification and Application of Psychiatric Principles in the Nursing Care of Maternity Patients, New York, American Nurses Association, 1962.

Rosengren, W. R.: Social instability and attitudes toward pregnancy as a social role, Social Problems 9:371-378, Spring, 1962.

Rubin, Reva: Basic maternal behavior, Nurs. Outlook 9:683-686, November, 1961.

———: Puerperal change, Nurs. Outlook 9:753-755, December, 1961.

———: Maternal touch, Nurs. Outlook 11:828-831, November, 1963.

———: The family-child relationship, Nurs. Outlook 12:36-39, September, 1964.

Selye, Hans: The stress syndrome, Am. J. Nurs. 65:97-99, March, 1965.

Smith, Reginald, and M. Juan, Sister: Postpartum tub-baths, Am. J. Nurs. 64:135-136, September, 1964.

Stapp, C. C.: Postpartum management of bowel function, Clin. Med. 71:530-532, March, 1964.

Thaxton, Adele: Teaching expectant parents what they want to know, Am. J. Nurs. 62:112, May, 1962.

Tyler, E. T.: Oral contraceptives, Am. J. Nurs. 61:51-53, August, 1961.

The Womanly Art of Breastfeeding, Franklin Park, La Leche International, 1963.

Wooden, Howard: Impact of the industrial revolution on hospital maternity care, Nurs. Forum 1, No. 1:91-104, Winter, 1961-1962.

———: The family-centered approach to maternity care, Nurs. Forum 1, No. 2:61-77, Spring, 1962.

Ziegel, Erna, and Van Blarcom, C. C.: Obstetric Nursing, ed. 5, New York, Macmillan, 1964.

CONFERENCE MATERIAL

1. The patient's husband is severely injured the day after her infant is born. What provision can be made by the hospital to keep the patient informed about conditions at home and the care of her three other children?

2. What instructions should be given to the primipara and her husband concerning her care following delivery and discharge from the hospital? How can the public health nurse participate most effectively in this family's care?

3. What approach would you use to help a mother who was undecided about whether or not to breast-feed her infant?

4. Why is the postpartal examination im-

portant? What is the nurse's role in relation to the examination?

5. A mother tells the nurse that she wants to breast-feed her baby for 6 to 8 months because she knows that she cannot become pregnant so long as she is nursing. How can the nurse reply?

6. What are the pros and the cons of early ambulation for the maternity patient?

7. How can the nurse help a nursing mother so that she can make her limited food budget provide well-balanced meals for the family? The family consists of the mother, the father (employed as a factory worker) and two small children.

8. A young mother is concerned that her 2-year-old child will be jealous of the new baby. How can this problem be handled?

9. What health teaching would you consider necessary to include as you give a bath to a primipara the first morning after delivery? A multipara?

Study Questions

UNIT FOUR: NURSING IN THE NORMAL PUERPERIUM

Read through the entire question and place your answer on the line to the right.

1. Soon after the mother was normally delivered, she complained of feeling chilly. The nurse observed that she was having a chill. In addition to reporting this to the physician, which of the following measures would the nurse carry out?
A. Provide external warmth to the mother with blankets.
B. Give a heart stimulant.
C. Prepare to give oxygen.
D. Give a hot drink.
E. Place the mother in shock position.

Select the number corresponding to the correct letter or letters.
1. A only
2. A and C
3. A and D
4. B and E

3

2. If a mother making satisfactory progress has a pulse rate of 90 immediately before delivery, what average rate or rates would be considered to be favorable soon after delivery?
A. 60
B. 70
C. 80
D. 90
E. 100

Select the number corresponding to the correct letter or letters.
1. C only
2. A, B and C
3. C, D and E
4. All of them

2

3. The appearance of the lochial discharge normally changes during the process of involution. In the space provided after the descriptive phrase in Column 2, place the letter of the period of time in Column 1 that corresponds to it.

Column 1	Column 2	
A. First day	1. Clotted blood with strings of membrane	G
B. From 1 to 2 days	2. Brownish color; thin, scanty	D
C. From 4 to 7 days	3. Blood mixed with small amounts of mucus	B
D. From 8 to 14 days	4. Pinkish color; moderate amount	C
E. Third week	5. Yellow, creamish color	G
F. Seventh week	6. Dark-brown with occasional bright-red	G
G. Not at all	7. Characteristic stale odor	G
	8. Characteristic foul odor	G

346

4. A good understanding of the physiologic changes taking place in the mother during the puerperium is a basis for good nursing. Which of the following processes are believed to accomplish involution of the uterus?
   A. The contraction of stretched muscle fibers
   B. The elimination of endometrium along with blood and serous discharge
   C. The casting off of a portion of the spongy layer of the decidua
   D. The generation of new endometrial lining from the layer of decidua attached to the muscular wall
   E. The formation of new endometrium

Select the number corresponding to the correct letters.
   1. A, B and D
   2. A, C and D
   3. C and E
   4. All of them

5. The nurse should be able to evaluate the observations she makes of her patient's condition. Which of the following changes in the height of the fundus would you consider to be indicative of normal progress of involution?
   A. Twelve hours after delivery—1 cm. above umbilicus
   B. Second day after delivery—6 in. above pubis
   C. Fourth day after delivery—3 in. above pubis
   D. Eighth day after delivery—2 in. above pubis
   E. Tenth day after delivery—1 in. above pubis

Select the number corresponding to the correct letter or letters.
   1. A only
   2. A and C
   3. B, D and E
   4. All of them   **2**

6. Which of the following seem to be the advantages gained from early ambulation after delivery?
   A. Improves bowel and bladder function
   B. Mothers seem to regain their strength more readily
   C. Minimizes the chances of hemorrhage
   D. Hastens involution of the uterus
   E. Eliminates incidence of thrombophlebitis

Select the number corresponding to the correct letters.
   1. A and B
   2. A, C and D
   3. B, C and E
   4. All of them

7. Although the procedures for perineal care vary from hospital to hospital, in what respects do they all agree?
   A. Requiring the nurse to carry out surgical aseptic technic
   B. Endeavoring to protect the patient against infection from external sources
   C. Using forceps to handle sponges in cleansing vulva
   D. Requiring that each sponge be used for one stroke only
   E. Requiring that perineal pads be sterile when applied

Select the number corresponding to the correct letters.
   1. A and E
   2. A, B and C
   3. B, D and E
   4. All of them   **3**

8. To keep the nipples in good condition for breast feeding, which of the following should be included in their daily care?

A. Keep the nipples clean and dry.
B. Wash with warm water once a day.
C. Wash with mild antiseptic solution prior to each feeding period.
D. Cover the nipples and areola with clean plastic breast squares to prevent contamination.
E. If nipple is sore, discontinue breast-feeding until tenderness subsides.

Select the number corresponding to the correct letters.

   1. A and B
   2. A, C and D
   3. B, D and E
   4. All of them

Note: The key to the correct answers to these questions is given on page 597.

Nursing the Normal Newborn

Care of the Newborn Infant
Care of the Premature Infant

Physiology of the Newborn • Characteristics of the Newborn
The Environment of the Newborn • Nursing Care of the Newborn
Infant Feeding • The Primigravida and Her Newborn

Chapter 15

Care of the Newborn Infant

INTRODUCTION

The 10 most important months of a baby's life are the 9 months before he is born and the 1st month after birth. During pregnancy the baby has been protected and nourished by the mother, but at birth the baby becomes an "independent" individual and undergoes the most profound physiologic changes that are encountered at any period of life. Certain of these alterations are immediate, and others are delayed, but they are all permanent and therefore significant.

The first 4 weeks of life are termed the *neonatal period*. From the standpoint of maternity care, the infant is considered through this period.

Since these first days and weeks are so critical, the nurse is called on to give expert nursing care when she assumes care of the newborn. It is necessary for her to use the utmost care in handling the baby, keeping him warm and protecting him from exposure and injury. In addition to the physical care that she gives the infant, she must make accurate observations and record and report them. Her communication and teaching skills are utilized, since she must ensure the infant's future well-being by helping the parents to develop an understanding of their baby's needs and to acquire skill in his care. In this way she reinforces their concept of themselves as adequate parents. The nurse also must be aware that some parents need assistance in developing healthy attitudes regarding child-rearing practices, so that the infant can make a satisfactory emotional and social adjustment. A close parent-infant relationship must be fostered (and provision made for this in the hospital environment), and communication must be maintained between the nurse and the parents. Thus, the care of the newborn infant presents an interesting challenge to those in maternity nursing.

PHYSIOLOGY OF THE NEWBORN

Recent research[1] has indicated that the infant must pass through approximately 6 overlapping stages before he becomes entirely adapted to extra-uterine life. During these stages he is in a "transition" period which he must negotiate successfully if he is to survive and to develop normally. The 1st step or stage begins with labor, when the fetus receives the stimulation from the uterine contractions and the changes in pressure as the membranes rupture. As he passes through the 2nd step, he encounters a variety of foreign stimuli—light, sound, heat, cold, gravitation, etc. Next he must initiate the breathing of air. Stages 4 and 5 require profound changes and reorgan-

[1] Arnold, H. W., *et al.*: Transition to extra-uterine life, Am. J. Nurs. 65:77-80, October, 1965; Desmond, M. M., *et al.*: The clinical behavior of the newly born: Part I, The term baby, J. Pediat. 62:307-325, March, 1963.

351

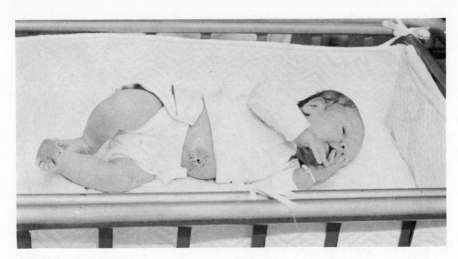

Fig. 15-1. A healthy newborn infant 4 hours after birth. *Note:* The umbilical cord has been clamped with a Hesseltine clamp (see Fig. 12-27B). (Mac-Donald House, The University Hospitals of Cleveland, Cleveland, Ohio)

ization in the functioning of the organ systems and metabolic processes. Here he must initiate respiration, change from fetal to neonatal circulation, alter hepatic and renal function and pass meconium. Stage 6 demands further reorganization of the metabolic processes to achieve a viable, steady state. This includes changes in blood oxygen saturation, reduction of enzymes, diminution in postnatal acidosis and recovery of the neurologic tissues from the trauma of labor and delivery. Since these changes take time, it is no wonder that the infant's natal day is so crucial to his life and future well-being.

Respiratory Changes

During fetal life, about the 4th month of pregnancy the infant apparently attempts respiratorylike movements. Some authorities feel that amniotic fluid is aspirated during this activity; others feel that the lungs actually manufacture amniotic fluid. At any rate, amniotic fluid seems to pass in and out of the lungs. Yet during gestation the lungs perform no other function.

Initiation of Respiration. With birth, however, profound changes occur. Now the lungs must exchange the oxygen and the carbon dioxide in the blood, work hitherto performed by the placenta. Exactly what initiates respiration is as yet unclear. It is believed to be a combination of physical, sensory and chemical factors, but precisely how each of these influences the other and to what degree is not known exactly. There is some evidence to indicate that the sudden change from the uterus to the air-breathing world produces enough physical stimulation to prompt respiration. It may be that the passive motion of the joints and the squeezing of the infant's thorax during delivery, as well as his spontaneous movements after birth, also contribute to minute ventilation and influence the other physical and sensory factors. It is worth noting in this regard that mothers of the various mammalian species, as they vigorously lick and cleanse their offspring after delivery, do, in fact, seem to apply a deliberate mechanical sensory stimulation to their young.

The chemical changes that occur in the blood as a result of the transitory asphyxia that occurs during delivery seem to be of paramount importance. These include a lowered oxygen level, an increased carbon dioxide level, and a lowered pH. If the asphyxia is prolonged, however, then depression of the respiratory center ensues rather than stimulation, and resuscitation is usually necessary (see Chap. 21). A vigorous infant often breathes seconds after birth and certainly within 1 minute of delivery.

A great effort is required to expand the lungs and to fill the collapsed alveoli. Surface tension in the respiratory tract as well as resistance in the lung tissue itself, the thorax, the diaphragm, and the respiratory muscles must be overcome. Moreover, any obstruction (i.e., mucus, etc.) in the air passages has to be cleared. The first active inspiration comes from a powerful contraction of the diaphragm, which creates a high negative intrathoracic pressure, causing a marked retraction of the ribs because of the pliability of the baby's thorax. This first inspiration distends the alveolar spaces which heretofore have been filled with fluid. Any remaining fluid that is left is reabsorbed rapidly if the pulmonary capillary blood flow is adequate, since it is hypotonic and passes easily into the capillaries. After several minutes of breathing, lung expansion should be complete.

Respiration in First and Second Periods of Reactivity. A healthy infant begins life with intense activity. This phase has been designated by some authorities as the 1st period of reactivity (see Suggested Reading). In this phase the infant exhibits outbursts of diffuse, purposeless movements which alternate with periods of relative immobility. At this time respiration is rapid (reaching as high as 80 breaths per minute), and there may be *transient* flaring of the alae nasi; retraction of the chest and grunting are not uncommon. Tachycardia also is present, at times reaching 180 beats per minute in the first minutes of life and thereafter falling to an average of 120 to 140 beats per minute.

After this initial response the baby becomes relatively quiet and does not respond intensely to either internal or external stimuli. He relaxes and may fall asleep. His first sleep occurs on an average of 2 hours after birth and may last anywhere from a few minutes to 2 to 4 hours.

When he awakes, he is again hyperresponsive to stimuli, and he begins his 2nd period of reactivity. His color may change rapidly (from pink to moderately cyanotic), and his heart rate responds to stimulation, becoming rapid. Oral mucus may be a major problem in respiration during this period. Choking, gagging and regurgitation alert the nurse to the presence of mucus, and appropriate intervention must be taken (see Chap. 21). Since the length of the 2nd period of reactivity is variable, the nurse must be particularly alert for the first 12 to 18 hours of the infant's life.

Character of Normal Respiration. As the infant adapts successfully to extra-uterine life, his respiration usually ranges from 35 to 50 breaths per minute. They are easily altered by internal and external stimuli. Normally, his respiration is quiet and shallow. This can be observed most accurately by watching the movement of the abdomen, since his respiratory activity is carried out largely by the diaphragm and the abdominal muscles. Periods of dyspnea and cyanosis may occur suddenly in an infant who is breathing normally (even after the transition period and after several days). This *may* indicate some anomaly or other pathologic condition and should be reported promptly. Therefore, the nurse should notify the physician if the respiration drops below 35 or increases beyond 50 when the infant is at rest, or if dyspnea or cyanosis occurs.

Circulatory Changes

The anatomic changes that occur with birth have been discussed previously in Chapter 4. The nurse will recall that a rapid change takes place, with oxygenated blood being distributed in a manner similar to that of circulation in an adult.

Total Blood Volume. The amount of time between birth and the clamping of the umbilical cord is an important factor in determining the amount of the infant's total blood volume. For instance, the baby receives an additional 50 to 100 cc. of blood if the cord is clamped and cut after pulsations have ceased. This is due to the fact that as the uterus contracts, it pumps blood from the placenta into the baby's circulation. The increased blood volume is quickly readjusted through the elimination of excess fluid.

The peripheral circulation of the newborn is somewhat sluggish. It is felt that this accounts for the residual cyanosis of the infant's hands, feet and circumoral area. The nurse will note that these areas often remain mildly cyanotic for 1 or 2 hours after delivery. The general circulatory lability probably accounts for the mottled appearance of the baby's skin when it is exposed to air and for the "chilliness" of the infant's hands and feet.

The pulse rate, like the rate of respiration, also is labile and generally follows a pattern similar to that of the respiration. When the respiration is rapid, the pulse tends to be rapid; similarly, when the respiration slows down, so does the pulse. As previously stated, the pulse is affected by both internal and external stimuli, and thus the nurse can be more accurate if she counts the *apical* pulse rate while the baby is quiet. The normal rate is usually 120 to 150 beats per minute, but it may rise to 180 with crying and other intense activity. When the infant is asleep, the rate may range from 70 to 90 beats per minute.

The blood pressure is characteristically low, being around 80/46 at birth and rising to 100/50 by the 10th day. Since the extremities of the newborn are so small, accurate auscultation is difficult. If any accuracy is to be obtained, proper equipment is essential. A cuff 1 inch wide should be used and should cover two thirds of the upper arm or thigh.

Erythrocyte Count and Hemoglobin Concentration. The newborn infant has a much higher erythrocyte and hemoglobin level than an adult. The erythrocyte level ranges between 5,000,000 and 7,000,000 per microliter, and the hemoglobin level is usually 15 to 20 Gm. per 100 ml. of blood. These higher rates are needed by the baby in utero for adequate oxygenation. After birth the need no longer exists, since the lungs are functioning, and a gradual decrease takes place, particularly during the 2nd and the 3rd weeks of life. There is usually a slight *increase* in these concentrations on the 1st and the 2nd postnatal days; this is due in part to the extra amount of blood received through delayed clamping of the cord and to the subsequent readjustment of the blood volume. The gradual decrease in the erythrocyte count and the hemoglobin concentration results in a "physiologic" neonatal anemia, which disappears spontaneously. Clinical symptoms usually do not appear (except in cases of nutritional problems and/or infection), and no therapy is needed. The lowest counts are reached when the infant is 3 months old, when the hemoglobin level ranges between 11 and 12 Gm. per 100 ml. of blood, and the erythrocyte count between 4,000,000 and 4,300,000 per microliter; after that there is a gradual increase.

PHYSIOLOGIC JAUNDICE. Another effect of the destruction of the red blood cells is the so-called physiologic jaundice which usually is seen on the 2nd or the 3rd day of life. It is thought that an increase in serum bilirubin results from the breakdown of the red blood cells, and this, together with a temporary inability to remove the bilirubin, results in the jaundice. The condition usually begins to sub-

side on the 6th or the 7th day, and it should disappear by the 2nd week of life. A bilirubin concentration of 13 mg. per 100 ml. of blood is beyond the physiologic limit and a total serum bilirubin above 18 to 20 mg. per 100 ml. is termed hyperbilirubinemia (see Chap. 21). Since the physiologic jaundice does not usually manifest itself until the infant is 2 or 3 days old, the nurse must be alert for any signs of jaundice before that time, especially in the first 24 hours of the baby's life. This latter type of jaundice is generally pathologic and should be reported immediately so that treatment can be instituted.

Blood Coagulation. Immediately after birth the intestinal tract of the infant does not harbor the bacteria necessary to help to synthesize the very important substance, vitamin K. In addition, other substances important in blood coagulation are manufactured in the liver and are under the influence of vitamin K; these substances are temporarily diminished. Thus the infant suffers from a transitory deficiency in blood coagulation. This condition occurs between the 2nd and the 5th postnatal days and returns to normal spontaneously in several more days. Some physicians feel that this deficiency can be minimized or prevented by the administration of a small dose of vitamin K_1 at the time of birth (see Chaps. 12 and 21).

White Blood Cells. The normal newborn has a wide range in the total number of white blood cells. A leukocytosis (15,000 to 45,000 cells per microliter) is present at birth, with polymorphonuclear cells accounting for a large percentage of the total count. During the first few days after delivery there is a considerable decrease in the total count, as well as a shift in the type of predominating cell. The polymorphonuclear neutrophils decrease, and the lymphocytes increase, so that by the end of the 1st week the lymphocytes predominate.

Temperature Regulation and Metabolic Changes

The temperature-regulating mechanism of the newborn infant is not fully developed at birth; thus his heat production is somewhat low, and he responds readily to environmental heat and cold stimuli. At birth his body temperature is assumedly the same or higher than that of his mother; however, with his entry into the air-breathing world, it may drop 1 or 2 degrees in spite of the application of external heat and blankets. With chilling the drop is even more precipitous and dangerous for the baby. If the infant is given adequate covering and protection, the temperature soon begins to rise, and it returns to normal in about 8 hours. The nurse should keep in mind how easily the infant responds to environmental cold and heat and avoid subjecting the baby to wide variations in temperature.

Basal Metabolism. Since the surface area of the newborn is large in comparison with his weight, his basal metabolism per Kg. of body weight is higher than that of an adult.

Thus his CALORIC REQUIREMENTS are high during infancy. About 50 to 55 calories per pound of body weight per day suffice in the beginning. However, because of the increase in activity during the neonatal period and the energy requirements needed for the baby's rapid growth at this time, an increase in the caloric requirements may be needed after several days. Caloric needs will vary a good deal, even for infants of the same age and weight.

Activity seems to be a determining factor. An infant who moves about a good deal, cries, etc., will need more calories than his more phlegmatic counterpart. The infant's caloric needs usually are based on weight-gain, well-being and satiety. A caloric intake of about 110 to 120 calories per Kg. of body weight per day (50 to 55 calories per pound per day) is usual after the first few days.

The infant's FLUID REQUIREMENT also is greater per Kg. of body weight than that of an adult. This is due to his increased muscular activity, caloric intake and basal metabolism.

Transitory Fever of the Newborn. This condition sometimes occurs between the 2nd and the 4th days of life. It is caused by a low fluid intake and the usual fluid loss that occurs in the immediate postnatal period. The temperature may rise as high as 38.9° to 40° C. (102° to 104° F.), the skin is dry, the fontanels may be depressed, the urinary output may be decreased, and a weight loss may occur. This condition is found most often in infants who do not take their feedings well (or who do not suck well) or in those who take only small, infrequent feedings. Both the fever and the sub-

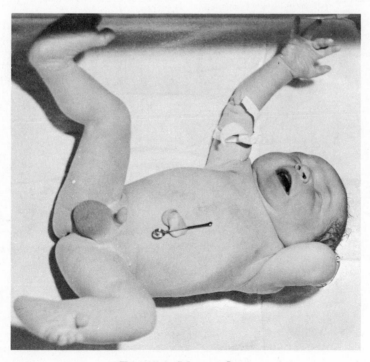

Fig. 15-2. Moro reflex.

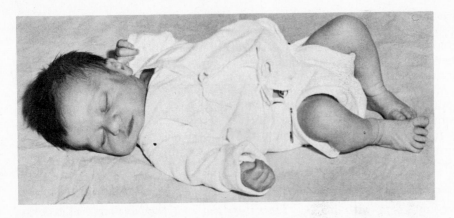

FIG. 15-3. Tonic neck reflex.

sequent side-effects can be remedied by increasing oral feedings, i.e, giving the baby water between milk feedings or administering parenteral fluids.

Neurologic Changes

The nervous system of the newborn is immature; that is, it is neither anatomically nor

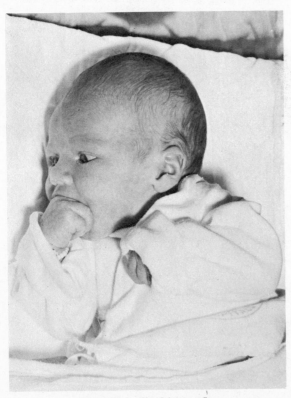

FIG. 15-4. Sucking reflex.

physiologically fully developed. Although all neurons are present, many remain immature for several months, and some, for years. Thus, the infant is uncoordinated in his movements, is labile in his temperature regulation, and has poor control over his musculature: he "startles" easily, is subject to tremors of the extremities, etc. During the neonatal period, however, development is rapid, and as the various nerve pathways controlling the muscles are used, the nerve fibers connect with one another. Gradually, more complex patterns of behavior emerge, and the higher cerebral levels begin to function.

Reflexes are important indices of the baby's normal development, for their presence or absence at certain times reflects the extent of normality in the functioning of the central nervous system.

The *Moro* or *startle reflex* (Fig. 15-2) indicates an awareness of equilibrium in the newborn. This reflex should be elicited when the baby is lying quiet. A sudden stimulus such as a change in position, a jarring of the crib, a jerking of the blanket or clothes, or even a loud noise (which jars his position) causes the baby to draw up his legs, to bring his arms forward in an embracing motion, and usually to cry. The movements should be symmetrical. If they are not, injury to the part that lags should be suspected. The Moro reflex should be present at birth; normally it disappears by 3 months of age. If it cannot be elicited at birth, edema of the brain may be present and/or injury to the brain. As the edema subsides, the reflex returns, and it should be demonstrable on the day following delivery. If frank brain damage has occurred, the reflex will be absent for several days; if the damage is not too severe, the reflex will return in 3 or 4 days. Occasionally, the reflex is present at birth but disappears over the first days. Increasing cerebral edema or slow intracranial hemorrhage then are suspected.

When the *tonic neck reflex* is elicited, the infant assumes a "fencing" position; that is, he lies on his back with his head rotated to one side. The arm and the leg on the side to which he is facing are partially or completely extended, and the opposite arm and leg are flexed (Fig. 15-3). This reflex also disappears in a few months, since it is another manifestation of the immaturity of the newborn's nervous system.

Several reflexes are involved in feeding. The *rooting reflex* causes the baby to turn his head toward anything that touches his cheek. This is helpful when he is searching for food. Brushing his cheek with the mother's breast, for example, enables him to find the nipple for nursing. The *sucking reflex* (Fig. 15-4) stimulates sucking movements whenever anything brushes the infant's lips. Normally, this reflex is present at birth and accompanies the *swallowing reflex*, absence of which indicates im-

maturity, narcosis, brain injury or retardation. Moreover, if it is not stimulated, it ceases to exist. The *gag reflex* operates when the infant takes more into his mouth than he can swallow. He can cough or hiccup a little if fluid does go "down the wrong way."

Since the infant is not well coordinated, he may have difficulty in bringing several of these reflexes into play at the proper moment, and he will need help from his mother or nurse. For instance, he may succeed in finding the nipple when he attempts to nurse, but if he gets the nipple under his tongue, successful sucking and swallowing are inhibited. It is important that the mother understand these feeding reflexes, so that she can help her infant. Often the inexperienced mother, in her anxiety to assist the infant to nurse, attempts to turn his head toward the breast by pushing on his cheek. The rooting reflex therefore is elicited, and the infant promptly turns his head in the opposite direction. This causes no end of consternation for both mother and baby.

The *grasp reflex* (Fig. 15-5) is present at birth in both the hands and the feet. The infant will grasp any object placed in his hands,

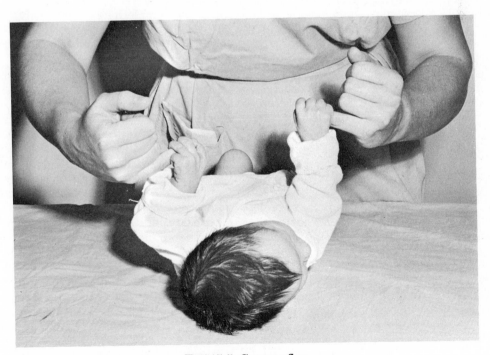

FIG. 15-5. Grasp reflex.

cling briefly, and then let go. Even at birth he may be able to hold onto an adult's forefinger so securely that he can be lifted to a standing position. Although the baby cannot actually grasp with his feet, stroking the soles causes the toes to turn downward as though trying to grasp. The grasping movements are a reflex action at birth, but with practice and experience they soon become voluntary and purposeful.

The *stepping* or *dancing reflex* is another action that is present at birth but soon disappears. This reflex causes the infant to make little stepping or prancing movements when he is held upright with his feet touching a surface. After this reflex diminishes, the infant will not attempt stepping motions until he is ready to stand and to walk. However, he does exercise the leg muscles a great deal and seems to derive a great deal of enjoyment from waving and kicking his legs about.

The next group of reflexes might be termed protective since they are necessary and at times essential to the preservation of the newborn's safety. The *blinking reflex* occurs when the infant is subjected to a bright light. The *cough and the sneeze reflexes* clear his respiratory passages. The *yawn reflex* draws in additional oxygen. These, together with the infant's ability to cry when uncomfortable, to withdraw from painful stimuli, to resist restraint, etc., are all defensive measures. As the baby grows and develops, these together with the other reflexes mentioned either diminish or become more highly developed according to the need. Thus, the infant's behavior patterns become more complex and highly developed.

Gastrointestinal Changes

It is well for the nurse to remember that the newborn, to be able to swallow, must have his food placed well back on his tongue, since he does not have the ability to transfer food from his lips to his pharynx. This means that the nipple should be placed well inside the infant's mouth. Sucking is facilitated by strong sucking muscles and ridges or corrugations in the anterior portion of the mouth. In addition, the *sucking pads* (deposits of fatty tissue in each cheek) prevent the collapse of the cheeks during nursing and further make sucking effective. This fatty tissue remains (even when fat is lost from the rest of the body) until sucking

is no longer essential to the baby's getting food. The salivary glands are immature at birth and manufacture little saliva until the infant is about the age of 3 months.

Stomach, Intestines, Digestion. The capacity of the newborn's stomach is rather difficult to measure, since the feedings may empty easily into the duodenum even before the feeding is completed. The capacity has been estimated to be approximately 50 to 60 cc. The cardiac sphincter is not as well developed as the pyloric sphincter, and hence the baby should be "bubbled" several times during the feeding so that any swallowed air can be eructed.

The newborn's intestinal tract is proportionately longer than that of an adult. Although it contains a large amount of secretory glands and a large surface for absorption, its elastic tissue and musculature are poor and not fully developed. Furthermore, nervous control is variable and inadequate. Nevertheless, the infant digests and absorbs a tremendous amount of food in proportion to his body weight.

Most of the digestive enzymes seem to be present and adequate, with the exception of pancreatic amylase and lipase. These last are somewhat deficient for several months but eventually reach a normal amount. The infant can digest simple foods more easily, but has a difficult time with the more complex starches. Protein and carbohydrates are easily absorbed, but fat absorption is poor.

REGURGITATION; VOMITING. The nurse and the mother will note that often the baby regurgitates (spits up) soon after a feeding. Sometimes regurgitation happens as long as 60 minutes after a feeding. This occurs because of the imperfect control of the cardiac sphincter and the immaturity of the nervous control. Activity also seems to be implicated, since the more active infant tends to spit up more often and for longer periods than the more quiet infant. The condition can be minimized by bubbling the infant well during and after feedings and by avoiding overfeeding. Handling the infant gently (and as little as possible) after feedings and placing him on his right side with his head and trunk elevated slightly also are helpful measures.

Occasionally, actual vomiting occurs during the first several days after birth. It is felt that this may be due to the secretions and material that were swallowed by the infant during delivery. Another cause is the swallowing of air by the infant during a feeding. This condition should subside within 2 or 3 days (with proper feeding, bubbling and positioning) and requires no special treatment. If the condition persists, however, or if the vomiting is of a projectile nature, then the physician should be notified immediately (see Chap. 21).

Stools. The baby's stools change daily during the first week of life, and their changes and amount should be recorded accurately (see p. 383).

Kidney Function and Urinary Excretion

The kidneys of the newborn function quite efficiently at birth. During fetal life, even though the placenta takes care of waste excretion, they become functional, and urine can be found in the bladder of the fetus as early as the 4th month of gestation. Excretion begins during the 9th week of gestation. Since the baby has urine in his bladder at birth, he may void at delivery; but sometimes urination is delayed for as long as 12 to 24 hours. Voidings during the first days after birth may be scanty and somewhat infrequent (unless edema is present) until feeding increases the fluid intake and consequent output. The number and the amount of voidings gradually increase until the infant is urinating as many as 30 times a day after the immediate postnatal period (see p. 384). With the development of bladder control, the frequency again decreases. The urine of the newborn (after the first voiding) has a high specific gravity and may appear to be quite cloudy due to the mucus and urate content as well as its high concentration. As the infant takes an increasing amount of fluid, the specific gravity gradually drops, and the cloudiness disappears, leaving the urine the usual straw color and almost odorless. Uric acid excretion is high in the newborn period, and this substance, when excreted on the diaper, may appear as reddish or "brick-dust" stains. Since the material looks like blood, it is sometimes thought that the infant is suffering from hematuria (see p. 384).

Changes in Hepatic Function

During fetal life the liver has performed an important role in blood formation, and it is thought that it continues this function to some degree after birth. Later in the neonatal period it produces substances that are essential in the coagulation of the blood (see p. 354). If the mother's iron intake has been adequate during pregnancy, enough iron will be stored in the infant's liver to carry him over the first months of life when his diet (primarily milk) is iron-deficient. About the 5th month, however, the baby's iron reserve is depleted, and unless foods containing iron are given, a deficiency will ensue.

CHARACTERISTICS OF THE NEWBORN

Immediately after birth or within the next few hours the physician will give the infant a complete physical examination. This usually includes: head (fontanels, overriding of skull bones), eyes, mouth (palate, gums, tongue), heart, lungs, abdomen, extremities, genitalia and anus. The measurements of the infant are noted, such as the circumference of the head and the shoulders, and the weight and the length. The average full-term boy baby weighs from 7 to 7½ pounds (about 3,300 Gm.) at birth; girl babies weigh a little less. The average length of a full-term infant at birth is about 20 inches (51 cm.).

The physician will scrutinize the infant carefully for any deformity (e.g., cleft palate, clubfoot), injury (e.g., cephalhematoma, fracture of the clavicle) or abnormality (e.g., tonguetie, phimosis). If a malformation or an injury is found, the physician will advise concerning the infant's care and will assume the responsibility for telling the parents about their baby.

General Appearance

The nurse should be familiar with the characteristics of the normal newborn so that she can distinguish them from the abnormal. For example, certain symptoms which might be cause for concern in an older child, e.g., rapid rate and rhythm of respiration, when observed in a newborn infant, may merely represent normal neonatal physiology. Also, it is well for the nurse to take a look at him from the standpoint of how he appears to his mother. The healthy newborn infant has many characteristics which momentarily may look unusual to her. The nurse should be ready to

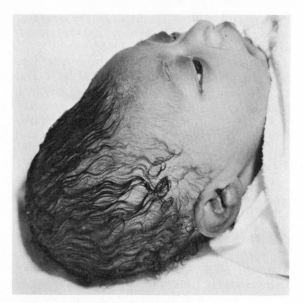

Fig. 15-6. Molding of the head.

talk with the mother about her baby and to answer her questions. A daily inspection sponge bath affords the nurse an excellent opportunity to observe the infant's anatomy and behavior, and thus to become familiar with the infant (see p. 380).

Position and Movements. The newborn infant usually lies with his arms and legs flexed, or tending to imitate the position that he has been accustomed to in utero. When the infant is awake, he sucks, yawns, sneezes, blinks and stretches. His movements for the most part are purposeless. For the first day or two he sleeps most of the time, but even while he is relaxed and quiet, he occasionally may exhibit some coarse, jerky movements. During the first few weeks of life he may lie with his head turned to one side and the arm and leg on that side extended, while the other arm and leg are drawn up (tonic neck reflex). If he is awakened suddenly or startled by jarring or a loud noise, he will thrust his arms out in an "embracing motion" (Moro reflex).

Head. The infant's head is large, comprising about one quarter of his size, and with cephalic presentations may initially appear to be asymmetrical because of the molding of the skull bones during labor. The suture lines between the skull bones and the anterior and the posterior fontanels can be palpated easily (Fig.

5-1). When the nurse's hand is passed over the fontanels, the areas should feel soft but neither bulged nor depressed. The anterior fontanel, the diamond-shaped and larger of the two (normally 2 to 3 cm. wide and 3 to 4 cm. long), may feel smaller for the first several days when there is marked overriding of the skull bones. The posterior fontanel is triangular in shape and is located between the occipital and the parietal bones. It is smaller than the anterior fontanel and may be almost closed at birth. Occasionally, the scalp is covered with a thick growth of hair which sheds for the most part before the permanent hair appears.

The face is small and round, and the lower jaw appears to recede.

Eyes and Visual Perception. The eyes are closed much of the time but will open spontaneously if the infant's head is lifted (a valuable point to remember when one wants to inspect the eyes). Recent research[2] has indicated that the infant from birth can see and discriminate patterns as the basis for form perception. This capacity is rather limited by imperfect oculomotor coordination and inability to accommodate for varying distances. Moreover, the eye, the usual pathways and the visual part of the brain are poorly developed at birth. Nevertheless, although the baby's vision is much less acute than an adult's, a good deal of visual experience is possible for him. Visual patterning seems to be particularly stimulating or interesting to him, more so than color or brightness alone. For instance, he will show a preference for a face or a solid object rather than a blob of light or a bright color. Thus, even the newborn sees a patterned and organized world which he explores discriminatingly (albeit with his limited means). When and how his visual contact with environment makes a lasting impression on his behavior remain topics for future research. Most mothers do not realize that their infant can see as well as he does, and they appreciate being informed of this fact. In addition, some mothers become exceedingly anxious when they observe strabismus or nystagmus in their infants, but they should be reassured that this

[2] Fantz, R. L.: Pattern discrimination and selective attention as determinants of perceptual development from birth *in* Kidd, A. H., and Rivoire, J. L. (eds.): Perceptual Development in Children, New York, International Universities Press, 1965.

lack of coordination is normal during the first few months of life.

All babies' eyes are blue or a slatey gray color at birth. By the time that the infant is 3 months old, they have achieved their permanent color, although complete pigmentation of the iris does not occur until the infant is about 1 year of age. Since the lacrimal glands are not functioning at birth, the baby does not shed tears when he cries. Tears do not appear for several weeks and sometimes for several months. There may be some edema of the lids and/or purulent discharge caused by the silver nitrate (see p. 375). The changes in the vascular tension of the eyes during delivery sometimes cause small areas of subconjunctival hemorrhage. These areas disappear spontaneously in 1 or 2 weeks and are not significant.

Ears and Hearing. The ear and the nerve tracts for hearing are anatomically mature at birth, and the newborn can hear after his first cry. Hearing apparently becomes acute within several days as the eustachian tubes become aerated, and the mucus in the middle ear disappears.

Lips, Mouth, Cheeks. The lips are sensitive to touch, and any stimulation of this nature usually elicits the sucking reflex. Moreover, the rooting reflex is well developed, so that when the cheek is stroked on one side the infant will turn his head in that direction. In conjunction with sucking, a labial tubercle may be present on the center of the upper lip, as well as the sucking pads (fat) in the cheeks. At this time the tongue does not extend far beyond the margin of the gums because the frenum is normally short. A mother's concern that her baby is tonguetied is usually unwarranted.

Body; Skin. The infant's neck is short. His chest is round and slightly smaller in circumference than his head. The breasts may be engorged initially and may even secrete "witch's milk." This condition, like menstruation, a vaginal tag or enlarged labia in girl babies, is due to a hormonal factor and without interference will disappear spontaneously. In boy babies the scrotum appears to be relatively large, and the prepuce is long and adherent to the glans penis (this separates in several months). The abdomen is round and protruding due to the relative size of the abdominal organs and weak muscular structures.

The respiratory movements are largely diaphragmatic, and breathing is rapid, shallow and irregular.

The infant's skin appears to be thin and delicate and is often dry and peeling. The baby's color may be pink, reddish or pale, becoming very ruddy when he cries. Initially, the hands and the feet are quite blue, due to the sluggish peripheral vascular circulation, but this cyanosis of the extremities soon disappears, often within a few hours. Vernix caseosa, a white cheesy material which has been a protection to the skin while the fetus is floating in amniotic fluid in the uterus, may be apparent, particularly in the creases of the body. Also, on the body there may be large areas of fine downy hair called lanugo. Milia may be present on the nose and the forehead, and small flat hemangiomas may be apparent on the nape of the neck, the eyelids or over the bridge of the nose. These so-called "stork bites," clusters of small capillaries, usually disappear spontaneously during infancy.

In nonwhite infants, dark bluish areas are usually apparent on the buttocks or the lower back. These "mongolian spots" have no relationship to mongolism and will disappear spontaneously during late infancy. A pilonidal "dimple" resulting from an irregular fold of skin sometimes is seen in the midline over the sacrococcygeal area.

Miscellaneous Conditions

At times the following conditions are seen in the normal newborn infant. Although they are not serious, they do represent some deviation from what is "usual." Moreover, they often cause concern in the parents; thus the nurse should be familiar with them so that she can answer any questions that the parents may have and give appropriate reassurance.

Icterus Neonatorum. This is an exceedingly common condition during the 1st week of life and, as the name implies, is characterized by jaundice. Physiologic jaundice is dependent on the normal neonatal rise in the serum bilirubin level (see p. 354). It makes its appearance, as a rule, on the 2nd or the 3rd day of life and disappears without treatment about the 6th or the 7th day. Almost 1 baby in 3 shows icterus, which often is due to physiologic jaundice. Most authorities attribute it to inadequate

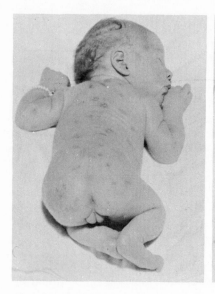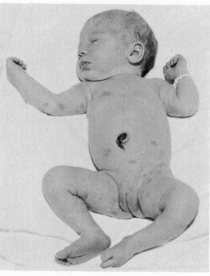

Fig. 15-7. Erythema toxicum. This "newborn rash" develops more frequently on the back, the shoulders and the buttocks. (MacDonald House, University Hospitals of Cleveland)

liver function and the destruction of red cells which takes place during the 1st week of life. The mother may be assured that the condition is due to a normal process and will clear up within a few days.

Erythema Toxicum. Sometimes referred to as the newborn rash, erythema toxicum is a blotchy erythematous rash which may appear in the first few days of life (Fig. 15-7). The erythematous areas, which develop more frequently on the back, the shoulders and the buttocks, have a small blanched wheal in the center. The cause of this skin disturbance is obscure, and no treatment is necessary. The

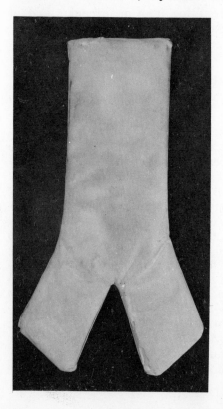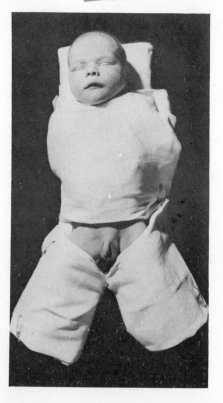

Fig. 15-8. Preparation of the infant, restrained for circumcision. (*Left*) Board, padded and covered with oilcloth, as used in many hospitals for circumcision. (*Right*) The infant, restrained on the board with towels, ready for circumcision.

Fig. 15-9. Technic of circumcision, using hemostat, scalpel and sutures. After cleansing penis and surrounding area, the prepuce is stripped back with the help of a partial dorsal slit (A to D). The prepuce is now clamped and excessive prepuce cut off (E). The suture material used is plain 00 or 000 catgut in a very small needle (F and G), but some physicians prefer silk.

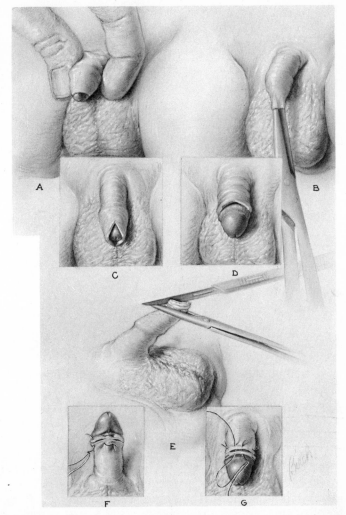

Fig. 15-10. Technic of circumcision with Yellen clamp. After cleansing area and stripping back prepuce as shown in Figure 15-9, the cone of the Yellen clamp is placed over the glans and the prepuce put on a stretch with sutures (A). The prepuce is now drawn through the beveled hole of platform (B). Screwing down clamp crushes prepuce, producing hemostasis. Three to 5 minutes of such pressure is necessary to prevent subsequent bleeding. The excess of the prepuce is then cut away (C) and the clamp removed (D). (Yellen, H. S.: Am. J. Obst. & Gynec. 30:146)

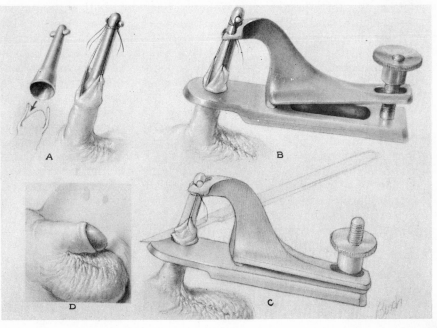

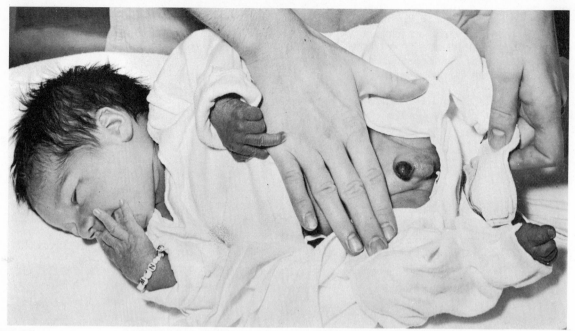

FIG. 15-11. Postcircumcision inspection for bleeding.

rash is transient and likely to change appreciably within a few hours, and it may disappear entirely within a day or so.

Milia are pinpoint-sized pearly white spots which occur commonly on the nose and the forehead of the newborn infant. When touched gently with the tip of the finger, these spots feel like tiny, firm seeds. They are due to retention of sebaceous material within the sebaceous glands, and if they are left alone, will usually disappear spontaneously during the neonatal period. Mothers often mistake milia for "whiteheads" and may attempt to squeeze them if the nurse or the physician has not warned them against such practice.

Phimosis. In many male infants the orifice in the foreskin of the penis is so small that the foreskin cannot be pushed back over the glans. This condition is known as phimosis. Although it is rarely of sufficient degree to obstruct the outflow of urine or to cause any immediate symptoms, it is undesirable because it prevents proper cleanliness. Phimosis may be corrected either by stretching the orifice of the foreskin with a hemostat, or by circumcision. Both of these procedures are carried out by the physician, but sometimes the nurse is asked to stretch the foreskin gently every day

after having first received detailed instructions from the physician. Preparation of an infant for circumcision, two common methods of performing the operation, and also postcircumcision inspection are depicted in Figures 15-8 to 11.

Breast Engorgement. Engorgement of the breasts is common during the neonatal period in both male and female infants (Fig. 15-12). It is due to the same causes that bring about mammary engorgement in the mother—that is, endocrine influence. In the case of the infant, its breasts have been acted on throughout pregnancy by the estrogenic hormone which passes to it through the placenta from the mother. This is the same hormone which prepares the mother's breasts for lactation. When it is withdrawn after birth, changes in the infant's breasts take place similar to those in the mother.

Mammary engorgement in the newborn subsides without treatment, but sometimes it persists for 2 or 3 weeks.

Menstruation occasionally occurs in newborn girls and is due to estrogenic hormone, as just described. It usually amounts only to slight spotting and need cause no special concern.

Fig. 15-12. Hypertrophy of breast in infant developing in the neonatal period.

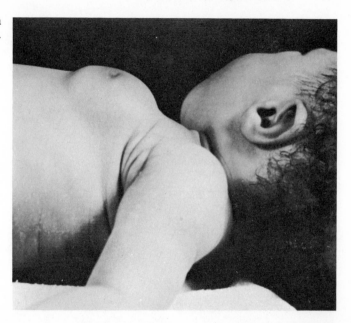

THE ENVIRONMENT OF THE NEWBORN

Prevention of Infection

The prevention of infection is of paramount importance in caring for the newborn. Everyone who is in contact with infants must assume this responsibility; this includes parents as well as personnel. Staff should take special care to instruct parents so that their activities conform to the prevention of infection. The basis of "good" technic in handling the infant is thorough hand washing with an antiseptic detergent or a soap (or detergent) containing hexachlorophene. Some institutions require scrubbing with a brush; others feel that detergent, water and friction are sufficient. Whichever the procedure, meticulous hand washing is essential, whether the infant is cared for in the central or regular nursery or in a rooming-in situation. The parents and the staff should be especially careful to wash their hands before a feeding and after a diaper change. The parents will need instruction about the importance (and technic) of proper hand washing, and reinforcement should be given as necessary during the hospital stay.

As with personnel in the delivery room (see Chap. 12), all nursery staff should have a pre-employment physical examination and a yearly physical examination thereafter to minimize the possibility of spreading infection from the staff among the newborn. In addition, any staff member who contracts *any* infection, i.e., respiratory, gastrointestinal, skin lesions, etc., should remain away from the nursery and contact with the newborn until the infection is gone *completely*.

If the mother manifests signs of infection and has been in contact with her infant, the infant will be isolated from the other babies (usually in the isolation or observation nursery) and will be removed from the mother's presence until her disorder is treated and cleared. Since the mother may be concerned about being separated from her baby and miss him, the importance of the precautions should be explained thoroughly. If the mother is concerned about continuing breast-feeding (and her condition permits), her breasts can be pumped to ensure stimulation and a continued supply of milk. Her milk is discarded, however, as an added precaution, until her infection subsides. The mother who has not had contact with her infant before she evidences signs of infection, also will be separated from her infant, and the foregoing explanation and management of feeding is applicable to her also.

Babies who are delivered outside a hospital environment are not admitted to the regular newborn nursery. They usually are cared for in

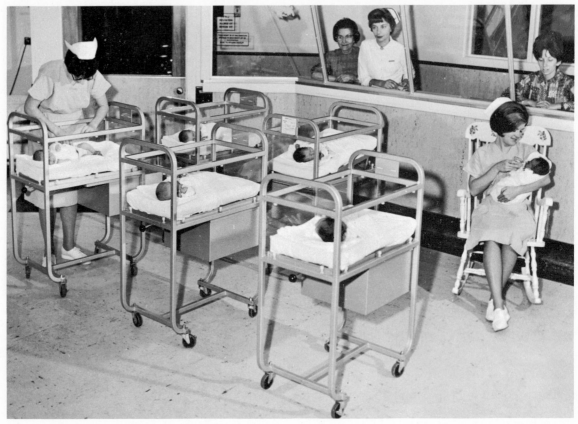

Fig. 15-13. The central nursery. (MacDonald House, University Hospitals of Cleveland, Cleveland, Ohio)

the observation nursery or with the mother in a rooming-in situation.

To further reduce the hazards of infection from outside sources, the number of visitors may be restricted in the maternity area, and no visitors are allowed in the nursery proper. Children also are excluded from the maternity unit, since various infections and particularly communicable diseases are so prevalent among them. To ensure cleanliness further, members of the staff wear special gowns when they care for infants. These gowns should be short-sleeved so that a thorough scrub or wash may be given the hands, the forearms and the elbows, and the gowns should be changed for each "shift" and more frequently if soiled. Masks are no longer worn, since they must be changed every 20 to 30 minutes to be effective, and, in fact, they can become a reservoir of bacteria when not applied and changed prop-

erly. Occasionally, the mother will be instructed to wear a mask in tending the baby if she has had a recent cold, or if she develops a cold when she goes home. The nurse should make certain that she understands the principles underlying the application and the wearing of the mask and especially that she be aware of how her hands can be contaminated in adjusting and tying it. Even at home a clean mask should be worn each time the need arises, and the mother should be instructed to wash her hands each time after she adjusts it.

Types of Care for the Newborn

The Central Nursery System. The central or general newborn nursery on the postpartal division is designed for the care of a variable number of healthy newborn infants (Fig. 15-13). In this system the infants are brought to their mothers at certain specified times during the day—generally for feeding and/or visiting. The staff assumes the responsibility for all the care of the babies. Some authorities feel that the separation of mother and child (and husband) in this manner results in an unnatural fragmentation of the family at a momentous time for building family unity (see Suggested Reading). Also with the emergence of the many drug-resistant organisms that abound in the hospital environment, the danger of epidemics (whenever a large aggregate of persons collect) is enhanced. Certainly, in a central nursery system the contact among the mother, the infant and the father is not as extensive as it would be in a rooming-in plan.

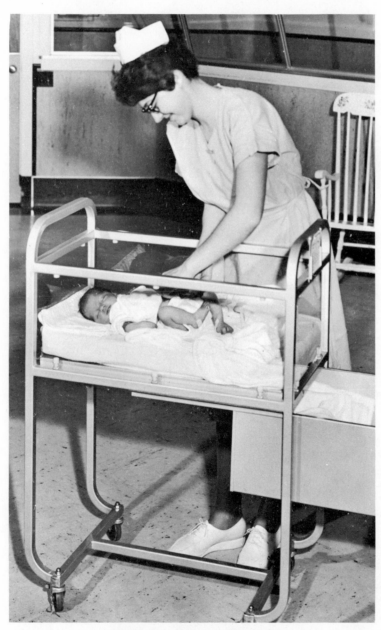

Fig. 15-14. Self-contained crib.

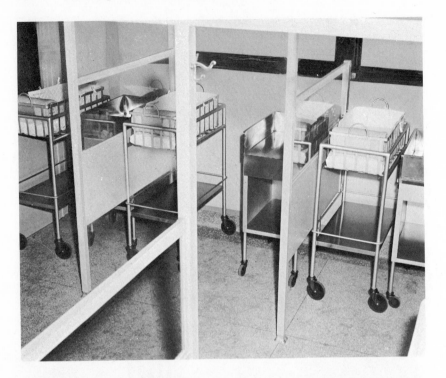

FIG. 15-15. Observation nursery with cubicles which provide complete isolation for each infant. Each unit is complete, containing all the equipment necessary for the care of the baby. (Margaret Hague Maternity Hospital, Jersey City, N. J.)

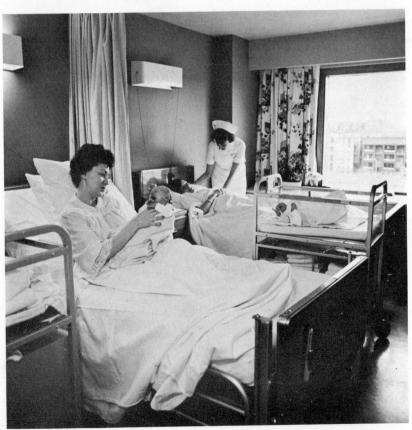

FIG. 15-16. Rooming-in 2-bed unit. (Cleveland Clinic, Cleveland, Ohio)

Fig. 15-17. Rooming-in unit. Mother feeding her baby. (Cleveland Clinic, Cleveland, Ohio)

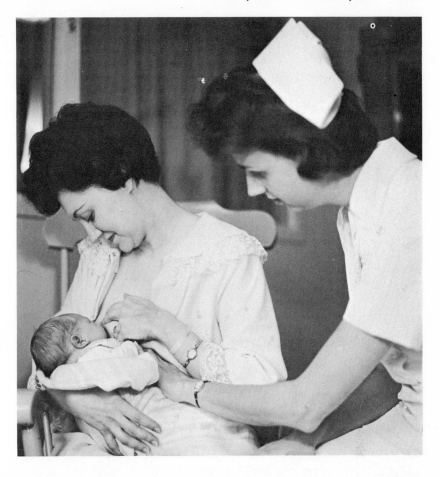

However, the hospital's physical plant may make a central nursery arrangement the only type feasible. Moreover, some mothers prefer the type of care that is given under a central nursery system for a variety of reasons. At any rate, some type of central nursery usually is found in most hospitals. Control of the physical facilities and stringent personnel policies accomplish a good deal of protection of the newborn so managed. For instance, cribs should be placed at least 2 feet apart with 3-feet-wide aisles between the cribs. Limiting the number of infants in a nursery from 8 to 12 also is helpful. Requiring all personnel to put on clean gowns before entering the nursery, limiting the number of individuals who may enter the nursery, and requiring strict adherence to nursery aseptic technic on the part of nursery personnel, all aid in protecting the infants. Washing the hands and arms to the elbows and scrubbing the fingernails thoroughly be-

fore entering the nursery, as well as washing the hands carefully before and after handling each baby, afford additional protection.

The central nursery is a so-called "clean" nursery. But it must be understood that there is a difference in nursery technic between what is considered to be "nursery clean" and what is considered to be "baby clean," i.e., what is clean for an individual baby. There should be no common equipment, such as a common bath table, used in providing care for the babies. There should be provisions in the nursery so that individual technic can be followed. Each infant should have his own crib and general supplies (Fig. 15-14), so that he can be given such care as his daily inspection bath or be diapered or dressed in his own bed. Most cribs are constructed with a built-in cabinet for the infant's own supplies (clean diapers, shirts and linens) and a drawer to hold the containers for cotton balls, safety pins, ther-

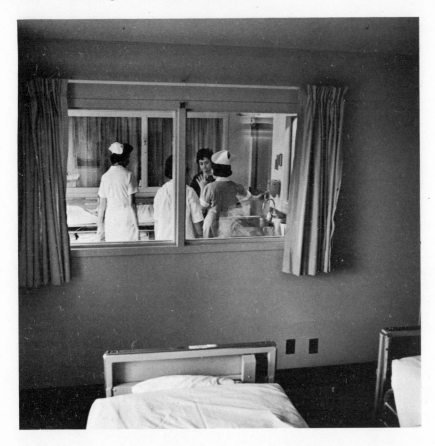

mometer, etc. When such cribs are not available, improvised units for the infant's crib should be obtained so that individual-care technic can be carried out.

If there is any evidence of a questionable infection at the time of delivery, if the infant is born on the way to the hospital, or if the infant is suspected of having an infection of the eyes, the skin, the mouth or the gastrointestinal tract, the infant should not be admitted to the central nursery.

Observation Nursery. Maternity hospitals should have an observation nursery where infants suspected of developing an infectious condition may be kept until the presence or absence of infection is determined (Fig. 15-15). When a definite diagnosis of infection is made, the infant must be transferred immediately to an isolation nursery away from the maternity division.

Aside from the fact that infants in the "suspect" or observation nursery must be

segregated apart from others, and naturally require closer supervision and care because of suspected infection, their nursing care otherwise should be like that given a healthy newborn infant.

Rooming-in. This term has been applied to the plan of having the new infant share his mother's hospital unit so that they may be cared for together. This type of arrangement has come to mean much more than caring for the mother and the infant in the same unit of space. Rather, it implies an attitude in maternal and infant care that supports parental education and is based on recognition and understanding of the needs of each mother, infant and family. Rooming-in often is discussed as if it were a modern innovation. Historically, however, all mothers back to paleolithic times "roomed-in" until the central nursery was instituted during the first 2 decades of the 20th century (see Suggested Reading). Nevertheless, rooming-in as it is practiced today does represent a departure from

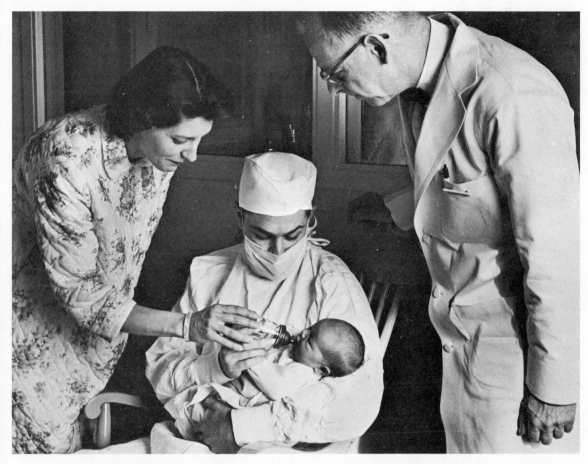

Fig. 15-19. Rooming-in unit. Mother is assisting father to feed his baby as physician observes. (Cleveland Clinic, Cleveland, Ohio)

the concept of the "traditional" central nursery.

Attitudes in maternal and infant care have changed, in part because of increased insight into the needs of the mother, her baby and the family as a unit. Rooming-in plays an important part in the family-centered approach to maternity care, for it not only provides an environment which fosters a wholesome, natural mother-child relationship from the very beginning, but it also affords unlimited opportunities for the parents to learn about the care of their baby.

To have a rooming-in program function successfully requires administrative planning and sound preparation of the entire hospital staff and the parents who use it. Generally, it demands a different architectural arangement.

Adequate space must be allowed for the mother's unit to accommodate the regular equipment needed for her, as well as that needed for the infant's care. Different physical plans for rooming-in arrangements have been developed, some units to accommodate one mother, others for as many as 4 of them. Each rooming-in unit should have an adjoining nursery and its own workroom. Where it has not been feasible to make major changes in the physical plan of a maternity hospital to provide for continuous rooming-in, some hospitals have adopted a modified rooming-in program, providing extended time for the mother and her baby to be together during the day but otherwise utilizing the central nursery.

The newborn infant must be protected from sources of infection regardless of where he is

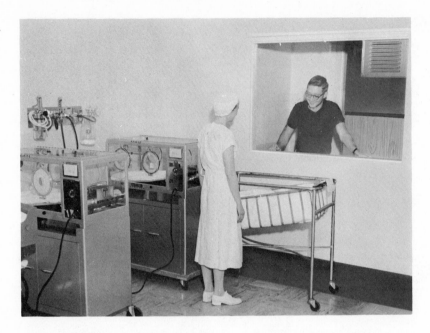

FIG. 15-20. A father sees his new baby immediately after delivery through the viewing window of the receiving nursery. The crib is tilted to keep the infant in Trendelenburg position for the first 12 hours after delivery. (MacDonald House, The University Hospitals of Cleveland, Cleveland, Ohio)

cared for. The same basic principles for asepsis employed in the nursery must be followed in infant care in the rooming-in unit. Some years ago Dr. Edith Jackson said that it was possible to provide "the essential psychological satisfactions" which the mother and baby derive from a rooming-in experience "without losing the hard-won safeguards to physical health."[3] This has been demonstrated, for epidemic infections, such as diarrhea and skin infections, which sometimes occur in large hospital nurseries have not been observed in rooming-in programs.

Individual mothers must be taken into consideration as to whether or not they should have rooming-in. Some mothers will want to have their babies with them most of the time so that they can get to know them and learn to care for them under the guidance of the nurses and the physicians. Other mothers may not want rooming-in, particularly multiparas, because they feel that this is an opportunity for rest and freedom from responsibility. Many mothers feel that they would enjoy rooming-in but hesitate because they do not feel sufficiently able to assume the care or the responsibility for the baby at this time. These mothers need help, of course, to understand that the

nurse is there to help them, and that they do not have to take over any more of the infant's care than they feel able or want to do. It is interesting to note that research[4] has indicated that these negative feelings and qualifications are not as significant or widespread as one might think.

Nurses with understanding and interest often can anticipate the mother's needs and desires and can be of invaluable help to her. Much of the practical care of the new baby must be learned by the new mother during her brief hospital stay to supplement the theoretical knowledge she has gained during the antepartal period. At this time the mother usually needs close supervision and guidance from the nurse so that she may develop confidence in her own ability to handle and care for her baby. The father, also, may share in some of these experiences and learn much about his baby and his baby's care. With this kind of preparation, parents of first babies in particular do not feel so helpless when they return home. These shared experiences undoubtedly contribute to an excellent foundation for stable and secure family relationships.

[3] Jackson, E. B.: Should mother and baby room together?, Am. J. Nurs. 46:17, 1946.

[4] Ringholz, Sharon, and Morris, M.: A test of some assumptions about rooming-in, Nurs. Res. 10: 196-199, Fall, 1961.

NURSING CARE OF THE NEWBORN

Initial Care

In the delivery room the initial care has been given to the infant's eyes and the cord, and appropriate identification has been added. The baby should be watched to see that he is kept warm (a most important detail), that respiration is normal, that color is good and that there is no bleeding from the cord (see Chap. 12).

It is customary in many maternity hospitals today to provide a "receiving" nursery on the labor and delivery division so that closer supervision and care for the infant may be assured immediately following the delivery (Fig. 15-20).

Observations

The infant's natal day, as previously stated, is the most hazardous during the postnatal period. Therefore, it is important that the nurse take particular care with her observations during the first 24 hours of the baby's life. The receiving or transition nursery in the labor or the nursery sections affords an excellent physical environment (similar to that of recovery room care for adults) for the extensive observations that are necessary (see Suggested Reading). "High-risk" babies (infants who have been exposed to or have experienced a prolonged labor, difficult labor, fetal distress, maternal complications during pregnancy and/or labor, respiratory distress, etc.) especially need intensive observation and often special equipment for their care, such as incubators, suction equipment, etc.

Behavior and Physiologic Responses. Because these are indicative of normal reactions in the newborn, they should be observed and recorded, as well as any abnormal signs. For instance, the frequency and the type of cry are important, since the infant aerates his lungs in this way. Moreover, the type of cry may be indicative of cerebral damage (see Chap. 21). In a vigorous, normal infant the cry should be lusty and should occur especially when the baby is handled or moved. If this does not happen, and the infant seems "sleepy" or depressed, it may be necessary to stimulate him to cry every hour or more frequently, depend-

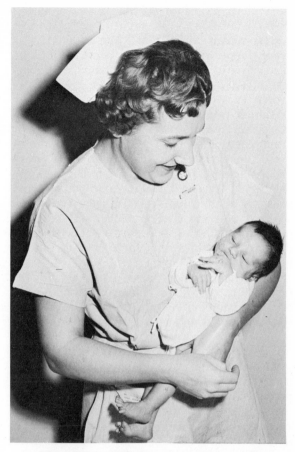

Fig. 15-21. Assessing the mother's understanding is a natural part of the verbal exchanges that accompany baby care or carrying the baby. Here, as always, tender loving care is the basis to all else.

ing on the degree of depression. This response may be aroused by changing his position or rubbing his back, head or feet. Occasionally, with a drowsy infant it becomes necessary to slap or rub the soles of the feet *gently* to elicit the necessary cry. The time of the baby's first stool and voiding should be noted, for this will give an indication of proper excretory function. It is sometimes necessary for the nurse to check with the delivery room records to see whether the infant voided or defecated at delivery. Finally, the newborn's general activity, muscle tone and reflexes (especially the Moro and the sucking reflexes) should be observed. A healthy infant will be active, evidence good muscle tone and respond with behavior appropriate to the various reflexes (see pp. 356-358).

Respiration and Color. These should be given close attention, for they are good indices of whether or not the newborn is experiencing respiratory insufficiency. Dyspnea, rapid respirations exceeding 50 breaths per minute, and persistent cyanosis should be reported to the physician. Since mucus in the nasopharynx often causes respiratory distress, the nurse should be particularly watchful for its presence. Gagging, vomiting, breath holding, retraction of the head, choking and cyanosis are all signs of the presence of mucus. It is particularly prone to develop in the 2nd period of reactivity following the first sleep. Postural drainage and the technic for aspirating mucus are explained in Chapter 21.

Condition of the Cord. This should be noted; any oozing or hemorrhage should be reported immediately, and the cord should be reclamped or retied as indicated. Oozing more often occurs between the 2nd and the 6th hours of life and frequently is associated with crying or the passage of meconium.

The baby's skin should be observed also for pallor and jaundice as well as cyanosis. Pressing the skin with a finger often enables clearer visualization of jaundice. The blanching that occurs with the maneuver provides a contrast that shows up the icteric color more clearly.

The significance of pallor and jaundice in the first 24 hours is explained in Chapter 21.

The infant's temperature should be checked frequently (every hour), and particularly if external heat is being applied. Even though the infant's temperature may have been quite low at first, he responds readily to external changes in temperature. Therefore, care must be taken that he does not become overheated.

Continuing Care

Cleansing. The daily cleansing of the infant affords the nurse an excellent opportunity for making the observations that are necessary during the immediate postnatal period. The materials used for the bath, its frequency, etc., may vary from institution to institution. Several decades ago the daily soap and water and oil baths were replaced with merely wiping off excess vernix with dry or slightly moist cotton balls. The diaper area was cleansed as necessary. However, in view of the increase in staphylococcal infections in newborn nurseries, the American Academy of Pediatrics recommends a sponge bath with a liquid detergent containing 3 per cent hexachlorophene after birth and every other day thereafter. A sponge bath is necessary until the cord drops off. In most institutions the suggestions of the Academy of Pediatrics are adhered to. On

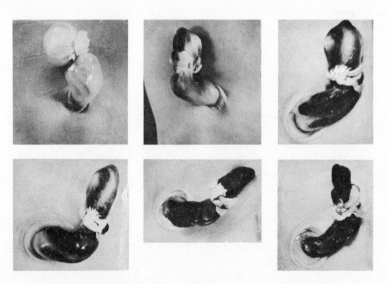

FIG. 15-22. The umbilical cord drying.

alternate days the diaper area and other soiled areas are cleansed with warm water as necessary. Thus some cleansing of the infant occurs daily, and the nurse should utilize the opportunity to inspect the baby thoroughly.

Assessing the Mother's Understanding. In the verbal exchanges with the mother during the daily care of the baby it is important that the nurse assess the mother's understanding and her skill in caring for her infant. Any basic principles or procedures related to infant care that the mother will find necessary and useful should be part of the nurse's teaching plan for the mother during her hospital stay. A referral to a public health agency may be necessary to ensure appropriate follow-up, particularly if the mother is inexperienced. The following principles of care can be conveyed easily to the mother (and the father when he is present).

Eyes. In the daily care of the baby no spe-cial treatment other than necessary cleansing with sterile water is given the baby's eyes unless there is a discharge. Any redness, swelling or discharge should be reported and recorded on the chart. There may be some reaction from the medication used for prophylaxis against ophthalmia neonatorum, but the physician will prescribe treatment if necessary.

Cord. Babies do not receive a tub bath until the cord has separated, and the umbilicus has healed. A cord dressing is considered to be unnecessary in most hospitals since exposure to the air enhances drying of the cord; nevertheless, it is still used in some institutions. If a cord dressing is used, it is removed when it becomes soiled, or when the baby is taken to the nursery for its initial bath. If the cord is left exposed to the air, some physicians prefer that the base be wiped with alcohol daily to encourage drying further and to discourage the possibility of infection.

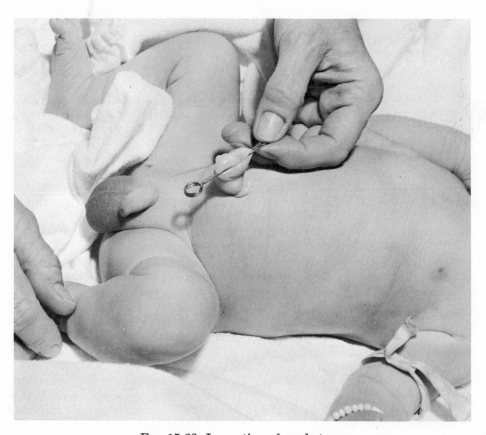

FIG. 15-23. Inspection of cord stump.

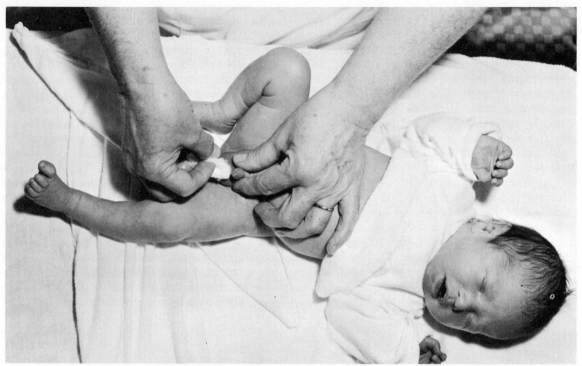

FIG. 15-24. Retracting foreskin for cleansing penis (uncircumcised). (MacDonald House, University Hospitals of Cleveland, Cleveland, Ohio)

No attempt should be made to dislodge the cord before it separates completely. If there is a red inflamed area around the stump or any discharge with an odor, this condition should be recorded and brought to the physician's attention immediately. The cord usually becomes detached from the body between the 5th and the 8th days after birth, but its detachment may be delayed until the 12th or the 14th day without causing any concern (Fig. 15-22). When the cord drops off, the umbilicus is depressed somewhat and usually free from any evidence of inflammation. No further treatment is necessary, except to keep the part clean and dry. When inflammation is present, the physician will give specific orders for care.

Adherent Foreskin. In a male infant, adhesions between the prepuce and the glans penis are very common. The foreskin may be extended beyond the glans. Reduction to a very small opening is spoken of as phimosis (see p. 364). A curdy secretion, called smegma, may form in considerable amount and collect under the prepuce behind the glans. Also, small amounts of urine may be retained. Any of these conditions favor irritation and, if found, should be reported to the obstetrician. He may perform the delicate operations of separating the adhesions, stretching the prepuce or circumcising the baby.

The manipulation following dilation and retraction is difficult at first, and should be done gently. The foreskin must be replaced immediately; if not, edema may result, rendering the replacing difficult.

Care Following Circumcision. When the newborn infant is circumcised, the main principles of postoperative care are to keep the wound clean and to observe it closely for bleeding (Fig. 15-11). For the first 24 hours the area is covered with a sterile gauze dressing to which a liberal amount of sterile petrolatum has been added.

Mothers are naturally anxious about their babies at this time, so, as soon as it is feasible after the circumcision has been done, the nurse should take the baby to his mother for a brief visit. She can be reassured that the procedure has not been very painful for her child. The infant will cry during the operation, but this is due as much to the necessary restraints as to the discomfort. Occasionally, a local anesthetic will be used, but generally the procedure is performed without it. Thus, the infant may be fed immediately after the circumcision, and both mother and baby seem to enjoy the comfort that the feeding and cuddling bring. It is unwise, however, to keep the baby away too long from the careful observation of the nurse.

The infant's diaper should be applied so that only one layer of the material covers the penis. This lessens the danger of masking any bleeding that might occur. In changing the infant's diaper the nurse should hold his ankles with one hand so that he cannot kick against the operative area. Unless the physician orders otherwise, the circumcision dressing can be removed postoperatively when the infant voids for the first time. If a length of petrolatum gauze was applied firmly to the site of operation, the physician may wish it to be left in place for 24 hours. Cleansing must be done gently but can be accomplished as necessary with cotton balls moistened with warm tap water. A fresh sterile petrolatum dressing usually is applied to the penis each time the diaper is changed for the first day. The penis must be observed closely for bleeding, and during the first 12 hours should be inspected every hour. It is advisable to place the infant's crib where he can be watched conveniently. Moreover, to keep all the nursing personnel alerted, some signal, such as a red tag, can be attached to the identification card on the crib. If bleeding occurs, usually it can be controlled with gentle pressure. Some physicians leave a p.r.n. order for local application of Adrenalin 1:1,000 solution to the bleeding point; but if bleeding persists, the physician should be notified immediately.

Since the length of the maternity stay has been considerably shortened, circumcision may be done on the 2nd or the 3rd postnatal day or even before the baby leaves the delivery room. To overcome the transitory coagulation deficiency, some physicians administer vitamin K_1 at birth. Sometimes the operation is performed on the day preceding discharge; therefore the nurse should ascertain the physician's wishes for aftercare and make certain that the mother knows how to care for her newly circumcised infant. Generally, the care will be the same as that described.

Care of Girl Babies. Similar adhesions sometimes are found about the clitoris in female infants and, when observed, should be reported to the obstetrician. The smegma which may accumulate between the folds of the labia should be gently and carefully cleansed with moistened cotton balls, using the front-to-back direction and a clean cotton ball for each

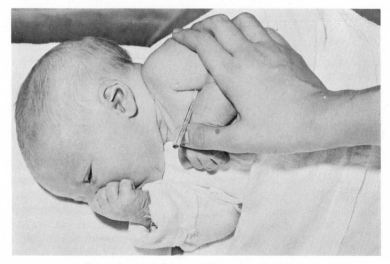

FIG. 15-25. Taking axillary temperature.

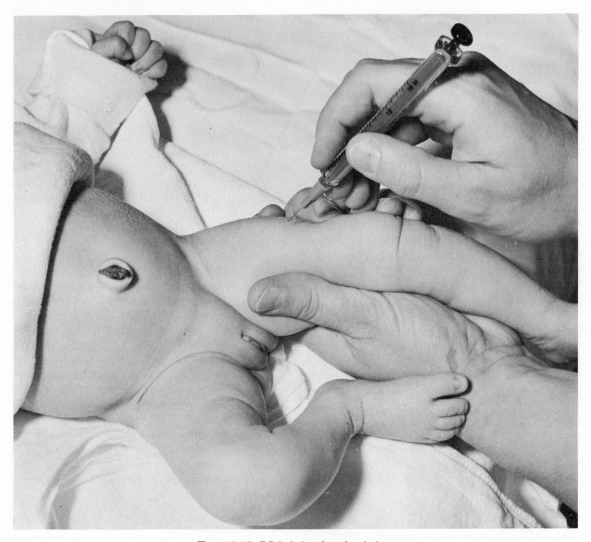

Fig. 15-26. I.M. injection for infant.

stroke. Occasionally, a slight bloody discharge may come from the vagina (see p. 364). This usually is due to a hormonal reaction and rarely reappears; cleanliness is the only treatment necessary. Very infrequently, the discharge may be caused by injury; if the discharge persists, it should be reported to the doctor.

Weight. The baby should be weighed on the birth date and every day or every other day thereafter. If the infant remains in the hospital longer than 5 days, he should be weighed at intervals prescribed by the medical staff. His weight should be recorded accurately.

During the first few days after birth the in-fant may lose 5 to 10 per cent of his birth weight. This is due partly to the minimal intake of nutrients and fluid and partly to the loss of excess fluid from his body. About the time the meconium begins to disappear from his stools, the weight commences to increase and in normal cases does so regularly until about the 10th day of life, when it may equal the birth weight. Then the baby should begin to gain from 4 to 6 ounces per week during the first 5 months. After this time the gain is from 2 to 4 ounces weekly. At 6 months of age the baby should be double his birth weight, and he should triple it when a year old. This is one way to note the baby's condition and progress, and when the baby is not gaining, that fact should be reported to the physician. Besides gaining regularly in weight and strength, the baby should be happy and good-natured when awake and inclined to sleep a good part of the time between feedings.

Pulse and Temperature. The clinical record of a normal baby should show a variation in pulse of 120 to 150. Only experience can teach a nurse to count an infant's pulse rate accurately (see p. 353). Touching his wrist will generally startle him and noticeably accelerate the heart beat. The pulse can always be felt at the temporal artery to best advantage, particularly during sleep. The rectal temperature may normally vary a whole degree (see p. 354). A premature baby, who may have a temperature below that of a normal baby, will stabilize his temperature within 24 to 72 hours somewhere between 96° and 98° F., depending on his weight—the smaller the baby, the lower the temperature will be.

Crying. After the baby is born and has cried lustily, he becomes quiet and usually sleeps. After the eyes, the cord and the skin have received the necessary care, he is dressed and placed in a warm crib and usually does not cry unless he is wet, hungry, ill or is moved. A nurse soon will learn to distinguish an infant's condition and needs from the character of his cry, which may be described as follows. A loud, insistent cry with drawing up and kicking of the legs usually denotes colicky pain; a fretful cry, if due to indigestion, will be accompanied by green stools and passing of gas; a whining cry is noticeable when the baby is ill, premature or very frail; a fretful, hungry cry, with fingers in the mouth and flexed, tense extremities, is easily recognized; and there is a peculiar, shrill, sharp-sounding cry which suggests injury. A nurse should make every effort to recognize any deviation from the usual manner in which a baby announces his normal requirements. Moreover, she should convey this information to the mother, since it is essential that the mother learn to interpret her infant's cues. The newborn has only his posture and his voice at this time to inform others of his needs.

"HYPERTONIC" BABIES. Occasionally, the nurse will find that an infant seems to be fussy from birth. He appears very active, startles easily, cries readily and more frequently (and apparently for no reason), is alert and awake much of the time and in general does not fit the usual pattern of activity, feeding and sleeping described. Some physicians term these babies "hypertonic"; that is, they do not seem to be able to relax as well as other infants. The parents, particularly, may find their adjustment to their new baby difficult and anxiety-provoking until they are informed (or learn by trial and error) that this is "normal behavior" for this child. All too often they assume they must be doing something "wrong" since in spite of their efforts their baby remains fussy, tense and crying. The nurse can be very helpful to the parents in giving them anticipatory guidance about their baby's behavior and helpful ways in which he can be soothed. She should inform the physician of her observations so that he may advise the parents appropriately. These infants usually respond favorably to being held securely. Thus, wrapping them snugly with a receiving blanket, cuddling them securely, changing their position slowly and surely rather than quickly, all help to allay undue tenseness. Of course, rocking the baby and walking with him are particularly successful measures, but no parent can or should do this over protracted periods of time.

Any new activity or procedures should be introduced to this kind of infant slowly. For instance, when he is given a tub bath for the first time, he should be placed in a small amount of water very slowly and each lower extremity immersed gradually. This will help him to be less frightened and startled. The parents should not consider an occasional evening out a luxury; rather it should be considered a necessary item in the care of their baby. These infants do place greater demands on their parents than do infants of a more placid nature, and a short time away from the baby does wonders in restoring the perspective and good humor of the parents.

Care of the Skin. The skin is thin, delicate, extremely tender and very easily irritated. Since the skin is a protective covering, breaks in its surface may initiate troublesome infection; hence skin disturbances constitute an actual threat to the baby's well-being.

The new baby does not perspire, usually, until after the 1st month, and he does not react to cold by having "goose flesh." In warm weather, or if the baby is dressed too warmly, he may develop prickly heat, a closely grouped pinhead-size rash of papules and vesicles, on the face, the neck and wherever skin surfaces touch. Fewer clothes and some control over the room temperature will help to relieve the discomfort.

BATHING. In the majority of hospitals today, elaborate procedures for bathing the infant have been discarded. It is recommended, as previously stated, that the skin be cleansed every other day with sterile cotton or a soft washcloth, warm water and a hexachlorophene detergent (see p. 374). Blood is removed from the skin after the delivery, but no attempt is made to remove the vernix caseosa thoroughly unless it is stained with blood or meconium. The vernix caseosa serves to protect the skin and disappears spontaneously in about 24 hours. If it remains in the creases and folds of the skin longer than 2 days, it is apt to cause irritation. In this case gentle wiping usually removes it sufficiently. On the alternate days that the hexachlorophene bath is given, an inspection bath should be given, at which time the infant can be "spot cleansed" as needed with the moistened cotton balls. The use of strong soap, oil and baby powder is discouraged by many pediatricians because of the sensitivity of the newborn's skin. The nurse should pay particular attention to cleansing (and dry-

ing) the scalp and all creases at the neck, behind the ears, under the arms, the palms of the hands and between the fingers and the toes, under the knees, the soles of the feet, and in the groins, the buttocks and the genitals.

Basic Principles. Each nurse will develop her own manner of bathing the newborn according to her manual dexterity, the size and the activity of the infant, and the facilities available. Several basic principles should be observed.

First, all equipment, clothing and supplies should be assembled so that the infant never is left alone or exposed unduly. Safety pins should be closed and placed out of the reach of the baby. Receptacles for soiled clothing, cotton balls, etc., should be available.

Second, care should be taken so that the environment is free from drafts and warm enough (i.e., 75° to 80° F.). The nurse should not have to interrupt the bath to close a door or a window. The water for the bath should be about 98° to 100° F. Water that feels warm to the elbow is approximately that temperature.

Third, in giving the bath the nurse should proceed from the "cleanest" areas to those that are "most soiled." Thus, the eyes are bathed first, then the face, ears, scalp, neck, upper extremities, trunk, lower extremities,

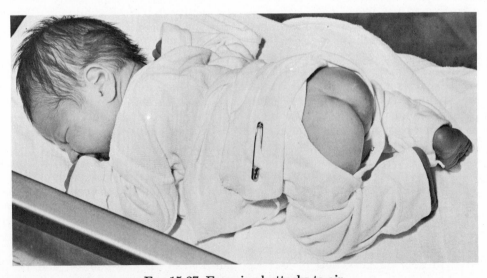

FIG. 15-27. Exposing buttocks to air.

and finally the buttocks and the genitals. Each of these in turn is washed, *rinsed well* and dried. To prevent undue exposure, a portion of the infant can be undressed at one time, bathed and then redressed.

Finally, *the infant never should be left alone*, even on a large work area; one hand should be kept on him at all times.

Demonstration and Practice. Each mother should have an opportunity to observe a demonstration of a sponge bath and, if at all possible, to give a bath to her infant. The various principles enumerated above can be conveyed to the mother readily. In addition, the nurse should explore with the mother what facilities are available in the home so that the necessities can be met and undue expense and difficulty avoided. For instance, a large drainboard which can be washed and padded adequately (and is a comfortable height for han-

dling the infant) can be utilized for the bath area. A large pan or basin does very well for the bathtub in the early weeks; it should be kept only for the baby's use. Thus, the extra expense of special equipment can be minimized.

THE CORD TIE should be left in place until the cord drops off; the clamp is removed in 24 hours, provided that the umbilical stump has dried sufficiently. The nurse should observe whether the skin is clear, pink, cyanotic, blotchy or jaundiced and if there is dryness present.

BUTTOCKS. Sometimes, despite good nursing care, the infant's buttocks become reddened and sore. A diaper rash may occur which is caused by the reaction of bacteria with the urea in the urine. This in turn causes an ammonia dermatitis. The most important prophylaxis lies in keeping the diaper area clean and dry. Sometimes, petroleum jelly, baby oil or a

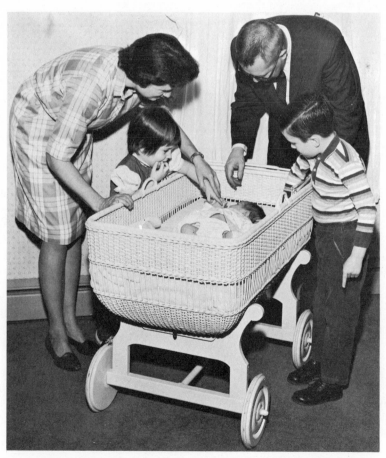

FIG. 15-28. The new baby comes home to his family.

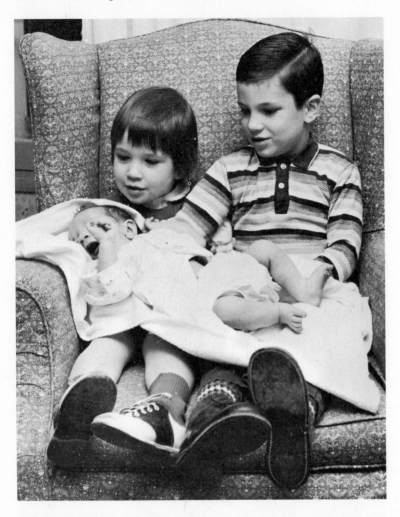

FIG. 15-29. The children wanted to hold their new brother. Sitting in the armchair and holding the baby are Kathy, age 2½ years, and Flip, age 4½ years.

bland protective ointment, such as vitamin A and D ointment, is prescribed by the doctor. Pastes may not be advised, because they are much more adhesive than ointments and thus create cleansing problems.

A simple treatment which is often effective is merely to expose the infant's reddened buttocks to air (Fig. 15-27) and light several times a day, using care to keep the infant covered otherwise. Warm daylight may be all that is necessary, although the use of a "lamp" treatment is more effective and at the same time provides a measure of warmth. An ordinary gooseneck lamp with a screened bulb (no stronger than 40 watts) can be placed on the table so that it is a foot or more away from the infant's exposed buttocks. The light may be used for 30 minutes at a time. Because the skin is already irritated, the nurse should

exercise care not to burn it further by using too strong a bulb or placing the light too close.

If the condition occurs at home, the treatment described above also is appropriate, and the mother can be so instructed. Boiling the diapers is another effective measure, since this destroys the bacteria. However, many of the detergents and conditioners nowadays have antibacterial agents in them; these may be effective in washing the diapers. Care should be taken to rinse the diapers thoroughly, since the residue of the detergent, etc., in itself can be irritating. In this respect the modern diaper services have very effective facilities; many sterilize diapers and entire layettes as part of the service.

Sleeping. After the profound experience of being born, the baby will need rest and sleep with as little handling as possible. If he is well

Fig. 15-30. Father gives the baby his bottle as Kathy and Flip help.

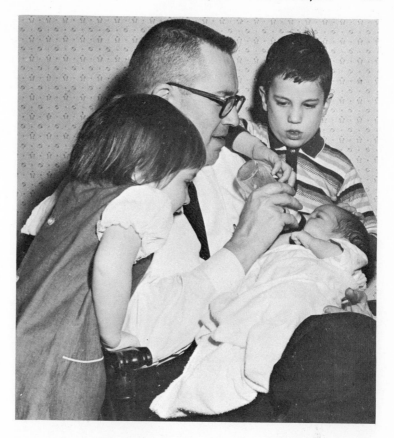

and comfortable, he usually sleeps much of the time and wakes and cries when he is hungry or uncomfortable. He may sleep as much as 20 hours out of 24 (although this varies considerably from infant to infant). It is not the sound sleep of the adult; rather he moves a good deal, stretches, and at intervals awakens momentarily. Since he responds so readily to external stimuli (and this may make him restless), his clothing and coverings are important. They should be light in weight, warm but not too warm, and free from wrinkles and "bunches." His position should be changed frequently when he is awake. He can be placed on either side or on his abdomen, especially when he is ready for sleep. If he is positioned on his back, then someone should be present, for if the baby regurgitates, he is more likely to aspirate in this position. As he gets older and learns to roll over, he will assume the position that he likes most for sleep.

Intestinal Elimination. During fetal life the content of the intestines is made up of brownish-green tarlike material called meconium. It is composed of epithelial and epidermal cells and lanugo hair that probably were swallowed with the amniotic fluid. The dark greenish-brown color of the meconium is due to the bile pigment. During fetal life and for the first few hours after birth the intestinal contents are sterile. Apparently, there is no peristalsis until after birth, because normally there is no discoloration of the amniotic fluid.

Stools. For the first 5 or 6 days, the stools gradually change from meconium to transitional stools (after which they become the regular milk stools). During this time the color of the stools changes from tarry black to a greenish black, to greenish brown, to brownish yellow and thence to greenish yellow. The transitional stools are composed of both meconium and milk stools; hence their variation in color. After the transitional stools the color gradually changes to a soft yellow of a smooth pasty consistency with a characteristic foul odor if the infant is formula-fed. Stools of

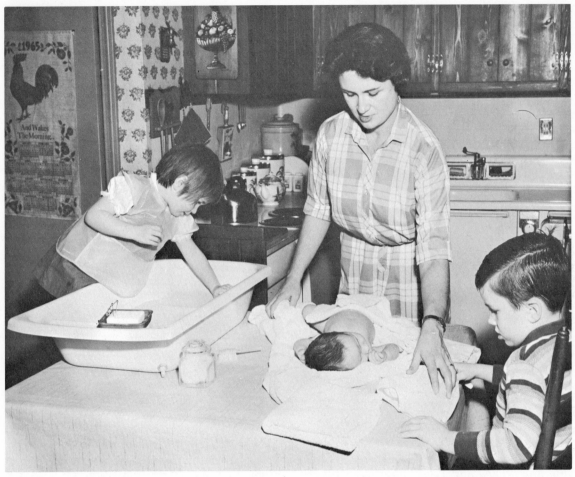

FIG. 15-31. Bath time for the baby. Kathy and Flip are allowed to help.

breast-fed infants tend to be golden yellow and of mushy consistency. Most newborns pass the first stool within 12 hours of birth—nearly all have a stool in 24 hours. If an infant has not passed a stool by this time, intestinal obstruction must be considered as a possible reason for the delay, and the baby must be observed closely. The number of daily stools on about the 5th day of life is usually 4 to 6. As the infant grows, this number decreases to 1 or 2 each day. The type of stool may be influenced by the mother's diet. However, there may be slight variations from the normal, which may have little significance if the baby appears to be comfortable and sleeps and nurses well. If the baby's stools have a watery consistency, are of a green color, contain much mucus, and flatus is being passed, the condition may be evidence of some digestive or intestinal irritation and should be reported to the physician. The number, color and consistency of stools should be recorded daily on the baby's record.

Urinary Elimination. Urinary activity of the fetus is evidenced by the presence of urine in the amniotic fluid. The baby usually voids during delivery or immediately after birth, but the function may be suppressed for several hours. However, if the baby does not void within 24 hours, the condition should be reported to the physician, as retention of the urine may be due to an imperforate meatus. After the first 2 or 3 days the baby voids from 10 to 15 times a day. When the urine is concentrated, red or rusty stains on the wet diaper may be due to uric-acid crystals in the urine.

INFANT FEEDING

The Newborn's Ability to Handle Food

One of the major physiologic adaptations which the infant must make in the transition from intra-uterine to extra-uterine life concerns the source of his nourishment and the ability to take food into his body, to digest it and to assimilate it. During prenatal life the nutritive substances for growth and handling of waste products are provided for via the placental circulation (see Chap. 4). Thus, prior to birth the gastrointestinal tract has not been required to utilize muscle, chemical or absorptive activity in handling food. Clement Smith makes the analogy that the digestion and the absorption of food is, like the respiration of air, a function that the infant has had no opportunity of practicing during its fetal career.[5] Following delivery not only must the gastrointestinal tract begin abruptly to process a rather large amount of food, but the infant must begin to suck and swallow to take the food into his stomach. The infant's capacity to take the food in and digest it is adequate when the food is appropriate, i.e., breast milk or milk formula, and when it is appropriately given.

Certain important considerations in relation to the development of the infant's digestive apparatus and infant feeding will be recalled here, because they have a direct bearing on feeding practices. The student is urged to utilize the appropriate references in the Suggested Reading at the end of the chapter for more thorough study, as well as to build on content in normal nutrition, physiologic chemistry, etc., covered in background courses.

SUCKING AND SWALLOWING REFLEXES. The infant's ability to take in food through his own efforts demands the ability to suck and to swallow. At birth the sucking and swallowing reflexes are already present, and normally they are quite strong. It is known that the swallowing reflex, as well as peristaltic movements in the stomach, become active during the last 2 months of fetal development, because bits of vernix caseosa and lanugo are found with other debris in the meconium stool. The nurse who has witnessed the birth of babies

[5] Smith, C. A.: The Physiology of the Newborn Infant, ed. 3, p. 228, Springfield, Thomas, 1959.

can easily recall how the infant is able to swallow mucus, and how sometimes, even while the initial care is being given in the delivery room, the infant will begin to suck on anything that gets near his mouth.

STOMACH AND INTESTINES. At the time of birth the infant's stomach is small, its capacity is approximately 50 to 60 cc., but it is capable of considerable dilatation. During feeding the infant's stomach is able to stretch to at least 3 or 4 times its approximate capacity. It is not merely distended by the amount of food taken in, i.e., milk, but also by the amount of air the infant swallows as he sucks the milk or cries. In the act of crying the infant tends to gulp in air.

The gastric musculature is somewhat deficient at birth. In contrast, the glandular structures in the mucosa are present, although shallow in contrast with those of the adult. The relatively greater length of the intestinal tract and the weakness of the abdominal musculature to serve as a supporting structure explain in part the reason that considerable distention of the stomach is possible.

Although gastric digestion is not considered to be a factor of primary importance to the nutrition of the newborn infant, many of the findings reported by Clement Smith in his textbook could be useful in the consideration of infant feeding schedules. For example, the stomach empties more slowly in the newborn period than any other time in life. However, the distended stomach is able to adjust its content by promptly emptying some or all of its content into the duodenum. A number of the studies on gastric motility have demonstrated wide individual differences in emptying time. The major portion of the feeding usually leaves the stomach in less than 3 or 4 hours, although the greater portion of this occurred $1\frac{1}{2}$ to 2 hours after the meal. In some instances the emptying time of the infants' stomachs took more than 8 hours. It was found also that the introduction of a second feeding before the stomach was empty caused portions of the first feeding to remain somewhat longer in the stomach than if the stomach was emptied from the last feeding before the next was offered. Another important finding is that human milk leaves the stomach somewhat more rapidly than cow's milk, although a formula made of cow's milk which has been boiled leaves the stomach more rapidly than that which is fed without this additional preparation.

Infant Nutrition. In the last several decades progress in scientific developments has made artificial feeding (formulas) so much like human breast milk in chemical composition that they are, in fact, almost identical. Although it is generally considered that the best food for the baby is that designed by nature—human breast milk—the individual differences in mothers and babies must be considered in the practical situation. It is the mother who makes the decision of how she wants to feed her baby, and the nurse should support her in this decision.

Some advantages of feeding breast milk are: it is exactly the correct chemical composition for babies, is constantly available (and no preparation is necessary), is at an even temperature, is free from bacteria, and causes a lower incidence of allergy.

In artificial feeding the differences in caloric allowances required for various infants will depend on: (1) the individual nutritional needs and (2) the infant's rate of growth. All of the infant's nutritional needs, except that for growth, can be met by providing 33 calories per pound per day. When the component necessary for growth is added, approximately 42 calories per pound per day will be required. One might anticipate that by the time some infants are 10 to 14 days old, they may consume 55 calories per pound per day, but this should not be followed rigidly.

Self-regulatory Feedings. A permissive feeding regimen for newborns means that babies should be offered as much formula or feeding as they seem to want and should not be forced to take the amount prescribed unless forcing has been specifically ordered by the responsible physician.

The variation in baby readiness and the desirability of individualizing the time of starting feedings needs to be stressed. The time of initiating feedings will depend on evidence of the infant's hunger and the readiness of the baby. Once the first feeding has been offered, the routine or prescribed schedule for offering feedings should be followed.

The permissive feeding regimen for breast-fed newborns may require even more flexibility. A mother who is breast-feeding may desire to begin breast-feeding her baby before the time specified by hospital routine for the first water feeding, as sometimes happens when the nursery requires that the first feeding be water and given by the nurse prior to other feedings. Unless there is a maternal complication or contraindication, every baby should visit his mother at each feeding time, starting with the first feeding of "breast" or "bottle," but excluding the 2 A.M. feeding period for the first visit unless the mother wants to see her baby at this time.

Composition of Human Milk. Breast milk, as it leaves the mother's breast, is a sterile fluid. It should have an alkaline or possibly a neutral reaction, but never an acid reaction. Colostrum cells should be absent after the 12th day, and the fat globules should be small, numerous and of uniform size.

Milk is a natural emulsion and consists of about 10 per cent of solids and 90 per cent of water. The solid substances are fat, sugar, proteins and salts. The fat of milk is the cream, the sugar is the kind known as "lactose," or "milk-sugar," and the protein makes up the bulk of the curd.

Artificial Feeding

Today, more infants in American hospitals are artificially fed than breast-fed. In artificial feeding it is necessary to modify the milk to approximate as nearly as possible the chemical and the physical characteristics of human milk. When human milk and cow's milk are compared, the difference in fat and protein content needs to be considered. Cow's milk is diluted, and therefore carbohydrate is added to the newborn infant's formula. It is generally accepted that even normal fat in milk (3.5%) is poorly tolerated. Thus, cow's milk is diluted essentially to lessen the fat component of the formula. In addition, when whole milk is diluted, the casein curd is more flocculent in the infant stomach and thus aids in the digestion of milk. In diluting the formula the carbohydrate of milk also is diluted inadvertently and should be restored to the original amount (4.5%) or more to furnish additional calories for optimal nutrition and weight gain. The added carbohydrate may be in the form of granulated sugar, corn syrup or a commercially prepared carbohydrate modifier. Added

TABLE 11. COMPARATIVE DATA ON RELATIVE COMPONENTS IN HUMAN MILK, COW'S MILK AND
EVAPORATED COW'S MILK IN NORMAL DILUTION (ACCORDING TO NELSON)*

	NORMAL DILUTION		APPROXIMATE PERCENTAGE COMPOSITION IN NORMAL DILUTION (GRAMS PER 100 ML.)			
TYPE OF MILK	*Ratio*	*Cals./oz.*	*Protein*	*Fat*	*Carbo-hydrate*	*Minerals*
Human milk, average	undiluted	20	1.1	4.5	6.8	0.2
Cow's milk, market average	undiluted	20	3.3	3.5	4.8	0.72
Cow's milk, evaporated (Standard brands)	1:1	22	3.6	4.2	5.3	0.75
Commercial premodified milks:						
Modified milk, Baker†	1:1	20	2.2	3.3	7.0	0.6
Bremil, Borden	1:1	20	1.5	3.5	7.0	0.5
Carnalac, new formula, Carnation	1:1	20	2.28	2.69	8.23	0.5
Modilac, Gerber	1:1	20	2.15	2.6	7.6	0.37
Enfamil, Mead†	1:1	20	1.5	3.7	7.0	0.35
Similac, Ross†	1:1	20	1.7	3.4	6.6	0.38

* Nelson, W. E. (ed.): Textbook of Pediatrics, ed. 8, p. 139, Philadelphia, Saunders, 1964.
† Also available in powdered form.

carbohydrate permits normal metabolism of fats, allows protein to be used to build new tissues instead of serving to provide calories, and encourages normal water balance.

The physician will prescribe the formula for the infant and give specific directions concerning its use. Various milk formulas are used today: diluted pasteurized milk with added carbohydrate, diluted evaporated milk with or without carbohydrates added, fresh skimmed milk, powdered skim milk, or one of the brands of prepared milk preparations (see Table 11). Of these milk formulas, the most widely used formula is diluted evaporated milk with added carbohydrate. It should be noted that evaporated milk has several advantages: It is safe because it is sterilized in an unopen can, it is convenient to store, the cost is relatively low, and the formula is simple to prepare. An evaporated milk formula for the newborn infant is usually made up of one part evaporated milk diluted with two parts of water and carbohydrate in sufficient amount to meet the required calories.

At the present time, commercially prepared formula in disposable bottles, complete with nipple, is available and, in fact, used in many hospitals today. The variety of these formulas available tends to increase almost daily. There are two advantages in being able to purchase prepackaged sterilized formula: It is a time-saving device for the mother, and such a formula does not have to be refrigerated. The major disadvantage of such formulas is that at the present time the cost to the individual consumer is almost prohibitive. It is anticipated, however, that in the very near future competition among the various companies will bring the price down to a point at which parents can afford to buy prepackaged sterilized formula without causing an undue strain on the family's budget.

Essential nutritional requirements are a basic consideration in the computation of a formula for the newborn infant. Certain "rules of thumb" concerning nutrients and formula computation are as follows:

1. *Proteins.* One and one half ounces of cow's milk per pound of body weight equals 1.5 Gm. of protein per pound, which equals one tenth of body weight.

2. *Carbohydrates.* One tenth ounce per pound of body weight equals 1 ounce per 10 ounces of milk prescribed, which also equals 1 per cent of the body weight. One third of the carbohydrate should be derived from the milk of the mixture, and the remainder added in the form of starch or sugar. Later in the first year the carbohydrate is given in the form of a starch cereal, and the carbohydrate in the milk formula may be reduced at that time.

3. *Fats.* Anywhere from 3 to 5 per cent is included, no specific amount being stipulated. If

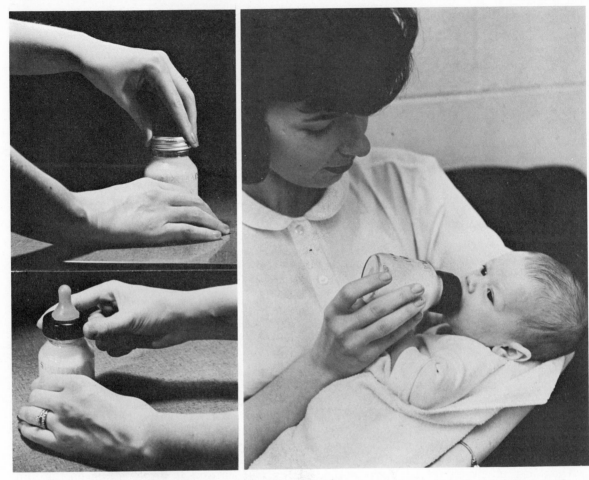

Fig. 15-32. The ready-to-use commercially prepackaged sterilized formula provides a safe, simple 3-step feeding for the convenience of the mother at home. At feeding time, (*left, top*) remove lid, (*left, bottom*) apply sterilized nipple, and (*right*) feed the baby. (Ross Laboratories, Columbus, Ohio)

the fats are restricted, a larger amount of protein or sugar, or both, is required for energy sources. The suitable quantity of fat is supplied in amounts of milk which furnish the required amounts of protein. An excess of fat is not to be desired.

4. *Minerals.* An adequate mineral-salt intake is supplied to any infant when 1½ ounces of milk per pound of body weight are given. Enough iron is stored in the liver of the normal infant (from the hemoglobin breakdown after birth) to suffice until about the 4th or 5th month. This deficiency is usually made up by the addition of the solid food supplements (egg yolk, fortified cereals, vegetables and fruit) which are usually added before this time, except in the completely milk-fed infant who refuses or is not offered these iron-containing foods in the first year.

5. *Water.* The requirement for water varies from 10 to 15 per cent of the body weight, or may be expressed as 1½ to 2½ ounces per pound of body weight. This is supplied in the milk itself, in the diluent of the milk mixture, and supplemented to instinctive demands by offerings of water and fruit juices between feedings.

6. *Calories.* The average requirement for growth in the first year is 50 calories per pound of expected weight, two thirds of this caloric need being supplied by the milk and one third by the added carbohydrate.[6]

Formula Computation. A simple problem with which to apply the basic rules of formula computation would be the food needs of an infant

[6] Meyer, H. F.: Infant Foods and Feeding Practice, p. 72, Springfield, Thomas, 1960.

weighing 10 pounds at 2 months of age, having weighed 6 pounds at birth. This infant would probably take 3 oz. more than his age in months (2) which would be (2 months plus 3 equals 5) 5 oz. per feeding. In 24 hours he probably would be satisfied with five feedings; hence, he would need 25 oz. in a total 24-hour period.

a good size to use and should be graduated in ounces and half ounces so that it will be possible at all times to know exactly how much food the baby has taken. A sufficient number of bottles and nipples should be sterilized to supply the feedings for the 24-hour period. It is always safer to have 1 or 2 extra bottles and

EXAMPLE—WHOLE MILK MIXTURE

1½ oz. whole milk per lb. of body weight (10 lb.)—
1 oz. CHO [carbohydrate] per 10 oz. milk used—
Diluent to make up total 24-hour amount—

5 feedings of 5 oz. each—

Milk, 15 oz. = 300 cal.
Cane sugar, 1½ oz. = 180 cal.
Water, 10 oz.
25 oz. = 480 cal.

Calorically, this should effect normal growth since it provides 48 calories per pound. Should it not provide normal weight increase of about 5 to 7 oz. per week, or should the infant fail to be satisfied by evidencing signs of hunger, the milk proportion could be increased, or the total amount be enlarged, or additional CHO added, or all of these could be changed to fit the infant's needs.

In calculating a formula with evaporated milk and a corn syrup for the same hypothetical infant, the construction would be as follows:

nipples in reserve in case of breakage (Fig. 15-34).

The shape of the bottle should be such that every part of the inner surface can be reached with a brush to facilitate cleaning.

The holes in the nipple are usually small, but they may be made the required size by heating a fine sewing needle with its eye fixed in a cork (used as a handle). The point is held in the flame until red hot, then accurately

EXAMPLE—EVAPORATED MILK MIXTURE

1 oz. evaporated milk per lb. body weight—
1/10 oz. CHO per lb. body weight—
Diluent to make up total 24-hour amount—

5 feedings of 5 oz. each—

Evap. milk, 10 oz. = 440 cal.
Corn syrup, 1 oz. = 120 cal.
Water, 14 oz.
25 oz. = 560 cal.

With this mixture the calories are increased to 56 per pound, which might easily be tolerated by said infant, especially if he were active and hungry and needed more food.[7]

Directions for Making Formula. The hands should be washed before assembling the equipment. All equipment used for the preparation of the formula should be kept separate (Fig. 15-33). If bottled milk is used, the outside of the bottle should be washed with soap and cool water as soon as received, and the bottle should be placed in the refrigerator. If canned milk is used, the top of the can should be washed with soap and water, using friction, and then thoroughly rinsed. Hot water should be poured over the top just before it is opened. All equipment should be washed thoroughly in warm soapy water and rinsed well so that no milk film remains to hold bacteria.

Bottles and Nipples. The 8-ounce bottle is

[7] Meyer, *op. cit.,* p. 75.

plunged into one of the three holes and withdrawn quickly. The procedure needs practice before holes of proper size can be made. Some nipples have crucial incisions instead of punctured holes to prevent them from clogging.

The test of proper hole size is made by holding the bottle, filled with milk and with the nipple attached, upside down. The milk should escape drop by drop, and if it runs in a stream, the hole is too large. The objection to the large hole is that the baby nurses too rapidly, which causes indigestion, colic and other disorders. If the stream is very rapid, the baby may have difficulty in swallowing.

Aseptic Method. In this method the bottles, nipples, nipple caps and equipment used in making the formula are sterilized before the formula is prepared. The mother will need a glass or enamel pitcher in which to mix the formula, a measuring cup, measuring spoons, tablespoon (to mix the formula), funnel (de-

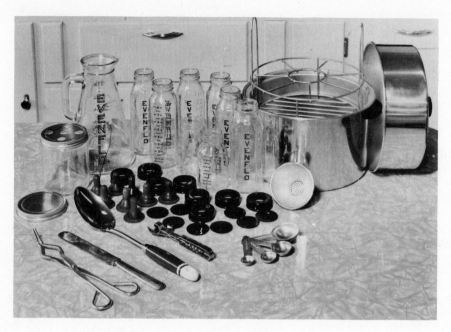

FIG. 15-33. Formula equipment. Sterilizer with bottle rack and tight-fitting lid; six 8-ounce nursers (for formula) and two 4-ounce nursers (for water and orange juice) complete with nipples, caps and sealing disks; quart-size formula pitcher with clearly marked graduations; nipple jar with perforated (for sterilizing) and solid lids; long-handled tongs; table knife; long-handled mixing spoon; can opener; set of measuring spoons and a funnel-strainer. (Pyramid Rubber Company, Ravenna, Ohio)

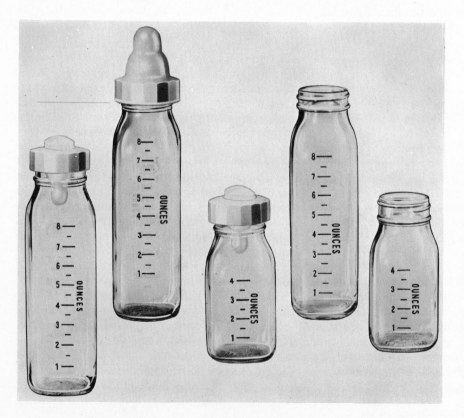

FIG. 15-34. A modern "nurser" for formula feeding is a complete unit consisting of a wide-mouthed bottle, nipple and screw-top all-in-one. It is safe and convenient because the cap seals the nipple and formula against contamination until used. During the feeding the collar can be screwed tighter or looser to regulate the rate of flow of the formula. (Davol Rubber Company, Providence, R. I.)

Fig. 15-35. Electric model of "Baby-All" formula and sterilizer outfit which may be used for regular or terminal sterilization. A nonelectric model is also obtainable. (Sanit-All Products Corporation)

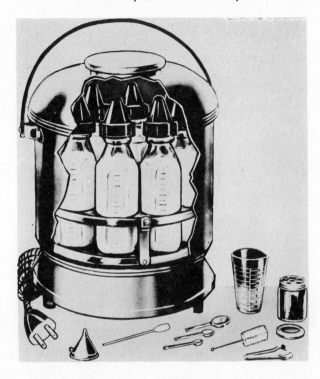

pending on the size of the bottle mouth), can opener (if canned milk is used) and some kind of tongs that can be sterilized. The tongs will be used as a forceps to handle the equipment. These items, together with the bottles, caps, and nipples are placed in a large pan or sterilizer half full of water and boiled vigorously for 10 minutes. The equipment and the bottles, nipples, etc., may be done separately if the sterilizer cannot accommodate such a large load. Care should be taken to place the forceps in such a way that the handles can be reached easily after sterilization. If the mother must reach into the water for them, then she contaminates the water and hence the materials being sterilized. After sterilization the formula is made according to directions. A specific amount of the formula is put into each bottle. The bottles are then nippled, capped and refrigerated.

Terminal Sterilization. In this method the formula is prepared under a clean but not aseptic technic. The equipment, bottles, nipples and nipple caps are washed thoroughly but are not sterilized. The formula is prepared and poured into the bottles, and the nipples and the caps are applied loosely. They then are placed in the sterilizer, covered with a

tight-fitting lid and sterilized by having the water boil rapidly in the bottom of the sterilizer for 25 minutes. In this method, formula, bottles, nipples and protectors are all sterilized in one operation. Before the formula is refrigerated, the screw collar should be made secure. The majority of hospitals use the autoclaving method, but in the home the procedure immediately above is used. In each method the formula must remain sterile and the nipple untouched and sterile until it reaches the baby's mouth.

There is a variety of bottles and nipples on the market, many of them sold as "units" (bottle, nipple and nipple protector) (see Fig. 15-34).

Hunger. If the baby is not getting enough food, he will wake before his regular nursing time and be obviously hungry. He will cry and fret, refuse water with apparent disgust, and when a feeding is offered, seize the nipple ravenously and nurse with great vigor. Often for the very young infant, increasing the amount of feeding is all that is necessary. For an older infant, increasing the concentration of the formula and/or its amount may be necessary. Solids sometimes are introduced at this time to help allay the hunger. Occasion-

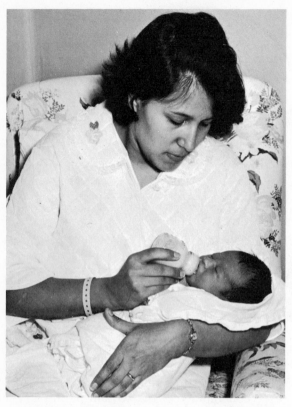

FIG. 15-36. The correct way to hold the baby's bottle.

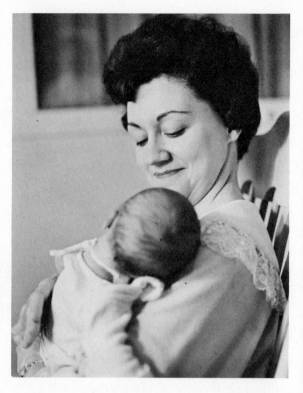

FIG. 15-37. Bubbling the baby. (Cleveland Clinic, Cleveland, Ohio)

ally, a baby appears to be hungry between feedings when in reality he is only thirsty. He may be given a small amount of tepid boiled water to satisfy his thirst.

Bubbling. After 5 minutes or so, or in the middle and at the end of each feeding, the infant should be held in an upright position and his back *gently* patted or stroked (Fig 15-37). Pounding the baby on the back vigorously is neither effective for bubbling him nor conducive to his well-being. The change in position (from semireclining to upright) is the important factor in eliciting a bubble. Often holding the infant upright and pressing him against the breast is all that is necessary. Because the new infant's gastrointestinal tract is labile, milk may be eructated with gas bubbles. Care should be taken to ensure adequate "bubbling" before the infant is placed back into the crib, thus preventing milk regurgitation.

Regurgitation. Regurgitation, which is merely an overflow and often occurs after nursing, should not be confused with vomiting, which may occur at any time and is accompanied by other symptoms. This regurgitation is the means of relieving the distended stomach and usually indicates that the baby either has taken too much food or has taken it too rapidly.

Assisting the Mother Feeding Her Infant

The feeding of the baby is one of the first tasks which must be achieved in the mothering role. The young inexperienced mother undoubtedly will need guidance, assistance and emotional support in feeding her new baby whether she feeds him by breast or by bottle. The help given by the nurse in the first feeding experiences not only helps the mother to deal with her anxiety in handling the new baby and in coping with the manipulative problems related to feeding him, but it lends her the emotional support that she so desperately needs in surmounting her own stress in the situation. The mother who has never handled a small infant before, being confronted with a sleepy or a squirmy infant, can feel all the more inadequate as she realizes that the responsibility to nourish this "bundle of joy" is hers.

The environmental climate surrounding the feeding of the baby should be peaceful and unhurried (Figs. 14-10, 11). The mother should be rested and ready. She should not have been rushed through a previous task, such as the morning bath or other daily care routine procedures, to meet a deadline imposed by the baby's feeding schedule. The nurse who brings the baby to his mother should avoid hurrying him to his mother's bedside, pushing the crib into the room, and leaving at once with the remark, "I'll be back to give you your baby as soon as I get the other babies out." Meanwhile, the mother looks at her hungry fretful baby in his crib, and often she is afraid to pick him up lest she be reprimanded for failing to wait for the return of the harassed nurse.

Expanding Contacts With the Baby. When babies are kept on a routine feeding schedule in the conventional maternity hospital, the mother's contacts with her baby are sometimes limited to the feeding period. It is unfortunate when the mother feels she must begin to feed her baby the moment she takes him into her arms. Feeding often takes up most of the time mothers and infants are together in the hospital, leaving little opportunity for their getting acquainted otherwise. Smith has described a plan whereby the demand feeding regimen to meet the needs of the individual baby was successfully achieved in a maternity hospital.[8] To provide some flexibility in the routine schedule, babies easily could be brought to their mothers at least 15 minutes before the feeding time and left with them for a similar period of time afterward, if the mothers so desired, without disrupting hospital routine. This plan would relieve some of the mother's stress at the beginning of the feeding period by allowing her more freedom to hold the baby leisurely, look at him or fondle him as she chooses. For mothers who are breast-feeding, this contact would have a positive effect on the let-down factor.

[8] Smith, C. S.: Demand feeding in the newborn nursery, Nurs. Outlook 6:514-515, September, 1958.

Getting Insight into the Mother's Goals and Problems. One must always bear in mind that each mother has her own goals in each new maternity experience. The astute nurse will utilize opportunities to assist the mother in achieving the mother's goals in accordance with the mother's individual capacity. Some time spent in purposeful conversation with the mother in addition to the time when her baby is with her may help the nurse to gain further insight into the mother's concerns. Even when hospital staffing is limited, the nurse who organizes her activities thoughtfully usually can find the "extra" time to accomplish what she considers to be the most important components of patient care.

One of the most obvious ways for the nurse to support the mother in the feeding experience is to stay with the mother until both mother and baby are settled, and then, in leaving the bedside to let the mother know that she is immediately available. The nurse who takes time to listen to what the mother is saying and to observe the interaction between the mother and baby often can identify problems that the mother is experiencing.

For example, the nurse left Mrs. Bee comfortably feeding her 2-day-old son. When she returned to the room 10 minutes later, Mrs. Bee looked up and said, "He only sucked for 2 minutes and now he's asleep. Look at him. Is his skin a little yellow? I can't make him take any more." Most mothers will verbalize their concerns, though they may not ask directly for help. In this instance the nurse responded with concern, "You wonder if he's had enough to eat?" The mother responded as she looked down at the baby, "Yes," and then went on to talk about her awkwardness in handling the baby and the bottle at the same time. She said, "I wonder whether perhaps I have tired the baby."

The nurse meets the mother's concern half way by her inquiry. At the same time, she must use judgment not to create concerns that do not exist. Responding to the mother's remarks in a way that leaves the conversation open and encourages the mother to express her concerns is not only helpful to the mother but also likely to give the nurse important clues about what the mother at the moment feels are "problems." The words that the nurse uses to speak with the patient are important, but even more important is the feeling communicated in this interaction between two people.

THE PRIMIGRAVIDA AND HER NEWBORN

With the birth of her baby the mother must assume a new role, along with all its concomitant tasks and responsibilities. Moreover, these adjustments must be undertaken before physical and psychological restoration from pregnancy and labor is complete. Since the adaptation to motherhood usually evolves as a slow, often unconscious modification of the individual's attitudes and activities, the professionals who provide for the mother's and the infant's care in the hospital are not always cognizant of what mother and baby experience in the early days of homecoming.

The literature on the development of maternal behavior (see Suggested Reading) tends to support the fact that primigravidas are generally more awkward and anxious and have more early concerns about their abilities to care for their newborn than do multiparas. One cannot assume that because the newly delivered mother seemingly makes a "good adjustment" during the first days after birth in the hospital that the adaptation will be smooth and uncomplicated after she returns home. This early period of adjustment—particularly during the first week of the infant's life—is a crucial one. Thoughtful nursing intervention at this time can make a significant contribution to the welfare of the family. Therefore it becomes important to ask what the nurse in the hospital might do to prepare the mother more adequately for coping with problems that she may encounter on going home with her new baby.

Mothers' Concerns About Their Babies

Every new mother experiences concerns to some degree about caring for her newborn infant. The mother who has had other babies may feel quite confident in performing the mothering tasks for the baby, but at the same time she may wonder how on returning home she ever will be able to manage her time and energy to give all the children and her husband what they need and what she would like to give them. On the other hand, the mother with her first baby may have many early concerns about fulfilling the infant care activities, such as feeding and bathing the baby, if she has had little or no experience.

Feeding the Baby. This is a major area of concern during the first weeks.[9] Adams found that the mother's questions usually were related to the amount and the frequency of feeding. The first days after delivery the mothers were asking how to prepare formula, but by the end of the week they were more interested in getting answers to questions about how to feed the baby, how often to feed and the amount of feeding. Mothers who were breast-feeding wanted to know about the adequacy of their milk supply. "Is he getting enough?" was a frequent question.

Bathing the baby is another task that mothers must learn to carry out, one that often causes concern. At first the task itself seems most important, thus, how to bathe the baby, i.e., the procedure, seems most urgent. But after new mothers have had some experience in handling their infants, they are more interested, as homegoing approaches, in learning how they are going to hold a squirming, soapy baby during his bath, and how to bathe him in a tub.

The baby's crying is of greater concern to mothers after the first week of life. When the baby spends most of his time in the hospital nursery, the mother may not get a chance to hear him cry, and she may wonder whether he can. One mother was ready to go home from the hospital (on her 5th postpartal day) and had never heard her baby cry. As the nurse wheeled his crib into the room that morning, the baby was crying lustily from hunger. The mother's face lighted up with great satisfaction as she said, "Now I *know* he can cry!" Mothers want to know why the baby is crying. With appropriate anticipatory guidance in the hospital, they can be helped to learn about the infant's communication through crying and how to interpret various kinds of crying.

Other Areas of Concern. "Concerns," aptly defines Adams, "are areas of special interest or worry to mothers as indicated by questions pertaining to particular areas of care." Other

[9] Adams, Martha: Early concerns of primigravida mothers regarding infant care activities, Nurs. Res. 12, No. 2:72, Spring, 1963.

questions they ask are related to care of the navel and/or circumcision, sleeping, taking the baby outdoors for the first time, hiccups, weight gain, rashes. Fathers, too, have concerns about tasks they must learn, particularly how to hold and to handle the new baby.

The Relation of Teaching to Areas of Concern. An understanding of how new parents view their problems with infant care activities must underlie any preparation for teaching mothers and helping them to learn about their babies and their care. The small group demonstrations of the infant bath and formula preparation are rather basic, but they need to include time for mothers' questions to be answered. There is a real need to have small group discussion conferences for new mothers, where they can initiate the conversation in the presence of a professional nurse who can act as a discussion leader or resource person.

Clinical Study: A Nurse and a New Mother

A clinical study in maternity nursing was carried out for the purpose of studying the nurse-patient interaction and nursing intervention with a young primigravida during the early puerperium.* There was conscious evaluation of the nurse-patient interaction by the nurse during the relationship. Also, there was an attempt to apply psychosocial concepts to this situation by reflecting on the psychodynamics of behavior. Because Olive Rich's writings have particular significance for maternity nurses, she has graciously consented to share them with the authors for use in this textbook (see Suggested Reading).

The Clinical Experience

The patient selected, a 24-year-old primigravida, had no major complications during pregnancy, labor or delivery. The nurse had daily contacts with the patient for 7 days, beginning with the day of delivery and extending through the day of discharge. The nature of the contacts varied. At times the contact was solely for verbal and nonverbal interaction; at other times other facets of nursing care were included, e.g., assisting the mother with breast-feeding and teaching her

* Part of a pilot project supported by Grant STIMH 7988-03 from the National Institute of Mental Health, United States Public Health Service.

how to carry out manual expression of breast milk. After the discharge of the mother from the hospital the nurse had three significant contacts with the patient in her home and three significant contacts by telephone. In the course of this experience there was only one direct interaction of the nurse with the patient alone. The patient had the same roommate throughout her hospital stay, and at home her mother and mother-in-law were both present—the latter intermittently—during the first two contacts with the nurse.

This clinical nursing study is directed to an examination of the possible dynamics involved when a patient who has made a good adjustment in the hospital suddenly encounters major problems on arriving home with her new baby. During the early postpartal days the patient's behavior was assessed by several staff members in the hospital setting as confident, mature, "doing just fine," and physically able and calm. In contrast, after the first 52 hours at home the young mother found herself fatigued and depressed. As she summarized it: "I just wasn't prepared for all this."

So that the student can understand and evaluate the nursing intervention, a fairly detailed description of the patient in the hospital and on the nurse's first visit to the home will be presented. As a further basis of understanding, concepts of the psychodynamics of pregnancy and childbearing as presented by selected authors will be discussed. Application will be made to this unique patient situation in the areas in which data are available. Finally, there will be some evaluation of the means of nursing intervention that were utilized and some reflective questioning about what other measures might have been of further help in preparing this mother for being at home with her baby.

The First Seven Days

The nurse's first contact with Mrs. X was on the afternoon of her day of delivery. Although Mrs. X had been in labor for more than 24 hours and had not slept for about 36 hours, she was sitting up in bed, making preparations to have her baby for a visit. She had seen her baby briefly on two previous occasions but had not held him. The nurse brought the baby from the nursery, placed him in his mother's arms, and waited for her comments. At first she looked and looked, not touching the baby's face but holding him quite securely.

PATIENT: "I don't know why, I expected him to be a towhead. I was when I was born. (*After a pause*) I don't see any forceps marks. They've trimmed his fingernails. Are his eyes blue?"

NURSE: "Most babies' eyes tend to be more

blue than brown at first. What color would you say your eyes are? Your husband's eyes?"

PATIENT: "Mine are hazel. His are brown."

NURSE: "It is possible that you could each have the characteristic of blue eyes to pass on to a child."

PATIENT: "He looks like his daddy."

NURSE: "What part of him? Can you tell?"

PATIENT: "No, not really. His nose maybe."

NURSE: "You can unwrap him if you'd like."

PATIENT: "He has big feet. Look at his long toes."

Mrs. X continued for about the next 30 minutes to hold the baby quite comfortably and to comment about him in a similar vein. Little pauses threaded her observations as she went on: "He was a very active baby when I was carrying him. What's he doing? Is he hiccupping? What can he really see? He has a nice pink color. Does he have a bridge in his nose? I was born without one. Has he been given water yet? His ears are so big! At least they seem to be, in relation to his head."

The questions and comments were stated rather matter-of-factly with a certain objectivity and a seeming lack of involvement, as though she were commenting on any baby in the nursery. Mrs. X did not speak to the baby, kiss him or show much change in voice or face during the first prolonged encounter with her baby. The nurse remained with the mother the entire time and offered once to take the baby back to the nursery, assuming that she might be tired, but she wanted to keep him longer. In this one contact with the baby, the mother displayed facets of maternal behavior as described by Rubin.[10]

These observations of the mother's first holding of the baby are presented in considerable detail because they introduce Mrs. X's continued relationship with her baby as the nurse saw it in the hospital. Mrs. X, of course, gained skill in handling the baby but continued to relate to him in a matter-of-fact manner. No spontaneous expression of delight in her child was observed.

Mrs. X made an apparently rapid physical recovery from childbirth. Even on the day of delivery she was able to sit on her episiotomy and did not complain of perineal pain. The gastrointestinal and urinary systems readily assumed normal functioning. The mother made no complaint of afterpains, even when nursing the baby. She had only minimal engorgement of the breast tissue and only occasional nipple tenderness during her 7 days in the hospital. Mrs. X's perception of her postpartal status was similar to this. On the day after delivery she was sitting on the side of her bed, with her legs hanging down. The nurse attempted to intervene.

[10] Rubin, Reva: Basic maternal behavior, Nurs. Outlook 9, No. 11:683-685, November, 1961.

NURSE: "Some mothers like to sit that way for feeding their babies. But they don't think about the fact that they've no backrest and no support for their arms, and that their feet hang down without support. They don't understand why they're tired until after it happens. Wouldn't you like to lie down in your bed or sit in the arm chair for feeding the baby?"

PATIENT: "No, I'm just fine. I feel good. I felt just fine all during pregnancy. You know, I worked until the 7th month."

On another occasion:

NURSE: "I see you have skimmed milk."

PATIENT: "That was my only problem during pregnancy—weight gain. I must have gained 30 to 35 pounds."

Other persons commented about Mrs. X's well-being. Her mother said, "I'm proud of how well she's done." The obstetrician spent a minimal amount of time with her during his hospital rounds. She had few questions and had "no problems." The pediatrician commented, "That's the kind of mother it takes to be successful with breast-feeding—one who's calm and doesn't get all flustered." Her roommate, who had a 16-month-old child whom she had breast-fed for several months, commented, "She's *so* mature." Whenever other nurses were asked about Mrs. X, they would report, "Oh, she's doing real well. She's just fine."

Mrs. X appeared to adjust with minimal difficulty to her first mothering task, that of feeding the baby. The baby nursed the first time the breast was offered and at fairly frequent intervals during the prelactation period. Mrs. X didn't appear to be upset about some of the baby's sleepy times during this period. She would hold the baby but not overstimulate him or urge him to nurse. There were no problems concerning the configuration of the breast or nipple for breast-feeding. About the 3rd postpartal day Mrs. X had some engorgement, and by the next day she had milk enough to affect a gain in the baby's weight. He continued to gain, and she was kept informed about his daily gain in weight until they were discharged from the hospital.

Although the nurse observed that Mrs. X did not express much spontaneous delight in her baby, the following interaction should be noted:

PATIENT: "Will the baby be coming to me at 2 o'clock this morning?"

NURSE: "You don't have milk yet, do you? There's no reason to disturb your rest until you have milk for the baby. Do you want to tell the nursery nurse, or should I?"

PATIENT: "I think I would like to have him—just to hold him."

NURSE: "Are you sure you don't need the rest? The purpose for bringing him at 2 A.M. is for his feeding and your comfort in relieving the milk, once it comes in. You may have him, if this is what you wish."

PATIENT: "I would like to have him."

Mrs. X said that she could use the signal system to call for anyone or to ask for anything during her hospital stay, but that it wasn't necessary; she had whatever she needed. From observation and discussion it seemed that Mrs. X was offered the "usual" guidance given to a new mother by the nurses. She had some assistance the first few days during the feeding periods, and she was included in a demonstration class for mothers on bathing the baby. She was presented with the possibility of her baby's being in her room for 2 to 3 hours in the afternoon for an "extended visit." (During this time the mother has the opportunity to observe her baby, to diaper and dress him, and to feed him if she desires.) Mrs. X took advantage of the extended visit during the last 2 afternoons she was in the hospital.

There were several instances of cues which verbally portrayed some of Mrs. X's need for instruction and guidance. The following exchange occurred in the first meeting:

NURSE: "I would like to help you with getting acquainted with your baby and with being a new mother."

PATIENT: "Sure. I don't know very much."

Several days later:

PATIENT: "I don't know just what I'm supposed to eat when I'm breast-feeding."

Then, several days later:

PATIENT: "They're going to bring him in to be with me from 1 to 4 tomorrow afternoon. I can diaper him and dress him. I need this kind of opportunity."

And still later:

NURSE: "Some doctors have printed instructions about their views of baby care."

PATIENT: "I hope mine does. There's so much I need to know."

On the second day of the extended visit experience the nurse came into the room and found the babies of both mothers asleep.

PATIENT: "I've had a busy time changing diapers and shirts."

NURSE: "What went on?"

PATIENT: "Well, he was messy before the feeding, so I changed him. Then I nursed him for 5 to 6 minutes, and he needed changing again. I had his clean diaper partly on him, and he voided all over his shirt and diaper. So I changed his shirt for the first time. There are three dirty diapers and a dirty shirt in the paper sack. They should have brought me a shopping bag!"

This was stated with a bit of humor accompanied by a moderate degree of frustration in the voice. (The nurse did not attribute any particu-

lar significance to these comments at this time.)

The patient expressed some concern and frustration about the length of her labor.

PATIENT: "Just how do you tell how long labor is? I had my first contraction at 3 A.M. on Sunday, and the baby wasn't born until 5 A.M. on Monday."

NURSE: "It's hard to judge when labor begins. Some of the early contractions are helping to thin and soften the cervix—and are useful. We call that prelabor. They don't accomplish anything very dramatic, though."

PATIENT: "I had a lot of back pain. I finally called the doctor, and he said to come into the hospital. But they slowed down when I got here. It would have been easier to stay at home longer. I had hardly dilated at all when I got here. If I'd been home, I could have been up and around. I was lucky, though. I was able to be up to the bathroom. There's no place to walk. I guess they don't like you walking up and down the corridors up there. The doctor had to give me something to stimulate labor, but then it wasn't too long—about 3 or 4 hours."

NURSE: "I don't know how one prepares a first-time mother for labor. Was it anything like you expected?"

PATIENT: "You can read a lot, and people can tell you. But you don't really know what to expect until you experience it yourself. I'm glad it's over, though, because I didn't know what it would be like."

NURSE: "I think mothers have two kinds of feelings about labor. They're eager to have it begin—"

PATIENT: "They're anxious to have the baby here."

NURSE: "They're tired of carrying that heavy uterus around. It's awkward."

PATIENT: "That never bothered me. I always felt fine."

NURSE: "Was that your main impression, that labor was long, and there was a lot of back pain?"

PATIENT: "Yes. I had no pains in the front, only pain in the back. I don't remember too clearly, because they gave me some medication to sleep. Dr. O said it would be a long time."

On another occasion (following the attendance of both patients in the room at the baby bath demonstration on Mrs. X's 4th postpartal day):

PATIENT: "They used the baby of another one of Dr. O's patients, one who delivered just 50 minutes after I did. There was a sort of race to see who'd get to the delivery room first."

NURSE: "You made it."

PATIENT: "Yes, but she'd come in only a few hours before."

NURSE: "And you'd been at work for at least 20 hours."

PATIENT: "Yes, and then some. I hope it won't be so long the next time. It shouldn't, should it?"

NURSE: (*To patient's roommate*) "Is it, Mrs. A? Was it as long this time"

PATIENT'S ROOMMATE: "No, but I have rather short labors. My first was only 8½ hours, and this one was 5 hours."

NURSE: "That's right. You're the one who has babies quite easily."

PATIENT: "You're lucky!"

Further discussion about labor continued (not all included here).

NURSE: "At least you're ready to have one more."

PATIENT: "Yes."

PATIENT'S ROOMMATE: "When I had my first baby, I said on the delivery table, 'Well, I'm ready to have another.' "

PATIENT: "I don't think I'd have said that."

NURSE: "But by the fourth day you are ready."

PATIENT: "Maybe even two days ago I'd have said it."

In summary, the nurse's evaluation of the patient at the time of homegoing was as follows:

1. She experienced a minimal amount of (physical) discomfort, less than what the nurse had observed in the immediate puerperium of a primipara in a long time.

2. She was concerned about her baby's welfare, although she related to him with some degree of objectivity and distance. She proceeded with the mothering skills of feeding, dressing and handling him with considerable naturalness and lack of apparent frustration. She didn't request much assistance from the nursing or medical staff in relation to her care or the baby's.

3. She seemed to have realistic plans for managing when she went home. Her mother-in-law lived with them and could assist with cooking, cleaning and answering the telephone. Her mother would come at intervals to assist with the laundry and heavier duties. Her husband would be there evenings and nights, and she would take care of herself and the baby.

The more dominant themes would lead one to assume that she would manage at home in a similar manner with maturity, calmness and matter-of-factness. The nurse herself would always have assumed so, had she not been privileged to see Mrs. X at home on the 9th postpartal day.

After First 52 Hours at Home

The nurse called the X residence about 6:15 P.M. on the day after the mother's discharge from the hospital. This time was selected to fit into the family's usual 5:15 P.M. dinner hour, as described by Mrs. X during her hospital stay. The purpose of the nurse's call was to determine whether this would be a suitable time to visit the family at home. Mrs. X's mother-in-law answered the telephone but soon called her son, because Mrs. X was feeding the baby.

PATIENT'S HUSBAND: "Hello."

NURSE: "Good evening. How's the new father?"

HUSBAND: "Pretty good."

NURSE: "I had mentioned to your wife that I might stop today, but that I would call first to see how things were going."

HUSBAND: "She's running a little behind schedule. We're going to have our dinner as soon as she's finished feeding the baby."

NURSE: "Perhaps I should wait and come tomorrow—or another time."

HUSBAND: "The baby was kind of fussy around 2."

NURSE: "2 P.M.?"

HUSBAND: "No, 2 A.M. this morning. I guess she was up most of the night with him."

NURSE: "Has she had any rest today?"

HUSBAND: "Not too much. Her mother said she would come over for a while this evening."

The conversation continued a short while. The nurse indicated that she would call again the next day to ascertain an appropriate visiting time. The nurse telephoned about 1:30 P.M. the following day.

PATIENT: "How are you?"

NURSE: "How are *you* is the question."

PATIENT: "I guess I'll survive."

NURSE: "You guess you'll survive?"

PATIENT: "I've just finished feeding him. He seemed hungry. He nursed for about 20 minutes. I'm getting him settled now."

NURSE: "How did it go last night?"

PATIENT: "He slept real well from about 11 P.M. to 2:15 A.M."

NURSE: "That was over 3 hours."

PATIENT: "Then he had a fussy period after I fed him. He didn't go back to sleep until about 4:30. I gave him some water. He took about 2 ounces. Then I had to wake him about a quarter to 8."

NURSE: "That was pretty good. He slept more than 3 hours *that* time."

PATIENT: "My husband was up with me, too."

There was further telephone discussion about feeding, and the nurse made arrangements to come for a visit within the next few hours.

Mrs. X was seated in an armchair. The front of her dress was open, but the brassière was in place. The baby was dressed in a kimona and wrapped in a receiving blanket. Mrs. X looked pale and tired. She didn't look up right away. The nurse sat down on a hassock near the mother's chair.

NURSE: "How are things going by now?"

PATIENT: "I just wasn't prepared for all this. I felt so good in the hospital."

PATIENT'S MOTHER: (*Rubbing lotion on creases of infant's arms and legs*) "I told Mary when she was pregnant that she ought to go to some classes, and she said, 'What do I want to go to classes for?'"

NURSE: "I don't really know *how* parents can be prepared for these early days. Classes help some, but perhaps one needs to experience them. I don't know if you can really get prepared!"

PATIENT'S MOTHER: "I think he's growing. I think I can see him growing."

NURSE: "You think you can see him change each day?"

PATIENT'S MOTHER: "Yes, I think I'm enjoying the baby more than Mary. She's so tired—and she has the responsibility."

Mrs. X excused herself. While she was gone, her mother commented:

PATIENT'S MOTHER: "She hasn't had much sleep. She's very tired. Everything's so new to her. I came over Monday night a while so she could get some rest. Now I helped with the laundry and bathed the baby just before his feeding."

Mrs. X returned with her mother-in-law and introduced her to the nurse. She sat down in the living room now, where the four adults were seated, and where the baby was asleep in his bassinet.

NURSE: (*To patient*) "I see you have something here to drink."

PATIENT'S MOTHER: "She's not eating very well. Says she's not hungry. I made her a steak sandwich for lunch. She only ate half of it—and some salad and some milk."

NURSE: "When you're so tired, it's hard to be interested in food."

PATIENT: "I just have to force myself. I'm not hungry."

NURSE: "What about fluids? Are you drinking plenty?"

PATIENT: "I'm drinking quite a bit. Milk, fruit juices, water."

NURSE: "How has today gone in comparison with yesterday?"

PATIENT: "Everything's so new. Things all seem to come at once. I don't know where to start. I've never been around babies much. Some people have younger brothers and sisters; others have baby sat. I never did much of that, at least not with such a small baby. Not even with my niece and nephew. My sister-in-law was so pro-

tective that even my mother couldn't get close to the baby."

NURSE: "There are a lot of young women who haven't had the benefit of caring for small babies."

PATIENT: "Everything's so new. I just want to do the right thing." (With this statement her eyes became watery and red, and the tears nearly spilled over.)

MOTHER-IN-LAW: "Mary's doing a fine job."

NURSE: "You had some question last night about how long the baby was nursing, and how to keep him awake. How has this been today?"

The discussion continued with details for feeding and other events surrounding the baby.

PATIENT: "Last night my husband said, 'You're never going to breast-feed another baby!'"

NURSE: "Why do you think he said that?"

PATIENT: "He compares our baby with my brother's child, who takes 8 ounces from the bottle and sleeps all night. He forgets that he's a 2-month-old baby!"

The discussion focused for a while on bathing the baby.

PATIENT: "I haven't done that yet. I'll need to take hold. There's so much I don't know about. It's different seeing it done than doing it."

NURSE: "Perhaps right now, if you're tired, it's just as well to let someone else bathe him. *You're* the only one who can feed him. Others can do some of the other things."

PATIENT: "I'm used to work. It's not that. I worked in an office for 6 years. I began to work even when I was in high school, when I was 15. You grow up fast under those circumstances."

NURSE: "You probably needed to have things pretty carefully scheduled, to work full time and to manage a house and take care of your husband."

PATIENT: "You can say that again."

NURSE: "Now you have a squirming, crying bundle that doesn't fit into any schedule. Remember, Dr. M said he's not even sophisticated enough to know he shouldn't have his fussy periods at night."

PATIENT: "If you only knew when it would *end*, you know—not even on the day, but which *week*."

NURSE: "If there were only some limits which you could count on, you mean, knowing that sleeping through the night would happen by such and such a time."

PATIENT: "It's not knowing that's hard."

Further conversation revealed that Mrs. X had expressed some of her feelings by crying, and that her husband had found her weeping when she'd gotten up to be with the baby during a fussy time at night. The nurse gave some guidance about scheduling, feeding, placement of the baby's crib, and she answered questions of Mrs. X and her mother. It was near the dinner hour, and the nurse made plans to visit again in a few days.

Just by chance Mrs. X's mother met the nurse in a distant part of the hospital. The following remarks are excerpts from the mother's comments: "My daughter was so sure of herself during pregnancy. I wanted her to go to prenatal classes to learn about babies, but she didn't want to. . . . She feels so inadequate. I wasn't prepared for her depression. She seems to feel so inadequate about the bath."

The expressed concerns of Mrs. X's mother added weight to the previous question of what was happening to cause such a marked change in Mrs. X's behavior and performance in her new role. What facets of nursing care in the hospital could have been utilized to prepare Mrs. X more adequately for coping with problems on her return home?

At the beginning of the third day, 52 hours after she returned home, Mrs. X seemed to experience the low point of her "depression." The following day the baby began to sleep longer between feedings. Mrs. X began to get more rest, her appetite improved, she felt stronger, and she bathed her baby. There were still frustrations and problems to be handled, but they seemed to be more manageable. For instance, on Monday of her 2nd week at home, the nurse telephoned at 3:30 in the afternoon to see whether she might stop for a visit. Mrs. X said that everything was topsy-turvy, and that she was still trying to get herself dressed. However, she had bathed the baby, and she was preparing dinner. The following week the nurse made her third visit to the home. It was her first contact with the patient alone. Although the nurse was aware that the "right moment" had probably passed for helping Mrs. X with the distress she expressed by nearly crying, she did introduce the subject. The following interaction occurred with some expression of feeling, but there was no weeping or overt manifestation of anxiety as the "first 52 hours" were discussed.

NURSE: "You've been home a little more than a week now. Is it what you expected? Anything like what you envisioned it would be?"

PATIENT: "I had *no* idea what to expect. I was never with small babies. I just didn't know how much time and work a baby would take. It's a 24-hour responsibility."

NURSE: "Those first days must have been pretty difficult. You must have felt a bit helpless at not knowing what to do when the baby cried."

PATIENT: "Yes, they were. Sunday wasn't so bad. I'd just come home, and people were around. My mother was here. But then Monday mother had to work, and my husband went to work, I was alone with the baby except for my mother-in-law. I knew how to change a diaper, but that was about all. I wanted to do the right thing for the baby."

NURSE: "I'm sure a mother wants to respond to her baby's needs, but deciding what is the right thing is hard. It is a lot of responsibility, to be a mother, a parent."

PATIENT: "I think we're getting acquainted. I can tell his cry when he's hungry; I can tell when he has gas by the way he draws up his legs."

NURSE: "You are more certain about making decisions as to what to do for him? You can decide when he needs milk—or water?"

PATIENT: "Yes. This week is so much better than last."

NURSE: "Did other things bother you those first days—beside not knowing what to do with the baby? The house?"

PATIENT: "Well, yes. I do have certain ways of doing things, and when other people help, they can't know how you do them. I've always been very healthy."

NURSE: "So you're not accustomed to having people help you?"

PATIENT: "No, I've always been quite independent. I've worked since I was 15. I worked until my 7th month of pregnancy. I felt so well in the hospital."

NURSE: "Yes, we kept talking about that, and kept looking for some problems, but—"

PATIENT: "There weren't any. Not even my stitches hurt after the 2nd day."

NURSE: "When you came home, you hit a low point."

PATIENT: "I wasn't prepared for being so depressed. I guess it's called the 'baby blues.'"

NURSE: "Some people have this experience in the hospital. Did it happen to you there?"

PATIENT: "Not really—maybe only once. One evening my husband didn't come to see me because he wasn't feeling well, but he didn't tell me until later. That upset me, because I wish he'd tell me. Maybe I could do something to help him."

NURSE: "You probably haven't felt so helpless in a long time as you did those first several days."

PATIENT: "No, I haven't. If we have another baby, I'd know more what to expect. . . ."

It may be helpful to have further information about Mrs. X and the significant people in her environment. Mrs. X is the younger of two children born to parents of different religious faiths. Although her father is in the family picture, Mrs. X did not once refer to him. Mrs. X's mother, on the other hand, has played an active role. She visited her daughter in the hospital and assisted her daughter with household tasks on the days in which she was not working. The mother commented that her daughter has always been a "good girl," and that she never had to worry about her when she was out on a date. If she were going to be late, she'd always call. Some of the interactions previously shared might provide some clues about her opinion of her daughter's adequacy as a mother.

There is little information about Mrs. X's brother except that he has been to college, is married, is the father of two children, and lives with his family in a nearby suburb. On the other hand, Mrs. X mentioned twice that she had gone to work when she was 15 (there are gaps in information here as to the reason for working and the nature of her work). On graduation from high school Mrs. X went to work as a bookkeeper and continued to work in that position through the 7th month of her pregnancy.

Mr. and Mrs. X have been married for several years. Mr. X, who is 9 years older than his wife, has been employed as a craftsman with the same company for the past 13 years. Mrs. X spoke with delight in her voice and her face when she told that her husband was thinking of painting a banner with the words "Welcome home, Mary and Johnny." On the day of discharge from the hospital, when the nurse first saw them together, they seemed to relate with warmth but with a certain self-consciousness and reserve. He was attentive in helping her into the car.

The nurse observed the new parents together briefly on two occasions in their home. On the day Mrs. X was so depressed, she eagerly listened for sounds of the car as the time for her husband's homecoming drew near. When he did come into the living room, she immediately offered to get his slippers. On another occasion he slipped his arm around her waist as she was in the kitchen warming a bottle of water for the baby. The X's are not in financial distress; they have two cars, hospitalization insurance, more than adequate equipment for the baby, and are buying a new suburban home.

They are eager to move into their new home. The advent of the baby has crowded them, since Mr. X's mother also lives with them in their 2-bedroom house. This necessitates placement of the baby's equipment in their bedroom and the baby in the living room. Mr. X's mother is an elderly woman who has a serious chronic illness. Mrs. X expressed her desire to contribute toward making a home for her mother-in-law and making her life as pleasant as possible. She commented several times on how well she and her mother-in-law got along. When the nurse was in the home, Mrs. X's mother-in-law was friendly and courteous, but she kept busy with her household tasks instead of joining in the conversation.

Comments and Conclusions

The concept that pregnancy is a period of disequilibrium and maturational crisis needs to be reiterated to professionals working with women during the childbearing cycle. This may need special emphasis in relation to the woman who has an uncomplicated pregnancy and childbirth experience, since it is usually the woman with problems and complications who occupies the major portion of the nurse's attention. Pregnancy involves profound physiologic and psychological changes. An intensive longitudinal study of 15 women during pregnancy and the 1st year after delivery was conducted by Bibring *et al.* in Boston. The theoretical framework on which the study is based is as follows:

Pregnancy is a crisis that affects all expectant mothers, no matter what their state of psychic health. Crises, as we see it, are turning points in the life of the individual, leading to acute disequilibria which under favorable conditions result in specific maturational steps toward new functions. We find them as developmental phenomena at points of no return between one phase and the next when decisive changes deprive former central needs and modes of living of their significance, forcing the acceptance of highly charged new goals and functions. Pregnancy as a major turning point in the life of a woman represents one of these normal crises, especially for the primigravida who faces the impact of this event for the first time. We believe that all women show what looks like remarkable, far-reaching psychological changes when they are pregnant. The outcome of this crisis, then, has profound effects on the early mother-child relationships.[11]

The final results of the study have not been published, but they may contribute significantly to understanding the nature of the crisis and the maturation expected.

Bibring states that the crisis does not end with the birth of the baby but continues into the puerperium and perhaps beyond:

The findings that crisis continues, more or less

11 Bibring, Grete, *et al.*: A study of the psychological processes in pregnancy and of the earliest mother-child relationships, Psychoanal. Stud. Child 14:25-26, 1959.

so, beyond parturition offer strong support in favor of the proposition that the frequent problems in the early mother-child relationship are partly due to an as yet incomplete reorganization of the mother's psychic equilibrium at the time of delivery.[12]

Deutsch agrees that the crisis period extends beyond the delivery of the baby.[13]

Pregnancy and childbirth could be discussed much more extensively as a general crisis, but it may be more helpful to investigate some of the possible components of the crisis and to reflect on those which may be applicable to Mrs. X's situation. The first several posthospital days illustrate an obvious crisis period for Mrs. X.

Components of the Crisis Situation

A very complex component of the crisis and disequilibrium has to do with the relationship of psychosexual development and maternal feelings.

Deutsch[14] writes extensively about motherhood, pregnancy, confinement and lactation in relation to Freud's concepts of psychosexual development. For example, breast-feeding the baby may arouse the erogenous area of the nipple and create sexual sensations. The nursing mother may be confused by the aroused sexual feelings and the feelings of love and responsiveness as she nurses her baby.

There is limited data from which to assess Mrs. X's situation in regard to the psychosexual component. Mrs. X appeared to be rather matter-of-fact about the process of breast-feeding. She would prepare the nipple for feeding in the presence of her roommate and the nurse, and she allowed the nurse to touch her breast to assist the baby in obtaining proper grasp of the areola. She practiced the technic of manual expression of breast milk at the same time her roommate was practicing, although a certain degree of privacy was planned during this teaching-learning experience.

Mrs. X did not ask questions of the nurse or the obstetrician concerning the appropriate time for renewing sexual intercourse in relation to the process of vaginal and perineal healing. The nurse introduced the subject, and Mrs. X seemed to appreciate the guidance offered, since the obstetrician had not included this in his homegoing instructions.

On three different occasions the subject of subsequent pregnancies and child spacing was indirectly introduced by giving information in relation to breast-feeding and ovulation. Mrs. X did not pursue the topic with further discussion or questions. She seemed to remain somewhat guarded and reserved in all of the relationships, and thus one would expect that she would maintain this reserve in the area of psychosexual material.

Closely aligned with the psychosexual component of the crisis is Caplan's description of the change in equilibrium between the ego and the id. He likens the usual relationship of id and ego to an iceberg, the portion above the surface being the ego and the portion below the surface being the id. During pregnancy the iceberg turns upside down and allows id material to come to the surface rather easily. Fantasies and wishes are consciously expressed with a relatively minimal production of anxiety.[15]

Caplan describes the pregnant woman as a kind of battery that needs to be charged. If those significant to her are not able to meet her needs for being nurtured, she may have more difficulty in extending herself to her child during those early months when the child has many needs but gives little to the mother in response to the fulfillment of those needs.

Rubin analyzes the passive and the dependent phases of the puerperium. These were discussed in Chapter 14.

There is very little data about Mrs. X's period of pregnancy except that she felt fine and continued to work until the third trimester of pregnancy. One would, however, question the degree to which she was allowed to be dependent and to receive care during the early puerperium in the hospital. She did "take in" rest and food, but on the day after delivery she was already taking her own bath in the shower. She had no obvious or particular reasons to request or demand nursing or medical care. One could question whether she might have been better fortified to cope with the baby at home if there had been more attention to the "battery-charging" process.

There are clues that Mrs. X is a "giving" per-

---

[12] *Ibid.*, p. 20.

[13] Deutsch, Helene: Psychology of Women, p. 261, New York, Grune & Stratton, 1945.

[14] *Ibid.*

[15] Caplan, Gerald: Concepts of Mental Health and Consultation, Children's Bureau Publication No. 373, p. 51, Washington, D. C., 1959.

son who does not ask much for herself. She was accustomed to giving herself to a job and to her family. She invested herself in her mother-in-law to provide "pleasant moments" for a woman with a serious illness. She invested herself in her husband in proper feeding ("He's not been served a TV dinner since we were married!") and in caring ("Would you like your slippers?"). She might well have had some conflicting feelings about the reversal in role with these significant people. It might have been easier for her to receive care from hospital personnel, because helping is an expected part of their function; but to receive care from those to whom she usually extended herself was quite a different situation.

Another component of the crisis of childbearing is the inescapable revival of feelings about the woman's relationship with her own mother. This relationship is always influenced by guilt feelings. The degree to which further independence from her mother is sought is somewhat in direct proportion to the extent of her guilt feelings. She is caught between two poles: that of needing her mother or a mother substitute in providing care and guidance in the new role of motherhood, and that of asserting that she is now the mother.

The fate of the identification with the mother is another factor that determines the course of pregnancy. In every instance the capacity for motherhood is related to this identification. The ego of the pregnant woman must find a harmonious compromise between her deeply unconscious identification with the child, which is directed toward the future, and her identification with her own mother, which is directed toward the past. Wherever one of these identifications is rejected, difficulties arise. In the first case the fetus becomes a hostile parasite, in the second the pregnant woman's capacity for motherhood is weakened by her unwillingness to accept her identification with her own mother.[16]

Many questions could be raised about Mrs. X's mother's advice that she attend some classes during pregnancy and her daughter's expressed lack of need and interest in attending prenatal classes. The question of why Mrs. X refused to attend classes has many facets. It is interesting to note the mother's response on the "52nd hour," the day of frustration and depression: "I told her when she was pregnant she ought to go to some classes." Perhaps Mrs. X did not need to depend on her mother too much during pregnancy or in the hospital period. She did indeed need her

mother in the early days at home. She needed her to do the laundry, to bathe the baby, and to give guidance in understanding the needs of her child. How could Mrs. X work through becoming a "coequal" with her own mother in terms of motherhood when she felt so helpless and inadequate in meeting her baby's needs?

Mrs. X's responses in "I just wasn't prepared for this. . . . I just want to do the *right* thing," may communicate something of ego inadequacy in relation to motherhood. She once commented ironically, "They call babies a bundle of joy!"

She was afraid to do certain things for the baby. The day after she had bathed the baby for the first time:

PATIENT: "It wasn't so bad once I did it. I just was afraid to be by myself to bathe him. I was afraid I wouldn't know what to do—like I couldn't get under one of his arms. So my sister-in-law says, 'Just skip it this time.'"

NURSE: "You were afraid you might hurt him."

PATIENT: "I had so much more confidence after I'd done it."

Something of the extent of her fear may be understood by the fact that it was 7 *days* after she had given the first bath that she ventured to give the bath when she was alone. Similarly, she waited to give vitamins to the baby until her husband was at home with her. This is quite in contrast with her observation of the nurse's handling of the baby when he was regurgitating some mucus on his first day of life. When the nurse asked her if she'd know what to do, she said: "Just turn him on his side to get the mucus out—so it doesn't get in his throat."

Perhaps it is somewhat artificial to attempt to describe components of a crisis experience. Certainly in the actuality of a situation these components overlap and merge. However, for the purpose of attaining a closer understanding of the patient in order to help her to achieve her goals, there is value in investigating all aspects of the situation. For practical purposes it might be said that Mrs. X's crisis is a fairly predictable one. Therefore, the nurse's anticipatory guidance will be of immense benefit to the new mother during a necessarily critical period of her life.

SUGGESTED READING

General

Adams, M. M.: Appraisal of the newborn, Am. J. Nurs. 55, No. 11:1336-1337, November, 1955.

---

16 Deutsch, *loc. cit.*, p. 145.

American Academy of Pediatrics: Standards and Recommendations for Hospital Care of Newborn Infants, rev. ed., Evanston, The Academy, 1964.

Arnold, H. W., *et al.*: Transition to extra-uterine life, Am. J. Nurs. 65, No. 10:77-80, October, 1965.

Berrien, C. D.: Evaluating the newborn, Nurs. Outlook 9:93-96, February, 1961.

Blake, Florence, and Wright, F. H.: Essentials of Pediatric Nursing, ed. 7, Philadelphia, Lippincott, 1963.

Bowlby, John: Maternal Care and Mental Health, Geneva, World Health Organization, 1952.

Buchanan-Davidson, D. J.: What we can learn from meconium, Am. J. Nurs. 63, No. 7:112-113, July, 1963.

Buetow, K. C., *et al.*: Effect of maintenance of "normal" skin temperature on survival of infants of low birth weight, Pediatrics, 34:163-170, August, 1964.

Clifford, S. H., and Davison, E. C.: The origin of obstetric nurseries, J. Pediat. 44:205-212, February, 1954.

Davis, M. E., and Rubin, Reva: De Lee's Obstetrics for Nurses, ed. 17, Philadelphia, Saunders, 1962.

DeLamerens, S., *et al.*: Neonatal bilirubin levels after use of phenothiazine derivations for obstetrical analgesia, J. Pediat. 65:925-928, December, 1964.

Desmond, Murdina, *et al.*: The clinical behavior of the newly born, J. Pediat. 62:307-325, March, 1963.

Eisenberg, R. B., *et al.*: Auditory behavior in the human neonate: Preliminary report, J. Speech Hearing Res. 7:245-269, September, 1964.

Fantz, R. L.: Pattern discrimination and selective attention as determinants of perceptual development from birth *in* Kidd, Aline H., and Rivoire, J. L. (eds.): Perceptual Development in Children, New York, International Universities Press, 1965.

————: "The origin of form perception," Sci. Am. 204:66-72, May, 1961.

————: Visual experience in infants: decreased attention to familiar patterns relative to novel ones, Science 146, No. 3644:668-670, October 30, 1964.

Gryboski, J. D.: The swallowing mechanism of the neonate: I. Esophageal and gastric motility, Pediatrics 35:445-452, March, 1965.

Keitel, H. G.: Preventing neonatal diaper rash, Am. J. Nurs. 65, No. 5:124-126, May, 1965.

James, L. S.: The importance of observations of the newborn infant at birth, Bull. Maternal Infant Health 10, No. 1:17-23, 1963.

James, L. S., *et al.*: Respiratory physiology of the fetus and newborn infant, New Eng. J. Med. 271:1403-1409, December 31, 1964.

Jonas, G.: Retention of a plastibell circumcision ring. Report of a case, Obstet. Gynec. 24:835, December, 1964.

Levin, S.: Baby habits, genesis and ontogenesis. Speculation on prehistory, biblical history and some phenomena of babyhood, Clin. Pediat. 3:741-742, December, 1964.

————: A Philosophy of Infant Feeding, Springfield, Ill., Thomas, 1963.

Lipton, E. L., *et al.*: Swaddling, a child care practice: Historical, cultural and experimental observations, Pediatrics, 35:519-567, March, 1965.

MacCready, Jean: A Feeding Room for Babies, Am. J. Nurs. 64, No. 7:117, July, 1964.

Marlow, D. R.: Textbook of Pediatric Nursing, ed. 2, Philadelphia, Saunders, 1965.

Meyer, H. F.: Infant Foods and Feeding Practice, ed. 2, Philadelphia, Saunders, 1965.

Nelson, Waldo (ed): Textbook of Pediatrics, ed. 8, Philadelphia, Saunders, 1964.

Parmalee, A. H.: Management of the Newborn, ed. 2, Chicago, The Year Book Pub., 1959.

Parmalee, A. H., Jr., *et al.*: "Infant sleep patterns from birth to 16 weeks of age, J. Pediat. 65: 576-582, October, 1964.

Polgar, George: The first breath: A turbulent period of physiologic adjustment, Clin. Pediat. 2:562-571, October, 1963.

Riker, A. P.: Breastfeeding, Public Affairs Pamphlet No. 353S, New York, Public Affairs Pamphlets, 1964.

Ringholz, Sharon, and Morris, M.: A test of some assumptions about rooming-in, Nurs. Res. 10: 196-199, Fall, 1961.

Shipley, T., *et al.*: The human electroretinogram in the first day of life, J. Pediat. 65:733-739, November, 1964.

Silverman, W. A., and Parke, P. C.: Keep him warm, Am. J. Nurs. 65, No. 10:81-84, October, 1965.

Smith, C. A.: The first breath, Sci. Am. 109:27-35, October, 1963.

————: The Physiology of the Newborn Infant, ed. 3, Springfield, Thomas, 1959.

Stella, Sister Mary: A disposable nurser system, Am. J. Nurs. 63, No. 11:100, November, 1963.

Stembera, Z. K.: Umbilical blood flow in healthy newborn infants during the first minutes after birth, Am. J. Obstet. Gynec. 91:568-574, February 15, 1965.

Ziegel, Erna, and Van Blarcom, C. C.: Obstetric Nursing, ed. 5, New York, Macmillan, 1964.

The Mother and Her Newborn Infant

Adams, Martha: Early concerns of primigravida

mothers regarding infant care activities, Nurs. Res. 12, No. 2:72-77, Spring, 1963.

Barnes, G. R., Jr., *et al.*: Management of breast feeding, J.A.M.A. 151:192-199, January 17, 1953.

Bibring, G. L., *et al.*: A study of the psychological processes in pregnancy and of the earliest mother-child relationship, Psychoanal. Stud. Child 16:9-72, 1961.

Birchfield, Marilyn: A mother's views on breast feeding, Am. J. Nurs. 63, No. 3:88-90, March, 1963.

Blake, Florence, and Wright, F. H.: Essentials of Pediatric Nursing, ed. 7, Philadelphia, Lippincott, 1963.

Bowlby, John: Maternal Care and Mental Health, Geneva, World Health Organization, 1952.

Brazelton, T. B.: Early mother-infant adjustment, Pediatrics 32, No. 5:931-936, November, 1963.

Brody, Sylvia: Patterns of Mothering, New York, Internat. Univ. Press, 1956.

Caplan, Gerald: An Approach to Community Mental Health, New York, Grune & Stratton, 1961.

————: Concepts of Mental Health and Consultation, Washington, D. C., U. S. Children's Bureau, 1959.

Davis, A.: The Skills of Communication, Am. J. Nurs. 63:66-70, January, 1963.

Deutsch, Helene: Psychology of Women, vol. 2, Motherhood, New York, Grune & Stratton, 1945.

Disbrow, M. A.: Factors Involved in Successful Breast Feeding, U.S.P.H.S. Grant GN7901, unpublished, 1962.

Guillot, E. C.: Patterns of help for post-partum mothers, Children 11:147-151, July-August, 1964.

Heinstein, Martin: Influence of breast feeding on children's behavior, Children 10, No. 3:93-97, May-June, 1963.

Iorio, Josephine: Breast feeding mothers help each other, Am. J. Nurs. 64, Vol. 10:119-120, October, 1964.

Keane, Vera: Nursing care of the family after delivery, Bull. Am. Coll. Nurs. Midwifery 9, No. 3:56-63, Fall, 1964.

Lesser, M. S., and Keane, V. R.: Nurse, Patient Relationships in a Hospital Maternity Service, St. Louis, Mosby, 1956.

McElin, T. W., *et al.*: The microbiological environment of a rooming-in maternity, Am. J. Obstet. Gynec. 83:907-917, April, 1964.

Mead, Margaret: Cultural Patterns and Technical Change, New York, New American Library, 1955.

Mintern, Leigh, *et al.*: Mothers of Six Cultures, New York, Wiley, 1964.

Moore, Lucille, and White, G. D.: Comparisons of teaching methods in maternal and infant care, Nurs. Outlook 13, No. 5:74-76, May, 1965.

Murray, B. L.: A challenge for nursing in maternal-infant care, Bull. Maternal Infant Health 8, No. 1:15-19, 23, 1961.

Newton, Michael, and Newton, Niles: The normal course and management of lactation, Clin. Obstet. Gynec. 5:44-63, March, 1962.

Newton, Niles: Maternal Emotions, New York, Hoeber, 1955.

Newton, Niles, and Newton, Michael: Mothers' reactions to their newborn babies, J.A.M.A. 181:206-210, July 21, 1962.

Nursing instruction aids breast feeding, Hosp. Topics 38:73, May, 1960.

Rich, O. J.: Personal communication to authors, 1965.

————: Clinical Study of a Primipara's Initial Adaptation to Mothering, U.S.P.H.S. Grant STIMH 7988-03, unpublished, 1965.

Richardson, F. H.: The Nursing Mother, New York, Prentice-Hall, 1953.

Rose, P. A.: Identification and Application of Psychiatric Principles in the Nursing Care of Maternity Patients, Clinical Nursing Monograph, New York, American Nurses Assoc., 1962.

Rubin, Reva: Basic maternal behavior, Nurs. Outlook 9:683-686, November, 1961.

————: Puerperal change, Nurs. Outlook 9:753-755, December, 1961.

————: Maternal touch, Nurs. Outlook 11, No. 11:828-831, November, 1963.

————: The family-child relationship and nursing care, Nurs. Outlook 12, No. 9:36-39, September, 1964.

Sarto, Sister Joseph: Breast feeding—preparation, practice and professional help, Am. J. Nurs. 63, No. 12:58-60, December, 1963.

Selye, Hans: The stress syndrome, Am. J. Nurs. 65, No. 3:97-99, March, 1965.

Wessel, Morris: Maternal and child nursing—as a pediatrician sees it, Nurs. Outlook 11, No. 3:207-210, March, 1963.

Wiedenbach, Ernestine: Family-Centered Maternity Nursing, New York, Putnam, 1958.

Yarrow, L. J.: "Maternal care and infant behavior, Children 10, No. 1:32-34, January-February, 1963.

Causes of Prematurity • Causes of Premature Deaths • Description at Birth
Nursing Management • Parental Reactions • Growth and Development

Chapter 16

Care of the Premature Infant

INTRODUCTION

The prevention of premature birth is considered by many authorities to be the most important problem in obstetrics. Yet, despite the importance of this problem, little progress has been made in achieving a desirable reduction in the prematurity rate. For example, the incidence has not changed perceptibly in the last 75 years; it still remains about 7 per cent in the white race and 12 per cent in the nonwhite races. In addition, little definitive knowledge has been obtained about the causes of this phenomenon. Many factors, of course, are known to be associated with it, among them race, ethnicity, economic status, illegitimacy, maternal age, quality of antepartal care, social class and nutritional status.

The basic meaning of the word "prematurity" is underdevelopment, referring to the inability of the infant born prematurely to make an adaptation to extra-uterine existence to a degree comparable with the survival rates in mature infants. For the purpose of clinical evaluation, however, more stringent criteria have been developed—criteria which admittedly are open to challenge. Thus, a premature infant has been defined arbitrarily as any infant of single or multiple birth that is born prematurely, at term or even past term with a weight of 2,500 Gm. (5½ lbs.) or less. Such an infant is usually less than 48 cm. (19 in.)

in length and usually has been born prior to the 36th week of gestation.

Nonwhites, because they generally have smaller infants than whites, have a higher percentage of premature infants. Infants over this empirical weight, even though apparently born at full term, occasionally may be diagnosed by a physician as "premature" on the basis of other considerations, such as faulty maintenance of body temperature, particular feeding difficulties or certain physical characteristics. This may apply especially to infants born to diabetic or prediabetic mothers. Although the upper limit of weight has been established, the lower never has been accepted by any authoritative group, and the level at which a dividing line is drawn between abortions and premature infants remains a matter of personal or local preference. The lower limit will depend on the definition of abortion, but the 1,000 Gm. figure is the one most frequently used. If the baby is from 6 to 8 weeks or more premature, the diagnosis is comparatively easy because of weight, length and physical characteristics. The closer to full term the baby is, the greater are the chances for survival.

The nursing care that is required for premature infants and their parents presents an interesting challenge for the nurse. The situation is a poignant one, for the life of the infant often hangs in the balance, and the postpartal course is complicated by concomitant psychological disorganization. The nurse is one of the key persons who is responsible for a successful outcome for both infant and parents.

CAUSES OF PREMATURITY

Since more than half of the neonatal deaths in the United States are due to prematurity, and since these rates have remained constant for many years, the emphasis on preventive care must be stressed. If an equal amount of the money expended on premature care were applied to preventive care, it would be interesting to prognosticate the results. The causes of prematurity demand continued attention and research, since compared with the information now available about other aspects of obstetrics, a paucity of definite answers exists. However, it is known that multiple pregnancy is the most common single cause of prematurity. Other causes are chronic hypertension, toxemia, infectious diseases (such as syphilis), acute abdominal conditions resulting in surgical interference, cardiac and diabetic diseases and thyroid disturbances.

Pregnancy itself also has its contributing causes—malformation in the embryologic development, erythroblastosis fetalis dependent on the Rh factor and faulty nutrition of the fetus. Abnormalities of placental structure resulting in the rupture of the membranes, placenta previa, abruptio placenta and hydramnios may cause prematurity. Then, too, there is a fairly large group of premature births due to undiagnosed causes. Also, the associated factors mentioned earlier are not to be forgotten. All in all, the problem involves a variety of interrelated variables, some physiologic, some pathological, and some that defy such neat categorization.

CAUSES OF PREMATURE DEATHS

Along with the dramatic advances made in the reduction of maternal and infant mortality in recent decades has gone a commensurate reduction in the death rate of premature infants. However, the mortality of premature infants still is disproportionately high. By far the commonest cause of death among prematures is idiopathic respiratory distress syndrome (hyaline membrane disease). These terms are used to describe a syndrome of neonatal respiratory distress in which pulmonary hyaline membrane with atelectasis are the principal findings at autopsy. This condition is seen frequently also among infants who have been delivered by cesarean section and among babies of diabetic mothers. Other principal causes of death include anoxia, malformations, bronchopneumonia, septicemia and other infections and birth injuries (principally cerebral, for the blood vessels of the premature lack the supporting wall structure and are damaged very easily).

DESCRIPTION AT BIRTH

As there are many degrees of prematurity, so also there are various stages of anatomic and physiologic development. Many of the symptoms described below may vary in infants of approximately the same fetal age, depending on the cause of prematurity and the physical condition of the mother and the infant. At birth the premature baby lacks the subcutaneous fat which is deposited during the last 2 months of intra-uterine development. This gives the skin a transparent appearance with the blood vessels easily seen through the skin, which often is of a deep red color, sometimes with a cyanotic hue. These premature babies are prone likewise to develop icteric skin changes. Lanugo is usually abundant all over the skin surface but disappears within a few weeks.

The external ears and the nose are very soft, due to the underdeveloped cartilage. The ears lie very close to the head. The skull is round, in contrast with the long anteroposterior skull diameter of the full-term infant. The fontanels are large, and the sutures prominent. The fingernails and toenails may be immature, often not reaching the ends of the fingers and the toes.

The infant may be puny and small, or he may approximate full-term weight; yet the internal organs may be imperfectly developed, and these babies appear to be reluctant to assume the responsibility to live. The respiration is shallow and irregular, due to the lack of lung expansion and proper gaseous exchange. There are often periods of apnea. Due to the irregular respiration and the poorly developed function of swallowing, there is danger of aspiration of milk or vomitus, causing cyanosis and predisposing to pulmonary infections. The premature baby regurgitates his food readily, because the stomach is tubular in form, and the sphincters are poorly developed. The urine is usually scanty.

The walls of the blood vessels are weak, and the tendency to hemorrhage is great. Since the central nervous system is not fully developed, the premature infant is sluggish, must be wakened to be fed, and the muscular movements are feeble. The temperature is usually subnormal and fluctuating, due to the underdeveloped heat-regulating center. The cry is monotonous, whining, "kittenlike" and effortless, showing a lack of energy. All these symptoms are evidenced in varying degrees, according to the stage of prematurity.

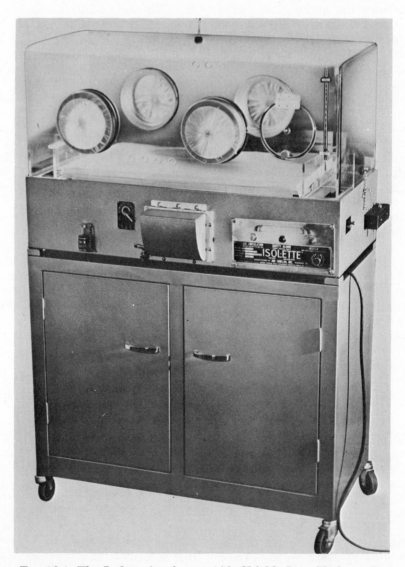

FIG. 16-1. The Isolette incubator. (Air-Shields Inc., Hatboro, Pa.)

NURSING MANAGEMENT

Since the life of the premature baby may depend on his nursing care, the nurse should realize the seriousness of this responsibility during this period of her nursing experience and make every effort to increase her knowledge and to develop her skill in caring for these infants.

Often, the first hours of the premature baby's life determine the outcome. He needs warmth, meticulous physical care, gentle handling, precise and careful feeding and protection from infection. It must be remembered always that the word "premature" means that this baby has arrived before he has had the opportunity to develop completely, and, if he is to live, this intricate development has to be completed against almost insurmountable odds—under conditions sometimes difficult even for the normal full-size baby.

Immediate Care

Since these infants come into the world "before their time," it occasionally falls to the nurse to assist with the delivery and/or the care immediately after the delivery. Even if the delivery has been effected under aseptic conditions, the care given a premature infant may differ from that given to the full-size baby, depending on his condition. For the very small and feeble premature baby, the urgency of providing immediate warmth, humidity and oxygen as indicated may precede the care of the eyes and completion of the care of the cord. Whenever possible, it is advisable to wait until the cord pulsation weakens before clamping it, so that the baby will benefit from the placental blood. The cord should be clamped or tied with special care because of the softness of the tissues, leaving space for a second ligature close to the body when the linen cord

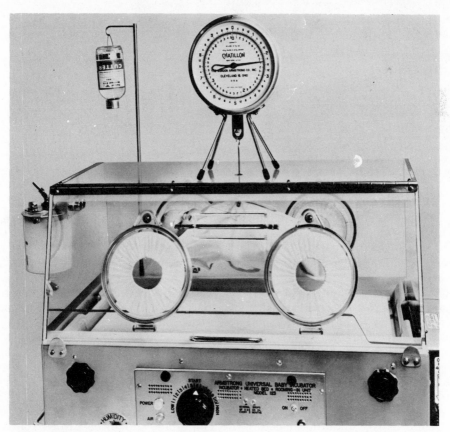

FIG. 16-2. The Armstrong Universal baby incubator. (The Gordon Armstrong Company, Inc., Cleveland, Ohio)

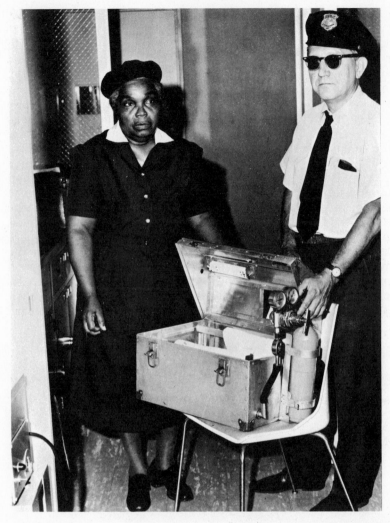

Fig. 16-3. Portable incubator, New York City Department of Health.

tie is used. The cord should be inspected at frequent intervals for bleeding, because prematurity is a predisposing cause of secondary hemorrhage. Since premature babies are also more susceptible to infections, asepsis is imperative. The head and shoulders should be level or slightly elevated but not in a head-down position. This is to prevent any undue pressure on the friable cerebral vessels.

As soon as the head emerges, the eyes should be wiped gently with moist sterile gauze. The instillation of prophylactic drops may have to be deferred until the condition of the baby warrants this treatment.

Because of the baby's underdeveloped and delicate structures, the resuscitation of the premature infant must be managed with extreme care and gentleness. Often the method of resuscitation will determine the baby's chances to live. The mucus should be removed from the nose and the throat with great care. Any injury to the delicate tissues is an avenue to trauma and infection which may lead to pneumonia.

Since the maintenance of body heat is so essential, a baby should be wrapped in a warmed blanket, and a heated bed or incubator (Figs. 16-1, 2) should be ready to receive him. When the baby's condition permits, his temperature and weight should be recorded. The infant should be turned gently from side to side periodically and occasionally stimu-

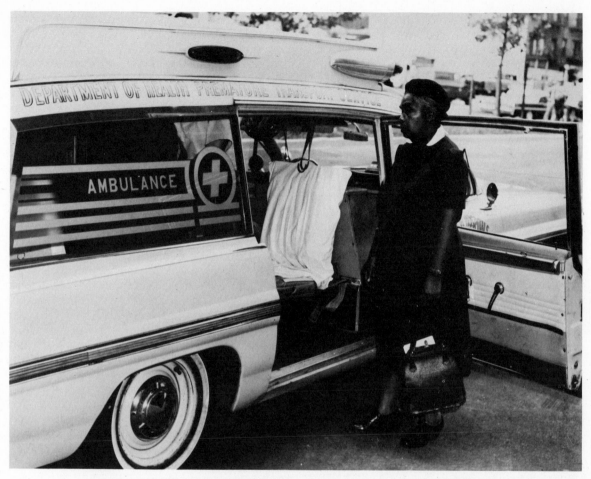

FIG. 16-4. Premature ambulance, New York City Department of Health.

lated to cry by very gentle *stroking* of the back. (These babies should be handled as little as possible.)

Continuing Care

Because of the nationwide interest in reducing deaths among premature infants, there have developed special premature nurseries and special premature referral centers in municipalities and other major health jurisdictions. Space is usually allotted in the hospital separate from the nursery for the full-term babies. Some centers concentrate on the care of the smaller babies. Generally, provision is made for the safe transport to and from the hospital (Figs. 16-3, 4). As discharge time ap-

proaches, plans are made for follow-up care in the home.

In these programs the premature infants spend the initial period in an incubator. During this time skilled medical and nursing care is aimed at maintaining adequate oxygenation, stabilizing the body temperature, safeguarding the baby against infection, supplying proper nutrition and feeding, maintaining a fluid and electrolyte balance and recognizing early abnormalities and infections.

Some hospitals have special premature nurseries which are air-conditioned in respect to temperature (85° to 90° F.), ventilation and humidity (50 to 65%) control. This may not be necessary where infants are "housed" in modern incubators. A study by Silverman and

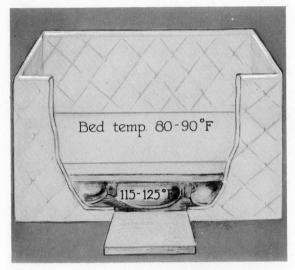

Bed temp. 80-90°F

115-125°F

FIG. 16-5. Homemade heated bed made from small canned goods box. The platform is 4 inches above the floor. The box is padded inside and outside with quilting. Three quarters of the bed is covered with a blanket. (Lundeen and Kunstadter: Care of the Premature Infant, Philadelphia, Lippincott)

his colleagues reported the following:

Survival rates of premature infants are higher in those kept at an incubator temperature of 89° F. during the first 5 days of life than those maintained at 84° F.[1]

In an emergency situation—for example, when the infant is born prematurely at home in an outlying rural area—some means to protect the premature must be devised until an incubator can be brought from the local health agency. An incubator can be improvised from a box or a cardboard carton (Fig. 16-5). Such a specially prepared bed may be heated by electricity from a wire-screened 25- or 40-watt light bulb, or, if electricity is not available, by the use of hot-water bottles, or heated bricks or sandbags.

A large majority of premature infants must receive oxygen initially because of respiratory difficulties or cyanosis. Nevertheless, this should not be used routinely and, except in an emergency, should always be prescribed by the physician. Oxygen therapy is often a lifesaving

[1] Silverman, W. A., Fertig, J. W., and Berger, A. P.: Pediatrics 22:876, 1958.

measure for the premature infant, but it must be used judiciously. The oxygen requirements for these infants vary, and thus it should be administered at the lowest concentration compatible with life. As a temporary measure, after necessary suctioning, the newborn may be given oxygen by mask or funnel placed over the infant's nose and mouth. The flow of oxygen should be set at a maximum of 3 liters when this method is used. When the premature infant is in an incubator, the lowest oxygen concentration to relieve the respiratory symptoms should be employed, if possible *not* over 40 per cent. Occasionally, higher concentrations are necessary, but in any case, oxygen therapy should be discontinued as soon as the infant can get along without it. One of the inherent dangers is the development of retrolental fibroplasia (see Chap. 21). Evidence has shown that there is a relationship between the use of relatively high concentrations of oxygen and the occurrence of retrolental fibroplasia.

The modern air-conditioned incubator is a miniature room in which the infant can live and be cared for under ideal atmospheric conditions, i.e., desirable levels of heat, humidity and oxygen. The very immature infant may require a completely air-conditioned environment, receiving heat, humidity and oxygen in the incubator, whereas an infant who is more mature may need only heat, and sometimes humidity. Many kinds of incubators are currently used, but the principle is the same, the difference being in the special construction details developed by various manufacturers.

The new incubators have controls on the outside of the unit to regulate atmospheric conditions accurately and to adjust the bed proper from the horizontal to the tilted positions (i.e., Trendelenburg and reverse-Trendelenburg positions). Special oxygen inlets provide either 40 per cent maximum concentration or high oxygen concentration in case it may be needed. Regardless of this, at regular intervals the nurse should check and record the oxygen concentration of the incubator with a reliable oximeter, i.e., an oxygen analyser, placed at the level of the infant's nose. The incubator can be ventilated with fresh air from the room through a large, replaceable air filter or through an outside air attachment when oxygen therapy is no longer required for the infant. Humidity can be controlled, and, by means of a nebulizer, supersaturated atmosphere can be created. Constant temperatures within the incubator can be regulated and maintained with a double-thermoswitch-controlled, sealed heating unit. Other features which are nontheless important to the nurse are that these incubators are so designed that the infant can be observed from all sides through transparent windows. Moreover, hand holes with air-tight doors and self-adjusting "sleeves" permit the nurses and the physicians to care for the infant without disturbing the atmospheric conditions. The incubators are made of stainless steel and plastic and constructed for easy removal of all essential parts, without tools, to permit proper cleansing and sterilizing.

Some persons have the impression that once the baby is placed in a good incubator, no further special precautions need be taken. This is a mistaken idea. Premature or underdeveloped infants require the most solicitous care in every way; merely to keep them in a proper atmosphere will avail nothing unless the other details of their care are executed carefully. The maintenance of asepsis in every detail is essential for these inadequately fortified babies. It is also urgent that doctors, nurses or anyone caring for a delicate premature baby should avoid contact with any possible source of infection which might be transferred to the baby.

Rest is a most important factor, and the baby must be shielded from excitement and disturbing influences. Light should be curtailed, and loud or sudden noises should be avoided. As long as the infant requires humidity or oxygen therapy, all routine care, such as feeding, altering his position, necessary changing of linen or cleansing his skin, etc., is given in the premature bed. The skin is extremely delicate and tender; and if diapers are used, they should be changed as soon as they become wet or soiled. Sometimes only a small pad is placed under the baby. Indeed, no clothing is really needed because of the controlled environment of the incubator. The skin does not require bathing or oiling if care is taken that body folds do not become irritated, and if the diaper area is kept clean and dry. If an incubator is not available, the baby is dressed in a jacket of cotton and gauze or flannel. The

weight and the temperature of the baby are both matters of importance and are carried out according to the hospital routine.

Feeding

In planning the feeding schedule for the premature infant, it is important to establish a food tolerance, since the intestinal tract (as well as other organs) is underdeveloped. The caloric needs of the premature baby are estimated according to the body weight. At first, the feeding should be in small amounts and then increased gradually to the amount that will produce a consistent gain, since vomiting, distention and diarrhea may be due to overfeeding.

According to some authorities, the general plan involves an initial period of rest, followed by small amounts of water at frequent intervals; gradual replacement of water feedings by milk feedings; gradual increase in amounts of milk and water at each feeding until caloric and fluid requirements are met. Some physicians advise adding a 5 per cent glucose solution to the drinking water.

In some areas of the country breast milk is considered to be the feeding of choice for premature infants. In other sections, however, modified formulas are preferred.

Prematures who weigh 3 pounds or less may be fed every 2 or 3 hours. Infants who weigh over 3½ pounds may be placed on a 4-hour feeding schedule. In addition to the feedings, premature diets usually include vitamin and iron preparations. These additions are introduced when the feeding and schedule are fairly well established, and the infant is able to tolerate them. The stomach of the premature baby needs rest between feedings as much as that of the full-term baby; therefore, the interval should be regulated accordingly. The schedule should be as near that of a normal infant as is compatible with his progress.

When a very small and weak infant is on a 3-hour feeding schedule, gavage feeding (Fig. 16-6) usually is indicated. It is common practice today to introduce a polyethylene retention catheter to the stomach rather than the gavage catheter at frequent intervals. The end to be introduced must be rounded and smooth (use very fine sandpaper and immerse the tip in melted wax). The distance between the

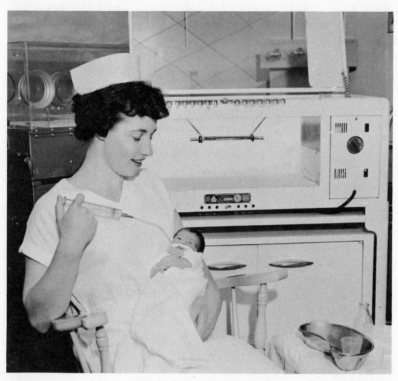

Fig. 16-6. Gavage feeding. When the premature infant does not require oxygen, the nurse can take him out of the incubator and hold him as she feeds him. (Babies and Childrens Hospital, The University Hospitals of Cleveland, Cleveland Ohio)

bridge of the infant's nose and the estimated area of the stomach should be measured and marked on the catheter. The tubing then is introduced into the lower end of the esophagus and may be left in place from 3 to 7 days. In some institutions only physicians pass the nasogastric tube; in others a skilled nurse is allowed to do this. A syringe usually is used to hold the milk for the feedings. No air should precede the milk. It should be introduced very slowly and at the correct temperature, while the infant is supported in a semireclining position. If the infant requires oxygen, he must be fed in the incubator. After the feeding the infant may need to be placed in the incubator with his head and shoulders slightly elevated. This guards against regurgitation and aspiration. When the infant is able to suck, gavage feeding may be discontinued in favor of a bottle with a small soft nipple. The infant will indicate his readiness for the bottle by consistently sucking on the tubing.

Currently in premature care, feeding by a medicine dropper usually is not used. When a medicine-dropper feeding is indicated for some specific reason, the glass tip should be protected by a small piece of rubber tubing which extends at least one quarter of an inch beyond the glass tip. When the infant is unable to suck, the swallowing reflex also is extremely weak. If a medicine dropper is to be used to feed such an infant, the procedure should be managed only by the most skilled practitioner, since aspiration can occur easily because of the poor swallowing reflex.

PARENTAL REACTIONS

The birth of a premature infant, as was mentioned earlier, causes a certain amount of disorganization in the parents before they are able to master their feelings and come to accept the event. Since the baby may be born before term, parents often are deprived of the last 6 to 8 weeks in which the final psychological (and sometimes material) preparation for the birth is made. None of the physical and emotional signs of approaching labor (enumerated in Chapter 12) may happen. These are helpful to the mother in alerting her to the near approach of another new phase in the childbearing process, and this awareness in turn assists her in achieving a psychological preparation. The result, then, may be a rather abrupt arrival of the infant, and the event may be surrounded by several anxiety-provoking features: an unattended delivery, a longer hospital stay for her baby and perhaps herself, separation of the infant and herself, and most heartrending of all, a delicate infant who may be in danger of death.

Guilt feelings and a certain amount of grieving in both parents are an invariable accompaniment. The parents ask themselves time and again such questions as: "What went wrong? What did we do? What made it happen? Can I really carry babies?" These guilt feelings and grief may be manifested in a variety of ways: general anger with the whole situation, self-depreciation, numerous complaints, blaming the spouse and/or attendants, insistent bids for reassurance and attention, profuse crying or extreme quiet and immobilization. Loneliness is also a problem, for the mother has no opportunity to see, hold, feed and examine her child as the other mothers have. We are all familiar with the wistful figure at the nursery window, gazing longingly through the glass, while the other mothers are occupied with feeding, changing and cuddling their infants. The loneliness continues when the parents go home without their infant, and because of the continued separation, the task of integrating the new member into the household is delayed. In addition, most mothers are concerned about whether they will be able to take adequate care of their babies when they do bring them home. The mother may still carry a picture of the frail infant surrounded by all the nursery paraphernalia and not realize that her baby will be reasonably mature when he is discharged from the hospital.

To cope with this concern, she may ask considerable questions while she is in the hospital and demand reassurance about the baby's condition; on the other hand, she may be quiet and uncommunicative, quite overwhelmed with the anticipated enormous responsibility. The economic drain on the finances cannot be overlooked, either; with medical and hospitalization expenses what they are today, the cost is considerable. Even for those who have adequate medical insurance, the maternity benefits are usually distressingly low. This, of course, adds to the general anxiety and strain of the situation.

Supportive Care. Although there is much that is specialized in the physical care activities for the premature infant, the mother's physical care remains generally the same as that for any normal postpartal course. Thus, the emphasis on care for these mothers should be 2-fold. (1) They need help to facilitate their emotional adjustment (this holds true for the father as well) and (2) to prepare for the care of the infant when they bring him home. The nurse will find Caplan's delineation of the mental hygiene activities of the nurse during pregnancy and the puerperium helpful in implementing these foci: (1) ego strengthening and general support, (2) mobilization of environmental resources of love and support, (3) anticipatory guidance, and (4) help in specific crises.[2]

The nurse can do much to strengthen the mother's ego by helping her work through her guilt feelings and grief and thus reinforce her concept of herself as an adequate, worthy person. To do this, the nurse must provide opportunities for the mother to ventilate her feelings and to question the situation. It is often difficult for the nurse to answer all the questions the mother and father ask her, especially if the prognosis for the baby is guarded. Yet, to avoid the questions or problems is to deprive the parents of a valuable avenue of coping with the problem. The fears and the fantasies engendered by not knowing are often worse than the facts, even though the facts are unfortunate. As the nurse listens to the mother and the father and reflects their concerns, she helps them to arrive at a clearer notion of the reality of the situation; thus they are able to separate fact from fancy and to work through to a more positive acceptance of their situation. The nurse can expect some negative feelings to be expressed, and the patient may go through a period of self-pity. An accepting, nonjudgmental attitude will help the patient to move to a more positive frame of mind.

Keeping the lines of communication open between the nursery staff and the patient is another useful supportive measure; the nurse on the postpartal unit can prepare herself with

[2] Caplan, Gerald: The mental hygiene role of the nurse in maternal and child care, Nurs. Outlook 2:14-19, January, 1954.

the latest reports regarding the baby's condition, so that she will have the information to give to the parents. Especially when the mother cannot be taken to see her baby in the premature nursery, it is very helpful if the nurse in the premature unit can make regular visits to the mother on the ward to inform her of her infant's progress. If circumstances within the unit prevent this, contact with the mother by telephone may be substituted. This two-way communication between the floor and the nursery helps the patient to feel that everyone is "tuned in" on her situation and concerned about her. It also gives her the opportunity to know the personnel who are responsible for the care of her baby, and this is reassuring in itself.

When the mother is able, she should be allowed to visit the nursery at least to observe her baby for a time. Some mothers find this difficult at first, especially if the infant is very small and/or ill. It is a wise nurse who allows the mother to indicate her readiness for such visits and gives appropriate encouragement as the mother is able to face the situation and take more responsibility.

Since the mother will be grieving to a certain extent and will be lonely, any environmental resources available that will convey love and support should be utilized. Certainly, her husband and available relatives are possible resources, as well as interested and empathic professional personnel. Often the latter, because they can be objective, are very helpful. Nurses must remember that the husband and wife must work through this mutual crisis, and even though they are both upset, they can gain strength and support from each other if they are helped to utilize positive coping mechanisms. If the family has a religious affiliation, their clergyman can lend valuable assistance also during this time.

All avenues of support should be explored with the parents. If the mother seems to benefit from visitors or visiting with the other patients, then there need be no restriction of visiting privileges. There is no reason to isolate a mother in a room by herself (even if there has been a fetal demise) without ascertaining whether the mother needs to be alone for a time. If possible, the same nurse should be assigned to her care, for if the mother is to work through her feelings, she must have time

to build a trust relationship, and this takes at least several encounters. Other personnel, such as the social worker, may be helpful if aid is needed financially, or strict budgeting is necessary. Another source of help that can prove invaluable is the public health or visiting nurse. The need for a referral for these patients and their infants never should be overlooked. Most patients are delighted to have someone to rely on during the first difficult days when they bring the baby home. Furthermore, some patients cannot make much progress during their short hospital stay in expressing their feelings and in working through the problem. Thus, they need a competent person when they return home to help them in this, as well as in making necessary arrangements in preparation for the baby's homecoming.

In making a referral, it is well to keep in mind the criteria for an appropriate referral, as stated by Wolff: it has merit; it is practical; it fits the patient's individuality; the right of the patient to say no is preserved.[3] The nurse should be particularly cognizant of the last point and present the referral as something that would be useful (describing its advantages), but allow the patient the option of making the decision. If there is refusal on the first try, the nurse always can reintroduce the topic later after the mother has had time to reconsider and is more aware of the factors involved in the home care of her baby. Although a nurse may know, as a professional, that follow-up is necessary, far more cooperation will be elicited from the parents if they have a choice in the matter.

Several hospitals are allowing the mothers to come into a portion of the premature unit to visit and feed their babies when the condition of the baby permits. At the same time they institute a counseling program on feeding and psychological aspects of care, which incorporates anticipatory guidance concerning the condition and the needs of the infants on arrival home. Coping with sibling rivalry also may be included. Appropriate reading material is given, and follow-up is done to see that the material is understood. This approach is very helpful, for it alleviates some of the separation and loneliness between mother and child and

3 Wolff, I. S.: Referral—a process and a skill, Nurs. Outlook 10:253-256, April, 1962.

later fosters self-reliance and confidence in the mother at home.

In implementing the final mental hygiene activity, the nurse will want to remember that the advent of a premature birth is a crisis in itself; however, the parents may have to adjust to various related crises, e.g., a sudden, downward turn in the baby's condition, financial embarrassment, unexpected developments regarding other children and relatives, etc. Thus, she should be prepared to help the parents to deal with these as they arise, and to seek appropriate resources for them if the matter lies beyond her competence. Her knowledge of the principles of communication and supportive care will be utilized here as they would be in any other crisis situation. Her willingness and ability to allow the parents to ventilate and work through their feelings about the situation is of prime importance. The nurse is one of the key persons in the care of the premature infant and his parents.

GROWTH AND DEVELOPMENT

Growth and development of the premature baby is primarily dependent on the degree of prematurity at the time of birth. Much will depend on the ability of the infant to meet the conditions attendant at birth and to adjust to the changes in his new environment. Those infants who react well to prompt treatment and care make their adjustment by the end of the 1st year. Others may require several years to match the "normal" child at that age.

The nurse often is asked if a premature baby ever will develop as well and become as strong and sturdy as one born at term. Although the premature baby is slower in regaining his birth weight, the average premature infant is likely to gain approximately the same amount of weight, i.e., an average gain of 13 to 15 pounds, as the full-term infant during the 1st year. Evidences of progress in his development are temperature stability, the increased vigor of his cry, stronger muscular activity, evidence of appetite and hunger, more normal periods of sleep, changes in the appearance and the characters of his skin due to the addition of the subcutaneous fat, the development of reflexes and general signs of health. Individual variations occur, of course, but the de-velopmental level achieved by the small premature infant during his 1st year generally will be lower than that expected for his chronologic age. Authorities differ in opinion concerning the length of time these infants may require to attain the physical and the intellectual developmental status of a full-size infant of comparable age. The World Health Organization's Expert Committee on Maternal and Child Health states:

It has been shown, for instance, that premature children may grow less quickly, have lower intelligence scores and more mental and physical handicaps than children of heavier birth weight. Again, the mechanism is by no means obvious and the specific influence of low birth weight is as yet unclear. Poor growth and development may merely be a reflection of an unfavorable environment.

The current definition of prematurity is based on the criterion of birth weight and there is no reason to suppose that children comparable in birth weight will also be comparable in viability or development.[4]

Parents of prematurely born infants invariably need special guidance and support to help them develop confidence in their ability to care for their baby, particularly in anticipation of taking him home from the hospital. The nurse has a real responsibility to help them so that they are adequately prepared for the baby's homecoming.

SUGGESTED READING

Blake, F. G., and Wright, F. H.: Essentials of Pediatric Nursing, ed. 7, Philadelphia, Lippincott, 1963.

Canice, Sister M.: Mothers in the nursery, Am. J. Nurs. 64:101, November, 1964.

Caplan, Gerald: The mental hygiene role of the nurse in maternal and child care, Nurs. Outlook 2:14-19, January, 1954.

Committee on the Fetus and Newborn, American Academy of Pediatrics: Standards and Recommendations for Hospital Care of Newborn Infants, rev. ed., Evanston, Illinois, 1964.

Cornblath, M., et al.: Research and nursing care in the premature nursery, Am. J. Nurs. 62:92-96, July, 1962.

[4] World Health Organization, WHO Expert Committee on Maternal and Child Health: Social Aspect in the Teaching of Obstetrics and Gynaecology, Technical Report Series, No. 266, p. 9, Geneva, 1963.

Corner, Beryl: Prematurity, London, Cassell, 1960.

Crosse, M. V.: The Premature Baby, London, Churchill, 1961.

Drillien, C. M.: The Growth and Development of the Prematurely Born Infant, Edinburgh, Livingstone, 1964.

Eastman, N. J.: The great deterrent: Prematurity, Bull. Sloane Hosp. Wom., Winter, 1964.

Follow-up of prematures *in* In the journals, Children 12:35, January-February, 1965.

Gunter, Laurie: Psychopathology and stress in the life experience of mothers of premature infants, Am. J. Obstet. Gynec. 86:333-340, June, 1963.

Hasselmeyer, E. G.: Behavior Patterns of Premature Infants, Washington, D. C., U. S. Department of Health, Education and Welfare, 1961.

Kaplan, D. M., and Mason, E. A.: Maternal reactions to premature births viewed as an acute emotional disorder, Am. J. Orthopsychiat. 30:539, July, 1960.

Lundeen, E. C., and Kunstader, R. H.: Care of the Premature Infant, Philadelphia, Lippincott, 1958.

Marlow, D. R.: Textbook of Pediatric Nursing, ed. 2, Philadelphia, Saunders, 1965.

Nelson, W. E.: Textbook of Pediatrics, ed. 8, Philadelphia, Saunders, 1964.

Owens, C.: Parents' response to premature birth, Am. J. Nurs. 60:1113-1118, August, 1960.

Parmelee, A. W.: Management of the Newborn, ed. 2, Chicago, Year Book Pub., 1959.

Petruska, Rita: A one page record for prematures, Am. J. Nurs. 63:67-68, March, 1963.

Silverman, W. A.: Dunham's Premature Infants, ed. 3, New York, Hoeber, 1961.

————: Diagnosis and treatment: Use and misuse of temperature and humidity in care of the newborn infant, Pediatrics 33:276-277, February, 1964.

Wolff, I. S.: Referral—a process and a skill, Nurs. Outlook 10:253-256, April, 1962.

Wortis, H., *et al.*: Development of lower-class premature children born in and out of wedlock, Social Work 9, No. 4:42-49, 1964.

CONFERENCE MATERIAL

1. What is the responsibility of the hospital and the nurse in preparing the mother to care for her baby after they leave the hospital?

2. What advice and help could you give the mother to help her to adjust the new baby in the home and to prevent (or deal with) sibling rivalry when there is a 2-year-old brother who is accustomed to having the undivided love and attention of his parents?

3. Compare the physiologic development of the premature infant with that of the normal full-term infant.

4. What are some other means which could be employed to supply external heat for the premature infant who requires it when a mechanical incubator is not available?

5. What information can you give parents about the "well-baby clinic" in your community?

Study Questions

UNIT FIVE: NURSING THE NORMAL NEWBORN

Read through the entire question and place your answer on the line to the right.

1. The neonatal period constitutes one of the most important periods of life because of the profound physiologic changes which occur. Which of the following statements concerning these alterations are correct?
   A. Certain of these physiologic changes are immediate; some are delayed.
   B. All of these physiologic changes are immediate.
   C. All of these physiologic changes are permanent.
   D. Certain of these physiologic changes are temporary.

Select the number corresponding to the correct letters.
   1. A and C
   2. A and D
   3. B and C
   4. B and D

_1_

2. Which of the following reasons best explain why the maternity hospital should adopt the rooming-in plan for the mother and her newborn?
   A. All mothers need the experience gained thereby.
   B. Selected mothers and babies may profit where the plan could be adopted.
   C. All mothers want this type of service.
   D. Most infants cry too much in a central nursery.
   E. All infants need this added attention.

Select the number corresponding to the correct letter or letters.
   1. A only
   2. B only
   3. A, C and D
   4. B, C and E

_2_

3. What type of initial bath usually is given the newborn infant?
   A. Tub bath
   B. Spray bath
   C. Oil bath
   D. Cleansing only as necessary with warm water and sterilized cotton
   E. Sponge bath with mild, unscented soap and warm water

_D_

4. What is the reason for selecting this method of skin care in the above question?
   A. The infant's skin must be washed thoroughly to prevent irritation.
   B. It stimulates the circulation.
   C. Special oils provide nourishment to the tissues.
   D. It is the best means of applying external heat.
   E. It lessens the danger of infection.

_E_

5. What is the usual procedure for the daily care of the genitals of the male infant who is not in need of circumcision?
   A. Wash externally with soap and water; otherwise let alone.

419

B. Retract and cleanse under the foreskin with cotton ball moistened with warm water. Replace foreskin over glans after cleansing.
C. Retract and cleanse under the foreskin with alcohol.
D. After cleansing, apply sterile petrolatum under the foreskin.
E. Stretch the prepuce and lubricate with mineral oil.

B

6. What is the principle underlying the concept of demand feedings for the newborn infant?
A. Maintaining a regular 4-hour schedule to establish eating habits
B. Feeding the infant every 2 to 3 hours to stimulate digestion
C. Fitting individual feedings to individual needs
D. Permissive feeding schedule causes less conflict with the mother's household activities.
E. More frequent feedings assure an adequate nutritional intake.

C

7. The young mother asks how she will know when her baby is hungry. Which of the following responses would be most appropriate for the nurse to reply?
A. "All crying indicates hunger."
B. "Feed the baby whenever he is awake."
C. "He will cry, fret and suck on anything in contact with his lips."
D. "Offer him water first; if he refuses the water, then feed him."

C

8. What is the established birth weight below which the infant is considered to need special premature care, regardless of whether or not he is born prematurely according to dates?
A. 4 pounds
B. 4½ pounds
C. 5 pounds
D. 5½ pounds
E. 6 pounds

D

9. The appearance of a healthy newborn infant's stools normally will change during the neonatal period. Which of the following types of stools, in sequence of appearance, would the nurse observe in the healthy infant?
A. Dark, tarlike
B. Clay-colored, soft
C. Mottled greenish-brown, soft
D. Smooth, yellow
E. Green, curdy

Select the number corresponding to the correct letters.
1. A and D
2. A, C and D
3. B, C and E
4. All of them

2

10. How does the composition of mother's milk compare with cow's milk?
A. Human milk contains more protein.
B. Human milk contains less protein.
C. Human milk contains more carbohydrate.
D. Human milk contains larger fat globules.
E. Human milk contains less iron.

Select the number corresponding to the correct letters.
1. A and C
2. A, C and E
3. B, C and D
4. B, D and E

3

11. Which of the following features are characteristic of the premature infant and distinguish him from the full-size infant?
A. The infant is usually puny and weighs less than 2,000 Gm.
B. The infant's head is proportionately large, his skull is round or ovoid in shape, and his facial features are small and angular.
C. The skin is soft, transparent and may be covered with lanugo.
D. These infants whimper and cry rather constantly, although the cry is weak.
E. The body temperature is unstable and thus responds rather readily to changes in the temperature of the environment.

Select the number corresponding to the correct letters.
1. A and B
2. B, C and D
3. B, C and E
4. All of them

_3_

12. When the mother learned that her premature infant was receiving gavage feedings she asked the nurse why this was being done. Which of the following reasons may be correct for the nurse to reply?
A. "This method of feeding your baby was indicated because he became exhausted when he tried to swallow."
B. "Feeding your baby this way prevents him from vomiting and thus eliminates the danger of his aspirating formula into his lungs."
C. "Feeding your baby this way conserves his strength and permits him to receive food into his stomach when sucking or swallowing may be difficult."
D. "He can be given his formula quickly this way and so he does not have to be handled as much."
E. "A tiny baby's resistance to infection is poor, so gavage feeding is really a protective measure against such infections as thrush, which he might acquire if he were bottle-fed."

Select the number corresponding to the correct letter or letters.
1. A only
2. C only
3. B, C and D
4. B, D and E

_2_

13. In caring for premature infants, which of the following precautions should be taken against retrolental fibroplasia?
A. The administration of oxygen should be discontinued as soon as feasible.
B. The concentration of oxygen in the incubator housing the infant should be tested periodically and kept at less than 40 per cent.
C. Daily determinations of the serum bilirubin level should be done when there is any indication of proliferation of the retinal capillaries.
D. High humidity should be maintained in the incubator constantly.
E. The infant's eyes should be protected from bright lights.

Select the number corresponding to the correct letters.
1. A and B
2. A, C and D
3. B, D and E
4. All of them

_1_

14. How can the public health nurse assist the family in the care and the supervision of the premature infant?
A. Visit the home before the infant leaves the hospital to evaluate the home situation and give anticipatory guidance to the parents as necessary.
B. Help the family to understand that the infant is still premature and must have the same kind of skillful, protective care in a sheltered environment similar to that in the hospital premature nursery.

C. Make daily visits to the home to bathe the infant, prepare the formula and, in general, give suggestions and guidance to the mother about her infant's care.
D. Visit the home again after the infant is discharged from the hospital to give the family guidance and assistance as necessary.
E. Help the family to understand that this infant requires a great amount of undisturbed rest and thus should not be held or cuddled as much as the full-size infant.

Select the number corresponding to the correct letters.
1. A and D
2. A, C and E
3. B, C and E
4. All of them

1

15. The premature infant has difficulty in regulating his body temperature because heat regulation is one of the least developed functions of his body. Which of the following conditions are responsible for this?
A. The surface area of the premature infant is relatively smaller than that of a normal full-term infant in proportion to body size.
B. Lack of subcutaneous fat which would furnish a measure of insulation
C. Limited ability to produce body proteins
D. Poor reflex control of skin capillaries
E. Frequent episodes of diaphoresis causing loss of body heat

Select the number corresponding to the correct letters.
1. A and C
2. B and D
3. B, C and E
4. All of them

2

Note: The key to the correct answers to these questions is given on page 598.

UNIT SIX

Operative Procedures in Obstetrics

Operative Obstetrics

Chapter 17

Operative Obstetrics

A number of special procedures which the physician may need to employ to assist the mother in labor and delivery come under the heading of operative obstetrics. These procedures include the induction of labor, episiotomy, the application of forceps and cesarean section.

EPISIOTOMY AND REPAIR OF LACERATIONS

Except for clamping and cutting the umbilical cord, episiotomy is the most common operative procedure performed in obstetrics. In view of the fact that this incision of the perineum, made to facilitate delivery, is employed almost routinely in primigravidas, the procedure has been discussed in the section on the conduct of normal labor (see Chap. 12).

Lacerations of the perineum and the vagina which occur in the process of delivery (see Fig. 12-38) have also been covered earlier in the text, because some tears are unavoidable even in the most skilled hands. The suturing of spontaneous perineal lacerations is similar to that employed for the repair of an episiotomy incision but may be more difficult because such tears often are irregular in shape with ragged, bruised edges.

FORCEPS

The common types of obstetric forceps are illustrated in Figures 17-1 to 4. The instrument, it will be seen, consists of two steel parts which cross each other like a pair of scissors and lock at the intersection. The lock may be of a sliding type, as in the first three types shown, or a screw type, as in the Tarnier instrument. Each part consists of a handle, a lock, a shank and a blade; the blade is the curved portion designed for application to the sides of the baby's head. The blades of most forceps (the Tucker McLane is an exception) have a large opening or window (fenestrum) in them to give a better grip on the baby's head, and usually they have two curves: a cephalic curve, which conforms to the shape of the baby's head, and a pelvic curve, to follow the curve of the birth canal. Axis-traction forceps, such as the Tarnier, are used less frequently today than formerly; this instrument has a mechanism attached below which permits the pulling to be done more directly in the axis of the birth canal.

The two blades of the forceps are designated as right and left. The left blade is the one which is introduced into the vagina on the patient's life side; the right blade goes into the right side. In the majority of hospitals today the nurse does not scrub for delivery but assists the obstetrician as a "circulating" nurse in the delivery room. However, if the nurse is ever expected to scrub and assist the obstetrician, she should articulate and disarticulate the forceps a few times and make sure that she knows which blade is which. Otherwise, this may prove to be rather confusing.

It may become necessary to deliver the baby by forceps because of reasons related to the mother's welfare (maternal indications), or because of conditions associated with the baby's condition (fetal indications). Among the more common maternal indications are: inability of the mother to effect delivery after 2 hours or so of complete dilatation of the cervix, maternal exhaustion, heart disease, toxemia of pregnancy and threatened rupture of the uterus. The chief fetal indication for forceps delivery is fetal distress, as shown by a slow, irregular fetal heart. Many obstetricians, however, deem it desirable to deliver almost all primigravidas with forceps in the belief that the operation spares the mother

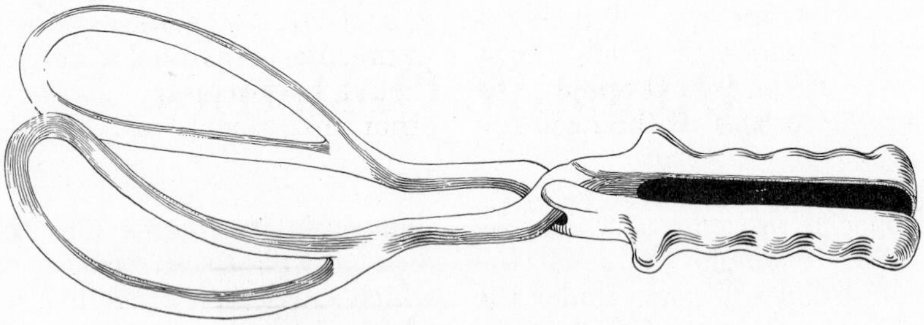

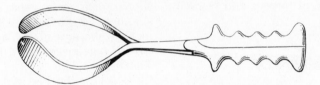

Fig. 17-1. Simpson forceps.

Fig. 17-2. Tucker McLane forceps.

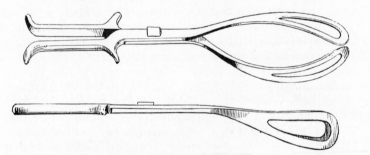

Fig. 17-3. Kielland forceps. (A) Front view; (B) side view.

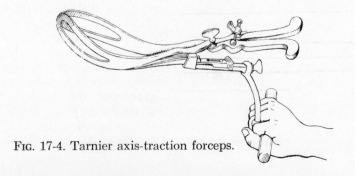

Fig. 17-4. Tarnier axis-traction forceps.

many minutes of exhausting bearing-down efforts and relieves pressure on the baby's head. This is usually referred to as "elective forceps."

Forceps operations never are attempted unless the cervix is completely dilated. In the vast majority of cases today, the procedure is carried out at a time when the baby's head is on the perineal floor (visible or almost so) and, as a rule, internal rotation has occurred so that the baby's head lies in a direct antero-posterior position. This is called *low forceps* and sometimes "outlet forceps." When the head is higher in the pelvis, with its lowermost point near the level of the ischial spines, the operation is called *midforceps*. If the head has

not yet engaged, the procedure is known as *high forceps*. High-forceps delivery is an exceedingly difficult and dangerous operation for both mother and baby and is rarely done. The obstetrician will inform the nurse of the type of instrument he wishes to use. Autoclaving is the usual type of sterilization employed, and several pairs of the generally approved forceps, each encased in suitable wrappings, are autoclaved and kept in the delivery room for immediate use. If the latter procedure is not done, most obstetricians will request that a pair of forceps be sterilized with the other instruments prepared for delivery in case they should be necessary in an emergency. The other instruments needed for a forceps de-

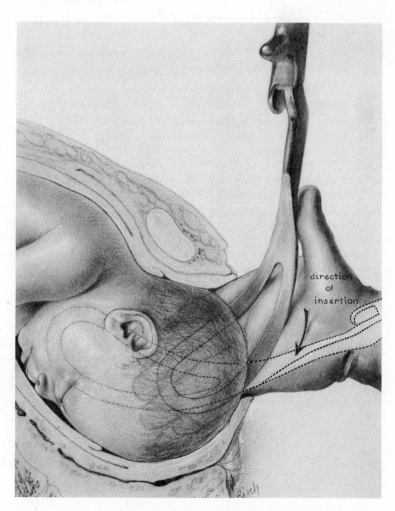

FIG. 17-5. Insertion of forceps blade.

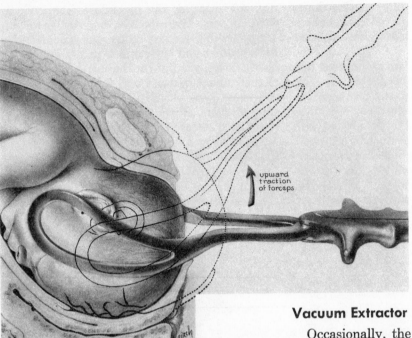

upward
traction
of forceps

FIG. 17-6. Applied forceps and direction of traction.

livery are the same as those required for a spontaneous delivery, plus those necessary for repair work (see Chap. 12).

Complete anesthesia is necessary, but in low-forceps deliveries it may be light, and in many institutions this type of operation is performed successfully under local infiltration anesthesia. The patient is placed in the lithotomy position and prepared and draped in the usual fashion. The obstetrician will first catheterize the patient. After checking the exact position of the baby's head by vaginal examination, he will introduce two or more fingers of his right hand into the left side of the vagina; these fingers will guide the left blade into place and at the same time protect the maternal soft parts (vagina, cervix) from injury. Taking the left blade of the forceps in his left hand, he introduces it into the left side of the vagina, gently insinuating it between the baby's head and the fingers of his right hand (Fig. 17-5). The same procedure is carried out on the right side, and then the blades are articulated. Traction is not continuous but intermittent (Fig. 17-6); and between traction, the obstetrician will partially disarticulate the blades in order to release pressure on the baby's head. Episiotomy is almost routine nowadays in these cases.

Vacuum Extractor

Occasionally, the nurse may see an instrument known as the vacuum extractor used in place of the forceps. The vacuum extractor consists of a cup that is applied to the fetal head and tightly affixed there by creating a vacuum in the cup through withdrawal of the air by a pump. Traction then can be exerted by means of a short chain attached to the cup, with a handle at its far end. The instrument inevitably causes varying degrees of injury to the fetal scalp, but these are rarely of a serious or a permanent nature. Nevertheless, for this and other reasons the vacuum extractor is not used extensively in the United States.

VERSION

Version consists of turning the baby in the uterus from an undesirable to a desirable position. There are three types of version: external, internal and Braxton Hicks.

External Version. This is an operation designed to change a breech presentation into a vertex presentation by external manipulation of the fetus through the abdominal and the uterine walls. It is attempted in the hope of averting the difficulties of a subsequent breech delivery. Obstetricians find the procedure most successful when done about a month before full term; it often fails, however, either be-

Fig. 17-7. Internal podalic version. Elbow length gloves are usually worn for this operation.

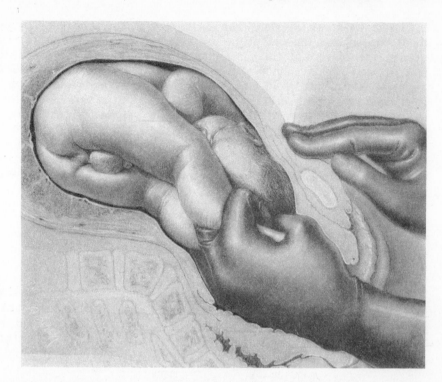

cause it proves to be impossible to turn the fetus around, or because the fetus returns to its original position within a few hours. Some obstetricians disapprove of it altogether.

Internal Version. Sometimes called internal podalic version, this is an operation designed to change whatever presentation may exist into a breech presentation (see Fig. 17-7). With cervical dilatation complete, the whole hand of the operator is introduced high into the uterus, one or both feet are grasped and pulled downward in the direction of the birth canal. With his external hand the obstetrician may expedite the turning by pushing the head upward. The version usually is followed by breech extraction (p. 489). Internal version finds it greatest usefulness in cases of multiple pregnancy in which the birth of the second twin is retarded.

Braxton Hicks Version. In this procedure, two fingers are introduced into a partially dilated cervix and, after manipulating the fetus to effect turning, one leg is drawn through the cervix. The operation is not designed to bring about immediate delivery and never is followed at once by extraction. Its purposes are either to compress the lower uterine segment with the infant's buttock (see pla-

centa previa, p. 463), or, more rarely, to stretch the cervix with the infant's thigh so that labor may be initiated. It is rarely used in modern obstetrics.

CESAREAN SECTION

Cesarean section is the removal of the infant from the uterus through an incision made in the abdominal wall and the uterus. The main indications for cesarean section fall into 5 groups: (1) disproportion between the size of the fetus and that of the bony birth canal, that is, contracted pelvis (p. 492), tumor blocking birth canal, etc.; (2) certain cases in which the patient has had a previous cesarean section, the operation being done because of fear that the uterine scar will rupture in labor; (3) certain cases of very severe toxemia of pregnancy, but rarely in eclampsia; (4) certain cases of placenta previa and premature separation of the normally implanted placenta; (5) miscellaneous complications.

Main Types of Cesarean Section

There are 4 main types of cesarean section.

Classic Cesarean Section. The incision is made directly into the wall of the body of the uterus; the baby and the placenta are extracted, and the incision is closed by three layers of catgut sutures (Figs. 17-8, 9). As a rule, classic cesarean section is employed only in those cases in which the operation is done prior to the onset of labor. At this time, the uterine contents are sterile, but after 6 or more hours of labor, particularly if the membranes have been ruptured, bacteria ascend from the vagina into the uterus and are potential sources of infection. When done after the patient has been in labor many hours, this type of operation is considered to be dangerous because of the ease with which infectious material during the puerperium may escape directly through the uterine wound into the peritoneal cavity. When any type of cesarean section is done prior to the onset of labor as the result of a prearranged plan, it is known as "elective" cesarean section. (As with "elective low for-

ceps," the obstetrician is not forced to perform the operation but elects to do it as the best procedure for mother and baby.)

Low Cervical Section. (Synonyms: 2-flap cesarean section; laparotrachelotomy.) The initial incision (the abdomen having been opened) is made transversely across the uterine peritoneum, where it is attached loosely just above the bladder. Two flaps of peritoneum are thus created. The lower flap and the bladder are now dissected off the uterus, and the uterine muscle is incised either longitudinally or transversely. The baby is ordinarily delivered head first, usually with forceps. After the placenta has been extracted and the uterine incision sutured, the lower flap is imbricated over the upper (Figs. 17-10, 11). This two-flap arrangement seals off the uterine incision and is believed to prevent the egress of infectious lochia into the peritoneal cavity. When low cervical cesarean was first introduced in this country by Dr. Alfred C. Beck,

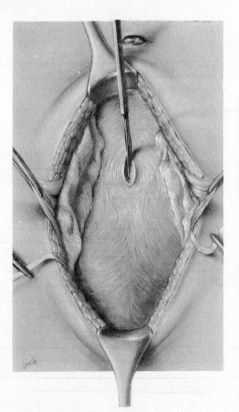 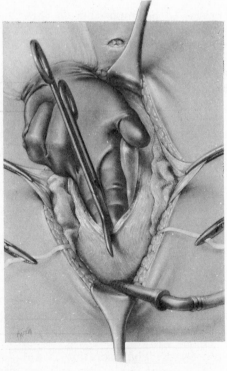

Fig. 17-8. Classic cesarean section. (*Left*) Uterus packed off with warm, moist gauze pads. Start of incision with knife. (*Right*) Continuation of incision with bandage scissors.

of Brooklyn, N. Y., about 1919, the operation was employed chiefly on patients who had been in labor for a number of hours, and it is undoubtedly safer than the classic procedure in such cases. But it has other advantages, and many obstetricians today prefer it in elective cases as well.

Extraperitoneal Cesarean Section. There are two extraperitoneal operations, one devised by Dr. W. Latsko, formerly of Vienna, Austria, and the other by Dr. E. G. Waters, of Jersey City, N. J. By appropriate dissection of the tissues around the bladder, access to the lower uterine segment is secured without entering the peritoneal cavity. The baby is delivered through a transverse incision in the lower uterine segment. Since the entire operation is done outside the peritoneal cavity, neither spill of infected amniotic fluid nor subsequent seepage of pus from the uterus can reach the peritoneal surfaces. Therefore, an extraperitoneal operation is thought to provide additional safety in cases of outright uterine infection.

Cesarean Section—Hysterectomy. (Synonyms: radical cesarean section; Porro operation.) This operation comprises cesarean section (usually classic) followed by removal of the uterus. Obviously, it is most undesirable in younger women, and obstetricians avoid it whenever possible. However, it may be necessary in certain cases of premature separation of the placenta and in patients with multiple fibroid tumors of the uterus. (See Moral Considerations, p. 455.)

Preparation

Preparations for cesarean sections are similar to those for any other abdominal operation, except that in these cases it includes preparations for the care of the infant. When the operation is an elective procedure, the patient is admitted 24 hours or more prior to surgery,

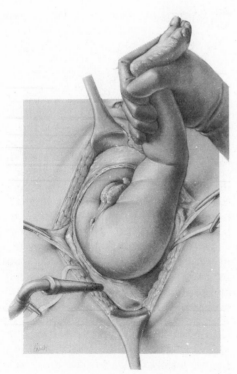

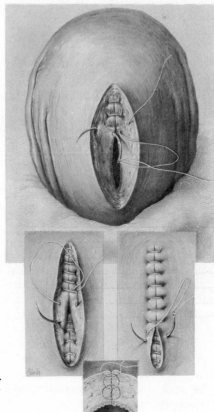

FIG. 17-9. Classic cesarean section. (*Left*) Delivery of infant. (*Right*) Method of suturing uterus.

Fig. 17-10. Low cervical cesarean section. (*Left*) High Trendelenburg position, bladder empty, with catheter in place. The peritoneum over lower portion of uterus is picked up with tissue forceps to determine how far up it is loosely attached to uterus. A transverse incision of the peritoneum, slightly concave downward, is to be made about 1 inch below the point where the peritoneum is firmly attached to the uterus.

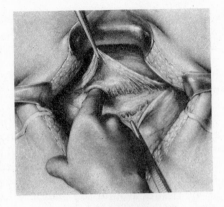

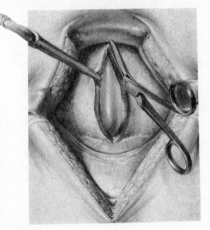

(*Right, top*) The lower edge of the incised peritoneum is picked up by the tissue forceps and gently stripped off the underlying uterine segment by finger dissection.

(*Right, bottom*) The upper flap of loose peritoneum has been stripped from the underlying muscle by finger dissection and is held back by a retractor. A small incision with a scalpel is made at the upper end of the lower uterine segment and carried downward with bandage scissors.

so that there is ample time for physical examination, routine laboratory studies, typing and crossmatching blood and other customary procedures. However, if there is an emergency, or if labor has started, then such preparations must be made with expediency. In any event, the usual hospital procedure should be followed.

Nursing Care

When the patient is admitted for an elective cesarean section, nursing care which is routine for any waiting mother, e.g., checking fetal heart tones and being alert to prodromal signs of labor, is employed. A short time before the operation the skin should be shaved to remove all hair from the abdomen and the vulva. The abdomen is shaved first, beginning at the level of the xiphoid cartilage and extending out to the far sides and down to the pubic area. Then the vulvar region is shaved. A retention catheter is inserted to ensure that the bladder remains empty during the oper-

ation, and it is unclamped during this procedure. The preoperative medication usually ordered is atropine. The use of narcotic drugs prior to delivery is avoided because of their depressant effect on the infant, but these medications should be readily available. Oxytocic drugs, i.e., oxytocin and ergonovine, should be ready in the operating room so that they can be administered promptly on the verbal order of the obstetrician when the infant is born.

In addition to the preparation of the operating room for the surgical procedure, preparation for the care of the infant must be accomplished. There must be a warm crib and equipment for the resuscitation of the infant. An infant resuscitator, such as the Kreiselman shown in Figure 12-13, is an efficient mechanical device, because it is equipped with heat, suction, oxygen (open mask and positive-pressure) and an adjustable frame to permit the proper positioning of the infant. Furthermore, such a resuscitator provides a convenient place to give initial care to the newborn. A competent person should be present at cesarean section to give the infant initial care and to resuscitate it, if necessary. This person may be a professional nurse, but in many hospitals today it is customary to have a pediatrician present so that he may "take over" the care of the infant as soon as it is born and thus free the obstetrician to devote all of his attention to the mother.

The obstetrician will direct the treatment of the mother, but usually postoperative care is the same as that following abdominal surgery. It is well to remember that the patient who has had a cesarean section has had both an abdominal operation and a delivery. The patient must be watched for hemorrhage, both from the abdominal incision and the vagina, and so the abdominal dressings and the perineal pad must be inspected frequently. If the abdominal dressings are bulky, it is impossible to palpate the fundus to see if the uterus is well contracted, but if the dressings are not massive, and do not extend above the level of

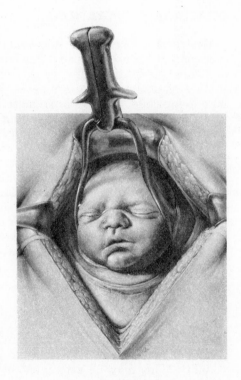

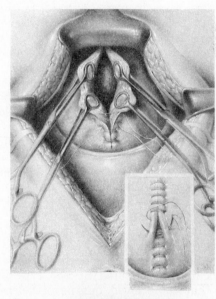

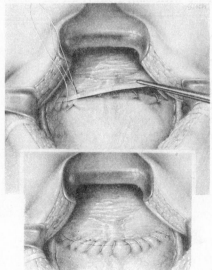

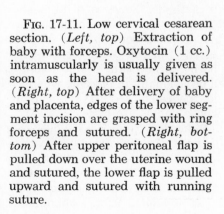

Fig. 17-11. Low cervical cesarean section. (*Left, top*) Extraction of baby with forceps. Oxytocin (1 cc.) intramuscularly is usually given as soon as the head is delivered. (*Right, top*) After delivery of baby and placenta, edges of the lower segment incision are grasped with ring forceps and sutured. (*Right, bottom*) After upper peritoneal flap is pulled down over the uterine wound and sutured, the lower flap is pulled upward and sutured with running suture.

the umbilicus, the nurse may feel the consistency of the fundus without difficulty. She should employ extreme gentleness if this is done in order not to traumatize the uterus, and remember that the uterus must not be massaged in the process. Oxytocics may be ordered to keep the uterus contracted and to control bleeding. The vital signs should be checked regularly until they have stabilized, and if there is any indication of shock or hemorrhage, it should be reported promptly. Although there may be no visible signs of external hemorrhage, one would suspect internal hemorrhage if the pulse rate becomes accelerated, the respiration increases in rate, or the blood pressure falls, bearing in mind, of course, that the drop in blood pressure could be due to the effects of some types of anesthetic drugs.

If the retention catheter is to remain in place until the following morning, it should be attached to "constant drainage" and should be watched to see that it drains freely. Intravenous fluids are usually administered during the first 24 hours, although small amounts of fluids may be given by mouth after nausea has subsided. A record of the mother's intake and elimination is kept for the first several days or until the need is no longer indicated.

Sedative drugs should be used to keep the mother comfortable and encourage her to rest. Her position in bed during the early postoperative hours may be dictated by the type of anesthesia that she received, but, nevertheless, she should be encouraged to turn from side to side every hour. Deep breathing and coughing should also be encouraged at this time to promote good ventilation. Today most mothers delivered by cesarean section are allowed early ambulation 12 to 48 hours following operation. It is felt that this contributes considerably to maintaining good bladder and intestinal function.

The patient's husband should be permitted to have a short visit with his wife as soon as it is feasible. The mother will be anxious to see her infant, too, and it should be brought to her as soon as she is able to see it. The nurse should remain with the mother while she has her infant with her.

An effort should be made to encourage breast-feeding, both because of the advantage to the infant and because the maternal proc-

esses need this stimulation. If the mother progresses satisfactorily, there should be no reason why the infant should not be put to breast after 24 hours and regularly thereafter.

The general care of the mother will be similar to that given any postoperative or postpartal patient. Daily breast care and perineal care are carried out per routine. The mother may have the afterpains, engorgement of the breasts and the emotional reactions which often accompany a normal delivery.

DESTRUCTIVE OPERATIONS

Destructive operations (designed for the most part to reduce the size of the baby's head and thus to expedite delivery) are rarely done in modern obstetrics and are *never* performed on a living child. Even in large maternity hospitals many years may pass without a single destructive operation. This salutary state of affairs is attributable in part to the widespread extension of prenatal care, in part to better management of women in labor, and in part to the availability of cesarean section, which makes it reasonably safe to effect abdominal delivery even in neglected cases. In the event that a destructive operation is necessary, the obstetrician will choose the necessary instruments.

INDUCTION OF LABOR

By the induction of labor is meant the artificial bringing on of labor after the period of viability. This may be attempted by medication, by instrumental means or by a combination of both methods. Toxemia of pregnancy is the most frequent reason for the procedure, since in this disorder continuation of pregnancy is often fraught with considerable danger to both mother and infant. Labor is also induced occasionally in patients who have gone beyond the calculated date of confinement and whose babies are large.

Medicinal Induction. Since it is believed that the intestinal peristalsis produced by a cathartic is somehow transferred to the uterus, with the consequent initiation of uterine contractions, castor oil has long been employed to induce labor. It is given in the amount of

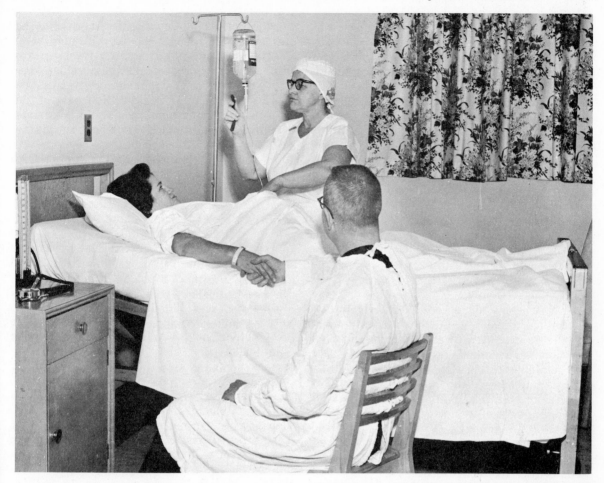

Fig. 17-12. Nurse checks rate of flow of intravenous oxytocin solution. (MacDonald House, University Hospitals of Cleveland)

1 ounce and followed by the administration of a hot soapsuds enema as soon as the castor oil has acted. While this is a harmless procedure, it usually fails and is employed less frequently today than it was formerly.

A much more efficient method for the induction of labor is the administration of oxytocin. The properties of this oxytocic agent and its use in the third stage of labor have already been discussed on page 274. For inducing labor, oxytocin may be administered intramuscularly, intravenously or intranasally.

Since oxytocin has dangerous potentialities when administered to a pregnant woman, the dosage used is always extremely small. The physician will specify the dosage to be employed and will make the injection himself. For the intramuscular administration of oxytocin, the dose is usually ½ to 3 minims (⅓ to 2 International Units). Because of the very small amount of solution to be given, the physician will want, as a rule, a tuberculin syringe for the injection and a small quantity of sterile intravenous saline solution for dilution of the oxytocin.

For the intravenous administration of oxytocin the physician will usually ask for a flask containing 500 cc. of 5 per cent glucose to which he will add the quantity of oxytocin which he wishes to use. The intravenous equipment is set up as usual so that the number of drops flowing per minute can be closely observed in the observation tube. This is extremely important, and the physician will specify the precise number of drops per minute which he wishes employed.

As already mentioned, the administration of oxytocin to a gravida carries certain hazards, and it is obligatory for her safety and that of the baby that a physician or a nurse be in constant bedside attendance to make certain that the number of drops flowing per minute does not change and to watch for certain untoward effects that may ensue. This is usually the responsibility of the physician, but occasionally it may fall to the nurse. If so, she must check the rate of flow of the oxytocin solution at frequent intervals to make certain that it remains constant. Whether oxytocin is administered intramuscularly or intravenously, the duration and the intensity of each uterine contraction must be watched closely and recorded, because any contraction lasting over 2 minutes indicates that the quantity of solution is too great, and the rate of flow should either be decreased or tentatively discontinued altogether. Furthermore, the fetal heart rate should be counted after each contraction and recorded. It will be recalled that the fetal heart tones should return to their normal rate and rhythm within 15 seconds or so after the termination of a contraction, and any persistence of fetal bradycardia is another indication for discontinuation of the oxytocin drip. In the event that the nurse should be left alone with the patient while the intravenous-drip oxytocin technic is being employed, and she observes any abnormalities in the uterine contractions or the fetal heart tones, she should turn off the solution *immediately* and report her findings to the physician.

The advantages of intravenous oxytocin over its intramuscular injection are severalfold. In the first place, it assures a uniform, although infinitesimal, concentration of the agent in the blood stream which can be maintained at the same concentration over long periods, whereas with intramuscular oxytocin there must necessarily be fluctuations in the blood and tissue concentration of oxytocin, depending on varying rates of absorption from time to time. Another advantage is that the oxytocin drip may be discontinued immediately in the event that untoward effects should be observed—an obvious safety factor.

Artificial Rupture of the Membranes. This is today the most common method of inducing labor. It is accomplished after placing the patient in the lithotomy position and carrying out antiseptic preparation of the vulva. The first two fingers of one hand are inserted into the cervix until the membranes are encountered. The cervix is stretched gently, and the membranes are stripped from the region of the internal os. A long hook, similar to one blade of a disarticulated vulsellum tenaculum, is inserted into the vagina, and the membranes are simply hooked and torn by the tip of the sharp instrument. As much fluid as possible is allowed to drain. Provided that the patient is near term, with other conditions favorable, artificial rupture of the membranes will almost always initiate labor within a few hours.

So far as the nurse is concerned, these obstetric operations do not differ greatly from any other surgical procedures. The direction of these operations is entirely the responsibility of the physician, and the nurse's share consists of these 3 responsibilities: (1) having everything in readiness beforehand, (2) giving reassuring advice to the patient and her family and (3) making sure that no opportunity is lost in rendering all possible assistance to the doctor.

SUGGESTED READING

Bishop, E. H.: Dangers attending elective induction of labor, J.A.M.A. 166:1953, 1958.

Bookmiller, Mae, and Bowen, George: Textbook of Obstetrics and Obstetric Nursing, ed. 4, Philadelphia, Saunders, 1963.

Brierton, J. F.: Rupture of the pregnant uterus, Am. J. Obstet. Gynec. 59:113, 1950.

Broomes, E. L. C.: Full term abdominal pregnancy with the delivery of a living child, J.A.M.A. 145:399, 1951.

Brundin, J., and Engstom, L.: Studies of diuresis during spontaneous and oxytocin induced labor, Obstet. Gynec. 16:577-580, November, 1960.

Chambers, W.: Nursing diagnosis, Am. J. Nurs. 62, No. 11:102-104, November, 1962.

Cosgrove, R. A.: Management of pregnancy and delivery following cesarean section, J.A.M.A. 145:884, 1951.

Danforth, D. N.: A method of forceps rotation in persistent occiput posterior, Am. J. Obstet. Gynec. 65:120, 1953.

Davis, M. E., and Rubin, Reva: DeLee's Obstetrics for Nurses, ed. 17, Philadelphia, Saunders, 1962.

D'Esopo, D. A., *et al.*: Elective induction of labor, Am. J. Obstet. Gynec. 89:561-567, July 1, 1964.

Eastman, N. J., and Hellman, L. M.: Williams Obstetrics, ed. 13, New York, Appleton, 1966.

Fish, Stewart: The Barton forceps, Am. J. Obstet. Gynec. 66:1290, 1953.

———: The Tucker McLane forceps: a history, Am. J. Obstet. Gynec. 65:1042, 1953.

Greenhill, J. P.: Obstetrics, ed. 13, Philadelphia, Saunders, 1965.

Hendricks, C. H.: Use of intranasal oxytocin in obstetrics, Am. J. Obstet. Gynec. 79:780, 1960.

Hendricks, C. H., and Pose, Serafin: Intranasal oxytocin in obstetrics, J.A.M.A. 175:384-387, February 4, 1961.

Hendricks, C. H., *et al.*: Effect of sparteine sulfate upon uterine activity in human pregnancy, Am. J. Obstet. Gynec. 91:1-10, January 1, 1965.

LaHaye, T. P., and Burkhart, F. L.: Sparteine sulfate as a myometrial stimulant with uterine activity monitored by the Lorand tokodynamometer, Am. J. Obstet. Gynec. 78:263, 1964.

Moon, R. E., and Wall, D. D.: Midforceps delivery, Am. J. Obstet. Gynec. 72:954, 1956.

Randall, J. H.: Newer trends in cesarean section, J. Iowa Med. Soc. 45:173, 1955.

Schaefer, George: Induction of Labor, Am. J. Nurs. 61, No. 9:89-92, September, 1961.

Spritzer, T. D.: Use of the vacuum extractor in obstetrics, Am. J. Obstet. Gynec. 83:307-310, 1962.

Swann, R. O.: Induction of labor by stripping membranes, Obstet. Gynec. 11:74, 1958.

CONFERENCE MATERIAL

1. A mother, Para 2, is admitted to the hospital at 42 weeks' gestation for induction of labor. Her membranes have been artificially ruptured and intravenous oxytocin has been started. Discuss the nursing care of this mother from this time until she is in active labor.

2. What specific nursing care would you give to a mother who sustained a third-degree perineal laceration as the result of a precipitous labor?

3. A 38-year-old gravida 5 had an uneventful pregnancy until the last trimester, when she developed pre-eclampsia. Now, at term, she is admitted to the hospital because of suspected abruptio placenta and, after consultation, is to have an emergency cesarean section. Discuss the nursing care of this mother from time of admission until she is taken to the operating room for surgery.

4. A primigravida, who has 3-year-old adopted twins, is delivered by low cervical cesarean section because of pelvic injuries received in an auto accident 6 years earlier. Discuss the nursing care of this mother following cesarean section.

Study Questions

UNIT SIX: OPERATIVE PROCEDURES IN OBSTETRICS

Read through the entire question and place your answer on the line to the right.

1. Which of the following structures are involved when an episiotomy is performed?
A. The vaginal mucosa
B. The levator ani muscle
C. The glans clitoris
D. The cardinal ligament
E. The fourchet

Select the number corresponding to the correct letter or letters.
1. A only
2. A and B
3. A, B and E
4. All of them

3

2. Obstetric forceps are frequently used to facilitate delivery. In which of the following conditions would it be indicated to deliver the infant by forceps?
A. The cervix fails to dilate completely.
B. The mother has heart disease.
C. The mother has a contracted pelvis.
D. Prolapse of the umbilical cord
E. Passage of meconium-stained amniotic fluid in vertex presentation

Select the number corresponding to the correct letters.
1. A and B
2. B, D and E
3. C and E
4. All of them

2

3. Which of the following principles should be observed in the use of intravenous oxytocin to stimulate labor?
A. The condition of the fetus must be satisfactory.
B. It should be used only in cases of secondary uterine inertia.
C. It should not be given to a multipara who has had 4 or more full-term pregnancies.
D. It should be used in cases of borderline pelvis.
E. A responsible person should be in constant attendance while the mother is receiving intravenous oxytocin.

Select the number corresponding to the correct letters.
1. A and B
2. A, C and E
3. B, D and E
4. All of them

2

4. What specific treatment should be included in the care given a mother who has had a repair of a second-degree laceration of the perineum?
A. Give daily routine perineal care.
B. Serve a soft diet until the 5th postpartal day.
C. Omit enemas until the 5th postpartal day.
D. Limit activities in regard to early ambulation.
E. Encourage the mother not to sit erect until wound has healed.

438

Select the number corresponding to the correct letter or letters.
1. A only
2. A, D and E
3. B, C and D
4. All of them

1

5. After a cesarean section, which of the following symptoms might indicate that the patient is having excessive bleeding?
A. Accelerated pulse and respiration and drop in blood pressure
B. Pain and tenderness in operative area
C. Abdominal distention
D. Sanguineous drainage from the abdominal wound and the vagina
E. Apprehension and restlessness

Select the number corresponding to the correct letters.
1. A and B
2. A, C and D
3. A, D and E
4. All of them

3

6. In caring for a mother who has been delivered by cesarean section, which of the following are usually employed to keep the uterus contracted and control bleeding?
A. Oxytocic drugs
B. Gentle massage of the fundus if it becomes relaxed
C. Icebag to the operative area
D. Pressure dressings and tight abdominal binder
E. Keep the patient flat in bed for the first 6 hours postoperatively.

Select the number corresponding to the correct letter or letters.
1. A only
2. A, C and D
3. B, C and E
4. All of them

1

Note: The key to the correct answers to these questions is given on page 598.

UNIT SEVEN

Maternal Disorders Associated With the Childbearing Cycle

Complications of Pregnancy
Complications of Labor
Complications of the Puerperium

Chapter 18

Complications of Pregnancy

INTRODUCTION

Regardless of the fact that from a biologic point of view childbearing is considered to be a normal reproductive process, the borderline between health and illness is less distinctly marked during this time because of the numerous physiologic changes that occur in the mother's body during the course of parturition. The importance of early and continued health supervision during pregnancy is paramount for the total well-being of the mother and her infant, for such preventive care makes possible the early detection of warning signals of potential pathologic conditions, so that serious problems may be averted or controlled by prompt treatment (see Chap. 8).

Certain "common complaints" are experienced by most expectant mothers to some degree; these are the so-called minor discomforts of pregnancy, which are not serious in themselves but nevertheless detract from the mother's feeling of comfort and well-being. Since these discomforts are usually related to normal physiologic changes occurring within the mother's body and are not in themselves pathologic, they have been included in the chapter on antepartal care (see Chap. 8). However, minor discomforts, if neglected, may lead to a major complication.

The maternal disorders associated with pregnancy may be considered from the standpoint of the complications of the pregnancy itself and from the standpoint of the complications that are related to the coincidental diseases which occur during pregnancy. There are only a few major complications of pregnancy, but they present a serious health problem, e.g., the toxemias of pregnancy. The coincidental diseases which may occur during pregnancy are those which might occur at any other time as well, because the pregnant woman is subject to any disorder or disease which might affect a nonpregnant person. However, when these illnesses arise coincident to pregnancy, the disorder is likely to complicate the pregnancy, the disorder itself may be aggravated by the pregnancy, or both effects may result (see p. 472).

Certain complications of pregnancy may seriously jeopardize the health of both mother and her unborn infant. Regardless of the dramatic progress made in reducing the maternal morbidity and mortality in this country during the last several decades, there are still substantial problems to be resolved. One of the major concerns today is related to the large proportion of women in our population who are receiving little or no antepartal care. In contrast with the pregnant women who receive more adequate health supervision, these women with inadequate antepartal care have a higher percentage of maternal complications and a higher maternal mortality rate. In addition, it is believed that their lack of antepartal care may contribute to complications affecting their offspring.

443

TABLE 12. INFANT DEATHS CAUSED BY NEONATAL DISORDERS ARISING FROM CERTAIN DISEASES OF THE MOTHER DURING PREGNANCY, UNITED STATES, 1963*

CAUSE OF DEATH†	NUMBER OF DEATHS		
	Total	With Immaturity	Without Mention of Immaturity
Certain Disease of Early Infancy:			
Neonatal disorders arising from certain diseases of the mother during pregnancy; attributed to:	741	466	275
Toxemias of pregnancy	245	157	88
Maternal diabetes	223	131	92
Maternal rubella	4	1	3
Toxoplasmosis	25	2	23
Other or unspecified diseases of mother during pregnancy	244	175	69

* Department of Health, Education, and Welfare: Vital Statistics of the United States 1963, vol. II, Part A, Table 1-20, Washington, D. C., U. S. Government Printing Office, 1965.

† Classified according to the Seventh Revision of International Lists, 1955.

A review of recent statistical data should serve to indicate some of the problem areas in maternity care (see Chap. 1). Disorders associated with pregnancy accounted for 51 per cent of the 1,466 maternal deaths which occurred in the United States in 1963. Of this number, 468 maternal deaths were due to complications of pregnancy, and 280 deaths were due to abortion. In addition, maternal complications during pregnancy influenced the infant mortality rates. It has been known that certain diseases of the mother during pregnancy may have a variety of antenatal influences on the fetus, resulting in postnatal manifestations of disease, deformity, premature births and stillbirths. The seriousness of this cannot be underestimated in view of the large number of infants whose lives are lost because of neonatal disorders arising from certain diseases of the mothers during pregnancy. Table 12 shows that 741 infant deaths in the United States in 1963 were due to such causes, the major problems being the toxemias of pregnancy and maternal diabetes.

TOXEMIAS OF PREGNANCY

"The toxemias of pregnancy are disorders encountered during gestation, or early in the puerperium, which are characterized by one or more of the following signs: hypertension, edema, albuminuria, and in severe cases, convulsions and coma."[1] Despite decades of intensive research, the cause of toxemia is still unknown. The name itself would give rise to the supposition that these conditions are due to circulating toxins in the blood, derived presumably from the products of conception; but this is probably not correct. Whether toxemia represents an exaggeration of the various physical changes which normally accompany pregnancy, or whether it depends on some entirely new deviation from the normal course of pregnancy is still one of the most important unsolved problems in the whole field of human reproduction.

The toxemias of pregnancy are a very common complication of gestation, being seen in 6 or 7 per cent of all gravidae. They rank among the three major complications (hemorrhage, puerperal infections and the toxemias of pregnancy) responsible for the vast majority of maternal deaths and account for some 1,000 maternal deaths in the United States each year. As a cause of fetal death they are even more important. It can be estimated conservatively that at least 30,000 stillbirths and neonatal deaths each year in this country are the result of toxemias of pregnancy. The great majority of these deaths are due to prematurity of the infant.

The huge toll of maternal and infant lives taken by the toxemias of pregnancy is in large

[1] Definition established by The American Committee on Maternal Welfare, April 1, 1952.

measure preventable. Proper antepartal supervision, particularly the early detection of signs and symptoms of oncoming toxemia and appropriate treatment, will arrest many cases and so ameliorate others that the outcome for baby and mother is usually satisfactory. The nurse is often the first to encounter the early signs and symptoms, not only in the hospital outpatient department but also on home visits, and it is of utmost importance that she be constantly on the lookout for them so that treatment may be instituted at the earliest possible moment.

Classification

The toxemias of pregnancy have heretofore been classified in many forms. In 1952 The American Committee on Maternal Welfare revised its classification as follows:

1. Acute toxemia of pregnancy
   A. Preeclampsia
      1. Mild
      2. Severe
   B. Eclampsia
2. Chronic hypertensive (vascular disease with pregnancy
   A. Chronic hypertensive vascular disease without superimposed acute toxemia
      1. Those cases in which hypertension was definitely known to exist before the onset of pregnancy
      2. Cases of early hypertension before the 24th week
   B. Chronic hypertensive vascular disease with superimposed acute toxemia
3. Unclassified toxemias

Acute toxemia of pregnancy is divided into two stages: *preeclampsia* (the nonconvulsive stage) and *eclampsia* (the convulsive stage). The condition is classified as *preeclampsia* when, after the 24th week of pregnancy, a gravida who previously has been normal in the following respects develops sudden elevation of blood pressure, albuminuria or edema (one or more of the symptoms). Certain criteria have been established to divide preeclampsia into two groups: "preeclampsia mild" and "preeclampsia severe," depending on the symptoms. In *preeclampsia mild*, the systolic blood pressure is found to be 140 mm. Hg or more, or is elevated 30 mm. or more above the

usual level; the diastolic pressure will be 90 mm. Hg or more, or is elevated 15 mm. or more above the usual level. Abnormal blood pressures must be observed on two occasions or more at least 6 hours apart, because a single reading may be misleading. The albumin in the urine is small in amount but must be of sufficient degree on 2 or more successive days. Persistent edema involving the hands and the face is present. The condition is classified as *preeclampsia severe* if any one of the following signs or symptoms is present: (1) a systolic blood pressure of 160 mm. Hg or more, or a diastolic pressure of 110 mm. or more; (2) marked albuminuria; (3) oliguria; (4) cerebral or visual disturbances; (5) pulmonary edema or cyanosis. Once the preeclamptic patient has a convulsion, she passes into the stage called *eclampsia*.

Chronic hypertensive vascular disease, sometimes called essential hypertension, is a disease which is not peculiar to pregnancy. When pregnancy aggravates the already existing hypertension so that the gravida with this chronic process develops an acute elevation of blood pressure and a significant degree of albuminuria, the condition is called *chronic hypertensive vascular disease with superimposed acute toxemia.* This disease is seen in all stages of gestation but is prone to occur between the 24th and 30th weeks. Furthermore, the symptoms may increase in severity to the stage of eclampsia.

Preeclampsia

As has been stated in the previous classification of the toxemias of pregnancy, preeclampsia is characterized by a sudden elevation in blood pressure, albuminuria and edema in a gravida who previously has been normal in these respects. It is the forerunner or prodromal stage of eclampsia; in other words, unless the preeclamptic process is checked by treatment or by delivery, it is more or less likely that eclampsia (convulsions and coma) will ensue. Characteristically, preeclampsia is a disease of the last 2 or 3 months of pregnancy and is particularly prone to occur in young primigravidae. The underlying disease processes of preeclampsia and eclampsia are probably identical, the chief difference being that

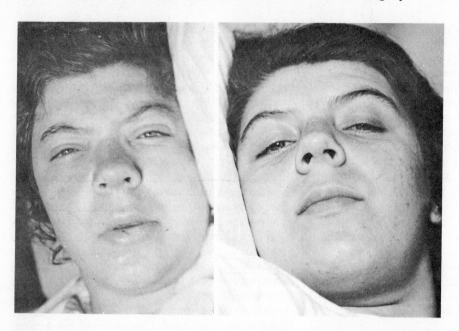

Fig. 18-1. (*Left*) Facies in preeclampsia. Note edema of eyelids and facial skin and general coarsening of features. (*Right*) Same patient 10 days after delivery.

the latter goes on to convulsions and coma, whereas the former does not.

Signs and Symptoms. The earliest warning signal of preeclampsia is sudden development of hypertension. Accordingly, the importance of frequent and regular blood pressure estimations during pregnancy cannot be emphasized too strongly. The absolute blood pressure reading is probably of less significance than the relationship it bears to previous determinations and to the age of the patient. For example, a rise from 110/70 to 135/85 in a young woman is a more urgent danger signal than a rise from 135/85 to 150/90 in a patient at 35.

The next most constant sign of preeclampsia is sudden, excessive weight gain. If cases of preeclampsia are studied from the viewpoint of fluid intake and output, it is at once apparent that these sudden gains in weight are due entirely to an accumulation of water in the tissues. Such weight gains, in other words, represent latent edema and almost always precede the visible face and finger edema which is so characteristic of the advanced stages of the disease. From what has been said, it is apparent that scales are essential equipment for good antepartal care. Weight gain of 1 pound a week or so may be regarded as being normal. Sudden gains of more than 2 pounds a week should be viewed with suspicion; gains of more than 3 pounds, with alarm. Weight increases

of the latter magnitude call for more frequent blood pressure determinations, and if these latter are also abnormal, hospitalization with intensive treatment is indicated. In investigating suspected edema, it is well to ask the patient if her wedding ring is becoming tight, since finger and facial edema is a more valuable sign of preeclampsia than is swelling of the ankles. In the facies of a patient with outspoken preeclampsia, the eyelids are swollen, and, associated with the edema, marked coarseness of the features develops (Fig. 18-1).

The sudden appearance of *albumin in the urine*, with or without other findings, always should be regarded as a sign of preeclampsia. Usually it develops later than the hypertension and the gain in weight and for this very reason must be regarded as being of serious omen when superimposed on these other two findings.

But the very essence of preeclampsia is the lightninglike fulminance with which it strikes. Although the above physical signs of preeclampsia usually give the physician ample time to institute preventive treatment, it sometimes happens that these derangements develop between visits to the office or the clinic, even though they be only a week apart. For this reason it is imperative that all expectant mothers be informed, both verbally and by some form of printed slip or booklet, in regard to certain danger signals which they themselves may recognize. Insofar as the toxemias of pregnancy are concerned, the following symptoms demand immediate report to the doctor: (1) severe, continuous headache; (2) swelling of the face or the fingers; (3) dimness or blurring of vision; (4) persistent vomiting; (5) decrease in the amount of urine excreted; and (6) epigastric pain (a late symptom).

It should be emphasized that the three early and important signs of preeclampsia, namely, hypertension, weight gain and albuminuria, are changes of which the patient is usually unaware. All three may be present in substantial degree, and yet she may feel quite well. Only by regular and careful antepartal examination can these warning signs be detected. By the time the preeclamptic patient has developed symptoms and signs which she herself can detect (such as headache, blurred vision, puffiness of the eyelids and the fingers), she is usually in an advanced stage of the disease, and much valuable time has been lost. Headache is rarely observed in the milder cases but is encountered with increasing frequency as the most severe grades are met. In general, patients who actually develop eclampsia often have a severe headache as a forerunner of the first convulsion. The visual disturbances range from a slight blurring of vision to various degrees of temporary blindness. Although convulsions are less likely to occur in cases of mild preeclampsia, the possibility cannot be entirely eliminated. Patients with severe preeclampsia should always be considered as being on the verge of having a convulsion.

Treatment. Prophylaxis is most important in the prevention and the control of preeclampsia. Since in its early stages preeclampsia rarely gives rise to signs or symptoms which the patient herself will notice, the early detection of this disease demands meticulous antepartal supervision. Rapid weight gain or an upward trend in blood pressure, although still in the "normal" range, are danger signals. Every pregnant woman should be examined by her obstetrician every week during the last month of pregnancy and every 2 weeks during the 2 previous months. The most promising prophylaxis of the disease lies in reduction of sodium intake and curtailing weight gain in all pregnant women. Finger edema is a frequent forerunner of preeclampsia, which may precede

the hypertension by several weeks and is a valuable warning sign.

AMBULATORY PATIENT. When the patient's symptoms are mild—i.e., there is minor elevation of blood pressure with minimal or no signs of edema and proteinuria—treatment may be instituted at home in the hope that symptoms will abate. During this period the patient should be examined by the physician at least twice a week, and she should be given a strict regimen to follow, as well as careful instructions in regard to symptoms to report promptly. The patient's activities should be restricted, and she should understand that bed rest during the greater part of the day is most desirable. Sedative drugs, such as phenobarbital, may be prescribed to encourage rest and relaxation, the dosage being dependent on the severity of the condition. Of major importance is a salt-poor diet. Therefore, the patient should be instructed so that she understands which foods have appreciable sodium content and therefore must be excluded from her diet, in addition to the fact that no salt may be added to her food in the kitchen or at the table. The diet should be well balanced but restricted in caloric content if the patient's weight gain indicates the need. It should contain ample protein, particularly lean meat, eggs and a quart of milk daily. Fluid intake should be maintained at 2,500 cc. daily; in hot weather, at 3,000 cc. Carbonated beverages should be avoided because of their sodium content.

The restriction of sodium in the diet of the preeclamptic patient is directed at reducing the edema. Even in normal nonpregnant persons an increased intake of sodium chloride causes water retention. Pregnant women, particularly gravidae suffering from preeclampsia, show a marked tendency to retain sodium, and there is reason to believe that this tendency of the tissues to retain sodium is closely correlated with their tendency to hold water. To superimpose still more sodium in the diet on this already existing sodium and water retention is obviously unwise.

By means of the above measures it is often possible to relieve the signs and symptoms of preeclampsia so that the patient proceeds to term satisfactorily.

HOSPITAL PATIENT. In the event that the patient's condition does not respond promptly to ambulatory treatment, she should be hospitalized without delay. A systematic method of study should be instituted upon admission to the hospital. A general physical examination and history should be obtained promptly, followed by constant vigilance for the development of such symptoms as headache, visual disturbances and edema of the fingers and the eyelids. Body weight should be obtained on admission and every other morning thereafter. Blood pressure readings should be taken every 4 hours except between midnight and morning, unless the midnight blood pressure has risen. Daily fluid intake and output records should be kept, and urine specimens sent to the laboratory daily for analysis for albumin and casts. Retinal examination is always included as part of the admission physical examination and is done every 2 to 3 days thereafter, depending on the findings. Blood chemical determinations are also included. Once the patient is admitted to the hospital, complete bed rest is essential.

Drugs and Diet. Even in milder cases, minimal doses of sedative drugs are helpful. Phenobarbital, 32 mg. (½ grain), may be given 4 times a day, or twice this dosage in cases of moderate severity. The dietary regimen previously described should be adhered to, or it may be indicated to restrict the sodium chloride to less than 3 Gm. daily. In such cases it may become necessary to substitute one of the commercial sodium-free milk powders in place of regular milk, since a quart of milk itself contains about 1.25 Gm. of sodium chloride. In many instances diuretics may be used routinely. Magnesium sulfate (epsom salts), 15 Gm., or citrate of magnesia, 200 cc., may be used every 2nd or 3rd day, although these merely increase water loss from the bowel, not sodium excretion. Ammonium chloride, 4 Gm. daily for 3 days, is frequently used. This may never be given for more than 3 days consecutively because of the acidosis which it tends to produce when it is used for longer periods.

Other diuretic drugs employed in the treatment of toxemias of pregnancy today are acetazolamide (Diamox), chlorothiazide (Diuril) and hydrochlorothiazide (Esidrix). The usual daily dose of acetazolamide is 250 mg., but since, like ammonium chloride, it produces a mild acidosis, it is not usually administered

for more than 5 days in a course. Moreover, this drug has a self-limiting effect and does not act as a diuretic after 2 to 3 days, although the medication may be resumed again after an interval of time. Chlorothiazide is used to diminish the fluid retention in toxemias of pregnancy and to control blood pressure. The usual adult dose to achieve diuretic results is 0.5 to 1.0 Gm. daily. Chlorothiazide increases the elimination of both sodium and water from the body without causing acidosis and is occasionally employed to relieve edema in normal pregnancy as well as in the toxemias. However, when dosage of the drug is adequate to increase the urinary output, potassium is also excreted. The potassium deficiency which will result can be avoided, of course, with the administration of potassium chloride, but a means more acceptable to the expectant mother would be to include foods rich in potassium chloride in her daily diet, for example, orange juice. It is well to instruct all patients on chlorothiazide therapy to drink 8 ounces of orange juice daily, since the potassium content is high and the sodium content low. A number of new compounds have been used effectively in recent years, for example, hydrochlorothiazide (Esidrix). They all resemble chlorothiazide in that they have both diuretic and antihypertensive effects, and they have the advantages of being effective over a longer period of time, of seeming to have a low incidence of side-effects and of producing a minimum of electrolyte imbalance when proper precautions are taken.

When severe preeclampsia exists, immediate and intensive medicinal therapy is imperative. Sedation is of major importance to forestall convulsions. The dosage of the drugs should be regulated so that they produce drowsiness and sleep from which the patient can be easily awakened. Morphine sulfate, 16 mg. (¼ grain) may be given hypodermically, followed by either paraldehyde per rectum or one of the barbiturates. If paraldehyde is employed, the dose should be about 10 to 15 cc., depending on the weight of the patient, and administered in 30 cc. of olive oil. Magnesium sulfate administered intramuscularly is another drug frequently chosen because it protects the patient with toxemia against convulsions during labor. In addition to its action as a vasodilator and diuretic, it has a sedative effect, because when given intramuscularly it acts as a central nervous system depressant. The tranquilizing drugs have been used effectively.

DELIVERY. Despite all efforts, the condition may persist to a marked degree, and in that event induction of labor may become necessary for the welfare of mother and infant. In occasional instances when the preeclampsia is severe and fulminating and conditions for induction of labor are not favorable, cesarean section may be the procedure of choice.

Postpartum. The signs and symptoms of preeclampsia usually abate rapidly after delivery, but the danger of convulsions does not pass until 48 hours have elapsed postpartum. Therefore, continuation of sedation throughout this interval is indicated. In the majority of cases the elevated blood pressure as well as the other derangements have returned to normal within 10 days or 2 weeks. In about 30 per cent of cases, however, the hypertension shows a tendency either to persist indefinitely or to recur in subsequent pregnancies. For this reason the prolonged follow-up of these patients is highly important.

Nursing Care. The nurse's responsibility in the detection and care of cases of preeclampsia is manifold. Since this complication of pregnancy is common and may occur antepartally, intrapartally or postpartally, it is important for the nurse to observe all maternity patients closely for the first indication of early symptoms, as well as to be quick to recognize and report any evidence pointing to an aggravation of the process. The early symptoms and the manifestations related to more severe preeclampsia, such as persistent headache, blurred vision, spots or flashes of light before the eyes, epigastric pain, vomiting, torpor or muscular twitchings, are all vastly important. Data collected in relation to these symptoms in addition to an accurate record of weight gain, fluid intake and elimination, diet and attitudes and behavior, when it is accurately recorded, can assist the physician in evaluating the symptoms and planning his course of therapy.

In setting the therapeutic atmosphere, the nurse should see that the environment is as comfortable and pleasant as possible. The patient should be in a single room, free from the stimuli of noise, strong lights and the presence of unnecessary equipment which might frighten her. To the best of her ability, the nurse must protect the patient from needless traffic into the room; otherwise, the coming and going of personnel to the bedside may be so constant that it could interfere with the efficacy of the treatment being carried out. Every effort should be exerted to relieve the patient's anxiety, which sometimes is brought about by apprehension regarding her illness or may be due to concern for the welfare of her family at home.

Regardless of the severity of the toxemia, certain responsibilities are carried out by the nurse. Medications ordered must be administered promptly, the prescribed diet should be supervised, a careful record of intake and elimination kept, blood pressure readings and basal weights taken, specimens collected and labeled accurately, and observations of slight symptoms or change in condition should be reported immediately, both verbally and on the patient's record. Since rest is a major consideration in the care of this patient, the nurse should plan a schedule of activities so that the patient is disturbed as little as possible. Medications, treatments and nursing procedures should be administered at the same time as far as the physician's orders will permit, but always with the thought in mind that only as much as will not overtire the patient should be planned for any one time. When any treatment is ordered, the procedure is best carried out after sedation has been administered. Before heavy sedation is initiated, any removable dentures or eyeglasses should be removed and stored in a secure place. If the patient is not in labor, the nurse must be alert to watch for signs of labor, particularly after sedation has been given. Any time an intravenous fluid is administered, if the physician has not specified the rate at which the fluid is to flow, it should be given slowly.

The nurse should see that the equipment necessary for the safe and efficient care of the patient is immediately available and in good working order. A padded mouth gag should always be ready for use at the bedside to prevent the patient from biting her tongue in the event that a convulsion develops. Trays for catheterization equipment and for the administration of special medications constitute part of the necessary equipment. Since water retention plays such a large role in the disease, and urinary output is likely to be diminshed, an indwelling bladder catheter may be ordered to ensure accuracy in obtaining output from the kidneys. Since the urinary output must be watched carefully, it is imperative to see that the retention catheter is draining properly at all times. In severe cases suction apparatus should be readily available for aspirating mucus, as well as equipment for the administration of oxygen, should symptoms such as cyanosis or depressed respiration indicate the need.

Eclampsia

Clinical Picture. As indicated, the development of eclampsia is almost always preceded by the signs and symptoms of preeclampsia. A preeclamptic patient, who may have been conversing with you a moment before, is seen to roll her eyes to one side and stare fixedly into space. Immediately, twitching of the facial muscles ensues. This is the *stage of invasion* of the convulsion and lasts only a few seconds.

The whole body then becomes rigid in a generalized muscular contraction; the face is distorted, the eyes protrude, the arms are flexed, the hands are clenched and the legs are inverted. Since all the muscles of the body are now in a state of tonic contraction, this phase may be regarded as the *stage of contraction*; it lasts 15 or 20 seconds.

Suddenly the jaws begin to open and close violently, and forthwith the eyelids also. The other facial muscles and then all the muscles of the body alternately contract and relax in rapid succession. So forceful are the muscular movements that the patient may throw herself out of bed, and almost invariably, unless protected, the tongue is bitten by the violent jaw action. Foam, often blood-tinged, exudes from the mouth; the face is congested and purple, and the eyes are bloodshot. Few pictures which the nurse is called upon to witness are so horrible. This phase in which the muscles alternately contract and relax is called the *stage of convulsion;* it may last a minute or so. Gradually the muscular movements become milder and farther apart, and finally the patient lies motionless.

Throughout the seizure the diaphragm has been fixed with respiration halted. Still no breathing occurs. For a few seconds the woman appears to be dying from respiratory arrest, but just when this outcome seems almost inevitable, she takes a long, deep, stertorous inhalation, and breathing is resumed. Then coma ensues. The patient will remember nothing whatsoever of the convulsion or, in all probability, events immediately before and afterward.

The coma may last from a few minutes to several hours, and the patient may then become conscious; or the coma may be succeeded by another convulsion. The convulsions may recur during coma, or they may recur only after an interval of consciousness, or they may never recur at all. In the average case, from 5 to 10 convulsions occur at longer or shorter intervals, but as many as 20 are not uncommon. Convulsions may start before the onset of labor (antepartum), during labor (intrapartum) or anytime within the first 48 hours after delivery (postpartum). About a fifth of the cases develop postpartally.

Upon physical examination, the findings of eclampsia are similar to those in preeclampsia, but exaggerated. Thus, the systolic blood pressure usually ranges around 180 mm. Hg and sometimes exceeds 200 mm. Hg. Albuminuria is frequently extreme, from 10 to 20 Gm. per liter. Edema may be marked but sometimes is absent. Oliguria, or suppression of urinary excretion, is common and may amount to complete anuria. Fever is present in about half the cases.

In favorable cases the convulsions cease, the coma lessens, and urinary output increases. However, it sometimes requires 1 or 2 days for clear consciousness to be regained. During this period eclamptic patients are often in an obstreperous, resistant mood and may be exceedingly difficult to manage. A few develop actual psychoses. In unfavorable cases the coma deepens, urinary excretion diminishes, the pulse becomes more rapid, the temperature rises, and edema of the lungs develops. The last is a serious symptom and usually is interpreted as a sign of cardiovascular failure. Edema of the lungs is readily recognizable by the noisy, gurgling respiration and by the large quantity of frothy mucus which exudes from the mouth and the nose. Toward the end, convulsions cease altogether, and the final picture is one of vascular collapse, with falling blood pressure and overwhelming edema of the lungs.

Like preeclampsia, eclampsia is a disease

of young primigravidae, the majority of cases occurring in first pregnancies. It is more likely to occur as full term approaches and is rarely seen prior to the last 3 months. Eclampsia is particularly prone to develop in twin gestations, the likelihood being about 4 times that in single pregnancies.

Prognosis. Eclampsia is one of the gravest complications of pregnancy; the maternal mortality ranges, in different localities and in different hospitals, from 5 to 15 per cent of such cases. The outlook for the baby is particularly grave, the fetal mortality being about 20 per cent. Although it is difficult in a given case to forecast the outcome, the following are unfavorable signs: oliguria; prolonged coma; a sustained pulse rate over 120; temperature over 103° F.; more than 10 convulsions; 10 or more Gm. of albumin per liter in the urine; systolic blood pressure of more than 200; edema of lungs. If none of these signs is present, the outlook for recovery is good; if two or more are present, the prognosis is definitely serious.

Even though the patient survives, she may not escape unscathed from the attack but sometimes continues to have high blood pressure indefinitely. This statement applies both to preeclampsia and eclampsia. Indeed, about 10 per cent of all preeclamptic and 5 per cent of all eclamptic patients are left with chronic, permanent hypertension. It is of even more importance to note that a still larger percentage of these women (about 50% of preeclamptics and 30% of eclamptics) again develop hypertensive toxemia in any subsequent pregnancies. This is known as "recurrent" or "repeat" toxemia. These facts make it plain that careful, prolonged follow-up of these mothers who have suffered from preeclampsia or eclampsia is imperative. Moreover, the prognosis for future pregnancies must be guarded, although, as the figures indicate, such patients stand at least an even chance of going through subsequent pregnancies satisfactorily.

Principles of Treatment. Since the cause of eclampsia is not known, there can be no "specific" therapy, and treatment must necessarily be empirical. By "empirical" treatment is meant the utilization of those therapeutic measures which have yielded the best results in other cases. It is thus based on experience. Since the experience of different doctors and

different hospitals varies considerably, the type of therapy employed from clinic to clinic differs somewhat in respect to the drugs used and in other details. However, the general principles followed are almost identical everywhere. For the nurse to memorize some particular regimen of therapy, as given in this textbook or as used in this or that hospital, will serve little purpose in her later career and conduces to an undesirable rigidity of attitude. However, she should grasp thoroughly the general principles involved. These are enumerated as follows:

1. PREVENTION. Let it be emphasized again that eclampsia is largely (but not entirely) a preventable disease. Vigilant antepartal care and the early detection and treatment of preeclampsia will do more to reduce deaths from eclampsia than the most intensive treatment after convulsions have once started.

2. CONSERVATIVE TREATMENT. Since eclampsia never occurs in nonpregnant women, nor in men, it is reasonable to believe that it must be due in some way to the pregnant condition. By the same token it might be concluded that the best way to treat eclampsia would be to terminate the pregnancy at once, that is empty the uterus. This was the therapy employed in the early years of the century and is known as the "radical treatment" of eclampsia; either the cervix was forcibly dilated and the baby extracted, or cesarean section was employed. The results were disastrous. A quarter to a third of the mothers died, often on the operating table from shock.

Dissatisfied with the poor results yielded by the radical treatment of eclampsia, about 1910, physicians began treating the convulsions with sedative drugs, ignored the pregnancy and allowed labor to start whenever it would. The most famous method of therapy of this sort is the Stroganoff regimen, based on sedation by means of morphine and chloral hydrate. The results were dramatic: the maternal mortality fell to 10 per cent, and the fetal mortality was no worse than before. Other physicians tried other sedative drugs and other means of combating the convulsions, but as long as they refrained from interfering with the pregnancy, the results were as good as Stroganoff's, that is, only 1 woman in 10 was lost. This program, whereby the eclamptic convulsions are treated by sedation or otherwise, the pregnancy ignored, and labor allowed to start when it will, is known as the "conservative treatment" of eclampsia. This is the policy generally followed today, because in the majority of cases it gives the best results.

Although the conservative treatment has shown itself to be the program of choice in most cases, hard-and-fast rules in eclampsia are unwise. Now and then cases occur in which cesarean section may be the best therapy.

3. SEDATION. The purpose of administering sedative drugs is to depress the activity of the brain cells and thereby stop convulsions. The drugs most commonly employed are described below.

Morphine. Because of its quick action and readiness of administration, morphine is usually the first drug which the eclamptic patient receives. Thus, it is often given at the patient's home to allay convulsions during transport to the hospital, or in the admission room of a hospital pending the institution of other types of medication. When given as a single initial dose, the amount ordered by the physician is likely to be large, from one quarter to one half a grain (0.016 to 0.032 Gm.), depending on the size of the patient. Morphine may also be administered during the subsequent course of the treatment, but the modern tendency is to rely on other drugs for the main sedative program.

Barbiturates. The more commonly employed of these are Luminal Sodium (0.3 Gm. subcutaneously) and Amytal Sodium (0.3 to 0.6 Gm. intravenously). The drugs produce sleep, muscular relaxation and lowering of the blood pressure.

Paraldehyde. Although pungent in odor and somewhat difficult to administer, paraldehyde is being used more and more in eclampsia. In this condition it is almost always given per rectum, diluted with an equal amount of olive oil, and in dosages which may range from 20 to 35 cc. of the pure paraldehyde, according to the severity of the disease and the size of the patient. Usually it is repeated from time to time, in somewhat smaller doses perhaps, in order to maintain a fairly deep narcosis.

Magnesium Sulfate. This is not only a central nervous system sedative (employed in tetanus) but it is believed to cause a dilatation of the peripheral blood vessels and thus lower the blood pressure. For these reasons

this drug is frequently used both in the treatment of preeclampsia and eclampsia. It may be given either intravenously or intramuscularly. When administered intravenously, it is sometimes given in amounts of 20 cc. of a 10 per cent solution and sometimes in a 2-cc. injection of a 50 per cent solution.

The intramuscular use of magnesium sulfate is more widely employed perhaps than the intravenous technic. Here the dosage varies considerably from institution to institution but may be given in amounts as large as 10 Gm. intramuscularly in a 50 per cent solution as an initial dose, followed by 5 Gm. every 6 hours. A 1 per cent concentration of procaine is frequently introduced in the injection solution to minimize discomfort following the injection. The initial dose is divided, 5 to 10 cc. being given into each buttock. In order to avoid tissue irritation as much as possible and to obtain wider dispersion, the needle is moved about while injecting the solution. After withdrawal of the needle the area is massaged with a dry warm pack, which then is taped over the injection site. These injections are always made by the physician.

Chloral Hydrate. As already mentioned, chloral hydrate in conjunction with morphine forms the basis of the Stroganoff treatment.

Other Drugs. Although the above principles of treatment may be regarded as more or less standard, the nurse will encounter many experienced obstetricians who secure good results with other procedures. Thus, in many hospitals various hypotensive drugs, such as Veratrone and Apresoline, are favored. These agents produce relaxation of the arterioles throughout the body and by thus reducing peripheral resistance to blood flow lower the blood pressure, often dramatically. They are frequently employed in combination with other drugs.

4. PROTECTION OF PATIENT FROM SELF-INJURY. The eclamptic patient must never be left alone for a second. When in the throes of a convulsion, she may crash her head against a bedpost or throw herself onto the floor; or she may bite her tongue violently. To prevent the latter injury, some device should be kept within easy reach which can be inserted between the jaws at the very onset of a convulsion. A piece of very heavy rubber tubing, a rolled towel or a padded clothespin is often

FIG. 18-2. Improvised mouth gag inserted between jaws of eclamptic patient to prevent tongue injury. (Putnam, Tracy J.: Convulsive Seizures, Philadelphia, Lippincott)

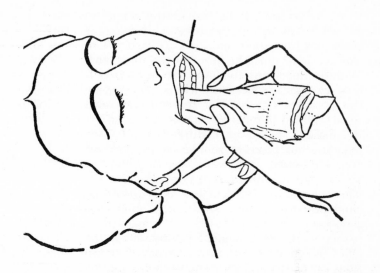

employed (Fig. 18-2). The nurse must take care in inserting it not to injure the patient (lips, gums, teeth) and not to allow her own finger to be bitten.

Eclamptic patients must never be given fluids by mouth unless thoroughly conscious. Failure to adhere to this rule may result in aspiration of the fluid and consequent pneumonia.

5. PROTECTION OF PATIENT FROM EXTRANEOUS STIMULI. A loud noise, a bright light, a jarring of the bed, a draft—indeed, the slightest irritation—may be enough to precipitate a convulsion.

6. PROMOTION OF DIURESIS. When an eclamptic patient begins to excrete substantial quantities of urine, the outlook is encouraging. Accordingly, efforts are generally made to stimulate renal activity. This is most often done by the intravenous administration of hypertonic glucose solution, usually about a 20 per cent solution in amounts ranging from 200 to 500 cc.

Nurse's Responsibilities in Eclampsia. The nurse's responsibilities in the management of a case of eclampsia are serious. Some of them have already been mentioned in the discussion of treatment. Although eclampsia usually is regarded as the climax to a mounting preeclamptic toxemia which has been present, the nurse must remember that it is occasionally observed as a fulminating case in an apparently normal woman who may develop severe symptoms in the span of 24 hours. In the event that

eclampsia occurs, the best quality of nursing care is necessary. The attack may come on at any time, even when the patient is sleeping. During the seizure it is necessary to protect the patient from self-injury. Never leave the patient for an instant unless someone is actually at the bedside to relieve you. Gentle restraint should be used to guide the patient's movements whenever necessary to prevent her from throwing herself against the head of the bed or out of it. Canvas sides, as well as pads at the head and the foot of the bed, are helpful. The padded mouth gag should be inserted between the upper and lower teeth at the onset of a convulsion to prevent the tongue from being bitten. Regardless of the fact that the nurse is exceedingly "busy" with the patient when a seizure occurs, she should make careful and complete observations of the duration and the character of each convulsion, the depth and duration of coma, the quality and the rate of pulse and respiration and the degree of cyanosis. A careful record should be kept so that this information can be used by the physician in treating the patient. During the coma which follows, care must be taken to see that the patient does not aspirate. It is understood, of course, that one never gives an eclamptic patient fluids by mouth unless it is certain she is fully conscious. The position of the patient in bed should be such that it promotes drainage of secretions and the maintenance of a clear airway. It may be necessary to raise the foot of the bed of the comatose patient a few inches to promote drainage of secretions from the respiratory passage. When this measure must be resorted to, it is particularly important to watch for signs of pulmonary edema, which would be aggravated by this position. The head of the bed may need to be elevated to relieve dyspnea. Even though the patient should be disturbed as little as possible, her position should be changed at hourly intervals.

The patient should be protected from extraneous stimuli. Light in the room should be eliminated except for a small lamp, so shaded that none of the light falls on the patient. Although the room should be darkened, the light should be sufficient to permit observations of changes in condition, such as cyanosis or twitchings. A flashlight, directed well away from the patient's face, may be used during catheterization and rectal installations and during the physician's examinations. Sudden noises, such as the slamming of a door or the clatter of a tray as it is placed on a table, and jarring of the bed must be avoided, because they are often sufficient stimuli to send the patient into convulsions. Only absolutely necessary conversation should be carried on in the room, and this should be in the lowest tones possible.

The fetal heart tones should be checked as often as time will permit. Also, the nurse must watch for signs of labor. In eclampsia this may proceed with few external signs, and occasionally such a patient gives birth beneath the sheets before anyone knows that the process is under way. Be suspicious when the patient grunts or groans or moves about at regular intervals, every 5 minutes or so. If this occurs, feel the consistency of the uterus, watch for "show" and bulging and report your observations to the physician. Convulsions which occur during labor may speed up this process, and more rapid preparation for delivery should be made. During the delivery, the same atmosphere of quiet should be maintained, and glaring lights should be kept away from the patient's face.

Throughout the care of the eclamptic patient a careful account of fluid intake and output should be recorded, along with all the other observations and pertinent data. And, since further complications of pregnancy may

occur in eclampsia, the patient should be observed for signs and symptoms of cerebral hemorrhage, abruptio placentae, pulmonary edema and cardiac failure.

Preeclampsia and eclampsia have been discussed in some detail because the nurse's role in the management of these conditions is extremely important.

Chronic Hypertensive Vascular Disease

As the name indicates, this disease is a chronic disorder of the vascular system associated with high blood pressure. In other words, these patients have a tendency to have hypertension, whether pregnant or not. Not infrequently the kidneys are also affected, with the result that albuminuria may be present as well as diminution in the excretory power of the kidneys. The age of these patients is usually in the 30's, most of them are multiparae with a number of children. The course of pregnancy in these chronic hypertensive women is often troublesome, the blood pressure showing a tendency to reach higher and higher levels as the last 3 months of pregnancy are reached. In general, the outlook for the baby is poor. The fetus often dies in utero. Following delivery, there may be a slight recession in the blood pressure, but it usually remains at a figure only slightly below that observed during pregnancy. Each subsequent pregnancy adds its increment to the hypertension, and, as a rule, the exacerbation in blood pressure occurs earlier and earlier in each succeeding pregnancy.

Aside from the high blood pressure, the signs and symptoms of hypertensive vascular disease may be surprisingly few. Headache is rather common, but even this complaint may be absent. The doctor's examination of the retina very often shows a narrowing of the arterioles, indicative of the fact that there is a generalized sclerosis of the small arterioles throughout the body.

In patients with chronic hypertensive vascular disease, we cannot prevent the occurrence of hypertension, since it was already present when conception took place. These patients already had the sclerosed, inelastic arterioles mentioned above, and it is understandable that the 50 per cent increase per minute output of the heart which pregnancy imposes (p. 117) will place a severe burden on such a vascular system. In the face of this chronic process and this burden imposed by pregnancy, very little can be done in such cases to relieve the hypertension. The physician will have a plan which he will discuss with the expectant parents. Hence, the problem is largely one of preventive medicine, in the sense that pregnancies either should be avoided altogether or limited.

Decision as to the best way of managing a case of hypertensive vascular disease will be made by the physician after taking into consideration a number of circumstances, such as the severity of the hypertensive process, the number of children in the family, the duration of the pregnancy when first seen, etc. If the process is mild, the pregnancy may be allowed to continue with the patient under close observation for signs of impending trouble. On the other hand, if the process is very severe, the mother's life may be at stake. In most cases in this group, the doctor may wish to

prevent further pregnancies and may recommend either ligation of the fallopian tubes or the use of some method of contraception.

Moral Considerations. The nurse should remember that such recommendations are not always acceptable to the patient, particularly if this involves ethical problems related to her religious beliefs. In such instances it is well to encourage the patient to discuss the problem with her priest or minister, as well as with her husband and her physician. Some pertinent references have been included in the suggested readings at the end of the chapter.

HEMORRHAGIC COMPLICATIONS

The causes of bleeding in pregnancy are usually considered in relation to the stage of gestation in which they are most likely to cause complications. Frequent causes of bleeding during the first half of pregnancy are abortion, ectopic pregnancy and hydatidiform

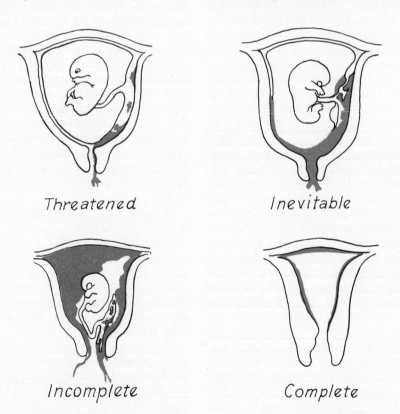

Threatened   Inevitable

Incomplete   Complete

Fig. 18-3. Stages of abortion. (Cooke, Willard R.: Essentials of Gynecology, Philadelphia, Lippincott)

mole. Although hydatidiform mole is a less common cause (it occurs once in about 2,000 pregnancies), it is nevertheless important, because uterine bleeding is its outstanding symptom. The two most common causes of hemorrhage in the latter half of pregnancy are placenta previa and abruptio placentae.

Abortion

Definitions. Abortion is the termination of pregnancy at any time before the fetus has attained a stage of viability, that is, before it is capable of extrauterine existence.

It is customary to use the weight of the fetus as an important criterion in abortion. Infants weighing 1,000 Gm. (2 lbs., 3 oz.) or less at birth possess little chance for survival, whereas those above this weight have a substantial chance of living. Thus, many authorities regard a pregnancy which terminates when the fetus weighs 1,000 Gm. (about 28 weeks of gestation) or less as an abortion. On the other hand, a small percentage of infants weighing 1,000 Gm. or less do survive. Modern advances in the management and care of premature infants have made it possible for smaller and smaller infants to survive, so fetuses weighing only 800 to 900 Gm. (1 lb., 13 oz. to 2 lbs.) may live. For this reason many authorities now maintain that fetal weight of 1,000 Gm. or less but more than 400 Gm. is classified as immature, and that fetal weight of 400 Gm. (about 20 weeks of gestation) or less constitutes an abortion. It is obvious, therefore, that how the termination of pregnancy is classified in different hospitals will depend wholly on the interpretation to which they subscribe. In summary, the following definitions are generally used. The termination of pregnancy at any time when the fetus weighs 400 Gm. or less is defined as an *abortion*. Infants weighing between 401 and 1,000 Gm. are called *immature*.

A premature infant is one born after the stage of viability has been reached but before it has the same chance for survival as a full-term infant. By general consensus, an infant which weighs 2,500 Gm. or less at birth is termed *premature*; one which weighs 2,501 Gm. (5½ lbs.) or more is regarded as *full term*.

It is well to remember that premature labor does not refer to abortion. *Premature labor is the termination of pregnancy after the fetus is viable but before it has attained full term*. Although the cause of many premature labors cannot be explained, the condition can be brought on by maternal diseases, such as chronic hypertensive vascular disease, abruptio placentae, placenta previa, untreated syphilis or a mechanical defect in the cervix.

As a measure to bring about greater uniformity in the interpretation of the terms "abortion," "miscarriage" and "viability," the World Health Organization, in 1950, introduced certain new definitions which, in effect, would substitute the term "early fetal death" for "abortion" and would tabulate all live births and fetal deaths in 4 groups, according to length of gestation.

Terminology of Abortion. The term "abortion" includes many varieties of termination of pregnancy prior to viability but may be subdivided into 2 main groups, namely, spontaneous and induced. *Spontaneous abortion is one in which through natural causes the process starts of its own accord. Induced abortion is one which is artificially induced, and may be in the form of either therapeutic abortion or a criminal abortion.* The laity, however, is inclined to associate the word "abortion" with instances in which criminal interference with pregnancy has been perpetrated, and to them, therefore, the term often carries a definite stigma. They employ the word "miscarriage" to designate spontaneous abortion, and the nurse will do well, in discussing the matter with patients or relatives to use that term.

In medical parlance the word "miscarriage" is rarely employed.

THREATENED ABORTION. An abortion is regarded as threatened if a patient in early pregnancy has vaginal bleeding or spotting; this may or may not be associated with mild cramps. The cervix is closed. The process has presumably started but may abate under suitable treatment (Fig. 18-3).

INEVITABLE ABORTION. Inevitable abortion is so called because the process has gone so far that termination of the pregnancy cannot be prevented. Bleeding is copious, and the pains are more severe. The membranes may or may not have ruptured, and the cervical canal is dilating.

INCOMPLETE ABORTION. An incomplete abortion is one in which part of the product of conception has been passed, but part (usually the placenta) is retained in the uterus. Bleeding persists until the retained secundines of the uterus have been passed.

COMPLETE ABORTION. Complete abortion is the expulsion of the entire product of conception.

MISSED ABORTION. In a missed abortion the fetus dies in the uterus, but, instead of being expelled, it is retained indefinitely. The term is generally restricted to cases in which 2 months or more elapse between fetal death and expulsion. During this period the fetus undergoes marked degenerative changes. Of these, maceration, or a general softening, is the most common. Occasionally it dries up into a leatherlike structure (mummification) and very rarely it becomes converted into stony material (lithopedion formation). Symptoms, except for amenorrhea, are usually lacking, but occasionally such patients complain of malaise, headache and anorexia. Hypofibrinogenemia, a hemorrhagic complication, may result (see p. 466).

HABITUAL ABORTION. By this term is meant a condition in which spontaneous abortion occurs in successive pregnancies (3 or more). This is a most distressing condition, some women having 6 or 8 spontaneous abortions.

THERAPEUTIC ABORTION. Therapeutic abortion is the instrumental termination of pregnancy by a physician because of some grave maternal disease which would make continuation of the pregnancy extremely hazardous to the mother. As a rule, one or more physicians are called into consultation to make certain that the procedure is absolutely necessary. Modern methods of antepartal care are making the necessity for therapeutic abortion relatively rare. The nurse must recall, moreover, that ethical principles of the Roman Catholic Church forbid the procedure, and that it may not be performed in hospitals of that faith.

CRIMINAL ABORTION. Criminal abortion is the termination of pregnancy without medical and legal justification. Since these operations always are performed surreptitiously, accurate figures concerning their frequency are difficult to secure, but the very minimum estimate is 100,000 annually in the United States, whereas some authorities put the figure at over half a million a year. This means that each year in this country between 100,000 and 500,000 potential lives are destroyed simply for "convenience," a frightful wastage of human life and a sorry reflection on our civilization. Quite apart from this destruction of fetal life, criminal abortion is one of the most common causes of maternal death. No reputable physician will induce an abortion without medical justification. Consequently, these clandestine operations usually are performed by hands which are not only unskilled but unclean. Fatal infections are common. Of those who survive many are left invalids, others permanently sterile. Most cases of so-called "infected abortion" are of this origin.

Every year huge quantities of castor oil, quinine and other "powerful" drugs are bought for the express purpose of interrupting early pregnancy. As a rule, these concoctions merely produce nausea and vomiting, while the pregnancy is not interrupted. However, certain of the patent medicines used for this purpose contain ingredients which act with such violence that hemorrhages into the bowel and the kidneys sometimes ensue, with results that may be exceedingly grave. The reputation of these drugs rests on the circumstance that the menstrual interval in the same woman often varies widely; a woman who has been accustomed to menstruate every 28 days may occasionally experience a 35-day cycle without apparent cause or detriment to health. If, in such a long cycle, when she thinks herself 5 or 6 days "overdue," she takes one of these medicines and starts menstruating the next day, naturally the drug is acclaimed as the benefactor. It is obvious that the same end would have been attained had she done nothing. At the present writing there is no drug known to the medical profession which will produce abortion in the human being, whether given by mouth or hypodermically.

Clinical Picture. About 75 per cent of all spontaneous abortions occur during the 2nd and the 3rd months of pregnancy, that is, before the 12th week. The condition is very common; it is estimated that about 1 pregnancy in every 10 terminates in spontaneous abortion. Almost invariably the first symptom is bleeding due to the separation of the fertilized ovum from its uterine attachment. The bleeding is often slight at the beginning and

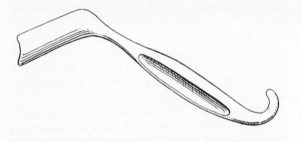

Fig. 18-4. Sims's speculum for inserting into the vaginal canal so as to expose the cervix to view.

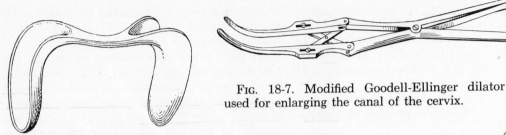

Fig. 18-7. Modified Goodell-Ellinger dilator used for enlarging the canal of the cervix.

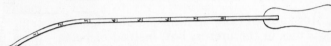

Fig. 18-8. Uterine sound.

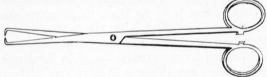

Fig. 18-5. Schroeder vaginal retractor for drawing back the vulvar or vaginal walls during an operation.

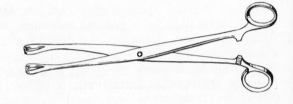

Fig. 18-9. Placental forceps with heart-shaped jaws.

Fig. 18-6. Bullet forceps used in grasping the lips of the cervix.

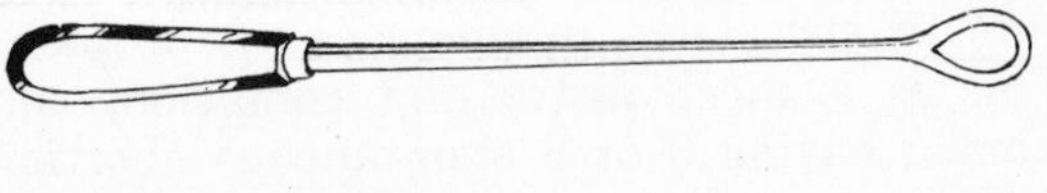

Fig. 18-10. Sims's sharp curette, a scraper or spoonlike instrument for removing matter from the walls of the uterus.

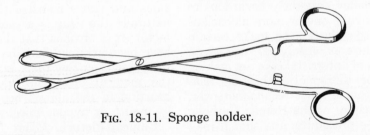

Fig. 18-11. Sponge holder.

may persist for days before uterine cramps occur; or, the bleeding may be followed at once by cramps. Occasionally the bleeding is torrential in nature, leaving the patient in shock. The uterine contractions bring about softening and dilatation of the cervix and expel the products of conception either completely or incompletely.

Causes. What causes all these spontaneous abortions—so tragic and shattering to so many women? If the evidence is reviewed with some perspective and with full fairness to all concerned, it is the inevitable conclusion that most of these abortions, far from being tragedies, are blessings in disguise, for they are Nature's beneficent way of extinguishing em-

FIG. 18-12. Hegar dilators, of graduated diameters from 5 to 12 mm. Larger sizes also are used.

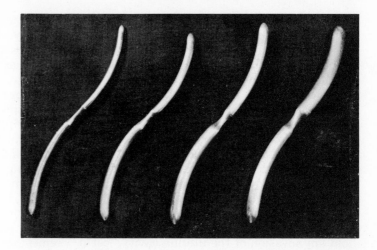

bryos which are imperfect. Indeed, careful microscopic study of the material passed in these cases shows that the commonest cause of spontaneous abortion is an inherent defect in the product of conception. This defect may express itself in an abnormal embryo, in an abnormal *trophoblast* (p. 75) or in both abnormalities. In early abortions, 80 per cent are associated with some defect of the embryo or trophoblast which is either incompatible with life or would result in a grossly deformed child. The incidence of abnormalities passed after the 2nd month is somewhat lower but not less than 50 per cent. Whether the germ plasm of the spermatozoon or the ovum is at fault in these cases, it is usually difficult, if not impossible, to say. Abortions of this sort are obviously unpreventable and, although bitterly disappointing to the parents, serve a useful purpose.

Spontaneous abortions may be due to causes other than defects in the product of conception. Severe acute infections, such as pneumonia, pyelitis and typhoid fever, often lead to abortion. Heart failure is another etiologic factor. Occasionally, abnormalities of the generative tract, such as a congenitally short cervix, produce the accident. Retroposition of the uterus rarely causes abortion, as was formerly believed. Many women tend to explain miscarriage on the grounds of injury of one type or another, or excessive activity. Different women exhibit the greatest variation in this respect. In some the pregnancy may go blithely on despite falls from second-story windows and automobile accidents so severe as to fracture the pelvis. In others a trivial fall or merely overfatigue seems to contribute at least to abortion. Since there is no way of telling who is susceptible and who is not it would seem prudent for every expectant mother to follow the dictates of common sense and avoid long automobile trips, lifting heavy weights and any form of activity which involves jolting.

Treatment. The severity of the symptoms manifested in threatened abortion will determine the treatment prescribed. If the patient is having only a slight vaginal bleeding or even spotting, without pain, she should be advised to stay in bed, eat a light well-balanced diet, avoid straining at bowel evacuation and the use of cathartics. If she appears to be apprehensive, a mild sedative may be given. She should be further advised to save all perineal pads, as well as all tissue and clots passed, for the physician's inspection. If the bleeding disappears within 48 hours, she may get out of bed but should limit her activities for the next several days. Stair climbing should be avoided for the first 24 hours and then resumed gradually. Coitus should be avoided for 2 weeks following the last evidence of bleeding. In cases in which pain accompanies the vaginal bleeding, the prognosis for saving the pregnancy is poor. Usually bleeding is observed first, and then in a few hours, sometimes days later, uterine contractions ensue. This is treated by absolute bed rest, narcotic drugs (paregoric, morphine, etc.) and some preparations of progesterone (see Chap. 3). When the pain and the bleeding increase, the patient should be hospitalized, if this has not already been done. If the abortion is incomplete, ordinarily efforts are made to aid the uterus in emptying its contents. Oxytocin may be administered, but if this is ineffectual, surgical removal of the retained products of conception should be done promptly, provided that the patient is afebrile and no other evidence of infection exists. Active bleeding may make this urgently necessary. Many times the tissue lies loose in the cervical canal and can be simply lifted out with ovum forceps; otherwise, curettage of the uterine cavity must be done. The instruments commonly used in completing an incomplete abortion are shown in Figures 18-4 to 12. If evidence of infection is present (fever, foul discharge or suspicious history of criminal abortion), the physician may prefer to withhold any invasion of the uterine cavity, lest it disseminate bacteria into the venous sinuses of the uterus and thence into the general circulation. Although the use of antibiotics has greatly reduced this hazard, it has not eliminated it entirely. On the other hand, bleeding and certain other circumstances may make removal of the uterine contents desirable despite the presence of infection. Complete abortion requires exactly the same care as that given during the postpartal period. As already indicated, habitual abortion may be helped by endocrine therapy as well as by meticulous attention to general hygiene, rest, vitamin requirements, etc.

Nurse's Responsibilities in Abortion Cases. Bleeding in the first half of pregnancy, no matter how slight, always must be considered as threatened abortion. The patient must be put to bed and the physician notified. An episode of this nature is indeed distressing to the expectant mother, many times alarming. The nurse should bear in mind that although the emotional support she gives her patient is important, she must never try to reassure her that "everything will be all right," because in fact the patient may lose this pregnancy. Perineal pads and all tissue and blood clots passed by the patient should be saved. The physician will wish to examine these to determine the amount of bleeding and, when tissue has been passed, to examine the products of conception to ascertain, among other facts, whether or not the abortion is complete. If bleeding is so copious as to be alarming, elevate the foot of the bed (shock position) while awaiting the physician's arrival. If surgical completion of the abortion is to be carried out, the same aseptic regimen is carried out as for delivery.

All cases of criminal abortion must be regarded as potentially infected, and strict antiseptic precautions must be carried out to prevent spread of infection to others. In regard to criminal abortion, the nurse can have only one attitude, to regard it as the murder of a potential human being and also as a procedure which kills thousands of mothers each year. In caring for a woman who has had a criminal abortion recently, or one whose history is suspicious, the nurse may find it difficult to handle her own feelings so that she does not reflect a judgmental attitude. It is helpful to remember that it is not within the province of the nurse to pass moral judgments as she gives nursing care. In such situations the nurse should direct her concern to the gravity of the patient's illness. Occasionally circumstances make it possible for the nurse to be of definite educational help on the question of the criminal abortion, both to her patients and to the public.

Incompetent Cervical Os

Recently, a mechanical defect in the cervix, incompetent cervical os, has gained recognition as a cause of late habitual abortion or premature labor. When repeated termination of pregnancy in the second trimester is due to an anatomic factor such as this, surgical treatment may make fetal salvage possible. One of the various treatments used to prevent relaxation and dilatation of the cervix when it is incompetent to carry on a "good" pregnancy is the modified Shirodkar technic.[2] In this, the vaginal mucous membrane is elevated and a narrow strip of some material such as Mersilene is carried around the internal os of the cervix and tied. Then the vaginal mucosa is restored to its original position and sutured.

The patient is kept in bed for the first several days postoperatively, often in Trendelenburg position initially, to prevent undue pressure on the cervix. The patient should be watched closely for signs of bleeding or labor. Demerol and Phenergan may be prescribed

[2] Durfee, R. B.: Surgical treatment of the incompetent cervix during pregnancy, Obstet. Gynec. 12:91, 1958.

Fig. 18-13. (a) Tubal abortion, showing passage of the products of conception, together with much blood, out the fimbriated end of the tube. (b) Rupture of tubal pregnancy into peritoneal cavity. There is an outpouring of blood into the abdomen from vessels at the site of the rupture.

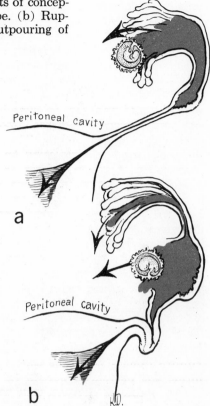

routinely for the first day, not necessarily for pain, but to keep the uterus quiet. Actually, these patients experience relatively little discomfort and usually feel quite well in a day or so. At the time of discharge, about the 5th postoperative day, the physician generally advises certain restrictions about coitus and the patient's daily activities. He frequently recommends at least one rest period in the horizontal position during the day. By and large, the expectant mother may resume a "normal" life during the rest of her pregnancy.

The nonabsorbable band is left in place until the patient is ready for labor. Then she may be delivered either by elective cesarean section or vaginal delivery. If the latter is the choice, the band must be cut and removed. Definitive cervical repair is done at a later date.

Ectopic Pregnancy

An ectopic pregnancy is any gestation located outside the uterine cavity. The majority of ectopic pregnancies are tubal gestations. Other types, which make up about 5 per cent of all ectopic pregnancies, are: interstitial (in the interstitial portion of the tube), cornual (in a rudimentary horn of a uterus), cervical, abdominal and ovarian gestations. About once in every 300 pregnancies the fertilized ovum, instead of traversing the length of the fallopian tube to reach the uterine cavity, becomes implanted within the wall of the fallopian tube. This condition is known as "ectopic pregnancy" (literally, a pregnancy which is out of place) or as "tubal pregnancy" or "extra-uterine pregnancy." Since the wall of the tube is not sufficiently elastic to allow the fertilized ovum to grow and develop there, rupture of the tubal wall is the inevitable result. Rupture most frequently occurs into the tubal lumen with the passage of the products of conception, together with much blood, out the fimbriated end of the tube and into the peritoneal cavity—so-called "tubal abortion." Or, rupture may occur through the peritoneal surface of the tube directly into the peritoneal cavity; and, again, there is an outpouring of blood into the abdomen from vessels at the site of rupture (Fig. 18-13). In either case, rupture usually occurs within the first 12 weeks.

Occasionally an ectopic pregnancy may develop in that portion of the tube which passes through the uterine wall, a type known as "interstitial pregnancy." In very, very rare instances, the product of conception, after rupturing through the tubal wall, may implant itself on the peritoneum and develop to full term in the peritoneal cavity. This extraordinary occurrence is known as "abdominal pregnancy." Surprisingly enough, quite a few living infants have been delivered in such cases by means of abdominal incision.

Ectopic pregnancy may be due to any condition which narrows the tube or brings about some constriction within it. Under such circumstances the tubal lumen is large enough to allow spermatozoa to ascend the tube but

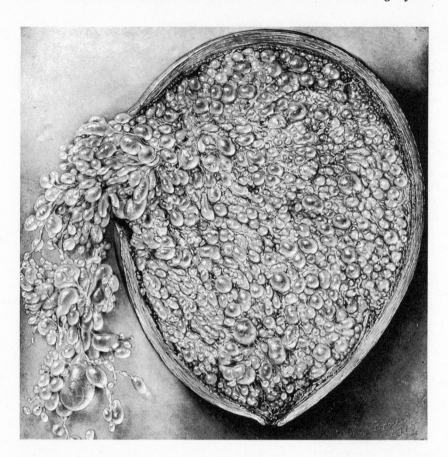

Fig. 18-14. Hydatidiform mole × ½. (Eastman, N. J.: Williams' Obstetrics, New York, Appleton)

not big enough to permit the downward passage of the fertilized ovum. Among the conditions which may produce such a narrowing of the fallopian tube are: previous inflammatory processes involving the tubal mucosa and producing partial agglutination of opposing surfaces, such as gonorrheal salpingitis; previous inflammatory processes of the external peritoneal surfaces of the tube, causing kinking, such as puerperal and postabortal infections; and developmental defects resulting in a general narrowing of the tubes.

In cases of ectopic gestation the woman exhibits the usual early symptoms of pregnancy and, as a rule, regards herself as being normally pregnant. After missing one or two periods, however, she suddenly experiences pain which is knifelike in nature and often of extreme severity in one of the lower quadrants. This is usually associated with very slight vaginal bleeding, commonly referred to as "spotting." Depending on the amount of blood which has escaped into the peritoneal cavity,

she may or may not undergo a fainting attack and show symptoms of shock.

Ectopic pregnancy is a grave complication of pregnancy and is an important cause of maternal death. Moreover, if a woman has had one ectopic pregnancy and subsequently becomes pregnant, she is more likely than in the case of the average woman to have another such accident.

In the vast majority of cases the tube has already ruptured, and the fetus is dead when the patient is first seen by the physician. It is indeed the rupture which produces the acute clinical picture. The treatment is removal of the tube, supplemented by blood transfusion.

During the transportation of such a patient to the hospital or in the interval when the patient is awaiting operation, the nurse can be of immeasurable assistance in combating the shock that is frequently present. Elevation of the foot of the bed and maintenance of body heat by means of hot-water bottles and blankets may help to save the patient's life.

Fig. 18-15. The 3 types of placenta previa, showing position of the placenta in relation to the internal os (B, C and D) contrasted with normal placental insertion (A). (*Below,* b, c and d) On vaginal examination the placenta can be felt during effacement and dilatation of the cervix in low implantation, partial and complete placenta previa.

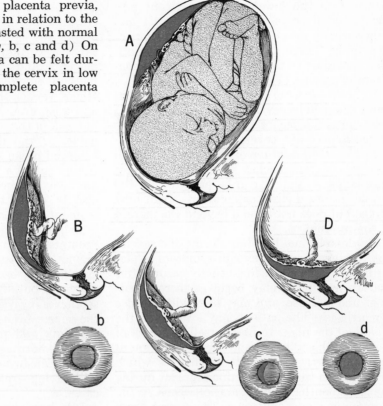

Hydatidiform Mole

Hydatidiform mole is a benign neoplasm of the chorion in which the chorionic villi degenerate and become transparent vesicles containing clear, viscid fluid. The vesicles have a grapelike appearance and are arranged in clusters involving all or part of the decidual lining of the uterus (Fig. 18-14). Although there is usually no embryo present, occasionally there may be a fetus* and only part of the placenta involved. Hydatidiform mole is rather an uncommon condition, occurring about once in every 2,000 pregnancies. The pregnancy appears to be normal at first. Then bleeding, a usual symptom varying from spotting to that of a profuse degree, occurs, so that one might suspect threatened abortion. If the patient does not abort, the uterus enlarges rapidly, and profuse hemorrhage may occur, at which time these vesicles may be evident in the vaginal discharge. Vomiting in

* See Moral Considerations, p. 455.

rather severe form may appear early. Severe preeclampsia, a complication which does not usually occur until the later months of pregnancy, may appear early in the second trimester. The treatment consists in emptying the uterus by dilating the cervix and carefully extracting the uterine contents. There is always great danger of injury to the uterine wall, which is weakened and of spongy consistency due to the growth of the mole. Some physicians advise hysterectomy. The follow-up care is very important because, although this is a benign process, extremely malignant chorioncarcinoma (formerly called chorionepithelioma) sometimes further complicates the picture.

Placenta Previa

Although abortion is the most frequent cause of bleeding early in pregnancy, the most common cause during the later months is placenta previa. In this condition the placenta is attached to the lower uterine segment (instead of high up in the uterus as usual) and either wholly or in part covers the region of the cervix. There are three types, differentiated according to the degree to which the condition is present (Fig. 18-15):

1. *Total placenta previa*, in which the placenta completely covers the internal os

2. *Partial placenta previa*, in which the placenta partially covers the internal os

3. *Low implantation of placenta*, in which the placenta encroaches upon the region of internal os, so that it can be palpated by the physician on digital exploration about the cervix, but does not extend beyond the margin of the internal os.

Painless vaginal bleeding during the second half of pregnancy is the main symptom of placenta previa. The bleeding usually occurs after the 7th month. It may begin as mere "spotting" and increase, or it may start with profuse hemorrhages. The patient may awaken in the middle of the night to find herself in a pool of blood. The bleeding is caused by separation of the placenta as the result of changes which take place in the lower uterine segment during the later months. This separation opens up the underlying blood sinuses of the uterus from which the bleeding occurs.

Fortunately, placenta previa is not a very common condition, occurring about once in every 200 deliveries. It occurs much more frequently in multiparae than in primigravidae. Placenta previa always must be regarded as a grave complication of pregnancy. Until recent years it showed a maternal mortality of approximately 10 per cent. Modern methods of management, plus the more liberal use of blood transfusion, have reduced this figure considerably. The outlook for the baby is always dubious, not only because the placental separation interferes with the infant's oxygen supply, but also because many of these babies are very premature when delivery must necessarily take place.

Treatment. There are two main forms of treatment: (1) pressure therapy exerted *per vaginum* and (2) cesarean section. The principle underlying the first of these is to compress the bleeding sinuses by exerting pressure on them and the overlying placenta. Depending on the nature of the case, the physician may choose to do this in one of several ways.

The method most frequently used at the present time is rupture of the membranes, which allows the head to gravitate downward and exert a certain amount of pressure on the placenta and the lower uterine segment. A method employed in the past was Braxton Hicks' version, by which the fetus was turned and a leg brought down so that a thigh and a buttock of the fetus compressed the lower segment, or the desired pressure therapy was achieved by an application of Willett's forceps to the infant's scalp with traction. Pressure methods of checking hemorrhage may serve also to dilate the cervix and to hasten the moment when delivery can be effected.

In present-day obstetric practice, however, "compression methods" of treating placenta previa (such as those described above) are losing favor, because cesarean section is usually safer both for mother and child. Cesarean section is invariably the treatment of choice in the severe forms of the complication, such as complete and partial placenta previa. As in other hemorrhagic complications of pregnancy, blood transfusion plays an important—often a lifesaving—role in the management of these cases.

Bleeding, shock and infection are the main dangers. Before the arrival of the physician, the nurse should keep a solicitous eye on the amount of bleeding and the pulse rate and watch for signs of oncoming shock (pallor, increased pulse rate, cold extremities, etc.). Should the bleeding be profuse, elevation of the foot of the bed and application of external heat may forestall shock. In determining the amount of bleeding, the patient should be instructed to report feeling the escape of fluid from the vulva. The nurse, in turn, should inspect the pad or bed frequently for hemorrhage.

One of the important facts about placenta previa to keep in mind is that a vaginal or a rectal examination may precipitate severe hemorrhage. Therefore, any patient who bleeds to any extent greater than "show" during the last half of pregnancy should never have a digital examination, either rectal or vaginal, at home. She should be sent to the hospital promptly, where everything is available for the immediate carrying out of any procedure that may be necessary for treatment. In the hospital, digital examination is performed only in the operating room, and then only after complete preparations are in readiness for carrying out abdominal and vaginal surgery as well as blood transfusion. This is usually referred to as the "double setup" (i.e., a setup for both vaginal and abdominal delivery).

Patients with placenta previa may later develop puerperal infection. This is understandable when one recalls that the open venous sinuses low down about the cervix are particularly accessible to infection and toxic conditions from any bacteria which might have been introduced into the vagina. Hemorrhage, moreover, lowers the patient's resistance to infection. It is essential, therefore, that meticulous attention be given to antiseptic and aseptic precautions in the handling of these cases.

Abruptio Placentae

Abruptio placentae (meaning that the placenta is torn from its bed) is a complication of the last half of pregnancy, in which a normally located placenta undergoes separation from its uterine attachment. The condition is frequently referred to as "premature separation of the normally implanted placenta"; other synonymous terms such as "accidental hemorrhage" (meaning that it takes place unexpectedly) and "ablatio placentae" (ablatio means a carrying away) are sometimes used. Bleeding may be apparent, in which case it is called *external hemorrhage*; or bleeding may be concealed, in which case it is called *concealed hemorrhage*. In other words, if a separation occurs at the margin, the blood is apt to lift the membranes and trickle down to the cervical os and thus escape externally. If the placenta begins to separate centrally, a huge amount of blood may be stored behind the placenta before any of it becomes evident (Fig. 18-16). Although the precise cause of the condition is not known, it is frequently encountered in association with cases of toxemia of pregnancy.

Premature separation of the normally implanted placenta is characterized not only by bleeding beneath the placenta but also by pain. The pain is produced by the accumulation of blood behind the placenta, with subsequent distention of the uterus. The uterus also enlarges in size as the result of the accumu-lated blood and becomes distinctly tender and exceedingly firm. Because of the almost woody hardness of the uterine wall, fetal parts may be difficult to determine. Shock is often out of proportion to blood loss, as manifested by a rapid pulse, dyspnea, yawning, restlessness, pallor, syncope and cold, clammy perspiration.

Clear-cut examples of this complication occur much less frequently than placenta previa and are uncommon.

Treatment consists either in cesarean section or in rupturing the membranes; but whatever course is indicated, the immense gravity of the situation demands the organized teamwork of physicians, nurses and laboratory technicians. Transcending all else in importance is therapy of the shock, which is almost invariably present. Where blood loss has been substantial, it should be replaced before proceeding with abdominal delivery. In less severe cases artificial rupture of membranes, when instituted promptly, may initiate labor, and vaginal delivery may be accomplished before the extent of detachment increases and the bleeding becomes more extensive.

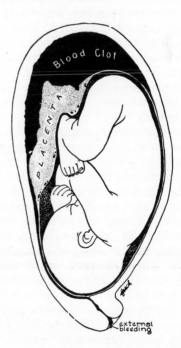

FIG. 18-16. Abruptio placentae with large blood clot between placenta and uterine wall.

Further Complications. In more severe cases a further complication may be encountered because of extravasation of blood into the uterine musculature and beneath the uterine peritoneum, so-called *"uteroplacental apoplexy"* or *"Couvelaire uterus."* Here the uterus remains flaccid, and, after either vaginal delivery or cesarean section, bleeding may be so profuse as to indicate prompt hysterectomy.

Another hemorrhagic complication which may follow in severe cases of abruptio is due to a deficiency in the fibrinogen level of the blood, so-called hypofibrinogenemia. It is well to remember that hypofibrinogenemia may be due to other complications, such as amniotic fluid embolism, missed abortion (after the 5th to 6th week) and septic abortion. The nurse should be aware of the possibility of this additional complication, particularly when the patient continues to bleed following delivery. The usual measures to stimulate uterine contractions prove to be of no avail, and even if hysterectomy has been performed, evidence of steady bleeding from the vagina continues. Needless to say, this must be reported promptly so that corrective measures may be begun immediately, in this case to restore the fibrinogen level of the blood. This could be accomplished eventually by blood transfusions but would require such a massive volume of blood that it would not be feasible in severe cases, whereas the administration of fibrinogen injected intravenously can promptly restore the deficiency.

Hemorrhage and/or trauma in labor must always be considered as predisposing factors to puerperal infection, and so the nurse must guard against infection and be alert for any symptoms. In many cases antibiotic therapy may be used as a prophylactic measure.

Outcome. Although abruptio placentae constitutes one of the gravest accidents which can befall a pregnant woman, the maternal mortality rate has been markedly reduced as a result of more intelligent management. The outcome for the infant depends to a great extent on the severity of the process. In the milder cases the infant may be born alive, but it is often born prematurely; in severe cases almost all infants die.

Mistaken Diagnosis of Hemorrhage

A false alarm concerning hemorrhage is sometimes due to a normal "show" at the beginning of labor. It simply means that dilatation of the cervix has begun, causing slight bleeding. No treatment is required. However, the nurse should reassure the patient and watch to determine whether or not the bleeding which is present is more than the normal show.

"Supine Hypotensive Syndrome"

Many pregnant women, if placed in the supine position in the last trimester, suffer a fall in blood pressure. In some of these women the drop is so great as to simulate shock due to blood loss. The chief cause of supine hypotensive syndrome is failure of venous return of blood from the legs and the pelvis as a result of the compression exerted by the enlarged uterus on the inferior vena cava. The condition can be corrected promptly by having the patient lie on her side rather than on her back.

BLOOD GROUPS AND THE RH FACTOR

Blood Groups

Following the discovery in 1900-1901 that certain antigens exist in human red blood cells, it became possible to divide all human blood into 4 main types or groups, now called A, B, AB and O, on the basis of the antigen or antigens within the erythrocytes. It was observed that the red blood cells of certain individuals became clumped (agglutinated) or dissolved (hemolyzed) when they were transfused into certain other individuals; thus no advantage was derived from the transfusion, and, moreover, injurious or toxic effects were induced due to the reaction of incompatible substances. In general,* an O person's blood may be given with safety to any one of the other 3 types (in the case of A-B-O genes, A and B are dominant over O). Therefore, O individuals are often called "universal donors." However, an O individual is least able to receive blood from the other 3 types; if transfusion is necessary, he should be given O blood. Any person of the other 3 blood types may be transfused with O type blood, but he is prefer-

* Important exceptions in O and other persons are concerned with the Rh situation, discussed later in this section.

ably transfused with blood of his own type, that is, A with A type, B with B type and AB with AB type. Thousands of tests show that about 40 per cent of our population are O type and about 40 per cent are A type.

These blood groups are not related to racial differences. All 4 types have been reported in all known nationalities, though they differ in proportions. In the United States the average for the white race is roughly 45 per cent O and 40 per cent A, but in the American Indians about 75 per cent are of O type and 25 per cent the A type.

It was once thought that blood from one member of a family would be compatible with that of any other member, but blood types may differ greatly within a given family. It is possible for a child born to an O and an AB parent to have A or B blood. For infant transfusion, the infant's blood should be cross-matched with that of the mother's blood type. At the time of delivery the infant cannot as yet produce antibodies.

The Rh Factor

Even carefully matched blood, e.g., A to A, or universal O to one of the other 3 types, has not always been free from undesirable effects. It is now known that there are several other antigens within erythrocytes, in addition to the 4 (A, B, AB and O) which resulted in the division of human blood into 4 major types. The most important of the recently discovered antigens is the Rh substance or factor. Its name is derived from the first two letters of the scientific term for the rhesus monkey, which always has the factor present in its blood. A person's Rh type depends on the presence or absence of the Rh antigen within the red blood cells. The Rh factor is an hereditary characteristic, transmitted according to the principles set forth in Mendel's law. About 85 per cent of our white population and slightly more of our Negro population are Rh positive. Therefore, such persons are said to be Rh positive (Rh+); persons lacking the Rh factor are called Rh negative (Rh−).*

When the blood of an Rh-positive person is introduced, through blood transfusion or otherwise, into the blood stream of an Rh-nega-

* Only about 7 per cent of Negroes and about 1 per cent of Chinese are Rh negative.

tive individual, the latter develops antibodies against the Rh factor present in the blood administered. Antibodies are substances which the body manufactures as a protective mechanism to counteract the effect of various kinds of new materials which may be introduced into the blood and the tissues. For instance, when bacteria gain access to the blood stream, antibodies against that particular kind of bacteria are usually developed and, sooner or later, destroy the bacteria. Accordingly, antibodies may be regarded as a sort of defensive army which the blood and the tissues muster against foreign invading forces. It is these antibodies which cure most infectious diseases, from the common cold to typhoid fever. Moreover, they often remain present in the blood and the tissues long after the disease has been combated successfully, making the person immune to that particular type of infection; in other words, should the same bacterium or material which incited the original manufacture of the antibodies be introduced again into the body, these defensive substances now stand ready to attack and destroy it.

Rh and Transfusions. As stated above, when an Rh-negative person is given a blood transfusion from an Rh-positive donor, antibodies are developed by the recipient against the Rh substance present in the administered blood. But, as is true when bacteria invade the body, these antibodies against the Rh factor do not form instantaneously but only after a period of time. Consequently, with the first transfusion, nothing out of the ordinary occurs. However, should this Rh-negative recipient receive at some later date another transfusion from an Rh-positive donor, antibodies probably will have been developed, and these will immediately attack the Rh factor. Since the Rh substance is an integral part of the red blood cells, this conflict causes a violent reaction in the blood stream with the destruction of many red cells. As the broken-down products of these fragmented red cells are disseminated throughout the body, they exert a poisonous effect, and, as a result, the recipient of the blood transfusion suffers a reaction usually manifested by a chill and fever but sometimes by more grave symptoms. In World War II, when many Rh-negative soldiers had to be given repeated blood transfusions, this Rh problem was a serious one. It was met by using Rh-negative donors for transfusions of

Rh-negative persons—in other words, by administering blood without any Rh factor in it to cause the trouble described above. Nowadays physicians and surgeons everywhere are careful to determine the Rh status of any prospective recipient of a blood transfusion; if it is negative, blood from an Rh-negative donor is employed.

Iso-immunization. Since it has been a rule for a long time that Rh-negative persons should never be transfused with Rh-positive blood, the number of expectant mothers who have developed Rh antibodies as the result of previous blood transfusions is becoming less and less. Today the main Rh problem is the formation of Rh antibodies as the result of the passage of Rh-positive fetal red cells across the placenta and into the blood of an Rh-negative woman. It is well-established that small numbers of fetal red cells do continually pass into the maternal circulation throughout the greater part of pregnancy. The process is tantamount to repeated minute transfusions. It is very clearly illustrated in Figure 18-17, which should be studied with care. When Rh antibodies are produced in this way, the process is known as *iso-immunization*.

Rh Differences in Mates. Since at least six sevenths of all persons, male or female, are Rh positive, Rh incompatibility is not as frequent as one might at first suppose. Even when an Rh-positive male parent mates with an Rh-negative female, there may be no erythroblastosis in the offspring, for the father may be *heterozygous* for Rh (has both Rh-positive and Rh-negative genes), and no difficulty occurs if the fetus has Rh-negative inheritance from both parents. The danger is much greater when the father is *homozygous* (has all Rh-positive genes), for the fetus will inherit the Rh-positive factor against which the mother produces antibodies, and these antibodies (as in the transfusion of incompatible Rh-positive blood to Rh-negative mothers) may lead to the destruction of the Rh-positive blood cells of the fetus. The danger to the fetus is increased with the ability of the mother's antibodies to pass through the placenta (Fig. 18-17).

In Rh differences in mates, as well as in blood transfusions, the reactions of the Rh-negative mother are slow, and 1 or even 2 normal births may occur before the mother has an infant with erythroblastosis. Once it occurs, all later pregnancies are risky, and future pregnancies may be contraindicated, because there is a substantial chance for the condition to recur in subsequent pregnancies.

Rh-Negative Pregnant Women. The present fund of knowledge concerning the Rh factor and erythroblastosis fetalis makes certain routines in antepartal management and care essential. Every pregnant woman should have her Rh type determined early in pregnancy. If the mother is Rh negative, it should be ascertained whether she has had previous blood transfusions, and the father's Rh type should be determined. If he also is found to be Rh negative, there will be no danger of hemolytic disease affecting this fetus, or subsequent ones, because the offspring will be Rh negative. In case the father is Rh positive, it should be determined whether he is homozygous or heterozygous for Rh. The Rh-negative mother's blood should be checked by laboratory tests several times during the first two trimesters of pregnancy to see whether her antibody titer is increasing, an indication of harmful reactions against Rh-positive factors. Only after the 34th week of gestation is it necessary to do this every 2 weeks. At the present time the Coombs' test is the one most frequently employed because it indicates the presence or the absence of Rh antibodies in the red blood cells. Moreover, it is considered to be the most sensitive test for the detection of Rh antibodies. With such checks, mating between an Rh-positive man and an Rh-negative woman may be perfectly safe, unless earlier Rh-positive blood transfusions complicate the situation. Even then, some degree of control is possible.

The nurse should bear in mind that when an Rh-negative woman's husband is Rh positive, this mother is often apprehensive about the outcome of her pregnancy. These patients must not be given any false hopes, but it is relatively safe to assume that when there is no serologic evidence to indicate sensitization, the prospects for normal childbearing for her are no different from those of an Rh-positive mother. However, this is not the case if the mother is sensitized, for then the outlook depends entirely on the severity of the manifestation in the individual.

As already indicated, certain cases of erythroblastosis fetalis may be prevented by proper investigation of the Rh type of women patients and any donors from whom they receive blood. During pregnancy, if the mother's antibody titer increases markedly, there is an additional problem in that the infant may be delivered prematurely by either induced labor or cesarean section. In such instances, a supply of

Rh-negative blood should be available for treating the infant, if born alive.

HYPEREMESIS GRAVIDARUM

A mild degree of nausea and vomiting, "morning sickness," is the most common com-

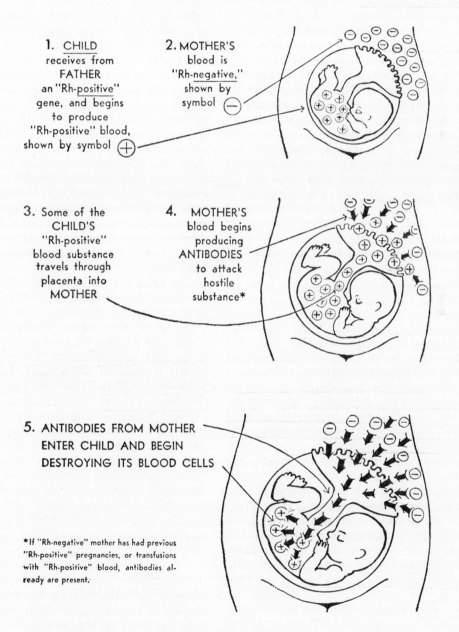

1. CHILD receives from FATHER an "Rh-positive" gene, and begins to produce "Rh-positive" blood, shown by symbol ⊕

2. MOTHER'S blood is "Rh-negative," shown by symbol ⊖

3. Some of the CHILD'S "Rh-positive" blood substance travels through placenta into MOTHER

4. MOTHER'S blood begins producing ANTIBODIES to attack hostile substance*

5. ANTIBODIES FROM MOTHER ENTER CHILD AND BEGIN DESTROYING ITS BLOOD CELLS

*If "Rh-negative" mother has had previous "Rh-positive" pregnancies, or transfusions with "Rh-positive" blood, antibodies already are present.

FIG. 18-17. Effect of the Rh factor. (Scheinfeld, Amran: The New You and Heredity, Philadelphia, Lippincott)

plaint of women in the first trimester of pregnancy. This manifestation is considered in the realm of a minor discomfort rather than a complication, and it usually responds to measures discussed in Chapter 8. It is uncommon today for this mild form of nausea and vomiting to progress to such serious extent that it produces systemic effects, i.e., marked loss of weight and acetonuria; but when it becomes thus exaggerated, the condition is known as hyperemesis gravidarum, sometimes called "pernicious vomiting." Because even the gravest case of hyperemesis starts originally as a simple form of nausea, all cases of nausea and vomiting should be treated with proper understanding and judgment, and none should be regarded casually. When simple remedies do not prove to be effective, and symptoms of hyperemesis appear to be imminent, the patient should be hospitalized for more intensive treatment. At the present time less than 1 pregnant woman in 300 has to be admitted to the hospital because of this complication of pregnancy, and, indeed, the grave cases of hyperemesis gravidarum are becoming rare. The recovery of those who are admitted to the hospital is usually rapid.

Cause

It is currently recognized that during pregnancy there are certain organic processes which are basic to all cases of vomiting, regardless of whether the symptoms are mild or severe. The endocrine and metabolic changes of normal gestation, fragments of chorionic villi entering the maternal circulation and the diminished motility of the stomach might well give rise to clinical symptoms.

It has long been thought that hyperemesis gravidarum is in large measure a *neurosis*. The term "neurosis," it will be recalled, is employed very loosely to designate a large array of conditions in which symptoms occur without demonstrable pathologic explanation, the symptoms being due, it is thought, to a functional disturbance of the patient's psyche. Some psychiatrists estimate that 40 per cent of patients who visit physicians belong in this neurotic class. As many examples show (quite apart from pregnancy), nausea is often psychic in origin. For instance, a repellent sight, an obnoxious odor or the mere recollection of such a sight or odor may give rise to nausea and even vomiting. Our general use of the adjective "nauseating" to depict a repulsive object is further acknowledgment that an upset mind may produce an upset stomach.

In all life's encounters there are probably few experiences which are at first more upsetting, mentally and emotionally, than the realization by a young woman that she is pregnant. At the onset are several weeks of anxious uncertainty before she can be sure of the diagnosis. Then, numerous adjustments must be made and plans changed. Emotionally, the implications of pregnancy extend far back into the past when she first met her husband, while its future ramifications are endless. The responsibilities entailed are plain enough, also, and seem, on first thought, perhaps more than can be assumed. These and a thousand other thoughts crowd themselves into the mind; and in women who cannot adjust themselves to all these new circumstances, it is understandable that the groundwork for an neurosis is laid. Beyond question, there is a large neurotic element in most cases of hyperemesis, a factor which looms large in the treatment of the condition.

The neurotic factor, on the other hand, is not the whole cause of hyperemesis, nor in all probability even the basic cause. As has been stated previously, in every case an important underlying organic process is also at work—either the dissemination of toxins into the maternal blood stream or some maladjustment of the metabolism to the changes wrought by the growing fetus. It is this toxic or organic element which is doubtless the fundamental cause of the disease. To what extent the patient reacts to this underlying process by vomiting seems to be determined in large measure by neurotic factors, that is, by her psychic and emotional stability and by the mental stress and strain which pregnancy has imposed.

Clinical Picture

The clinical picture of the patient suffering from pernicious vomiting varies in relation to the severity and the duration of the condition. In any event, the condition begins with a typical picture of "morning sickness." The patient experiences a feeling of nausea on arising in the morning, she may even be unable to retain her breakfast, but she recovers in a few hours and has no further episodes until the next morning. With the majority of these patients this pattern persists for a few weeks and then suddenly ceases.

A small number of patients who have "morning sickness" develop persistent vomiting which lasts for 4 to 8 weeks or longer. These patients vomit several times a day and may be unable to retain any liquid or solid foods, with the result that marked symptoms of dehydration and starvation occur. *Dehydration* is pronounced, as evidenced by a diminished output of urine and a dryness of the skin. In some instances slight jaundice may develop. Further results of dehydration may be observed in the patient's vital signs. The pulse is usually accelerated, often to 130 or over, and a low-grade fever may be present. The temperature seldom rises above 101° F. (38.4° C.), but it may persist despite therapy to combat dehydration.

Starvation, which is regularly present, manifests itself in a number of ways. Weight loss may vary from 5 pounds to as much as 20 or 30 pounds. This is tantamount to saying that the digestion and the absorption of carbohydrates and other nutrients has been so inadequate that the body has been forced to burn its reserve stores of fat in order to maintain body heat and energy. When fat is burned without carbohydrates being present, the process of combustion does not go on to completion. Consequently, certain incompletely burned products of fat metabolism make their appearance in the blood and in the urine. The presence of acetone and diacetic acid in the urine in hyperemesis is common. In severe cases considerable changes associated with starvation and dehydration become evident in the blood chemistry. There is a definite increase in the nonprotein nitrogen, uric acid and urea, a moderate decrease in the chlorides and little alteration in the carbon dioxide combining power. Then, too, vitamin starvation is regularly present, and in extreme cases, when marked vitamin B deficiency exists, polyneuritis occasionally develops, and disturbances of the peripheral nerves result.

The severe type of vomiting may occur in either acute or chronic form. With prompt, persistent and intelligent therapy, the prognosis of hyperemesis is excellent.

Treatment and Nursing Care

The principles underlying the treatment of hyperemesis gravidarum are as follows: (1) combat the dehydration by liberal administration of parenteral fluids; (2) combat the starvation by administration of glucose intravenously and thiamine chloride subcutaneously and, if necessary, by feeding a high-caloric, high-vitamin fluid diet through a nasal tube; (3) combat the neurosis by psychotherapy, sedatives and "isolation."

Although it may be necessary on occasion to treat cases of hyperemesis in the home, hospitalization is urgently desirable, because isolation from relatives, change of atmosphere and better facilities for intravenous medication confer unusual benefits in this condition. During the first 24 hours in the hospital it is customary to withhold all food and fluids by mouth in order to give the gastrointestinal tract as complete a rest as possible. Glucose solution, usually in 10 per cent concentration, is administered intravenously and, in addition, normal saline solution subcutaneously or intravenously. The total fluid intake should approximate or exceed 3,000 cc. in the 24 hours. The nurse must keep a careful record of the exact quantity of fluids given, the amount of urine excreted and the quantity of the vomitus. Sedation is accomplished either by Luminal Sodium hypodermically in dosage of 1 or 2 grains (0.06 to 0.12 Gm.) every 4 hours, or by the rectal instillation of some barbiturate drug such as Amytal Sodium, 3 grains (0.2 Gm.) every 6 hours. Thiamine hydrochloride, 50 mg. daily hypodermically, supplies the most urgent vitamin needs during the first 24 hours. All visitors are excluded during this period, including husband and relatives.

After such a regimen for 24 hours, dry toast, crackers or cereal are given by mouth in small quantities every 2 or 3 hours. Fluids are given on alternate hours in small amounts (not over 100 cc. at a time); hot tea and ginger ale usually are tolerated better than plain water. If no vomiting occurs, the amounts and the variety of the food are increased gradually until the patient is on a regular soft, high-vitamin diet. The intravenous administration of fluids may have to be continued for several days, depending on the oral intake.

The success of the treatment will depend in

large measure on the tact, the understanding and the attitude of the nurse. Although optimism must be the keynote of the nurse's approach to the patient, this must be coupled with a plainly avowed determination to conquer the complication. The patient must be led gradually to understand that, in the treatment of vomiting, the nurse knows no such word as "failure." Not a few of these patients are in psychological conflict because of family, financial or social difficulties, and many are averse to the whole idea of pregnancy. If one can only get to the root of these difficulties in a tactful, empathic way, and help the patient to become reconciled to becoming a mother, a great deal will have been accomplished.

The nurse must exercise great care in preparing and serving trays for patients suffering from hyperemesis. The portions should be extremely small and attractively arranged. Cold liquids such as ginger ale or lemonade must be ice-cold; and hot foods, such as soups, cocoa and tea, must be steaming hot, since lukewarm liquids may be nauseating. It is best not to discuss food with the patient, even when serving the tray, but simply to assume that she will enjoy it and talk about other matters. At all times keep the emesis basin out of view, since the sight of it may start vomiting. Likewise, the smell of food may be nauseating; accordingly, the patient's room should be kept well-aired and should be as far from the kitchen as possible.

If vomiting continues despite these measures, as it rarely does, the physician may institute nasal feeding. A small rubber tube (Levin tube) is inserted by the physician through a nostril and on down into the stomach. The tube is strapped to the patient's cheek, connected with an overhanging bottle and left in place. By this means, large amounts of vitamin-rich liquid foods may be administered. The secret of success with nasal feeding lies in very slow but constant introduction of food into the stomach. The apparatus should be so arranged that the number of drops per minute passing through the tube can be counted. This should not exceed 50 per minute. Even this slow rate, it may be noted, yields about 200 cc. per hour.

Even the most severe cases of hyperemesis usually will respond favorably to the treatment described if patience and persistence are exercised; but, in extremely rare instances, the patient may continue to vomit despite all efforts, and such grave signs may develop that the physician is forced to the conclusion that further continuation of pregnancy will be at the cost of the woman's life. The following signs are grave omens and, especially when several are present, may call for therapeutic abortion if it has been decided that the mother is to be removed from danger: (1) jaundice; (2) delirium; (3) steadily rising pulse rate to levels of 130 or above; (4) fever of 101° F. (38.4° C.) or above which persists despite liberal fluid intake; and (5) hemorrhages in the retina, as observed by the physician during ophthalmoscopic examination. (See Moral Considerations, p. 455.)

COINCIDENTAL DISEASES AND PREGNANCY

During pregnancy every effort should be made to improve the general physical condition of the mother and to decrease any attendant strain and depletion of her energy due to illness. When chronic conditions, such as cardiac disturbances or kidney disease, are present, the pathologic condition should be checked early in pregnancy and preferably beforehand. This is really a part of the general health control of the individual.

The pregnant woman is quite naturally subject to diseases, both medical conditions and those requiring surgical intervention, which affect the nonpregnant woman. Any disease that affects the individual's health adds inevitable complications in pregnancy. The pregnancy may be jeopardized by the disease; or the disease process may be aggravated by the pregnancy, and at this time a latent condition may even become active.

One cannot group the adverse effects of coincidental complications of pregnancy wholly into these two specific categories, for one or the other, or both, may occur. A number of diseases in which either one of these effects, or both, may be seen includes rheumatic heart disease, diabetes mellitus, chronic hypertensive vascular disease, pyelonephritis, pneumonia and untreated syphilis. In addition to these mentioned, other general physiologic disturbances and infectious diseases and their relations to pregnancy are discussed briefly on the following pages.

General Physiologic Disturbances

Anemia. During pregnancy the blood volume is increased (p. 116). Because of this hydremia, hemoglobin estimations in gestation are likely to be lower than ordinarily considered as normal. This is not a true anemia, since the total amount of hemoglobin in the body remains the same, and sometimes the condition is referred to as the "pseudoanemia of pregnancy." Hemoglobin standards which have been established for nonpregnant women, i.e., 12 to 15 Gm. per 100 cc. of blood, are applicable for normal pregnant women also. The diagnosis of true anemia is made when the hemoglobin falls below 12 Gm., or the hematocrit below 35 per cent.

The hemoglobin levels of pregnant women fall as the result of a number of factors. Most of these cases represent a true anemia due to iron deficiency. The need of the fetus and the growing uterus for iron, inadequate iron intake in the diet and a low hemoglobin level at the start of pregnancy combine to bring about this anemic state. It is encountered more commonly in Negro women than in white women.

The symptoms are few, but some of these patients complain of becoming tired easily; many are pale; and in a few the pulse rate is fast. Because of the rather frequent occurrence of anemia in pregnancy, hemoglobin determinations are a routine part of antepartal care. The treatment consists of an iron-rich diet (emphasis on liver, meat, eggs, spinach, etc.) supplemented by the administration of some iron compound such as ferrous sulfate. In patients with anemia who do not tolerate orally ingested iron well, as shown by gastrointestinal disturbances, or in whom rapid effects are desired, injections of intramuscular iron in the form of Imferon are most helpful.

Cardiac Complications. Rheumatic heart disease is a serious complication of pregnancy. Heart lesions, especially those of the mitral valve, may be greatly aggravated by pregnancy. Constant medical supervision of the pregnant woman with any degree of cardiac involvement, however mild, is imperative, for,

fortunately, much can now be done to aid cardiac patients. If the patient has placed herself under medical care at the beginning of gestation, and if the physician has made a proper and thorough examination of all her organs at that time, he will be in a position to administer promptly such treatment as may be necessary. In this day of heart specialists, the specialist and the obstetrician must work hand in hand; and each in his own province is of the greatest help to the other. It is also absolutely essential to have close cooperation between the patient and the physician. In this situation the nurse may play an important part—by helping the patient to understand and to observe with care the primary principles of antepartal care.

The treatment of heart disease in pregnancy is governed to a large measure by the functional capacity of the heart. Rest probably will accomplish more than any other single measure, and the amount of rest needed will naturally vary with each individual, some patients having to be kept at rest a great part of the time. Strenuous activity and undue excitement must be avoided during pregnancy. The great majority, however, may safely indulge in moderate activity, and all should be in the fresh air as much as possible. Upper respiratory infections play great havoc in patients with heart disease and may even precipitate heart failure; accordingly, the nurse should advise all such patients to take special precautions against catching cold—that is, they should avoid large gatherings and people known to have sore throats, colds, etc. All of these safeguards will be advised by the physician, but the nurse may aid greatly in helping the patient to carry out his instructions.

Although heart failure usually occurs suddenly, the onset may be gradual. The nurse should be alert to particular signs and symptoms which may be warning signals and report her observations to the physician promptly. Such symptoms include sudden limitation in the patient's ability to carry on her usual household activities, increased dyspnea on exertion, tachycardia, coughing or attacks of smothering with the cough. It is well to remember that serious cardiac lesions complicating pregnancy may predispose to premature labor or may be responsible for premature death. In the past many cardiac patients have had their pregnancies terminated by therapeutic abortion, but today many such pregnancies are carried to a happy completion by providing thorough medical supervision and nursing care during pregnancy and labor. However, these successes should not lead us to forget that, if not adequately cared for, even mild cardiac disorders as well as the severe types result in definite invalidism or even death.

Diabetes. Diabetes mellitus is a serious complication of pregnancy, because 15 to 20 per cent of the infants of diabetic mothers are lost either in utero or during the early neonatal period. This is more than 5 times the usual perinatal death rate. Diabetes exerts a deleterious effect on pregnancy for several reasons:

1. The disease is more difficult to control during pregnancy because of changes in sugar tolerance. Hence, the dosage of insulin has to be regulated with extreme care and changed from time to time to prevent episodes of hyperglycemia on the one hand and hypoglycemia on the other. Hyperglycemia is very detrimental to the fetus because of the accompanying acidosis.

2. Toxemia of pregnancy is several times more frequent than in nondiabetic gravidas.

3. The infants are frequently excessive in size, and sometimes they are huge. As might be expected in such cases, mechanical difficulties in labor may result.

4. Hydramnios is frequent.

5. Congenital malformations are more common.

6. The neonatal period is associated with special hazards, i.e., respiratory difficulties, hypoxia and hypoglycemia. In fact, despite their large size, these babies frequently behave like premature infants and require incubator care (see Chap. 21).

The main objective in the management of diabetes complicated by pregnancy is rigid control of the disease. For this reason diabetic gravidas must be seen by the physician more often in pregnancy than usual and often are admitted to the hospital for short periods for various kinds of regulation. Although opinion varies about the desirability of cesarean section in diabetic pregnancies, this method of delivery is employed in a substantial proportion of the cases. As already stated, the babies require special pediatric and nursing care.

Provided that the diabetes is well controlled, the outlook for the mother is excellent.

Urinary Tract Infection. Inflammation of the ureter and the pelvis of the kidney is not uncommon during pregnancy. It seldom occurs earlier than the 4th month, and occasionally an acute attack of great severity occurs in the puerperium, in which case care will be required to distinguish it from puerperal infection. It is due to several causes, each of which may aggravate the condition. Among the possible causes are mechanical pressure on the ureters, hormonal effects acting on the tonus and peristalsis of the ureters, improper intestinal elimination, an increase of colon bacilli, and certain displacements of the bladder due to pregnancy itself. The symptoms may be gradual and slight, or quite acute in their onset, with chills and high temperature, 103° or 104° F. (39.4° or 40° C.). The patient often complains of frequency of urination, pain in the kidney region and malaise. In the acute form the patient is seized suddenly with acute abdominal pain, sometimes attended with chills or shivering; after a few hours the abdomen may become distended, and vomiting may occur. The pain, diffused at first, usually localizes in the right side. It is necessary for the nurse to secure definite instructions from the physician concerning the treatment; but rest, forced fluids and a bland, nonirritating diet (chiefly milk) may be advised in the interim. Heat over the kidneys will relieve pain.

DRUGS. The main aim of treatment in urinary tract infection is to rid the urine and the urinary tract of bacteria. During recent years the treatment of infections of the urinary tract has been revolutionized by the introduction of the sulfonamide group of drugs. The fluid intake is maintained between 2,500 and 3,000 cc. daily. The physician will follow the results of treatment not only by means of the temperature chart but also by thorough and repeated examinations of the urine. These examinations will entail both a microscopic study of the number of pus cells present and a survey of the bacteria yielded on culture. Accordingly, the nurse will be asked to secure frequent catheterized urine specimens. Follow-up of these cases is highly important and must be carried out not only during the remainder of pregnancy but also for several months after delivery, until it is certain that the urine is sterile, and x-ray studies of the kidney reveal a normal state.

Ptyalism. Although this is one of the rarer complications of pregnancy, it is one which is most annoying to the patient and very stubborn in resisting treatment. It is due entirely to altered innervation or changes in nerve control and is characterized by an enormously increased secretion of the salivary glands. Women at times have been known to discharge as much as 2 quarts of saliva daily from this cause. This complication, if it occurs at all, usually appears in the early months of pregnancy and lasts a considerable time, but, fortunately, it is inclined to cease spontaneously. It is seen in highly nervous women of low vitality and is likely to cause great mental depression and interfere with nutrition.

The treatment consists in building up the general health and the administration of such medication as may be prescribed by the physician. The use of astringent mouthwashes often contributes to the patient's comfort. Any treatment may seem to be inadequate, and the condition is most disagreeable.

Infectious Diseases

Certain infectious diseases have no proved specific ill effect on the mother or the baby, but, if possible, any communicable disease should be avoided during pregnancy, for even mild diseases add strain at this particular time.

With infectious diseases two types of effects may occur: (1) on the mother and (2) on the fetus. The diseases which often have serious effects on the infant are discussed in Chapter 21. Among those directly affecting the mother are the following.

The Common Cold. The susceptibility to acute upper respiratory infections is apparently greater during pregnancy. Therefore, the pregnant woman should make every effort to avoid contacts with these infections. When she does acquire a cold, prompt medical attention is usually desirable, because the common cold often precedes more serious conditions affecting the upper respiratory tract. Prescribed medication should be used in preference to the various antihistamine drugs obtainable without a prescription. Rest in bed helps the individual and aids in checking the spread of the disease.

Pneumonia. Pneumonia, which may follow the common cold, can frequently lead to complications of pregnancy. The pneumonia organisms, especially streptococci, also may infect the uterus, causing puerperal infections. Prompt use of penicillin and other antibiotics is most helpful. Since antibiotics have been employed, the occurrence of abortion and premature labor is less common.

Influenza. Serious complications may follow influenza, especially in the pneumonic type in which pregnancy is sometimes interrupted. Sulfa drugs and such antibiotics as penicillin usually are given to help forestall pneumonia, but they do not control the influenza virus.

Measles. Ill effects are not commonly noted in pregnancy, but pregnant mothers who contract measles are said to be more likely to have premature labors. No other definite effects are reported, although eruptions have been noted on infants at birth.

German Measles. Rubella, or German measles, is caused by a virus—distinct from the virus of measles (rubeola). German measles produces most serious effects on the mother's unborn infant if it occurs in the first trimester of pregnancy. These infants are often afflicted with congenital malformations such as cataracts, deafness, heart lesions and mental defects (see Chap. 21). There are no antiserums against German measles. At one time gamma globulin was considered by some to be a wise precaution for pregnant mothers. However, it is now believed that gamma globulin does not protect either the mother or the fetus from rubella. If it is given early enough, it may suppress the rash. Rubella virus has been found to be present in the blood even in the absence of the rash.

Typhoid fever, which is now relatively rare in this country, may cause serious complications in pregnancy, resulting in abortion, prematurity and infant mortality. Immunization is not contraindicated during pregnancy, and antityphoid vaccine should be administered when necessary.

Brucellosis (Undulant Fever, Malta Fever). These debilitating diseases in humans are contracted mainly from unpasteurized milk. In this country today, conditions for the production and the processing of milk are set by U. S. Public Health Service standards. When these diseases are seen, the bacteria have been found in the human placenta, but abortion in humans is very infrequently traced to this organism, although brucella bacteria do cause abortion in cattle. Good results have been attained with Aureomycin and also with combined streptomycin-sulfadiazine.

Scarlet Fever. There seems to be greater susceptibility to scarlet fever during the puerperium. The cause is a streptococcus, and so the risk of developing puerperal fever is clear. Antibiotics are effective in treating the disease, but sometimes abortion is caused by scarlet fever contracted during early pregnancy, due to the mother's high fever.

Erysipelas. This disease, usually caused by streptococci, may be very serious at any time, but in pregnant women there is the danger of developing puerperal fever. Care must be taken to avoid transferring streptococci from any local lesions to the genital area. Strict isolation is essential. Appropriate drugs (penicillin, sulfa drugs, etc.) should be used if necessary. The streptococci may pass through the placenta and cause the death of the fetus.

Smallpox. Cases of abortion and prematurity increase with the severity of the attack, especially with the hemorrhagic type. As in measles, small pox may be transmitted through the placenta, for eruptions may be present in live births.

Malaria. In more severe cases of malaria the incidence of abortion and premature labor is increased. Prompt therapy is of utmost importance. Malaria organisms have been found in the blood of the cord and the fetus; they are frequently found in the placenta, although no ill effects have been noted on the infants. Quinine or the newer related drugs, such as Atabrine, should be administered to women with malaria history to prevent recrudescence during pregnancy and the puerperium. The decrease in malaria reported (1951) by the Communicable Disease Center of the U. S. Public Health Service makes malaria much less important as a complication of pregnancy.

Tuberculosis. The average case of tuberculosis in itself has only a slight effect on the course of pregnancy, since it rarely predisposes to abortion, premature labor or even stillbirth. (Fortunately, the disease is seldom acquired congenitally, although a small number of authentic cases have been reported in which, in addition to a tuberculous condition of the placenta, tubercle bacilli were found in the cord blood, together with tuberculous lesions in the baby.) Medical opinions differ, but the consensus is that pregnancy does not exert an adverse effect on tuberculosis. Some authorities think that this disease becomes aggravated by pregnancy, and that only a patient in an arrested case should consider becoming pregnant. Pregnancy is undertaken with some risk, for although a tuberculous lesion may remain latent for an indefinite time, provided that the natural resistance is not overtaxed, it must be noted that pregnancy is one of the factors often responsible for overtaxing the resistance sufficiently to convert a latent, inactive lesion into an active one. Maintenance of the proper hygiene, nutrition and excellent surroundings so that health is conserved in every possible way will do much to prevent activity in a latent focus. Other authorities deny that the tuberculosis is necessarily aggravated by pregnancy, basing this belief on statistics of a large series of tuberculous patients who have progressed satisfactorily in pregnancy.

The symptoms of tuberculosis in pregnancy do not differ materially from those that accompany the disease in other conditions. During the early months of gestation the characteristic anemia and general malnutrition of tuberculosis are usually pronounced, but in the latter months there is often considerable improvement. Too often, however, this is followed by a rapid decline after delivery.

Treatment will depend on the type of involvement as well as on the particular stage of pregnancy. Prophylactic treatment is most important since it offers most chance of success. The patient must be given every medical and hygienic advantage, wholesome food (milk is of very great value), fresh air and sunshine and absolute rest. Any cough or rapid loss of weight should be reported. It is rarely indicated for the physician to interrupt the pregnancy. When a tuberculous patient reaches term, the labor is made as easy as possible to conserve her strength. Under no circumstances should a tuberculous woman be allowed to nurse her baby, for the baby's sake as well as for her own. Months of careful follow-up treatment will be necessary. The patient should not consider becoming pregnant again until a sufficient time has elapsed to establish a reasonable certainty that her disease has been arrested.

It is in the group in which tuberculosis is unsuspected that tragedies occur, many of which could be avoided. Therefore, a complete medical history always should be taken. Exposure to tuberculosis in the family, a history of hemoptysis, pleurisy, or fistula in ano, and a cough or loss of weight over a period of time suggest strongly the presence of possible tuberculosis. These danger signals are of the utmost value, and if heeded will often enable the physician to recognize tuberculosis symptoms developing during pregnancy which he otherwise might attribute to the pregnancy itself.

Examinations of the chest (roentgenographic) and the sputum (microscopic) should be done routinely in suspected cases. The newer antibiotics (streptomycin, hydrostreptomycin, neomycin) should be available if need is indicated. There may be undue alarm due to confusion of tuberculosis with the milder disease, histoplasmosis, unless expert testing (skin and sputum) facilities are available.

Poliomyelitis generally does not complicate pregnancy or delivery, except in the very unusual cases in which respiratory paralysis develops; in these rare cases cesarean section has given satisfactory results. Fortunately, the fetus rarely contracts the disease. Of about 80 cases reported during pregnancy, less than one fifth occurred in the first trimester. A milder form of infection of poliomyelitis is attributed to a different virus, the Coxsackie virus, which produces less paralysis but is often unrecognized.

The Venereal Diseases

The huge increase in the prevalence of venereal diseases during the past decade has aroused the concern of physicians, nurses and public health officials. Syphilis among teenagers has shown an increase of 230 per cent between 1956 and 1964, according to a report of the United States Communicable Disease Center. The number of reported cases in the infectious stage of syphilis has climbed steadily from a low of 6,399 in 1956 to 22,969 in 1964 —more than a 3-fold increase. Dependable

data on the prevalence of gonorrhea are more difficult to obtain, but all the evidence suggests a comparable increase in that disease.

Syphilis. In the early decades of the century syphilis was the most common cause of stillbirth, and the recent upsurge in its prevalence proves the obvious threat that stillbirths from this cause likewise will increase. Hence, it is essential that all physicians and nurses be alert to this threat and take vigilant steps to meet it.

SYPHILIS AND PREGNANCY[*]

Causative Organism. Syphilis is a specific infectious disease caused by a spirochete, *Spirochaeta pallida* or *Treponema pallidum*, discovered by Schaudinn and Hoffmann in 1905.

Types of Syphilis. Syphilis in any individual may be acquired or congenital. The acquired form is usually transmitted by sexual intercourse; however, other forms of personal contact may transmit the infection, such as kissing, an examination of the patient by a contaminated physician and the nursing of the newborn by an infected person. Congenital syphilis is a term applied to syphilis transmitted to the child before birth. An infected mother may transmit syphilis to the fetus through the placenta. Such transfer may occur from mothers whether they were syphilitic at the time of conception or whether they acquired syphilis during early pregnancy.

In this discussion of syphilis and pregnancy, we may focus our attention on three points: (1) the detection of syphilis in the pregnant mother; (2) the treatment of such infected mothers; and (3) the prompt detection of syphilis in the baby after birth.

Diagnosis of Syphilis in Pregnant Mothers: Clinical Symptoms. In syphilis there is usually a primary lesion or hard chancre located where there was a defect in the surface epithelium, allowing the entrance of the spirochete. In women, the initial lesion of syphilis is less easily observed than in men, and, unless seen on the vulva, is usually unnoticed. In a large proportion of recently infected women, no evidence of a scar of a chancre of the genitals may be seen. The secondary manifestations, likewise, are often unnoticed. The skin eruptions are mild and disappear rather rapidly. On the other hand, the presence of condylomata lata may cause the patient to consult her physician.

Previous Pregnancy History. The history of previous pregnancies is most significant in indi-

[*] By William T. Daily, M.D., Department of Obstetrics and Gynecology, The Long Island College Hospital, Brooklyn, N. Y.

cating syphilis in the mother. In a series of pregnant syphilitic women studied, a large proportion of pregnancies failed to go to term, ending in a miscarriage, in a premature, a full-term stillbirth, or in the birth of a syphilitic infant. Abortion in the first trimester of pregnancy is noted but slightly more frequently than in ordinary pregnancy; on the other hand, interruption of pregnancy during the 5th, 6th or 7th month is common.

Blood Tests. Blood tests constitute the most common and important method of detecting syphilis. The importance of blood tests is evident when we realize that syphilis complicating pregnancy in a primigravida is seldom recognized until the damage is done, unless the practice of making routine serologic tests is followed. The advantage of this third method of detecting syphilis is shown by the fact that out of 144 pregnant women thus shown to have syphilis, only 6 gave evidence of a primary lesion, and the history and physical examination were suggestive of syphilis in but 34 patients in the series. Without the blood tests, over 100 of these mothers would have failed to receive the necessary treatment.

The tests devised by Wassermann, Kahn, Kline, Mazzini and the U. S. Public Health Service test V.D.R.L. are the ones now most frequently used in this country. If the blood test is found to be positive or questionable, the test is repeated to make sure that any possible laboratory error is eliminated. Should a test be positive, treatment is inaugurated, even though there are no other indications of syphilis (lesions, pregnancy history). . . .

Several types of tests are used to determine the condition of the infant.

1. The cord blood test should be made on every suspicious or treated case. However, this test is not wholly reliable; but a positive cord blood test indicates the need for close follow-up and frequent examinations.

2. The placenta may furnish suspicion, if not evidence, of pathologic changes. The normal placenta at full term weighs about 500 Gm. Normally, the relative weight of the baby to placenta is about 6:1. The placenta of syphilitic infection is larger, heavier and paler than normal. Since a premature placenta is relatively heavier than a placenta at term, and because many syphilitic babies are born prematurely, this may account for the too common opinion regarding the great size and weight of a syphilitic placenta. Histologically, the chorionic villi are greatly enlarged; they show diminished branching and they are more club-shaped. On cross section, the vessels are seen to be diminished in number and stenosed or obliterated by endoarteritic changes. The

stroma is more granular, and the stroma cells lose their normal stellate appearance. The villi, due to their greater size or thickness, approach each other, reducing the intervillous spaces. Syphilis of the placenta is not a common lesion, and many hesitate to make a positive diagnosis unless the spirochete is seen in microscopic darkfield examination.

3. The umbilical cord vein, in an area near the placenta, may be scraped and studied for spirochetes under a darkfield examination.

4. An x-ray examination of the long bones, especially the lower and upper ends of the femur, upper fibula and tibia, and the upper humerus and lower radius, is most valuable in determining the syphilitic condition of the infant. The usual lesion is an epiphysitis.

5. Blood tests may also be used. The newborn baby of a treated mother should be referred to a pediatrician familiar with the treatment of syphilis in the newborn about the 6th week after birth, for repeated serologic and x-ray examinations.

Conclusion. Syphilis of the newborn is preventable, and, if a child is delivered with the infection or succumbs to its virulence, either before delivery or neonatally, two and only two persons are largely responsible: first, the mother for her failure to be examined early in her pregnancy, and, secondly, the physician (or clinic) whom she consults, if he neglects to take routine serologic tests and which, if positive, he fails to treat intensively.

TREATMENT OF SYPHILITIC MOTHERS. The present-day treatment of syphilis in pregnancy consists in the intensive administration of penicillin as soon as the disease is recognized. The earlier in pregnancy therapy is started, the better are the results. The course of treatment consists of the administration of approximately 6 million units of penicillin, given over a period of 10 days. It is well established that this dosage is several times that necessary to protect the baby from syphilis, and it is believed to be enough to cure the mother also; but it is quite possible that further experience will result in a still higher dosage to make certain of permanent maternal cure. The intensive treatment schedule has posed a difficult problem for these patients, but it has been met in many cities by special treatment centers.

Penicillin, with rare exceptions, has been free from serious toxic effects. The frequent injection schedules formerly used have now been replaced by schedules permitting 1, 2 or 3 injections a week for 1 to 2 weeks. This relatively short treatment period with its freedom from severe toxic reactions has a great advantage over the previously accepted 1 to 2 years of arsenical and bismuth therapy. . . . Penicillin also possesses the ability of being filtered through the placenta and consequently can act as a very potent agent in the treatment of congenital syphilis in utero. Unfortunately, failures do occur as the result of relapse or reinfection, and this accounts for most of the rare instances of congenital syphilis resulting from treated mothers.

Gonorrhea. This disease should be studied by the nurse with the other infectious diseases; but, because of the consequences of gonorrheal infection to the mother at the time of labor and during the puerperium, as well as the risk of permanent injury to the baby's eyes at the time of birth, this disease is of special concern to the maternity nurse.

The disease is due to a microorganism, known commonly as the gonococcus organism (*Micrococcus gonorrhoeae* or *Neisseria gonorrhoeae*). It may affect any mucous membrane, e.g., that of the eye, but usually attacks the mucosa of the genital tract, particularly the opening of the bladder and the crypts around the cervix, causing a catarrhal discharge of pus. It is called a venereal disease simply because the usual mode of transfer of this infection is by sexual intercourse. The infection often extends into the uterus and the tubes, causing a very serious localized peritonitis, and may cause sterility by a mechanical blocking of the tubes. Gonorrhea is not commonly considered to be a fatal disease, in the sense that a high proportion of the cases terminate in death, but in the list of diseases causing chronic ill health, especially in the female sex, gonorrhea is most important.

Gonorrhea does not greatly modify the course of pregnancy, and its existence is often unsuspected by the patient. The vaginal discharge may increase, as it normally does during pregnancy, and, with the local congestion of the venous system, the patient may have some irritation in the vulvar region. Pregnancy may act as a barrier to the ascent of the gonococcus, and thus the fetus may be protected during development. The patient may abort, but more commonly she carries the

baby to full term and delivers normally. However, after delivery, conditions are quite different. Even when a patient has had a normal labor, the cervix is dilated, and the minute tears and abrasions offer many avenues for the spread of the infection, and the lochial discharge makes an ideal culture medium for the bacteria. This condition may lead to the development of a form of puerperal fever.

It is now routine practice to obtain a specimen of vaginal secretions for culture on the first antepartal visit. In the female, the diagnosis of gonorrhea is confirmed by culturing the organisms from fresh vaginal secretions.[3] If the culture is positive, penicillin is given promptly, for it yields dramatic results in treatment of this disease. Cure may be effected by a single intramuscular injection of suitable dosage of penicillin in at least 90 per cent of the cases. In chronic cases 1 or 2 repeated doses may be necessary.

Gonorrhea is not hereditary, but, if a woman is infected at the time of her confinement, the organism may get into the baby's eyes and cause blindness. This infection of the eyes is called ophthalmia neonatorum. The prophylactic treatment of the baby's eyes at this time never should be neglected (see Chap. 12).

SUGGESTED READING

Abramson, Julius, and Tenny, Benjamin: Cardiac disease in pregnancy, New Eng. J. Med. 253: 279, 1955.

Alter, N. M., and Cosgrove, S. A.: Hydatidiform mole: practical considerations, Obstet. Gynec. 5:755, 1955.

Bartholomew, R. A., *et al.*: The mechanisms of bleeding during pregnancy, Am. J. Obstet. Gynec. 66:1042, 1953.

Baruey, G. G., and Strauss, Anselm L.: The social loss of dying patients, Am. J. Nurs. 64:119-121, June, 1964.

Berger, Max, and Caranagh, Denis: Toxemias of pregnancy, Am. J. Obstet. Gynec. 87:293-305, October 1, 1963.

Black, M. E., and Miller, Max: Management of diabetes and pregnancy. Clin. Obstet. Gynec. 1: 229, 1958.

Borell, Ulf, *et al.*: Effect of uterine contractions on the human uteroplacental blood circulation,

[3] U. S. Public Health Service Publication No. 573, 1958.

Am. J. Obstet. Gynec. 89, No. 6:881-890, August 1, 1964.

Brown, A. A., and Podair, Simon: Venereal disease—a renewed challenge, Public Affairs Pamphlet No. 292A, New York, Public Affairs Pamphlets, 1964.

Bunim, J. J., and Appel, S. Baer: Pregnancy and rheumatic heart disease, J.A.M.A. 142:90, 1950.

Burt, K. L., Donnelly, J. F., and Fleming, S. P.: Acute toxemia of pregnancy associated with organic heart disease, Am. J. Obstet. Gynec. 68:528, 1954.

Bysshe, S. M.: Premature separation of the normally implanted placenta, Am. J. Obstet. Gynec. 62:38, 1951.

Cherny, W. B., Carter, F. B., Thomas, W. L., and Peete, C. H., Jr.: Hypotensive drugs in pregnancy toxemia, Obstet. Gynec. 9:505, 1957.

Cianfrani, Theodore, and Conway, M. K.: Ectopic pregnancy, Am. J. Nurs. 63, No. 4:93-95, April, 1964.

Cosgrove, S. A.: Therapeutic abortion, J. Mich. Med. Soc. 55:795, 1956.

Davidson-Buchanan, D. J.: A drop of blood, Am. J. Nurs. 65, No. 7:103-107, July, 1965.

de Alvarez, Russell: Toxemias of pregnancy, Am. J. Nurs. 54:1486, 1954.

Deschin, Celia: Teen-agers and venereal disease, Children 9:144-148, July-August, 1962.

————: VD and the adolescent personality, Am. J. Nurs. 63, No. 11:59-62, November, 1963.

Eastman, N. J.: Williams Obstetrics, ed. 13, New York, Appleton, 1966.

Giblin, Elizabeth, and Osmond, Thelma: Nursing care in toxemias of pregnancy, Am. J. Nurs. 54:1488, 1954.

Glassberg, B. Y.: Venereal disease among adolescents, Nurs. Outlook 10:731-732, November, 1962.

Groasmun, Ruth: Nursing care of the pregnant diabetic, Am. J. Nurs. 58:102, 1958.

Guyton, A. C.: Textbook of Medical Physiology, ed. 2, Philadelphia, Saunders, 1961.

Hall, Madelyn: Caseholding in venereal disease research, Nurs. Outlook 10:727-728, November, 1962.

Hansen, R. R., and Taylor, E. S.: When the cervix is the cause of premature delivery, Am. J. Nurs. 60, No. 10:1454-1455, 1960.

Holman, Edwin: Medicolegal aspects of sterilization, artificial insemination and abortion, J.A.M.A. 156:1309, 1954.

Holmes, F.: Incidence of the supine hypotensive syndrome in late pregnancy; a clinical study of 500 subjects, J. Obstet. Gynec. Brit. Empire 67:254-258, 1960.

Horowitz, W.: Management of the pregnant patient with cardiac disease, New Eng. J. Med. 252:511, 1955.

Krug, E. E.: Pharmacology in Nursing, ed. 9, St. Louis, Mosby, 1963.

Larsen, G. I.: What every nurse should know about congenital syphilis, Nurs. Outlook 13, No. 3:52-55, March, 1965.

Lentz, J. W., and Hall, M. N.: Venereal disease control in the twentieth century, Nurs. Outlook 10:722-726, November, 1962.

Liley, A. W.: Liquor amnii analysis in the management of the pregnancy complicated by rhesus sensitization, Am. J. Obstet. Gynec. 82:1359-1369, December, 1961.

Lund, C. J.: Studies on the iron deficiency anemia of pregnancy, Am. J. Obstet. Gynec. 62:947, 1951.

McAllister, J. B.: Ethics with Special Application to the Nursing Profession, ed. 2, Philadelphia, Saunders, 1955.

McFadden, C. J.: Medical Ethics, ed. 4, Philadelphia, Davis, 1956.

Pearse, H. A., and Ott, H. A.: Hospital control of sterilization and therapeutic abortion, Am. J. Obstet. Gynec. 60:285, 1950.

Pedowitz, Paul: Placenta previa, Am. J. Obstet. Gynec. 92, No. 9:16-25, September 1, 1965.

Pedowitz, P., and Shlevin, Edmund: The pregnant diabetic patient, Am. J. Obstet. Gynec. 69:395, 1955.

Peel, Sir John: Progress in the knowledge and management of the pregnant diabetic patient, Am. J. Obstet. Gynec. 83, No. 7:847-856, April, 1962.

Pritchard, J. A.: Anemia in obstetrics and gynecology; an evaluation of therapy with parenteral iron, Am. J. Obstet. Gynec. 77:74, 1959.

Rauh, L. W.: Rubella and pregnancy, Ohio Med. J. 51:875, 1955.

Reid, D. E., et al.: Maternal afibrinogenemia associated with long-standing intrauterine fetal death, Am. J. Obstet. Gynec. 66:500, 1953.

Rosen, H.: Therapeutic Abortion: Medical, Psychiatric, Legal, Anthropological, and Religious Considerations, New York, Julian Press, 1954.

Rosenbach, L. M., and Gangemi, C. R.: Tuberculosis and pregnancy, J.A.M.A. 161:1035, 1956.

Rouse, G. P.: Pregnancy and diabetes, Am. J. Nurs. 58:100, 1958.

Rovinsky, J. J., and Guttmacher, A. F.: Medical and Surgical and Gynecologic Complications of Pregnancy, ed. 2, Baltimore, Williams & Wilkins, 1965.

Russell, K. P., et al.: Acute renal failure as obstetric complication, J.A.M.A. 157:15, 1955.

Schaefer, George, et al.: The pregnant woman with tuberculosis, Am. J. Nurs. 63, No. 8:68-73, August, 1963.

Semmens, J. P.: Placenta previa: the role of conservative management in a controlled study, Am. J. Obstet. Gynec. 77:63, 1959.

Smith, Kaighn: Cesearean section in the treatment of placenta previa, Am. J. Obstet. Gynec. 77:55, 1959.

Stevens, Dom Gregory: Principles of Ethics, ed. 5, Philadelphia, Lippincott, 1959.

Tatum, H. J.: The obstetric patient with toxemia, Clin. Obstet. Gynec. 7:233-248, March, 1964.

Taylor, Susan D.: Clinic for adolescents with venereal disease, Am. J. Nurs. 63, No. 11:63-66, November, 1963.

Webster, H. D., *et al.*: Ectopic pregnancy, Am. J. Obstet. Gynec. 92, No. 1:23-34, May 1, 1965.

Weil, R. J., and Stewart, L. C.: The problem of spontaneous abortion: psychosomatic and inter-personal aspects of habitual abortion, Am. J. Obstet. Gynec. 73:322, 1957.

Weiner, A. S., and Wexler, Irving B.: Heredity of the Blood Groups, New York, Grune & Stratton, 1958.

Wesselfoeft, Conrad: Acute infectious diseases in pregnancy, Ann. Int. Med. 42:555, 1955.

World Health Organization: Venereal Diseases: A Survey of Existing Legislation, Geneva, 1956.

Zuspan, F. P., *et al.*: Abdominal pregnancy, Am. J. Obstet. Gynec. 74:259, 1957.

———: Epinephrine infusions in normal toxemic pregnancies: II. Plasma glucose, nonesterified fatty acid, and epinephrine-norepinephrine alterations, Am. J. Obstet. Gynec. 92, No. 8: 1102-1106, August 15, 1965.

Chapter 19

Complications of Labor

INTRODUCTION

The opportunity labor affords to give nursing care in its broadest sense has been stressed in Chapter 12. The opportunity is present in an even greater degree in cases of complicated labor. The importance of supportive care of the highest caliber cannot be emphasized enough. Fortunately, the principles of care in these instances usually do not differ significantly from those in normal labor. Some modification, of course, will be necessary at times. Yet because of the stress of the situation, more is demanded of the nurse. Her observations, reporting, technical skills, physical and emotional supportive measures must all be brought into play and carried out with a fine degree of competence, for the labor experience is often prolonged and painful—for all those concerned: mother, father, nurse and physician.

Since modifications of care will be dealt with primarily in this chapter, the student is urged to review in Chapter 12 the basic concepts and components of nursing care during labor.

MECHANICAL DYSTOCIA

Occasionally the nurse will see instances in which hours and hours of labor pass without progress. In such instances there is obviously something wrong with the mechanics or "machinery" of labor. In other words, these are cases of dystocia (difficult labor) in which the mechanics of the process are at fault—cases of mechanical dystocia. But what precisely *is* wrong?

Reduced to its simplest constituents, the process of labor resolves itself into the propulsion by certain *forces* of an irregular object (the infant or *passenger*) through the birth canal (the *passage*). Only three factors are involved in labor therefore—the forces, the passenger and the passage. When, despite many hours of labor, the infant fails to come, one of these three factors or some combination of them must be at fault.

Let us make this clear by a homely example. If a person were trying to force his foot into a boot and was unable to do so, what could be the causes of his failure? First, he might not be pushing hard enough. (The forces are at fault.) Second, he might not be holding his foot in the correct position; the foot cannot be jammed in any way but must be flexed sharply so that the smallest diameters present themselves. (The position is faulty.) Third, the boot may be too small, or (what amounts to the same thing) the foot may be too big. (There is disproportion between the size of the foot and the boot.)

Likewise, when Nature tries to propel an infant through the birth canal and fails to do so, there can be only three causes of the failure —the same three. The forces are inadequate

482

(uterine inertia); or the position of the infant is at fault; or there is disproportion between the size of the infant and that of the birth canal.

Uterine Dysfunction

Definition. The nurse will recall that in normal labor a latent phase of several hours' duration occurs first, in which effacement and a small amount of dilatation take place. An active phase follows this, in which progressive, accelerated dilatation occurs. This is followed by a phase of deceleration or slowing just before full dilatation (see Chap. 10). A significant prolongation of any of these phases is known as uterine dysfunction.

Heretofore, the term "uterine inertia" was used to describe a dysfunctional labor. Inertia was classified as either primary or secondary. Primary inertia occurred at the onset of labor (i.e., the contractions were of poor quality and ineffectual) and was due to unknown causes. Secondary inertia occurred later in labor and was felt to be related to maternal exhaustion. However, increasing knowledge regarding uterine action and the phases of labor indicates that it would be more appropriate to discuss the topic in terms of dysfunction as it relates to the phases of dilatation. The two terms "inertia" and "dysfunction" are used interchangeably to some extent. If the word "inertia" is used, then primary inertia should refer to prolongation of the latent phase and secondary inertia should indicate a prolongation or abnormality of the active phase.[1]

Causes. The chief causes of uterine dysfunction are injudicious use of analgesia (i.e., excessive or too early administration of the drugs), minor degrees of pelvic contraction, and slight extension of the fetal head, e.g., occiput posterior positions. Other contributing factors include overdistention of the uterus, excessive cervical rigidity and maternal age. Often, however, the cause is unknown. More research must be done to obtain increased definitive knowledge concerning the etiologic factors in this condition.

Complications. The complications of uterine

dysfunction are unfortunate for both mother and infant. Fetal injury and death are the most serious outcomes of this disorder. For the mother, exhaustion and dehydration may occur if labor is allowed to become too prolonged. The nurse should watch for any elevation of the maternal temperature and pulse, for these are the clinical signs that herald the onset of secondary complications. Acetonuria is another sign of exhaustion and dehydration. These symptoms should be reported immediately. Generally, in patients having dysfunctional labor, supportive intravenous therapy and electrolyte replacement will have been begun before this syndrome occurs. Intrauterine infection is another common maternal complication in these types of labor; broad-spectrum antibiotics are the usual choice of treatment. It is particularly important not to allow intra-uterine infection to occur, since it contributes heavily to the increased perinatal mortality. In addition, dysfunctional labor appears to have some long-term consequences. Research[2] has indicated that difficult labors and deliveries have a deleterious effect on future childbearing. Apparently, the more difficult the labor and delivery, the less inclination there is to have future children. In addition, the fear and anxiety that are engendered by a complicated childbirth become a special concern of the health team if these patients do have subsequent children.

Types of Uterine Dysfunction. HYPERTONIC UTERINE DYSFUNCTION. There are two varieties of uterine dysfunction. The first of these is the hypertonic type. Its name is derived from the fact that the muscle of the uterus is in a state of greater than normal muscle tension, i.e., incomplete relaxation. In these instances the contractions are of poor quality in the latent phase of labor, and the force of the contraction also is distorted, that is, one segment of the uterus may contract with more force than another. Although these contractions are inefficient from the standpoint of accomplishing dilatation, they are extremely painful. It is particularly important to help these mothers to distinguish between the anticipation of pain and the actual pain (see Chap. 12), for as labor wears on, and no

[1] Eastman, N. J., and Hellman, L. M.: Williams Obstetrics, ed. 12, pp. 858-859, New York, Appleton, 1961.

[2] Jeffcoate, T. N., *et al.*: Inefficient uterine action, Surg. Gynec. Obstet. 95:257, September 4, 1952.

progress is made, the mother's strength and ability to cope with the contractions diminish, and hence the pain seems to be intensified. The anxiety and fear which are generated can easily lead to panic, which is detrimental to resumption of a successful labor course.

This matter of the intensity of labor contractions is something with which the nurse must familiarize herself so that she may report intelligently. At the height of an excellent uterine contraction it is impossible to indent the uterine wall with one's fingertips, and during a fairly good contraction it may be possible to cause some slight indentation; but if the uterine wall can be indented easily at the height of a contraction, it is a poor one. In evaluating the intensity of a labor contraction, reliance should be placed on this tactile examination and not on the amount of "complaining" done by the patient about her pain.

The nurse should be alert also to signs of fetal distress, since in hypertonic dysfunction fetal distress tends to appear quite early in labor.

Treatment for this type of dysfunctional labor generally consists of rest and fluids. When medication is indicated to produce the needed rest and relaxation, an injection of 16 mg. of morphine may be prescribed, because it usually stops the abnormal contractions. In addition, a 0.1- to 0.2-Gm. dose of a short-acting barbiturate may be administered. Intravenous fluids are utilized to maintain hydration and electrolyte balance, and in most instances normal labor resumes when the patient awakens.

Intrapartal Infection. Occasionally, however, some patients do not respond to this regimen, and labor becomes prolonged. In such patients who have been in labor for 24 hours or more or who have ruptured membranes (whether from uterine dysfunction or other causes), bacteria are likely to ascend into the uterus and give rise to infection. This is known as *intrapartal infection* and is a serious complication. It is signalized by a rise in temperature, often in association with a chill. Because of this danger, it is customary to take temperatures every 2 hours in patients whose labors have lasted more than 24 hours. Even an elevation of half a degree should be reported at once to the physician. Intrapartal infection is much more likely to occur if the membranes have been ruptured for a long time. As previously stated, treatment is usually in the form of antibiotics. Oxytocin also may be used in these cases in spite of its adverse effects (it tends to increase the hypertonicity of the muscle). However, only dilutions of two or three times the usual strength should be employed. Cesarean section is resorted to if fetal distress occurs.

HYPOTONIC UTERINE DYSFUNCTION. The second variety of uterine dysfunction has been designated as hypotonic. Here the tone or tension of the muscle of the uterus is defective or inadequate. In these cases the uterus contracts synchronously, but the force is inadequate to accomplish dilatation. This condition occurs in the accelerated or active phase, or even during the second stage of labor; the contractions become infrequent and of poor quality, and the uterus is easily indentable at the acme of a contraction. Signs of fetal distress usually do not appear until intrapartal infection has developed. Thus, it is important that the nurse be cognizant of the signs and the symptoms of both these secondary complications and report these accordingly.

Treatment. When hypotonic dysfunction is suspected, diagnosis should be confirmed by x-ray pelvimetry and sterile vaginal examination in order to ascertain accurate pelvic measurements, abnormalities of presentation and position, state of the cervix and level of the presenting part. It should be stressed that early diagnosis is a chief factor in reducing fetal death and injury. If a marked degree of disproportion exists (see p. 492), or if there is an uncorrectable malposition, then cesarean section will be employed to effect delivery. If these conditions are not present, then supportive therapy together with stimulation of the uterus will be the treatment of choice.

Explanations to Parents. It goes without saying that labors of this type are extremely discouraging for the mother and the father. The diagnostic procedures as well as the therapy will take a certain amount of time, and carrying out these measures will require patience and waiting on the part of everyone concerned. It is essential that the couple know and understand this fact. This will mean that the doctor or the nurse will spend sufficient time with the parents to explain what is happening in depth and in terms that are appropriate for them. It is very possible that repeated reinforcement of the explanations, progress, etc., will be needed. Feedback from the parents should be encouraged, so that their level of understanding and acceptance can be ascertained. The normal tension and anxiety found in any labor certainly will be intensified, and it is important that it not be compounded by fantasy or misunderstanding. Since dysfunctional labor is so variable, it is often impossible (and unwise) to give the parents any ironclad definite reassurances as to when effective labor will commence. Yet some kind of boundaries must be placed on when this ineffective phase will end, and progress will begin, so that the mother will have some goal to look forward to and to work for. Therefore, it is important to reassure the patient, reminding her that her case is not absolutely unique (patients think after many hours that theirs is the longest labor in obstetric history), that certain specific measures are known and can be taken to help effective labor to begin, and that she will be receiving competent medical and nursing care throughout her labor. If possible, the course of action should be explained by the doctor (or by the nurse with the doctor's permission), so that the parents can anticipate more realistically what is in store and therefore can be more reassured that certain definite measures are available to them and are being employed.

Further Treatment and Care. In addition, all the comfort measures which promote relaxation should be utilized. Sponge baths, various positioning, soothing backrubs, clean, dry linen, quiet conversation, reading or other diversionary activities as well as a quiet restful environment are all appropriate. However, the patient should not be isolated in a dark room on the premise that she should "sleep" or "rest"; any patient who is having a difficult or complicated labor should never be left alone unless she is actually sleeping, and then frequent observations should be made to see when she awakens. Human contact is one of the most important items of "treatment" in cases of complicated labor and should never be neglected. The presence of the same person, nurse and/or doctor, is very helpful for the reasons already mentioned in Chapter 12. Coaching the mother in breathing patterns and relaxation technics also will conserve her strength.

The doctor may want the patient to have fluids by mouth, or he may order intravenous infusions to maintain hydration and electrolyte balance. A total of 2,000 cc. or more of intravenous fluid may be given in 24 hours. Hot soapsuds enemas probably will be ordered from time to time in the hope of stimulating more effectual uterine contractions. In certain cases (in some it may be dangerous) the physician may ask that the patient be allowed to walk about, in the belief that this may favor

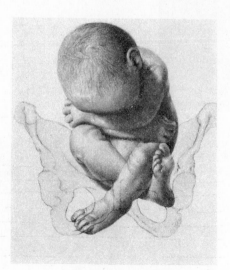

FIG. 19-1. Footling breech.

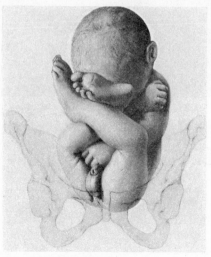

FIG. 19-2. Frank breech.

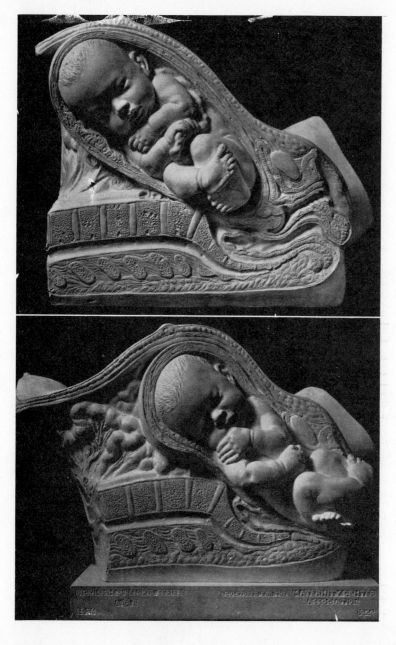

FIG. 19-3. (A, B) Delivery in footling breech presentation. (Dickinson-Belskie Breech Delivery Series, sculptured for the Maternity Center Association, New York)

descent of the head, which in turn will exert greater pressure on the lower uterine segment and thereby stimulate stronger contractions.

Rupturing the membranes often stimulates satisfactory labor. As previously stated, if there is no critical disproportion or uncorrectable malposition, and amniotomy fails to bring about desired results, then an intravenous infusion of oxytocin usually will be utilized to stimulate the uterus. It should be used with the utmost caution and in very small doses, for the employment of oxytocin in labor can be fraught with dangerous possibilities, i.e., tetanic contraction of the uterus with asphyxiation of the fetus and even rupture of the uterus. (Contractions are termed "tetanic" when the uterus stays contracted continuously with no regular periods of relaxation.)

Because it affords better control of dosage, the intravenous administration of oxytocin by

FIG. 19-3. (C, D) Delivery
in footling breech presentation.

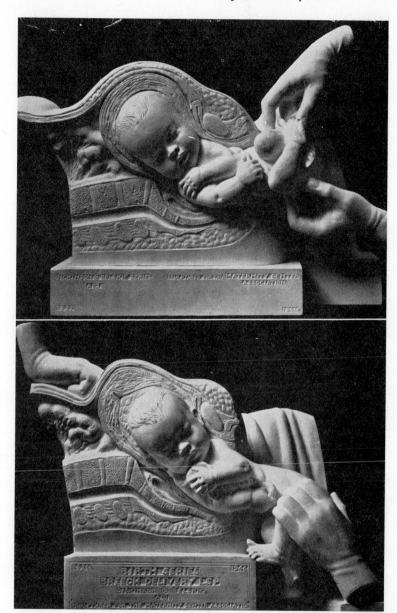

the continuous drip technic, as described on
page 435, is being used extensively in the treatment of dysfunctional labor. Sparteine sulfate
(Tocosamine) sometimes is used as an alternative to oxytocin to stimulate labor. It is
given in repeated doses until satisfactory
uterine action is achieved; however, there are
limits to the total dosage that can be used (see
p. 276). The intramuscular administration of
Tocosamine does not assure the precise and
controlled blood level of the drug that the

intravenous administration of oxytocin does.
In addition, the dosage cannot be discontinued or decreased readily, as can the oxytocin
infusion.

Abnormal Fetal Positions

Persistent Occiput Posterior Positions. As
stated on page 23 and illustrated in Figures
2-5 and 2-7, the fetal head usually enters the
pelvic inlet transversely and therefore must

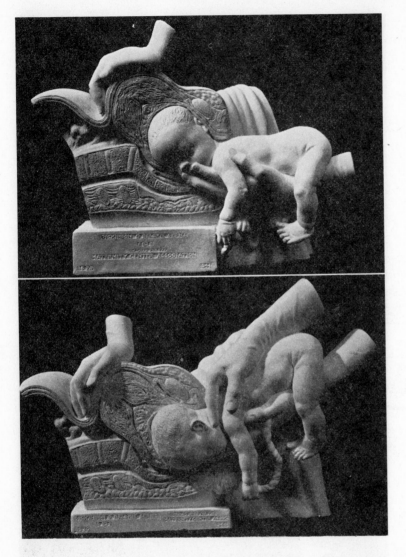

Fig. 19-3. (E, F) Delivery in footling breech presentation.

traverse an arc of 90° in the process of internal rotation to the direct occiput anterior position. In about a quarter of all labors, however, the head enters the pelvis with the occiput directed diagonally posterior, that is, in either the R.O.P. or the L.O.P. position. Under these circumstances the head must rotate through an arc of 135° in the process of internal rotation.

With good contractions, adequate flexion and a baby of average size, the great majority of these cases of occiput posterior position undergo spontaneous rotation through the 135° arc just as soon as the head reaches the pelvic floor. This is a normal mechanism of labor. It must be remembered, however, that labor is usually prolonged, and the mother has a great deal of discomfort in her back as the baby's head impinges against the sacrum in the course of rotating. Nursing intervention should be aimed at relieving the back pain as much as possible. Sacral pressure, backrubs and frequent change of position from side to side can be helpful, and they should be employed to the degree that seems to be well-tolerated by the patient. In a small minority of cases, however, perhaps 5 or 10 per cent, these favorable circumstances do not exist, and rotation may be incomplete or may not take place at all. If rotation is incomplete, the head becomes arrested in the transverse position, a condition known as *transverse arrest*. If anterior rotation does not take place at all, the occiput usually rotates to the direct occiput posterior position, a condition known as *persistent occiput posterior*. Both transverse arrest and persistent occiput posterior position represent deviations from the normal mechanisms of labor and may require operative delivery.

Breech Presentations. These are presentations in which the breech instead of the vertex presents at the pelvic brim. They occur in about 3 per cent of all term deliveries (see Chap. 5). In breech presentation the infant often passes meconium from his rectum during the course of labor, and after the membranes are ruptured, and the liquor amnii has escaped, the nurse may find the black, tar-colored material coming from the patient's vagina. She should make certain that the presentation is, in fact, a breech, for if such a phenomenon occurred in a vertex presentation, then it would be an indication of probable fetal distress.

Explanation and appropriate reassurance are important for mothers who have breech presentations, as they are for any patients having an abnormal presentation or complicated labor of any type. Many patients are steeped in old wives' folklore of the fearfulness of a "breech birth" and become exceedingly anxious and terrified as soon as they find out (or overhear) that theirs is this type of presentation; the same is often true of the husbands, and the anxiety and fear that are communicated from one partner to the other can impede the patient's working effectively with her labor. With modern obstetric technics and knowledge, labor need not be prolonged or exceptionally painful.

CLASSIFICATION. Breech presentations are classified as follows:

1. *Complete*, when the feet and the legs are flexed on the thighs, and the thighs are flexed on the abdomen, so that the buttocks and the feet present (see Fig. 5-6).

2. *Footling*, when one or both feet present through the cervix (Fig. 19-1).

3. *Frank*, when the legs are extended and lie against the abdomen and the chest, with the feet meeting the shoulders, and the buttocks present (Fig. 19-2).

DELIVERY. With strong contractions, particularly in multiparae, breech cases may be delivered spontaneously, or at least with very little aid by the attendant. The breech is pushed through the vulva as the result of the mother's bearing-down efforts and rises upward in front of the symphysis pubis. With the emergence of the trunk, the legs descend, the attendant simply receiving them and steadying the breech. With further bearing-down efforts, the shoulders are expelled; then, as the attendant holds up the body, the head is extruded with the face directed back at the perineum (Fig. 19-3 A to F).

However, in the majority of breech cases, especially in primigravidae, it is necessary for the physician to give more aid than is indicated above, and, as a rule, this amounts to extraction of the shoulders and the head after the umbilicus has appeared (Fig. 19-4).

Occasionally, cases of precipitate breech delivery may fall to the care of the nurse. These cases are uncommon and, when they do occur, seldom give rise to difficulty, because the very fact that they are precipitate presupposes a small infant, excellent expulsive forces and a capacious birth canal. As the breech emerges, it is received and is steadied with a sterile towel and sterile hands, and the mother is urged to bear down strongly. This usually will effect delivery of the shoulders in cases of this sort, but if it does not, the arm which is the more posterior is drawn out of the vagina by passing the first and the middle fingers over the infant's shoulder, down the arm to the elbow, and then drawing the forearm and the hand across the face and the chest and out. The other arm is delivered in the same way; and then, to favor the birth of the head, the body of the baby is raised upward in a vertical position. If there is any great delay, the nurse may place two fingers into the baby's mouth, with the trunk resting on the palm of the same hand and the legs straddling her forearm. Then, with the other hand, upward and outward traction is made on the shoulders, while firm downward pressure is made by an assistant on the lower abdominal wall. As with any other emergency delivery by the nurse, the nurse's composure and teamwork with the patient are important cornerstones to a successful outcome. (See Chap. 12.)

The great danger in breech delivery is to the baby as the result of the trauma which he may sustain in delivery. In footling presentations,

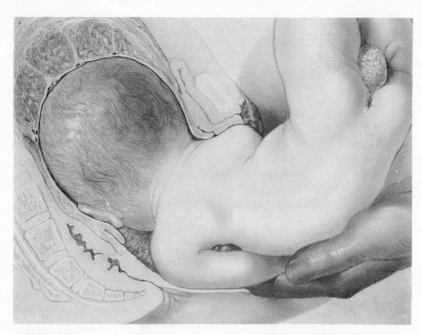

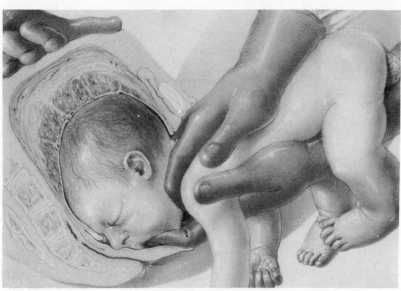

Fig. 19-4. (*Top*) Extraction of posterior shoulder in breech delivery. (*Bottom*) Extraction of head in breech delivery (Mauriceau maneuver).

prolapse of the umbilical cord (see p. 498) is common. Even in the most skilled hands, and considering only full-term infants, about 1 breech infant in 15 succumbs as the result of delivery. The danger to the mother is not appreciably greater than in vertex deliveries, but lacerations of the birth canal are more frequent.

Shoulder, Face and Brow Presentations. In shoulder presentations the infant lies crosswise in the uterus instead of longitudinally (see Fig. 5-8). This complication occurs about once in every 200 cases and is seen most often in multiparae. Not infrequently an arm prolapses into the vagina, making the problem of delivery even more difficult (Fig. 19-5). The physician usually will turn the infant in these cases, bringing a foot or both feet into the vagina, an operation known as "version" (p. 428). Shoulder presentation is a serious complication, occasionally causes rupture of the uterus (p. 496) and carries a much greater risk to the infant than either vertex or breech presentations.

Face presentations are also seen about once in every 200 cases. They usually terminate spontaneously, the face coming through the vulva with the chin anterior. As edema of the scalp is common in vertex presentations (caput succedaneum), so in face presentations the presenting part, the face, becomes greatly swollen and purplish. This disappears within a few days. Brow presentations are even more rare and are much more difficult to deliver because the largest diameter of the fetal head, the occipitomental, presents. They frequently convert themselves into face or occipital presentations; or the physician may convert them or perform version.

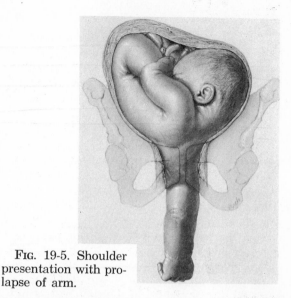

Fig. 19-5. Shoulder presentation with prolapse of arm.

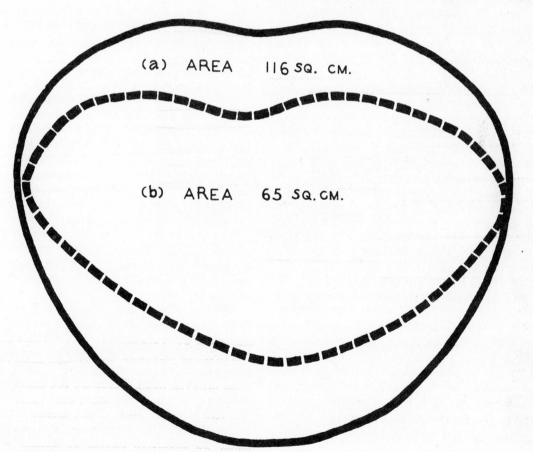

Fig. 19-6. Areas (actual size) of normal pelvic inlet (a) and contracted inlet (b). The extreme degree of pelvic contraction shown in (b) occurred in a 26-year-old Negro woman who had had severe rickets in infancy. This might have been prevented by giving cod liver oil in infancy and childhood. (J. H. H. 283193)

Disproportion

Contracted Pelvis. Disproportion between the size of the infant and that of the birth canal (commonly spoken of as cephalopelvic disproportion) is caused most frequently by contracted pelvis. The pelvis may be contracted at the inlet, the midpelvis or the outlet. In the case of inlet contraction the anteroposterior diameter of the inlet is shortened to 10 cm. or less, or the greatest transverse diameter is 12 cm. or less. The sacrum is broader and less concave from side to side, thinner from behind foreward and shorter from above downward. Figure 19-6 illustrates the shape of a contracted inlet as compared with that of a normal pelvic inlet. Inlet contraction is most often due to rickets, a fact indicating how much good may be accomplished by the prevention of rickets in infants and children through an adequate intake of vitamin D. Contracted pelvis due to rickets is much more common in the Negro race than in the white. In midpelvic contraction, the distance between the ischial spines is diminished; it is often found in conjunction with outlet contraction. In outlet contraction, the angle formed by the pubic rami is narrow, and the ischial tuberosities are close together; it thus resembles a male pelvis insofar as the outlet is concerned. This type of pelvic contraction occurs with equal frequency in the white and the Negro races, but its cause is not known. It is not only likely to hinder the egress of the infant at the outlet but also may be responsible for deep lacerations, since the narrow pubic rami tend to push the infant's head posteriorly in the direction of the rectum.

One of the main functions of antepartal care is to detect pelvic contraction during pregnancy, so that—long before labor begins—some intelligent decision can be reached about how best to deliver the infant. Of course, in such a case as that shown in Figure 19-6, cesarean section is obligatory. But all gradations of contracted pelvis are encountered, and, depending on the size of the infant and other factors, many patients with moderate degrees of the condition can be delivered vaginally without difficulty.

In doubtful cases the physician may give the patient a "trial labor," that is, 6 or 12 hours of labor to ascertain whether or not with adequate contractions the head will pass through the pelvis. For these patients labor may be even more anxiety-provoking than usual (depending in part on the extent and the depth of supportive antepartal counseling), and if cesarean section is the ultimate outcome, there may be a great deal of disappointment and perhaps even a feeling of failure. The warm empathic attitude of the nurse is particularly needed with these patients. Frequent reports on the progress of labor should not be overlooked when the progress is favorable; if it is not, then compensatory reassurance and anticipatory guidance regarding cesarean section may be given if the physician so desires. The health team does the patient a disservice in avoiding the subject if progress is not made in labor.

Oversize Baby. Excessive size of the infant is not commonly a cause of serious dystocia unless the fetus weighs over 4,500 Gm. (10 pounds). About 1 infant in 100 will fall in this class. The trauma associated with the passage of such huge infants through the birth canal causes a decided increase in fetal mortality; this has been estimated as 15 per cent (almost 1 in 6), in contrast with the usual death rate of 4 per cent for normal-size infants. Uterine inertia is frequent in labors with excessive-size infants, and at the time of delivery the shoulders may give great difficulty. Even though these infants are born alive, they often do poorly in the first few days because of cerebral hemorrhage and must be watched closely for signs of that condition (see Chap. 21).

One of the common causes of excessive-size infants is diabetes. Large infants are also more commonly seen in older multiparae and after prolonged pregnancies; the majority of such infants are boys.

Despite tales to the contrary, tremendously large infants—weighing over 13 pounds—are extremely rare and almost all are born dead. In 50,000 deliveries at the Johns Hopkins Hospital, there have been only two such cases. Both these infants were boys; the smaller, who weighed 13 pounds, 7 ounces, was the ninth child of a 34-year-old Negro woman; and the larger, 14 pounds, 4 ounces, was the seventh child of a white woman aged 44. The largest infant born at the New York Lying-In Hospital in 100,000 cases weighed 15 pounds. Although there may be rare exceptions, most stories that one hears of infants weighing over 15 pounds at birth are the result of either gross exaggeration or incorrect scales.

Hydrocephalus. Hydrocephalus, or an excessive accumulation of cerebrospinal fluid in the ventricles of the brain with consequent enlargement of the cranium, is encountered in 1 fetus in 2,000, approximately, and accounts for some 12 per cent of all malformations at birth. Associated defects are common, spina bifida being present in about one third of the cases. Varying degrees of cranial enlargement are produced, and not infrequently the circumference of the head exceeds 50 cm., sometimes reaching 80 cm. The amount of fluid present is usually between 500 and 1,500 cc., but as much as 5 liters has been reported. Since the distended cranium is too large to fit into the pelvic inlet, breech presentations are exceedingly common, being observed in about one third of such cases. Whatever the presentation, gross disproportion between the size of the head and that of the pelvis is the rule, and serious dystocia is the usual consequence. This is a tragic and serious complication of labor, and the obstetrician will find it necessary, as a rule, to puncture the cranial vault and aspirate as much of the cerebrospinal fluid as may be necessary to permit delivery. This procedure in itself does not injure the child. Nevertheless, fetal mortality is very high, 70 per cent (this percentage includes very mild forms of the disease).

Births of this type are a terrible tragedy for all concerned; the mother must undergo a difficult labor at great risk to herself, the husband will suffer with her, the fetus may expire, and the physician and the nurse must cope with a grave crisis with a poor prognosis. It is often difficult to describe the emotional climate at this time; perhaps it is impossible if one has not experienced a similar loss or disappointment. A state of emotional shock prevails, in which disbelief, noncomprehension and, sometimes, denial prevail. It seems to the husband and wife that the hopes and the dreams of 9 months and perhaps a lifetime lie shattered around them. This is a situation in which the nurse will be called on to exercise her nursing skill to the utmost, not only during labor but after the delivery, and particularly if there is an obvious abnormality, or if a fetal demise occurs. The components of care

that are useful in helping the parents in such a crisis are discussed fully in Chapter 21, Disorders of the Newborn.

HEMORRHAGIC COMPLICATIONS

Postpartal Hemorrhage

It has been said of the three stages of labor that the first stage is the most difficult for the physician and the nurse (because of the patience required during the long hours of waiting, that the second is the most difficult for the infant (because of the trauma and asphyxia it may undergo in passing through the birth canal); and that for the mother the third stage is the most dangerous because of the likelihood of postpartal hemorrhage and shock.

Definition and Incidence. The average blood loss postpartum is about 300 cc. The term "postpartal hemorrhage," as ordinarily used, does not refer to bleeding of this magnitude but only to excessive blood loss; and, by rather general consensus, when postpartal bleeding reaches 500 cc. or more, it is designated as "postpartal hemorrhage." Bleeding of this degree occurs in every 20 or 30 cases despite the most skilled care. Hemorrhages of 1,000 cc. and over are encountered once in about every 75 cases, whereas blood losses of even 1,500 and 2,000 cc. are encountered now and then. In other words, postpartal hemorrhage is a fairly common complication of labor. Moreover, it is one with which the nurse must be intimately familiar, because she will be expected to assume an important role in the prevention and treatment of the condition.

The Three Causes. In order of frequency, the three causes of postpartal hemorrhage are:

1. Uterine atony
2. Lacerations of the perineum, the vagina and the cervix
3. Retained placental fragments

Uterine atony is by far the most common cause. Again let us recall that the uterus contains huge blood vessels within the interstices of its muscle fibers, and that those at the placental site are open and gaping. It is essential that the muscle fibers contract down tightly on these arteries and veins, if bleeding is to be controlled. They must *stay* contracted down, for only a few seconds' relaxation will give rise to sudden, profuse hemorrhage. They must stay *tightly* contracted down, because continuous, slight relaxation gives rise to continuous oozing of blood, one of the most treacherous forms of postpartal hemorrhage.

Lacerations of the perineum, the vagina and the cervix are naturally more common after operative delivery. Tears of the cervix are particularly likely to cause serious hemorrhage. Bright red arterial bleeding in the presence of a hard, firmly contracted uterus (no uterine atony) suggests hemorrhage from a cervical laceration. The physician will establish the diagnosis by actual inspection of the cervix (retractors are necessary) and, after locating the source of bleeding, will repair the laceration.

Retained Placental Fragments. Small, partially separated fragments of placenta may cause postpartal hemorrhage by interfering with proper uterine contraction. Careful inspection of the placenta to determine whether a piece is missing will rule out or confirm the diagnosis; the treatment, obviously, is to remove the placental fragment. This is an uncommon cause of postpartal hemorrhage, but occasionally the nurse will encounter cases in which profuse bleeding occurs suddenly a week or more after delivery. These late hemorrhages are usually designated by the term "puerperal hemorrhage." They are almost always caused by a retained placental fragment.

Predisposing Factors. There are certain factors which predispose to postpartal hemorrhage, so that to a certain extent it may be anticipated in advance. Among these, one of the most important is the size of the infant. With a 9-pound infant, the chances of postpartal hemorrhage are 5 times as great as they are with a 5-pound infant. Excessive bleeding is twice as common in twin pregnancy. Hydramnios (excessive amount of amniotic fluid) is another predisposing factor. Other conditions in which postpartal hemorrhage is extremely frequent are premature separation of the placenta and placenta previa. Finally, operative delivery, particularly if a prolonged general anesthetic has been given, greatly increases the likelihood of this complication.

Clinical Picture. Excessive bleeding may occur prior to the birth of the placenta, but it is seen more commonly thereafter. Although it is occasionally torrential in character, the most common type is a continuous trickle—minute by minute. These small constant trickles are not alarming in appearance, consequently, no one may become alarmed, and no one may do anything. This is what makes this type of hemorrhage so treacherous. This fact has been emphasized particularly by Doctor Beecham, of Philadelphia, in his survey of 52 deaths from postpartal hemorrhage which occurred in that city. The average interval between delivery and death in this series was 5 hours and 20 minutes. Only 6 patients, 11.5 per cent, died within 2 hours of delivery, and none in less than 1½ hours. In other words, there would have been ample time for intensive treatment in any of these cases, had the attendant known how much blood was being lost.

Treatment. The first and most important thing to do is to grasp the uterus and massage it vigorously. This must be continued until the uterus assumes a woody hardness; if the slightest relaxation occurs, the massage must be reinstituted. In many cases the uterus stays contracted most of the time but occasionally relaxes; it is therefore obligatory to keep a hand on the fundus constantly for a full hour after bleeding has subsided. When the uterus is well contracted, care should be taken *to avoid overmassage,* because such practice contributes to muscle fatigue, which in turn further encourages uterine relaxation and excessive bleeding. Even then the danger is not over, since relaxation sometimes occurs 2 or more hours after delivery; in these cases the uterus may balloon with blood, with very little escaping externally. Accordingly, the consistency, size and the height of the uterus should be checked frequently until several hours have elapsed. Ordinarily, the height of the fundus after delivery will be about at the level of the umbilicus. If the uterus becomes distended with blood, or if the bladder becomes full and presses upward against the uterus, causing it to rise in the abdomen, then the fundus can be palpated several centimeters above the umbilicus. The nurse must make absolutely certain that she is actually massaging the uterus and not a roll of abdominal fat or a distended bladder (see pp. 277, 312). When properly contracted, the uterus should feel like a small- to medium-sized hard grape-

Fig. 19-7. Bimanual compression of uterus in treatment of postpartal hemorrhage.

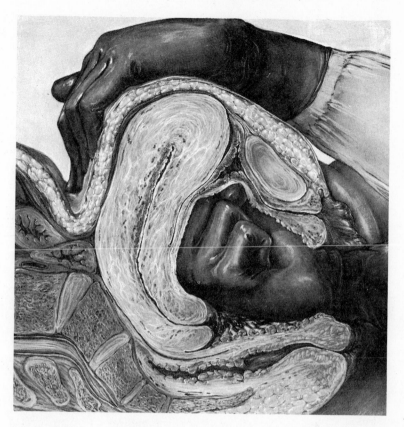

fruit. Frequently, a big, boggy, relaxed uterus is difficult to outline through the abdominal wall, and it may be necessary to push the hand well posteriorly toward the region of the sacral promontory to reach it. The very fact that the uterus is hard to identify usually means that it is relaxed. If the nurse is not sure that she is feeling the uterus, she should inform the physician at once.

ALLAYING ANXIETY. The frequent massage and deep palpation are often painful to the mother; at best they are disturbing, since they come at a time when the mother wants nothing more than to rest and sleep after her great effort. If she is awake and alert, then the continued attention and scrutiny may increase her anxiety. It must be remembered that apprehension is a natural concomitant of hemorrhage and shock. Therefore the nurse should take pains to make her observations as quickly and efficiently as possible and to allay the mother's (and father's) concern by appropriate explanation and reassurance.

This aspect of nursing care may be difficult to implement. If the mother or the father expresses concern and questions the activity by asking "What's wrong?" then say simply, "The uterus has a tendency to relax, and must be massaged so that it will contract down as it should." Usually, such a statement will suffice. This will indicate to the mother and father the reason for the continued activity without associating hemorrhage and its fearsome consequences with the actions of the attendants. If the mother drifts off to sleep between the nurse's observations, then the nurse should gently rouse her by speaking her name before she commences massage, so that the mother is not awakened abruptly to the painful sensation of someone squeezing her abdomen.

OTHER ASPECTS OF CARE. Vital signs will be required every 5 to 15 minutes, and any variation, however slight, should be reported immediately. One of the most perfidious things about postpartal hemorrhage is the fact that the blood pressure and the pulse may show only moderate alterations until a large amount of blood has been lost. Then, when the vascular system can no longer compensate for the diminished blood volume, the pulse increases rapidly, the blood pressure drops precipitously, and shock ensues.

One way that the nurse can keep a more accurate account of the blood loss is to keep a perineal pad count. In doing this she counts the number of pads saturated, how fully they are saturated, and the time it took for the saturation to occur. Thus, her nurse's notes might read: "Two pads ¾ saturated in 20 minutes." This type of report is more helpful to the physician than a more general, vague statement like, "Saturating perineal pads quickly."

If the bleeding occurs prior to delivery of the placenta, the physician may find it necessary to extract the placenta manually. (A change of gloves as well as gown may be called for to ensure strict asepsis, since the uterine cavity is to be invaded.) Oxytocics will invariably be requested, ergonovine or oxytocin or both intramuscularly. One or the other of these may be given intravenously by the physician.

If these measures fail to stop the bleeding, the physician probably will carry out bimanual compression of the organ (Fig. 19-7). This provides the most efficient means of massaging and compressing the uterus. Packing the uterus with gauze, a procedure once considered valuable to promote hemostasis in such cases, is seldom utilized today. It is considered by many authorities, e.g., Eastman, Hellman, Cosgrove, Leff and Berkeley, to be inadequate and conducive to infection. If shock threatens, the Trendelenburg position should be employed, external heat applied, and preparations for blood transfusion made.

In the handling of a case of postpartal hemorrhage, the nurse may be taxed to her utmost. The physician in charge may have to search for and suture a cervical laceration or start a blood transfusion or even resuscitate the infant; another physician may be needed to give the anesthesia. To the nurse, or nurses, will usually fall the important tasks of massaging the uterus, giving oxytocics, helping with the transfusion and caring for the infant. The nurse must be prepared to act quickly and efficiently if the lives of these bleeding mothers are to be saved.

If postpartal hemorrhage should occur after the physician has left, the nurse should grasp the uterus at once, press out as much blood as possible and begin vigorous massage, sending word, of course, to the physician. If massage fails to stop the bleeding, the physician usually will not object if the nurse gives the patient an intramuscular injection of ergonovine or oxytocin. If possible, this arrangement should be understood beforehand.

Late Postpartal Hemorrhage. Occasionally, postpartal hemorrhage may occur later than the first day following delivery. These late postpartal hemorrhages may take place any time between the 2nd and the 28th day, are usually sudden in onset and may be so massive as to produce shock; they are due almost always to retained placental fragments. Late postpartal hemorrhage is fortunately uncommon, occurring perhaps once in 1,000 cases. The physician probably will carry out instrumental dilatation of the cervix, followed by removal of the placental fragments either with a curet or ovum forceps.

Rupture of Uterus

Rupture of the uterus is fortunately a rare complication, but when it does occur, it constitutes one of the gravest accidents in obstetrics, since almost all of the infants and about a third of the mothers are lost. In this condition the uterus simply bursts, because the strain placed upon its musculature is more than it can withstand. It may occur in pregnancy but is more frequent in labor. In modern obstetrics the most common cause is rupture of the scar of a previous cesarean section. Accordingly, when observing labor in a patient who has had a previous cesarean section, the possibility of this accident always should be borne in mind. Other contributing factors include prolonged and/or obstructed labor, certain faulty presentations, multiparity, traumatic delivery, such as version and extraction, and the injudicious use of oxytocin in labor. When rupture occurs, the patient complains of a severe, sudden, lancinating pain during a strong labor contraction. The rupture may be complete or incomplete; pain and abdominal tenderness are always present in both cases. If there is complete rupture, regular contractions cease, since the torn muscle can no longer contract. There is an outpouring of blood into the abdominal cavity and sometimes into the vagina. The uterus may be palpated abdominally as a hard mass lying alongside the fetus. The patient soon exhibits signs of shock: her pulse is rapid and weak, her skin cool and clammy, her face may be pale and her nostrils dilated, a sign of air hunger. If the rupture is incomplete, the contractions may continue, and the signs of shock may be delayed, since the blood loss is slower. As soon as the diagnosis of rupture of the uterus is made, rapid preparations for an abdominal operation should ensue, since hysterectomy is the usual treatment. In addition, antibiotics are administered to combat infection, and blood transfusions are given to replace blood loss and to alleviate shock. Since this accident gravely compromises the lives of both the infant and the mother, early diagnosis, prompt treatment, blood transfusions and antibiotics are essential components in improving the prognosis.

AMNIOTIC FLUID EMBOLISM

At any time after the membranes have ruptured there is a possibility that amniotic fluid may enter the gaping venous sinuses of the placental site as well as the veins in the cervix, be drawn into the general circulation and in this way reach the pulmonary capillaries. Since the amniotic fluid invariably contains small particles of matter, such as vernix caseosa, lanugo and sometimes meconium, multiple tiny emboli may reach the lungs in this manner and cause occlusion of the pulmonary capillaries. This complication, amniotic fluid embolism, is almost invariably fatal and, as a rule, causes the death of the mother within 1 or 2 hours. Fortunately, this tragic condition is rare, occurring only once in many thousand labors.

The clinical characteristics of the condition are sudden dyspnea, cyanosis, pulmonary edema, profound shock and uterine relaxation with postpartal hemorrhage. A highly important feature of amniotic fluid embolism is a diminution in the fibrinogen content of the blood, or hypofibrinogenemia. The mechanism is similar to, if not identical with, that which occurs in abruptio placentae and missed abortion, as described on pages 457 and 465.

The treatment consists of oxygen therapy,

blood transfusion and the intravenous administration of fibrinogen, but, as indicated, this is usually futile.

ACCIDENTAL COMPLICATIONS

Lacerations of Perineum

Lacerations have already been referred to as a cause of postpartal hemorrhage. In addition, perineal tears may do great damage in destroying the integrity of the perineum and in weakening the supports of the uterus, the bladder and the rectum. Unless these lacerations are repaired properly, the resultant weakness, as the years go by, may cause prolapse of the uterus (called by the laity "falling of the womb"), cystocele (a pouching downward of the bladder) or rectocele (a pouching forward of the rectum). These conditions, which originate from perineal lacerations at childbirth, give rise to many discomforts and often necessitate operative treatment.

Because lacerations of the birth canal sometimes occur during the process of normal delivery, and are sometimes unavoidable even

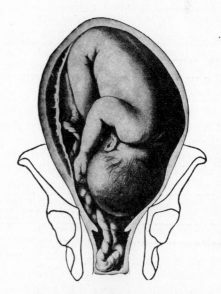

FIG. 19-8. Prolapse of the umbilical cord (Bumm). As the head comes down, the compression of the cord between the fetal skull and the pelvic brim will shut off its circulation completely.

in the most skilled hands, this subject has already been discussed in Chapter 12.

Prolapse of Umbilical Cord

In the course of labor, the cord prolapses in front of the presenting part about once in every 400 cases. It is a grave complication for the fetus, since the cord is then compressed between the head and the bony pelvis, and the fetal circulation is shut off (Fig. 19-8). The accident is usually due to premature rupture of the membranes when the head, the breech or the shoulder is not sufficiently down in the pelvis to prevent the cord from being washed past it in the sudden gush of amniotic fluid. After the membranes rupture, the cord comes down, and it may be either a concealed or an apparent prolapse. In the latter instance, the diagnosis is made when the cord is seen; but when the cord is not visible, the correct diagnosis will not be made unless the patient is examined and the cord is felt, or examination of the fetal heart reveals distress due to pressure on the cord. This is why it *must* be a routine practice to listen to the fetal heart sounds immediately after the membranes rupture and again in about 10 minutes.

If the nurse is alone with the patient, she should send immediately for the physician and then attempt to relieve the pressure on the cord by elevating the patient's hips, thus allowing the head to gravitate away from the pelvis. This takes place in either the "knee-chest position" (see Fig. 14-25) or the Trendelenburg position. In the home the latter is arranged by slipping the back of a straight-backed chair, covered with a flat pillow, under the buttocks and the shoulders, with the knees down over the rungs of the chair. In putting the patient in such a position, her hips must be kept raised above the level of her shoulders. If the patient is unable to remain in either of these positions very long, she may be put in the elevated Sims's position, that is, on her side with the hips elevated by pillows in order to raise the hips higher than the thorax. Any change in position must be carried out slowly!

If the physician is expected to arrive on the scene within the next 15 minutes, this is all that the nurse should do. If he can be reached by telephone in this period, instructions about further therapy should be sought. If no medical advice can be obtained at the end of 15 minutes, and the umbilical cord is protruding from the vagina, the nurse should protect the exposed cord with sterile wet saline dressings, if they are available. In handling the cord, great care must be exercised not to compress it. The nurse should *never* attempt to replace a prolapsed cord into the vagina.

This particular complication is not painful for the mother; however, it can be very frightening, for many patients realize it can result in their infant's death. Also whether they realize the grave implications or not, the various antic positions and quickened responses of the attendants give them an indication that all is not well. Therefore, again, the calmness, warmth and efficiency of the nurse can do much to reassure the patient that all possible measures are being taken to bring the situation under control. It goes without saying that these patients never should be left unattended, and the husbands, if they are present, should be treated with consideration. It is difficult, when any crises occur, to deal with the husband or relatives of the patient with appropriate thoughtfulness, since most of the energy is directed toward meeting the pressing (and often lifesaving) demands of the situation. However, it must be remembered that the patient and her husband are considered as a unit, and a few moments usually can be found to apprise the husband of what is being done for his wife.

Inversion of Uterus

Inversion of the uterus is a rare and highly fatal accident of labor in which, after the birth of the infant, the uterus turns inside out. Shock is profound, in many cases causing the death of the mother. This rare complication is mentioned here only to stress the two common causes: (1) pulling on the umbilical cord and (2) trying to express the placenta when the uterus is relaxed. In the former case, the traction on the attached placenta simply pulls the uterus inside out, while in the latter the hand pushes the relaxed muscular sac inside out. The umbilical cord *never* should be pulled on, and the uterus *never* should be pushed upon unless it is firmly contracted.

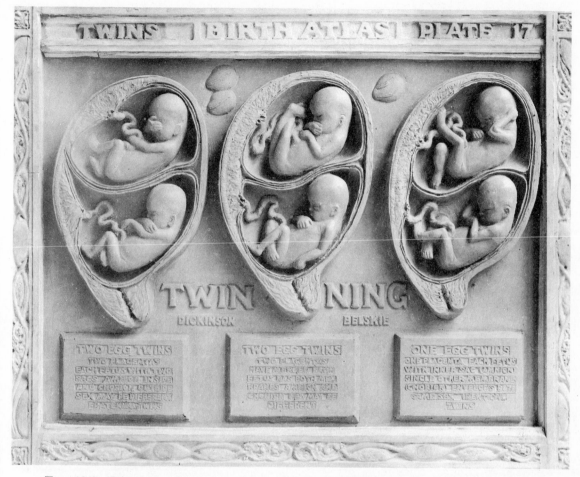

FIG. 19-9. One-egg and two-egg twins. (Dickinson-Belskie models, Cleveland Health Museum, Cleveland)

FIG. 19-10. Single- and double-ovum twin differences. A and B, double-ovum twins; there are two chorions; in B the two placentas have fused. C, single-ovum twins; there is only one chorion and one placenta.

MULTIPLE PREGNANCY

When two or more embryos develop in the uterus at the same time, the condition is known as multiple pregnancy. Twins occur approximately once in every 54 births in the white race and once in every 39 births in non-white races. Triplets occur approximately once in 9,400 births; and quadruplets, once in 620,-000. These statistics have been altered somewhat due to the recent advancements in hormone therapy for infertility. Over 40 cases of quintuplets have been recorded, but with a few notable exceptions, none of these infants has survived more than a few weeks. The Dionne quintuplets, the most familiar case, were exceptional in that they were the first to live to adulthood.

Heredity plays an important causative role in twin pregnancy, and if there are twins in the family of either the expectant mother or her husband, the likelihood of twins is greater.

Twins may be of two kinds: identical and nonidentical. Identical twins *are* identical because they come from a single egg; hence they are called "single-ovum twins." Fertilization takes place in the usual way, by a single spermatozoon, but then, very early in the ovum's development, it divides into 2 identical parts instead of continuing as a single individual. Such twins are always of the same sex and, as we have implied, show close physical and mental resemblances. Nonidentical twins come from the fertilization of two ova by two spermatozoa and are therefore known as "double-ovum twins" (Fig. 19-9). Such twins, according to chance, may be of the same sex or of opposite sexes; and the likelihood of their resembling each other is no greater than that of any brother and sister.

Single-ovum twins have 1 placenta and 1 chorion, but there are normally 2 amnions and 2 umbilical cords (Fig. 19-10). In double-ovum twins each fetus has its own chorion, amnion, cord and placenta, but the placentas may be partially fused. These double-ovum twins are much the more common of the two types, making up about 85 per cent of all twins.

In the majority of instances (but not all) it is possible for the physician to make a diagnosis of twins by abdominal examination during the last few months; in doubtful cases, a roentgenogram may be necessary to settle the question.

Twins are likely to be born about 2 weeks before the calculated date of delivery. Even though pregnancy goes to full term, twins are usually smaller than single infants by nearly 1 pound; however, the outlook for such infants, provided that the pregnancy continues into the last month, is almost as good as that for single infants.

The patient with a multiple pregnancy faces greater discomforts and greater hazards than does a woman with a single pregnancy. The latter weeks of a twin pregnancy are likely to be associated with heaviness of the lower abdomen, back pains and swelling of the feet and the ankles. Abdominal distention makes sleeping difficult, and therefore the doctor may prescribe a hypnotic. A well-fitting maternity girdle will make daytime more comfortable for her. Because of the excessive abdominal size, the patient may find that frequent small feedings are more suitable than the usual three larger meals a day. The nurse can be very helpful in giving the mother anticipatory guidance regarding these matters during the antepartal period.

Moreover, there are serious complications which these patients are particularly prone to develop: premature labors, toxemia and postpartal hemorrhage. Coitus probably will be restricted during the last 3 months of pregnancy to mitigate against the possibility of early labor. Also travel will be curtailed, since labor may begin at any time without warning, and delivery in strange surroundings may be hazardous. The mother will be encouraged to take frequent afternoon rests and to avoid activities involving physical strain.

The antepartal course of these patients should be followed with special care for signs of toxemia. Thus, the mother's antepartal visits usually will be more frequent to ensure meticulous supervision. A low-salt diet and diuretics will be ordered when indicated. In addition, iron may be prescribed, since anemia is usual in multiple pregnancy.

Postpartal hemorrhage is twice as common in twin pregnancy, although mechanical difficulties in labor are less frequent than might be expected. Uterine dysfunction, however, is encountered rather often. A spontaneous delivery is particularly desired in instances of twins, since this type of delivery results in less blood loss and maternal morbidity and a greater likelihood of healthy, undamaged infants.

At delivery, when the first baby is born, the physician usually has to rupture the membranes of the second twin. Then with combined vaginal and abdominal manipulation, he turns the infant to either a breech or a vertex presentation. *Judicious* abdominal pressure is used to propel the presenting part through the birth canal and effect either a spontaneous delivery or forceps or breech extraction. Occasionally, a version and extraction (see p. 428) may be necessitated if the vaginal and abdominal maneuvers are unsuccessful.

As soon as the second twin is delivered, the doctor will order an oxytocic to be given, and the nurse should assist the obstetrician in observing the fundus carefully for distention due to an accumulation of blood. An intravenous infusion of glucose usually will be administered prophylactically. To guard against uterine atony and blood loss, after the placentae are expressed, oxytocin will be added to the infusion to ensure a firmly contracted uterus.

NURSING CARE. As with any delivery, the nurse will have the responsibility of supportive care for the patient as well as assisting the doctor in whatever activities are indicated. Since these infants are apt to be small, oxygen and/or resuscitative measures may be necessary. The care will be similar to that for the premature baby (see Chap. 16). Any supplies and/or equipment that may be needed (resuscitator, oxygen apparatus, etc.) should be procured early in the delivery and kept in readiness (but out of the patient's sight, if possible). Maternal vital signs as well as the fetal heart tones should be checked frequently.

Two other points should be considered. Especially in the case of undiagnosed twins (i.e., the presence of twins is not discovered or suspected until labor and delivery), there is a decided psychological and economic (albeit somewhat delayed) shock to the parents. Emotionally, one additional child may be desired and acceptable; two may impose a burden, particularly if this pregnancy was to be "the last." The parents may wonder if they can manage the care of two newborn infants simultaneously. Problems may be compounded in feeding, especially if the mother is desirous of nursing her infant. In addition, two of everything must be provided, instead of one, and this additional cost may put a strain on the budget. In terms of long-range planning, the present housing may be inadequate, especially if the children are of different sexes and eventually will require separate rooms. The cost entailed in additional construction and/or new housing is considerable. None of these problems is insurmountable and can be worked through satisfactorily in time. Some parents need an understanding and empathic person to help them over the initial adjustment period. In some cases they may need the help of a social worker or a public health nurse to help them plan for the unexpected new baby. Many parents seem to adjust nicely with being able merely to ventilate their surprise (and, in some cases, chagrin). Certainly the professional nurse is able and qualified to give this type of support.

SUGGESTED READING

Bruce, Sylvia: Reactions of nurses and mothers to stillbirths, Nurs. Outlook 10:88-91, February, 1962.

Donnelly, J. F.: Toxemias of pregnancy, Am. J. Nurs. 61:101, April, 1961.

Eastman, N. J., and Hellman, L. M.: Williams' Obstetrics, ed. 13, New York, Appleton, 1966.

Filler, W. W., Filler, N. W., and Zinberg, S.: Sparteine sulfate in labor, Am. J. Obstet. Gynec. 88:737-746, March 15, 1964.

Goodrich, F. W., Jr.: Obstetrical hemorrhage, Am. J. Nurs. 62:96-98, November, 1962.

Hendricks, C. H., et al.: The pharmacologic control of excessive uterine activity with isoxsuprine, Am. J. Obstet. Gynec. 82:1064-1078, November, 1961.

Hutchinson, H. T., et al.: Effects of magnesium sulfate on uterine contractility, intrauterine fetus, and infant, Am. J. Obstet. Gynec. 88:747-758, March 15, 1964.

Morgan, H. S., and Kane, S. H.: An analysis of 16,327 breech births, J.A.M.A. 187:262-264, January 25, 1964.

Morrison, J. E.: Pathological anatomy of anoxia, Cereb. Palsy Bull. 3:559-565, December, 1961.

Pinto, R. M., et al.: Action of estradiol 17 on

activity of the pregnant human uterus, Am. J. Obstet. Gynec. 88:59-69, March 15, 1964.

Rubin, A., and Grimm, G.: Results in breech presentation—a 7-year study, Am. J. Obstet. Gynec. 86:1048-1049, August 15, 1960.

Skipper, J. K., *et al.*: Barriers to communication between patients and hospital functionaries, Nurs. Forum 11, No. 1:14-23, 1963.

Tucker, J. M.: Nursing care in obstetric hemorrhage, Am. J. Nurs. 62:98-99, November, 1962.

Willson, J. R.: Management of Obstetrical Difficulties, ed. 6, St. Louis, Mosby, 1961.

Puerperal Infection • Subinvolution of the Uterus • Hemorrhage (See Chap. 19) • Vulvar Hematomas • Disorders of the Breasts • Bladder Complications • Puerperal Psychoses (See Chap. 9) • Pulmonary Embolism

Chapter 20

Complications of the Puerperium

PUERPERAL INFECTION

When inflammatory processes develop in the birth canal postpartally, as the result of bacterial invasion of these highly vulnerable areas, the condition is known as puerperal infection. It is really a postpartal wound infection of the birth canal, usually of the endometrium. As is true of other wound infections, the condition often remains localized but may extend along various pathways to produce diverse clinical pictures. Febrile reactions of more or less severity are the rule, and the outcome varies according to the portal of entry, the type, the number and the virulence of the invading organisms, the reaction of the tissues and the general resistance of the patient.

Puerperal infection is one of the most common causes of death in childbearing. Frequently used (but less satisfactory) synonyms are puerperal fever, puerperal sepsis, puerperal septicemia and childbed fever.

Causative Factors

The vast majority of puerperal infections are caused by the streptococcus, but most of the well-known pathogenic bacteria—such as the staphylococcus, the colon bacillus and the Welch bacillus—may be responsible for the disease.

What are the sources of these bacteria? The late Dr. John Osborne Polak, of Brooklyn,

N. Y., used to teach that there are "eleven causes" of puerperal infection—the 10 fingers and the nasopharynx. He meant by this that the attendants themselves are most likely to carry infection to the parturient uterus. The physician may inadvertently do so in two ways. In the first place, gloved and sterile though his hands may be during the vaginal examinations or the operative manipulations, he may carry bacteria already in the vagina upward into the uterus. In the second place, his hands and the instruments he uses may become contaminated by virulent streptococci as the result of droplet infection, dispersed by himself or some of the attendants, and in this manner he may be responsible for introducing bacteria into the birth canal. Even in modern obstetrics, the latter is a very common mode of infection, and unless the utmost vigilance is used in masking all attendants in the delivery room (both nose and mouth) and in excluding therefrom all persons suffering or recovering from an upper respiratory infection, it is a constant source of danger.

Although a less common means of transfer today than a few decades ago, careless physicians and nurses have been known to carry bacteria to the parturient from countless extraneous contacts—from other cases of puerperal infection, from suppurative postoperative wounds, from cases of sloughing carcinoma, from patients with scarlet fever, from infants with impetigo neonatorum, from umbilical infections of the newborn and, finally, from the autopsy table. The physician himself may have the infection on his own person, such as an infected hangnail or felon.

Coitus late in pregnancy is more common than ordinarily believed and may introduce extraneous organisms to the birth canal or carry upward bacteria already present on the vulva or in the lower vagina.

During the second stage of labor, the chances of fecal matter being transferred to the vagina are great, another constant source of danger.

Following completion of the third stage of labor, the site of previous placental attachment is a raw, elevated area, deep red in color and about 4 cm. in diameter. Its surface is nodular, due to the presence of numerous gaping veins, many of which are occluded by clots. These form excellent culture media for bacteria. Furthermore, at this time, the condition of the entire endometrium is peculiarly favorable to bacterial invasion, since it is less than 2 mm. thick, is infiltrated with blood and presents numerous small wounds. Since the cervix rarely escapes some degree of laceration in labor, it is another ready site for bacterial invasion. Vulvar, vaginal and perineal wounds offer still other possible portals of entry.

Puerperal infection is much more likely to occur if the mother has had a traumatic labor or a postpartal hemorrhage. Therefore, hemorrhage and trauma must be regarded as important predisposing causes of this infection. Other causes in this respect are prolonged labor, prolonged rupture of the membranes, retention of placental tissue and pre-existing conditions, such as anemia, which lower the mother's general resistance to disease.

Prevention of Infection

The prevention of infection throughout the maternity cycle has been emphasized in foregoing sections as an important factor in the maintenance of health and the prevention of disease. During pregnancy, blood studies are done routinely and iron prescribed as necessary, not only for the immediate value but also because anemia predisposes to puerperal infection. A great deal of emphasis is placed on health teaching at this time, particularly in regard to general hygiene. The patient is advised to avoid all possible sources of infection. Some physicians advise against tub baths in the last weeks of pregnancy, because the bath water may introduce surface bacteria from the body into the vagina, particularly in multiparas. It is well for the nurse to recognize that this idea is still prevalent in many circles, although it is now believed to have little validity. The greatest hazard of tub baths in these last weeks of pregnancy arises because climbing in and out of the tub is awkward and sudden changes in balance might result in a fall and, thus, the likelihood of physical trauma. Coitus should be avoided during the last two months of pregnancy, and vaginal douches after the fifth month. Contacts with upper respiratory infections should always be avoided.

During labor, care should be exercised to limit bacteria from extraneous sources. In the hospital, cleanliness and good housekeeping are imperative, but, nevertheless, individual care technic reduces the chance of contamination from other patients. Each patient should have all of "her own" equipment, which includes her own bedpan. This bedpan should be cleansed after each use and sterilized once a day. Scrupulous hand washing on the part of all personnel after contacts with each patient will do much to prevent the transfer of infection from one patient to another. The strictest rules should be enforced for surgical cleanliness during labor and delivery. No one with an infection of the skin or the respiratory tract should work in the maternity department. The nasopharynx of attendants is the most common source of contamination of the birth canal. Masks usually should be worn any time that the external genitalia are exposed for examination or treatments, in the labor room as well as in the delivery room. To be effective, masks must cover the nose and the mouth and be clean and dry; thus they must be changed frequently and should not hang around the neck when not in use.

During the puerperium the same careful precautions should be carried out. For many days following the delivery, the surface of the birth canal is a vulnerable area for pathogenic bacteria. The birth canal is well protected against the invasion of extraneous bacteria by the closed vulva, unless this barrier is invaded.

Patients should be taught the principles of perineal hygiene and how to give themselves self-care. The nurse should remember never to use her fingers to separate the labia in giving perineal care, because this permits the cleansing solution to enter the vagina.

Types of Puerperal Infection

Generally speaking, puerperal infection can be divided into two main types: (1) *local processes* and (2) *extensions of the original process.* When a lesion of the vulva, the perineum, the vagina, the cervix or the endometrium becomes infected, the infection may remain localized in these wounds. However, the original inflammatory process may extend along the veins (the most common way) and cause thrombophlebitis and pyemia, or through the lymph vessels to cause peritonitis and pelvic cellulitis.

Lesions of the Perineum, the Vulva and the Vagina. These lesions are highly vulnerable areas for bacterial invasion in the early puerperium and so may become infected. The most common of these is a localized infection of a repaired perineal laceration or episiotomy wound. The usual symptoms are elevation of temperature, pain and sensation of heat in the affected area and burning on urination. The area involved becomes red and edematous, and there is profuse seropurulent discharge. If a wound of the vulva becomes infected, the entire vulva may become edematous and ulcerated. Infections involving the perineum, the vulva and the vagina cause the patient considerable discomfort and alarm. These local inflammatory processes seldom cause severe physical reactions, provided that good drainage is established, and the patient's temperature remains below 38.4° C. (101° F.). To promote good drainage, all stitches must be removed so that the surface is laid open. Because the drainage itself is a source of irritation and contamination, the wound must be kept clean and the perineal pads changed frequently. Care must be exercised in cleansing the wound to see that none of the solution runs into the vagina. It is understood, of course, that vaginal douches would never be given at this time. Treatments by such means as sitz baths or the perineal heat lamp are generally used for the relief of pain. Antibi-

otics or one of the sulfonamides is prescribed to combat the infection. If drainage is impaired, the patient not only will have more pain but also may have a chill, followed by a sudden elevation of temperature.

Endometritis. This is a localized infection of the lining membrane of the uterus. Bacteria invade the lesion, usually the placental site, and may spread to involve the entire endometrium. When endometritis develops, it usually manifests itself about the 3rd or the 4th day after delivery. In the milder forms the patient may have no complaints or symptoms other than a rise in temperature to about 38.4° C. (101° F.) which persists for several days and then subsides. On the other hand, the more virulent infections are often ushered in by chills and high fever, with a comparable rise in pulse rate. In the majority of severe cases the patient experiences a chilly sensation, or actual chills, at the onset and often complains of malaise, loss of appetite, headache, backache and general discomfort. It is not unusual for the patient to have severe and prolonged after-pains. The uterus is invariably large and is extremely tender when palpated abdominally. The lochial discharge is increased in amount and distinguished from normal lochia by its dark brown appearance and foul odor. If the infection remains localized in the endometrium, it is usually over in about a week or 10 days. But when extension of the infection occurs to cause peritonitis, pelvic thrombophlebitis or cellulitis, the disease may persist for many weeks, often with dramatic temperature curves and repeated chills.

TREATMENT depends on the severity of the condition. Mild cases with temperature under 100° F. and no chills are best handled by simple measures. Fowler's position facilitates lochial drainage. Ergonovine 4 times daily for 2 days promotes uterine tone, and forced fluids provide additional support. However, isolation is desirable to protect other patients and to afford the mother greater rest. In this group it is unnecessary to discontinue breast-feeding.

In severe cases breast-feeding is discontinued not only because it exhausts the mother but also because it is usually futile in the presence of high fever. In addition to the routine measures, antimicrobial drugs may be indicated.

Thrombophlebitis. This is an infection of

the vascular endothelium with clot formation attached to the vessel wall. It may be of two types: pelvic thrombophlebitis, an inflammatory process involving the ovarian and the uterine veins, or femoral thrombophlebitis, in which the femoral, the popliteal or the saphenous vein is involved. The latter type of thrombophlebitis is often spoken of as phlegmasia alba dolens (painful white inflammation) and also very frequently as "milk leg"—a term once given to the condition by physicians in the belief that it was due to the collection of milk in the affected leg. Early ambulation may be a factor in preventing this complication.

FEMORAL THROMBOPHLEBITIS. This condition presents a special group of signs and symptoms. It is a disease of the puerperium characterized by pain, fever and swelling in the affected leg. These symptoms are due to the formation of a clot in the veins of the leg itself, which interferes with the return circulation of the blood. When "milk leg" develops, it usually appears about 10 days after labor, although it may manifest itself as late as the 20th day. As in all acute febrile diseases occurring after labor, the secretion of milk may cease when phlegmasia alba dolens develops.

The disease is ushered in with malaise, chilliness and fever, which are soon followed by stiffness and pain in the affected part. If it is in the leg, the pain may begin in the groin or the hip and extend downward, or it may commence in the calf of the leg and extend upward. In about 24 hours the leg begins to swell, and although the pain then lessens slightly, it is always present and may be severe enough to prevent sleep. The skin over the swollen area is shiny white in color.

The acute symptoms last from a few days to a week, after which the pain gradually subsides, and the patient slowly improves.

The course of the disease covers a period of 4 to 6 weeks. The affected leg is slow to return to its normal size and may remain permanently enlarged and troublesome.

The prognosis is usually favorable. In some of the very severe cases, however, abscesses form, and the disease may become very critical or even be fatal. In very rare instances the clot may be dislodged and carried to the heart, causing instant death.

The treatment of femoral thrombophlebitis consists in rest, elevation of the affected leg, the use of icebags along the course of the affected vessels, analgesics, as indicated for the pain, and penicillin. Anticoagulants, such as heparin and Dicumarol, may be prescribed to prevent further formation of thrombi. A "cradle" should be used to keep the pressure of the bedclothes off the affected part. Under no circumstances should anyone rub or massage the affected part. The leg should be handled with the utmost care when changing dressings, applying a bandage, making the bed or giving a bath. As the acute stage subsides, nourishing food and the most carefully regulated hygienic conditions are needed to build up the patient's strength. As recovery is usually tedious, skillful nursing care is required to preserve the tissues of the body.

PELVIC THROMBOPHLEBITIS. This is a severe complication in the puerperium. The onset usually occurs about the 2nd week following delivery with severe repeated chills and dramatic swings in temperature. The infection is usually caused by anaerobic streptococci, and although it is difficult to obtain a positive blood culture, bacteria are present in the blood stream during chills. Penicillin therapy is used, because it is effective in treating most strains of this organism, and as long as the chills and the fever persist, blood transfusions may be given. Heparin and Dicumarol may be prescribed to prevent the formation of more thrombi. A further problem is likely to arise with metastatic pulmonary complications, such as lung abscesses or pneumonia.

These patients are usually mentally depressed and discouraged. If the nurse is conscious of this complication, she will make every effort to keep the patient contented and have her realize the value of immobilization, even though the convalescent period is prolonged. The nurse may also make suggestions to the family as to ways in which they may be helpful.

Peritonitis. Peritonitis is an infection, either generalized or local, of the peritoneum. Here, as a rule, the infection reaches the peritoneum from the endometrium by traveling via the lymphatic vessels; but peritonitis may result also from the extension of thrombophlebitis or parametritis. The clinical course of pelvic peritonitis resembles that of surgical peritonitis. The patient has a high fever, rapid pulse and, in general, has the appearance of being profoundly ill. She is usually restless and sleepless and has constant and severe abdominal pain. Hiccups, nausea and vomiting, which is sometimes fecal and projectile, may be present. Antibiotic therapy is given to combat the infection, analgesic drugs for discomfort and mild sedative drugs to relieve the restlessness and apprehension. If there is intestinal involvement, oral feedings are withheld until normal intestinal function is restored; meanwhile, fluids are administered intravenously. Blood transfusions and oxygen therapy may be indicated for supportive treatment. The record of intake and output must be kept, and, in order to be of value to the physician, the elimination of fluids from the skin by sweating should be noted accurately.

Pelvic Cellulitis, or Parametritis. This is an infection which extends along the lymphatics to reach the loose connective tissue surrounding the uterus. It may follow an infected cervical laceration, endometritis or pelvic thrombophlebitis. The patient will have a persistent fever and marked pain and tenderness over the affected area. The problem is usually unilateral but may involve both sides of the abdomen. As the process develops, the swelling becomes very hard and finally either undergoes resolution or results in the formation of a pelvic abscess. If the latter occurs, as the abscess comes to a point, the skin above becomes red, edematous and tender. Recovery is usually prompt after the abscess is opened.

Signs and Symptoms

It is highly important that the nurse recognize and report early signs and symptoms of puerperal infection so that proper treatment may be instituted without delay. When puerperal infection develops, one of the first symptoms usually seen is a rise in temperature. Although temperature elevations in the puerperium may be caused by upper respiratory infections, urinary tract infections and the like, the majority are due to puerperal infection. Puerperal morbidity is the term used to include all puerperal fevers. The Joint Committee on Maternal Welfare in this country has defined puerperal morbidity as a "temperature of 100.4° F. (38° C.), the temperature to occur on any two of the first ten days postpartum, exclusive of the first 24 hours, and to

be taken orally by a standard technic at least four times daily." The symptoms may vary, depending on the location and the extent of the infectious process, the type and the virulence of the invading organisms and the general resistance of the patient. The affected area is usually painful, reddened and edematous and the source of profuse discharge. The patient may complain of malaise, headache and general discomfort. As mentioned above, the temperature is elevated, and in the more severe infections, chills and fever may occur. In its typical form each of the clinical types of puerperal infection presents a very characteristic set of signs and symptoms, although occasionally one form of the disease is combined with another. The distinctions between these different types of infections are of importance, because the clinical course, the treatment and the prognosis depend on the particular form of infection. For this reason these aspects of the various puerperal infections have been discussed in the preceding pages.

Treatment

The use of the sulfonamides and antibiotic therapy has brought about radical changes in the treatment and the prognosis of puerperal infection. These drugs are effective in combating most of these infections, but, nevertheless, the management and the care of patients with puerperal infections are highly important and demand the utmost in skill. Penicillin is effective against the hemolytic streptococcus, the Welch bacillus and the staphylococcus. Since penicillin is not effective against the colon bacillus and certain strains of staphylococci, sulfadiazine or Gantrisin are usually prescribed for infections caused by these organisms. Resistant staphylococcal infections are often vulnerable to erythromycin used in conjunction with Gantrisin. The dosage of these drugs depends on the severity of the disease and the type of the offending organism. Wound cultures are frequently taken to gain information about the organism; and in severe cases blood cultures may be taken, but if they are to be of real diagnostic value they must be taken at the time of the chill. The infected lesions are treated the same as those of any surgical wound. Drainage must be established, and since this discharge is of a highly infectious nature, care must be taken to see that it is not spread, and that all contaminated pads and dressings are wrapped and burned.

The curative treatment, of course, will be directed by the physician, but good nursing care is essential. The patient should be kept as comfortable and quiet as possible, for sleep and rest are important. Conserving the patient's strength in every way, giving her nourishing food, increased amounts of fluids, fresh air and sunshine will help to increase her powers of resistance. To promote drainage the head of the bed should be kept elevated, a measure which also contributes to the patient's comfort.

Care must be exercised to prevent the spread of the infection from one patient to another. Isolation of infected patients from others is desirable in order to protect the healthy maternity patients. Ideally, the patient with puerperal infection should be away from the maternity divisions. If it is impossible to arrange for such complete segregation, the nurse must consider every patient with puerperal infection as "in isolation" and follow scrupulous technic accordingly. Regardless of the situation, the nurse who is caring for a patient with puerperal infection (or any infection, for that matter) should not attend other maternity patients. The hands of all attendants need special attention and should be scrubbed thoroughly after caring for a mother who has an infection. In certain cases strict isolation technic, with special gowns, masks and rubber gloves, is essential. Clean isolation gowns, masks and gloves should be available for all persons who attend the isolated patient and after being used should be left in the room and disposed of in special hampers or containers. Under no circumstances should this apparel be worn outside the patient's room. Since it is assumed that the nurses who care for these patients are fully acquainted with principles of good isolation technic, this aspect of care will not be pursued further here.

SUBINVOLUTION OF THE UTERUS

Subinvolution is the term used to describe the condition which exists when normal involution of the puerperal uterus is retarded.

The causes contributing to this condition may be (1) lack of tone in the uterine musculature, (2) imperfect exfoliation of the decidua, (3) retained placental tissue and membranes, (4) endometritis and (5) presence of uterine fibroids. Subinvolution is characterized by a large and flabby uterus; lochial discharge prolonged beyond the usual period, sometimes with profuse bleeding; backache and dragging sensation in the pelvis; and disturbance of health until corrected. Since this abnormality is the result of local conditions, an important phase of the treatment rests in correcting the causative factor. Oxytocic medication, such as ergonovine, may be administered to maintain the uterine tone and prevent the accumulation of clots in the uterine cavity, and hot vaginal douches may be prescribed for several days. When the condition is due to disturbances of the endometrium or retained secundines, dilatation and curettage may be necessary. If the uterus is displaced, it may delay normal involution and should be corrected by a suitably fitting pessary.

Early ambulation is believed to have decreased the incidence of subinvolution. And, since it is recognized that breast-feeding stimulates uterine contractions, the fact that a mother is not breast-feeding may be an influencing factor when subinvolution occurs.

HEMORRHAGE

These complications are discussed in Chapter 19.

VULVAR HEMATOMAS

Blood may escape into the connective tissue beneath the skin covering the external genitalia or beneath the vaginal mucosa to form vulvar and vaginal hematomas, respectively. The condition occurs about once in every 500 to 1,000 deliveries. These hematomas may develop shortly after labor, but more frequently they occur in the first few days of the puerperium. Vulvar hematomas manifest themselves by severe perineal pain and the sudden appearance of a tense, fluctuant and sensitive tumor of varying size covered by discolored skin. When the mass develops in the vagina, it may temporarily escape detection, but pain and inability to void shortly will lead the obstetrician to perform a vaginal examination, which will establish the diagnosis. Small hematomas are usually treated expectantly, but if they are large, incision and evacuation of the blood, with ligation of bleeding points, are required.

DISORDERS OF THE BREASTS

Certain aspects of many of the following subjects have been presented in Chapters 13 and 14. Here the discussion is centered on complications.

Engorgement of the Breasts

Any time after the 3rd postpartal day, after lacteal secretion has been established, engorgement of the breasts may occur. The onset is usually rapid, and, as the breasts become distended, dilated veins may be visible under the skin, and on palpation the breasts feel hard and nodular. This condition, commonly called "caked breasts" by the laity, is likely to occur in mothers who are breast-feeding as well as in those who are not. At one time it was believed that this was brought about because the lobules of the breast gland became overdistended with milk, but engorgement is really an exaggeration of the normal venous and lymph stasis of the breasts which occurs in relation to lactation (see The Breasts in Chap. 13). The breasts become tense and swollen for a day or so, with the result that the mother experiences throbbing breast pains which may extend into the axilla. The breasts are sometimes so immensely distended and painful that some analgesic medication, such as codeine, may be required. The condition may be relieved by supporting the breasts properly with a tight breast binder or brassière, worn day and night, and by applying icecaps at intervals over the affected areas. When the breasts are well supported, they are not only more comfortable but also, if pendulous, the support aids in preventing congestion caused by the interference with the circulation (see Fig. 14-8). Immediate treatment of engorged breasts is important, because if the condition is allowed to persist, it may threaten the mother's future milk supply. With prompt attention the engorgement usually subsides after 24 to 48 hours. If the mother is breast-feeding, the regular emptying of the breasts by suckling and adequate breast care then will be all that is necessary.

The mother who is desirous of breast-feeding may have additional problems when she is trying to nurse her infant. Because of the fullness of the breasts and the simultaneous flattening of the nipple, the infant may be unable to get a proper grasp on the areola and nipple. Sometimes the use of the breast pump at very low pressure, and for only a few minutes, prior to the feeding will bring the nipple out sufficiently to permit the infant to grasp it. It must be remembered that too vigorous use of the breast pump or frequent and prolonged nursing periods are irritating to the breast, as well as highly discomforting to the mother. When the engorgement is pronounced, it may be helpful to apply hot compresses to the breasts before the nursing period.

Drying Up the Breasts

When the mother is not breast-feeding, for one reason or another, measures must be taken to inhibit lacteal secretion. This is discussed in Chapter 14.

Abnormalities in Mammary Secretion

It is obvious to the nurse who has had experience taking care of new mothers and their infants that there are marked individual variations in the amount of milk secreted by the breast in almost every case. In most instances it depends on the degree of development of the glandular portions of the breast rather than on the individual's general health or the physical appearance of these organs. A mother with large, well-formed breasts may be eager to breast-feed her infant but produces such a meager quantity of breast milk that she is unable to do so. On the other hand, another mother with small, flat breasts may have a remarkably good milk supply and be able to suckle her infant successfully. Obese women with exceedingly large breasts, the bulk of which is fatty tissue, usually do not have a good supply of breast milk for their infants.

When there is an absolute lack of mammary

secretion, the condition is called *agalactia*. This condition rarely occurs and is seldom seen; in fact, one of the authors has seen it only once in 13 years. As a rule, there is at least a small amount of mammary secretion, but it is so scant that, despite all efforts to stimulate lactation, the quantity would be inadequate to supply the nourishment required for the infant. Since in the latter instance it is a case of hyposecretion rather than an absolute lack of it, perhaps in time it will be more properly called hypogalactia. One point should be made clear here. When one speaks of abnormalities in mammary secretions, this does not refer to temporary episodes which may momentarily affect lactation but in no way affect the mother's ability to continue with breast-feeding. For example, many new mothers, especially primiparas, who have been breast-feeding their infants quite successfully in the hospital find that when they are discharged home there is a sudden diminution in their milk supply. More than likely this is due to the anxiety and fatigue involved with the experience, because once they are settled and rested at home, the milk supply usually resumes normally. This happens so frequently that new mothers are warned that it may occur.

Occasionally the other extreme in lactation is observed, i.e., the mammary secretion is excessive, so-called *polygalactia*. When this secretion is so copious that it constantly leaks from the nipples, it is called *galactorrhea*. The latter condition is not common, but when it does occur, it may be hazardous to the mother's health if it continues over a prolonged period. The condition is best treated by measures which are similar to those used to "dry up the breasts," i.e., limit the fluid intake, use a tight breast binder and apply icecaps to the breasts, in this instance immediately after breast-feeding. In addition, the failure to empty the breasts completely at each feeding may help to check the excessive secretion.

Abnormalities of the Nipples

Variations in what is considered to be normal in the nipple, which is cylindrical in shape and projects well beyond the center of the areolar surface, are not unusual and present no difficulty until the mother wants to breast-feed her infant. The *flat nipple*, i.e., a slightly rounded projection above the breast surface, or the *depressed nipple*, i.e., one which is slightly depressed below the breast surface, are difficult for the infant to grasp with its mouth. The *inverted nipple* is the most pronounced variation, because this nipple is actually inverted, and in this state it is impossible for the infant to grasp it. When these abnormalities exist, the mother should begin corrective measures during pregnancy, such as described by Hoffman (p. 158). Afterward, the use of an electric breast pump or a rubber nipple shield at the beginning of each nursing period may be of value to help draw the nipple out. This may require considerable patience and persistence on the part of the mother, but with encouragement and help from the nurse, she may be successful. However, a real danger may arise if persistent efforts at breast-feeding are attempted and are unsuccessful, because the breasts become engorged and/or the nipples become sore, with resultant fissures or erosions on the surface. These raw, cracked surface areas make breast-feeding a very painful experience for the mother and, moreover, provide a portal of entry for pathogenic bacteria which may give rise to mastitis.

Mastitis

Mastitis, or inflammation of the breast, may vary from a "simple" inflammation of the tissues to a suppurative process which results in abscess formation in the glandular tissue. Mastitis is always the result of an infection, usually caused by *Staphylococcus aureus* or hemolytic streptococcus organisms. The disease in most instances is preceded by fissures or erosions of the nipple or the areola, which provide a portal of entry to the subcutaneous lymphatics, although under conducive conditions organisms present in the lactiferous ducts can invade the tissues and cause mastitis.

Symptoms. Puerperal mastitis may occur any time during lactation but usually occurs about the 3rd or 4th week of the puerperium. There is usually marked engorgement of the breast preceding mastitis, although engorgement per se does not cause the infection. When the infection occurs, the patient complains of acute pain and tenderness in the breast and often experiences general malaise, a chilly sensation or, in fact, may have a chill followed by a marked rise of temperature and an increased pulse rate. On inspection the breast appears hard and reddened. The obstetrician should be notified at once and treatment instituted promptly in the hope that resolution may take place before the infection becomes localized as an abscess.

Treatment. Puerperal mastitis is preventable, for the most part, by prophylactic measures. An important measure is initiated when the expectant mother learns about breast hygiene and begins to take special care of her breasts during the latter months of pregnancy (see Chap. 8). After delivery, appropriate breast care will further help to prevent the development of lesions, but if they do occur, proper treatment must be given promptly. Any time the mother complains of sore, tender nipples, they should be inspected immediately. At this time there may be no break in the surface, but if the condition is neglected, the nipple may become raw and cracked. The alert nurse often can detect even a very small crack in the surface of the nipple if she inspects it carefully. Once a break in the skin occurs, the chances of infection mount, because pathogenic organisms are frequently brought to the breast by the hands or may reach the breast from the patient's nightgown or bedclothes.

With early treatment by antibiotics or chemotherapeutic agents, the inflammatory process may be brought under control before suppuration occurs. Penicillin is effective in treating acute puerperal mastitis if the therapy is started promptly, and often symptoms subside within 24 to 48 hours. The breasts should be well supported with a tight breast binder or well fitted brassière. While the breasts are so painful, small side pillows used for support may give the mother some measure of comfort. Icecaps may be applied over the affected part, but if in time it becomes apparent that suppuration is inevitable, heat applications may be ordered to hasten the localization of the abscess. Most obstetricians advise that breast-feeding be discontinued immediately in cases of mastitis.

If the treatment outlined above is unsuccessful, measures will have to be taken to remove the pus when abscess formation occurs. The obstetrician may prefer in some cases to aspirate the pus rather than resort to incision and drainage. When incision and drainage are done, the abscess should be well walled off. The operation is performed under general anesthesia, so the nurse must prepare the patient for surgery accordingly. In operating the incision is made radially, extending from near the areolar margin toward the periphery of the gland, in order to avoid injury to the lactiferous ducts. After the pus is evacuated, a gauze drain is inserted. Following the operation the care of the patient is essentially the same as that for a surgical patient. Complete recovery is usually prompt.

Epidemic Puerperal Breast Abscess

During the last decade a type of puerperal breast abscess has been seen, both in this country and abroad, which is unlike the type described above. In this new manifestation the offending organism is also *Staphylococcus aureus*, but an antibiotic-resistant strain which has been identified by bacteriophage typing as 52/42B/80/81 and called the "epidemic" strain. Another difference is related to the portal of entry of these microorganisms. In these cases there is no history of nipple lesions, and the infection is introduced through apparently normal lactiferous ducts in the breast, not through the connective tissue. An infant who has been exposed to the epidemic strain of the staphylococcus, and has the organisms present in his nose and throat, can introduce the infection to the mother's breast in the process of nursing. Once these organisms are introduced into the mother's breast, milk provides a superb culture medium for them. Efforts to prevent puerperal mastitis cannot be limited to the care of the mother's breasts but must extend to the hospital nursery, where the infant may acquire the virulent organism. In the nursery such equipment as soap-solution containers, cribs, mattresses, blankets, linens and floors can harbor the organisms. Some methods to help control the spread of infection at its source include rigid nursery aseptic technic on the part of all personnel, measures to prevent the spread of organisms from infant to infant, such as proper spacing of cribs, and the exclusion of carriers from the maternity divisions as soon as they are identified. It should be remembered that in maternity hospitals the nasopharynx of newborn infants tends to become readily infected with *Staphylococcus aureus*, and, moreover, the infection may persist for some weeks after the infant leaves the hospital. Where intensive studies have been carried out and puerperal mastitis or breast abscess appeared after discharge from the hospital, the cultures of the mothers' nares on admission to the hospital did not show evidence of the epidemic strain of the organism. In these cases the infants were the source of infection, because the offending organism was cultured from the nose, the throat and the skin of the infants.

Symptoms. The symptoms of epidemic puerperal breast abscess develop slowly and subtly and usually appear about the 3rd or the 4th week after delivery. The condition is characterized by high fever; the breast becomes very tender, swollen and indurated and suppurates rapidly. The surface of the breast may not be consistently reddened because the abscess is often deep. In some cases the infection may involve more than one portion of the breast, or both breasts.

Treatment and Care. The underlying principles for the care of this form of breast abscess are essentially the same as those described in puerperal mastitis. Breast-feeding should be discontinued immediately, for obvious reasons. Since the offending organism here is antibiotic-resistant, the effects of antibiotic therapy are of questionable value. Nearly all of these infections are susceptible to chloramphenicol, erythromycin and bacitracin but have identical antibiotic sensitivity with resistance to tetracycline, streptomycin and penicillin. The staphylococcus develops antibiotic resistance easily. In the beginning, the treatment of these infections with erythromycin usually resulted in prompt improvement in the condition, but now erythromycin-resistant strains of coagulase-positive staphylococci have been isolated from infections of mothers and their infants. When suppuration occurs in the breast, incision and drainage are usually done as soon as localization of the abscess becomes evident, in order to limit the extent of tissue destruction. When this has been done, special measures must be employed for the control of infection. To protect the surrounding area of the breast, it should be washed with a soap containing hexachlorophene, because such cleansing reduces the occurrence of staphylococci to some degree. This soap is also advocated for hand washing and baths. When warm moist applications to the wound are prescribed, vigilance and care must be exercised so that the underlying skin does not become macerated. Aside from the unnecessary discomfort that this would cause the mother, such maceration would provide another portal of entry for microorganisms. When such infections occur, either in the mother or her infant, the nurse should emphasize health teaching in her care of the mother, not only concerning hygienic measures for the prevention of skin infections but also the urgency for prompt treatment of any member of the family if carbuncles, boils, burns or other skin lesions develop.

The *epidemiologic aspects* of antibiotic-resistant infections of infants and their mothers are far-reaching and a major problem, because when these infections occur, nearly all the hospitals in the community may be affected for varying periods of time. A few years ago this was considered a "hospital" infection, but now it may be found throughout a general community. Once the organism is introduced into a family, this organism can be the cause of disease in the family over a long period of time. For example, the infant may acquire the infection in the maternity nursery, 4 weeks later the mother may develop a breast abscess, and 5 months later the father may develop a boil—all caused by this epidemic strain of staphylococcus. Flaws in nursery "clean technic" in hospital nurseries have long been cited as the cause of spreading skin infections in the newborn, but when these epidemic infections have occurred in hospital nurseries, and the staff has scrutinized their technic and improved it wherever possible, the results have not been as gratifying as one would hope for, because the epidemics have disappeared and appeared again after a period of time. In fact, large numbers of infections have occurred despite meticulous nursery technic. It must be remembered that these infections are not confined to the maternity service but may be spread by carriers to or from other clinical services in the hospital as well as to other members of the family and the community. The infection is thought to be airborne and is easily spread by droplet contamination from the nasopharynx of carriers of these microorganisms. Scrupulous technic in giving patient care in the hospital is undoubtedly an important factor in prevention and control, both in the nurseries or on postpartal divisions, but this alone will not solve the problem. Washing with hexachlorophene has already been mentioned as a means to reduce the occurrence of staphylococcal infections, but this has not reduced the colonization of the organisms in the nasopharynx of individuals. The housekeeping functions which are routine in every institution are of vast importance, both from the standpoint of procedure and personnel, and should be investigated and improved as much as possible. The nurse will find it advantageous to pursue the current literature regarding antibiotic-resistant staphylococcal infections, because there is a wealth of information in the professional journals, and space here does not permit an adequate discussion of the subject. Some references have been listed in the Suggested Reading at the end of this chapter.

BLADDER COMPLICATIONS

The two most common bladder complications in the puerperium are retention of urine and residual urine. In the former, the patient is unable to void at all; in the latter, she is able to void certain amounts of urine but is unable to empty the bladder.

Retention of urine, or the inability to void, is more frequently seen after operative delivery. It often lasts 5 or 6 days but may persist for 2 weeks or longer. The main cause is probably due to edema of the trigone, which may be so pronounced that it obstructs the urethra. Very temporary urinary retention may be due to the effects of analgesia and anesthesia received in labor. As already stressed, the nurse should make every effort to have the patient void within 6 hours after delivery (see Chap. 14). If the patient has not done so within 8 hours, the physician usually will order catheterization. In some hospitals this is routine if voiding has not occurred within 8 hours postpartum. The nurse should remember that it may not be prudent for her to wait for a designated lapse of time to indicate when the bladder should be emptied; rather she must be observant for evidence indicating the degree of bladder distention, because the bladder may fill in a shorter span of time than has been specified, and this should be reported to the physician. At this particular period the bladder has increased capacity, and, because it is usually not as sensitive to distention as prior to pregnancy, overdistention and incomplete emptying may occur; thus the problem of residual urine frequently results. Repeated catheterization may be necessary for several days; or the physician may request the insertion of an indwelling catheter which will provide constant drainage.

When the mother continues to void small amounts of urine at frequent intervals, the nurse may suspect that these voidings are merely an overflow of a distended bladder, and that there is residual urine there. The physician will order catheterization for residual urine, and, to be completely accurate, this must be done within 5 minutes after the patient voids. If 60 cc. or more of urine still remains in the bladder after the patient has voided, it is usually considered that the voiding has been incomplete. It is not uncommon for the catheterization to yield 800 cc. or more of residual urine. Large amounts of urine (from 60 to 1,500 cc., as shown by catheterization) may remain in the bladder, even though the patient may think she has completely emptied her bladder when she voided. The condition is due primarily to lack of tone in the bladder wall and is more likely to occur when the mother's bladder has been allowed to become overdistended during labor. A distended bladder requires prompt attention because of the resultant trauma; moreover, it may be a predisposing cause of postpartal hemorrhage.

In many cases of residual urine the patient is without symptoms other than scanty urination, but in others there may also be suprapubic or perineal discomfort. The treatment of this condition is usually confined to catheterization after each voiding until the residual urine becomes less than 30 cc. In severe cases constant drainage by means of an indwelling catheter may be employed.

The normal bladder is very resistant to infection, but when stagnant urine remains in a traumatized bladder, and infectious organisms are present, there is danger of cystitis. When cystitis occurs, the patient often has a low-grade fever, frequent and painful urination and marked tenderness and discomfort over the area of the bladder. The physician will order a catheterized specimen of urine for microscopic examination, and if pus cells are present in association with residual urine, the diagnosis of cystitis is confirmed. Since it is important in the presence of bladder infection to avoid accumulations of stagnant urine in the bladder, an indwelling bladder catheter may be inserted. In addition, chemotherapeutic agents are prescribed, and fluids should be forced.

PUERPERAL PSYCHOSES

These are discussed in Chapter 9, The Mental Hygiene of Pregnancy and Childbirth.

PULMONARY EMBOLISM

Pulmonary embolism is usually due to the detachment of a small part of a thrombus which is washed along in the blood current until it becomes lodged in the right side of the heart. In many cases the thrombus originates in a uterine or a pelvic vein, although its origin may be in some other vessel. When the embolus occludes the pulmonary artery, it obstructs the passage of blood into the lungs, either wholly or in part, and the patient may die of asphyxia within a few minutes. If the clot is small, the initial episode may not be fatal, although repeated attacks may prove so. The condition may follow infection, thrombosis, severe hemorrhage or shock, and it may occur any time during the puerperium, especially after sudden exertion.

Symptoms. The symptoms of pulmonary embolism are sudden intense pain over the heart; severe dyspnea; unusual apprehension; syncope; feeble, irregular or imperceptible pulse; pallor in some cases, cyanosis in others; and eventually air hunger. Death may occur at any time from within a few minutes to a few hours, according to the amount or degree of obstruction to the pulmonary circulation. If the patient survives for a few hours, it is likely that she may recover.

Treatment. The treatment consists, first of all, in preventing the accident by careful attention to all details of surgical asepsis and to the proper management of labor and delivery. Following delivery, early ambulation may be an additional prophylactic measure, since circulatory stasis is undoubtedly a causative factor. In some instances it is almost impossible to prevent a fatal attack, because the patient may be recovering without elevation of temperature and without complications and yet, on the 7th or 10th day, suddenly cries out, passes into a coma and succumbs.

When embolism occurs, rapid emergency measures to combat anoxia and shock must be carried out promptly. Oxygen is administered without delay, and anticoagulants are given. Morphine may be helpful to relieve the patient's apprehension and usually is given. It is essential that the patient be kept absolutely quiet and on her back, for the slightest movement may cause fatal results. If the patient survives the attack, absolute rest is mandatory, in the hope that meanwhile the clot may be absorbed. Dicumarol therapy will be continued to prevent recurrent emboli. During this time the patient must be kept warm, quiet, comfortable and as free from worry as possible. She may be given a light, nourishing diet during early convalescence.

SUGGESTED READING

Adams, Ralph, *et al.*: Control of infections within hospitals, J.A.M.A. 169:1557, 1959.

Bhose, Lokenath: Postpartum eclampsia, Am. J. Obstet. Gynec. 89, No. 7:898-902, August 1, 1964.

Carrington, E. R., and Sivak, A. M.: Epidemic puerperal breast abscess: I. Preventive and therapeutic aspects; II. Nursing care, Am. J. Nurs. 58:1683, 1958.

Casady, G. U., *et al.*: Postpartum hypertension after use of vasoconstrictor and oxytocic drugs: Etiology, incidence, complications and treatment, J.A.M.A. 172:1011-1015, 1960.

Daniels, R. S., *et al.*: Severe postpartum reactions; an interpersonal view, Psychosomatics 5:21-26, January-February, 1964.

Douglas, R. G., and Birnbaum, S. R.: Intrapartum and puerperal infection, Clin. Obstet. Gynec. 2:693-704, September, 1959.

Eastman, N. J., and Hellman, L. M.: Williams Obstetrics, ed. 13, New York, Appleton, 1966.

Gibbs, C. E., and Misenhimer, H. R.: The use of blood transfusions in obstetrics, Am. J. Obstet. Gynec. 93, No. 1:25-31, September 1, 1965.

Goodrich, F. W., Jr.: Obstetric hemorrhage, Am. J. Nurs. 62, No. 11:96-98, November, 1962.

Greenhill, J P.: Obstetrics, ed. 13, Philadelphia, Saunders, 1965.

McElin, T. W., *et al.*: Puerperal hematomas, Am. J. Obstet. Gynec. 67:356, 1954.

Qureshi, M. A., and Hafner, C. D.: Postpartum intestinal volvulus, Am. J. Obstet. Gynec. 89, No. 8:1080-1081, August 15, 1964.

Ringrose, C. A. D.: A five-year study of massive obstetrical hemorrhage at the Royal Alexandra Hospital, Edmonton, 1958 through 1962, Am. J. Obstet. Gynec. 90, No. 2:232-235, September 15, 1964.

Russell, K. P., *et al.*: Coagulation defects, Clin. Obstet. Gynec. 3:703-717, September, 1960.

Shaffer, T. E., *et al.*: Staphylococcal infections in newborn infants: I. Study of an epidemic among infants and nursing mothers, Pediatrics 18:750, 1956.

Speert, Harold: Puerperal fever, Clin. Obstet. Gynec. 3:767-777, September, 1960.

Steiner, G. J.: Late postpartum eclampsia: report of a case, Obstet. Gynec. 24:594-596, October, 1964.

Taylor, E. S.: Intrapartum and postpartum hemorrhage, Clin. Obstet. Gynec. 3:646-665, September, 1960.

Thomas, W. O.: Postpartum hemorrhage and postpartum hematomas, Clin. Obstet. Gynec. 5:655-669, September, 1962.

Thompson, W. B., and Budd, J. W.: Erroneous diagnoses of amniotic fluid embolism, Am. J. Obstet. Gynec. 91, No. 5:606-620, March 1, 1965.

Tucker, J. M.: Nursing care in obstetric hemorrhage, Am. J. Nurs. 62:98-99, November, 1962.

Wysham, D. N., *et al.*: Staphylococcal infections in an obstetric unit: I. Epidemiologic studies of pyoderma neonatorum; II. Epidemiologic studies of puerperal mastitis, New Eng. J. Med. 257:304, 1957.

CONFERENCE MATERIAL

1. What provisions are made in regard to the care of the infant when the mother develops a puerperal infection in the hospital? At home? What are the implications for the nurse making a home visit?

2. As you consider the situation in which you are working, what measures could be instituted by the hospital or public health agency to further the prevention and the control of infection? What is the role of the nurse in this endeavor?

3. If the mother develops a rash 3 days after delivery and a diagnosis of scarlet fever has been made, what would you consider to be the method of managing this problem?

4. An infant has been exposed to infection caused by staphylococci of the epidemic strain while in the hospital nursery. What instructions should be given the mother concerning the prevention and the control of infection following their discharge from the hospital?

5. How do you account for the maternal mortality rate due to postpartal complications? What contribution can the nurse make toward improving these conditions?

6. If you have a patient whose pregnancy was complicated by cardiac disease (or tuberculosis, or syphilis or diabetes), and who is discharged from the hospital in satisfactory condition following delivery, what would be the responsibility of the hospital and the public health agency in the community for this patient's health supervision? Who has the responsibility for initiating referrals to related health agencies?

7. What routine procedures are employed in maternity care for the detection and the control of venereal disease? How would you go about finding out which states in the United States have legislation governing premarital and antepartal health examinations? What is the existing legislation in your state?

Study Questions

UNIT SEVEN: MATERNAL DISORDERS ASSOCIATED WITH THE CHILDBEARING CYCLE

Read through the entire question and place your answer on the line to the right.

1. Which of the following signs and symptoms should the nurse anticipate when a pregnant patient has a history of heart disease?
A. Dyspnea
B. Slow pulse rate
C. Decrease in blood pressure
D. Hemorrhage

Select the number corresponding to the correct letter or letters.
  1. A only
  2. B only
  3. A, C and D
  4. All of them

_____1_____

2. Which of the following factors influence the answer which you have given in Question No. 1?
A. Increased need for oxygen intake
B. Increased blood volume
C. Toxic damage to the heart
D. Failure of kidneys to excrete

Select the number corresponding to the correct letters.
  1. A and B
  2. A and C
  3. B, C and D
  4. All of them

_____1_____

3. Which of the following signs and symptoms would the patient with a ruptured fallopian tube manifest?
A. Hegar's sign
B. Intense pain
C. Profound shock
D. Irregular fetal heart tones
E. Vaginal bleeding

Select the number corresponding to the correct letters.
  1. A and B
  2. A, C and D
  3. B, C and E
  4. B, D and E

_____3_____

4. Which of the following factors must exist before an erythroblastotic infant can be produced?
A. Rh-negative mother
B. Rh-positive father
C. Rh-positive fetus
D. Rh-positive substance from the fetus must find its way into the mother's blood stream to build up antibodies.
E. Mother must have had a previous Rh-positive pregnancy or transfusion.

Select the number corresponding to the correct letters.
  1. A and D
  2. A, C and D
  3. B, C and E
  4. All of them

·_____4_____

516

5. What is the best known method to prevent erythroblastosis fetalis?
A. Early determination of Rh factor of parents
B. Transfusing the mother during pregnancy
C. Transfusing all Rh-negative fathers
D. Transfusing all Rh-negative babies
E. Repeated small transfusions of Rh-positive blood to the mother

Select the number corresponding to the correct letter or letters.
 1. A only
 2. A and B
 3. B, C and D
 4. C, D and E

1

6. Which of the following statements concerning diabetes complicated by pregnancy are correct?
A. The size of the placenta tends to be in direct relationship to the size of the infant.
B. Toxemia occurs more frequently than in nondiabetic pregnancies.
C. Deliveries are always performed by cesarean section, usually 2 weeks prior to term.
D. The fetus tends to be large.
E. Hypoglycemia occurs in the infant following delivery.

Select the number corresponding to the correct letters.
 1. A and B
 2. B, D and E
 3. B, C, D and E
 4. All of them

2

7. Which of the following are causes of bleeding in the first and second trimesters of pregnancy?
A. Menstruation
B. Abortion
C. Abruptio placentae
D. Placenta previa
E. Ectopic pregnancy

Select the number corresponding to the correct letters.
 1. A and B
 2. A, B and D
 3. A, B and E
 4. B, C, D and E

3

8. How is inevitable abortion distinguished from threatened abortion?
A. Dilatation of the cervical canal
B. Rupture of the membranes
C. Pain
D. Bleeding

Select the number corresponding to the correct letter or letters.
 1. A only
 2. B only
 3. A, B and D
 4. All of them

1

9. What is the effect of tetanic contractions on the pregnant uterus?
A. Descent and rotation are hastened.
B. Ruptured uterus is imminent.
C. Fetal distress may occur.
D. Uterine inertia may follow.
E. Perineal lacerations may occur.

Select the number corresponding to the correct letter or letters.
 1. A only
 2. B only
 3. A, C and D
 4. B, C and E

2

10. Insofar as the toxemias are concerned, which of the following symptoms during labor should be reported to the physician promptly?
A. Hard, painful uterine contractions
B. Epigastric pain
C. Dimness of vision
D. Headache
E. Decrease in urinary excretion

Select the number corresponding to the correct letters.
1. A, C and D
2. A, C and E
3. B, C and D
4. B, C, D and E

4

11. Which of the following conditions contribute to postpartal hemorrhage?
A. Toxemias of pregnancy
B. Overdistention of the uterus due to twins or hydramnios
C. Unwise management of the third stage of labor
D. Involution
E. Retained placental fragments

Select the number corresponding to the correct letters.
1. A and C
2. A, B and D
3. B, C and E
4. All of them

3

12. A patient in the first stage of labor develops secondary uterine inertia. Which of the following are important in the treatment of this condition?
A. Pitocin
B. Sedation
C. Fluids
D. Bed rest
E. Ambulation

Select the number corresponding to the correct letters.
1. A, B and D
2. A, C and E
3. B, C and D
4. B, C and E

3

13. To which of the following causes may urinary tract infections during the puerperium be attributed?
A. Poor hygiene
B. Urinary retention
C. Uterine inertia
D. Subinvolution
E. Trauma sustained during delivery

Select the number corresponding to the correct letters.
1. A and B
2. A, B and E
3. B, D and E
4. All of them

2

14. Which of the following are the chief dangers from sore, cracked nipples?
A. Infection of the infant from nursing
B. Invasion of bacteria resulting in abscess of the nipple
C. Invasion of bacteria through the nipple into the breast tissue
D. Formation of scar tissue which will prevent normal nursing thereafter
E. Formation of a permanent fissure in the nipple

Select the number corresponding to the correct letters.
1. A and C
2. B and C
3. B, D and E
4. B, C, D and E

2

15. Which of the following veins is likely to be involved in puerperal thrombophlebitis?
A. Splenic vein
B. Popliteal vein
C. Renal vein
D. Ovarian vein
E. Saphenous vein

Select the number corresponding to the correct letters.
1. A, B and D
2. B, C and E
3. B, D and E
4. All of them

3

16. In the spaces provided in Column 2, write the term or the phrase which best fits each statement in Column 1.

Column 1

A. A suppurative process in the glandular structure of the breast

B. A localized infection of the lining membrane of the uterus

C. An infection of the loose connective tissue which surrounds the uterus

D. Failure of the puerperal uterus to be restored to its normal proportions as rapidly as expected

E. Exaggeration of the normal venous and lymphatic stasis of the breasts following the development of lacteal secretion

Column 2

A. *Mastitis*

B. *Endometritis*

C. *Pelvic cellulitis or parametritis*

D. *Subinvolution*

E. *Engorgement*

Note: The key to the correct answers to these questions is given on page 598.

Abnormalities of the Fetus and the Newborn

Disorders of the Newborn

Parental and Staff Reactions to Defects and Disorders • Neonatal Respiratory
Distress • Injuries • Infections • Malformations • Inborn Errors of
Metabolism • Hemolytic Disease of the Newborn • Miscellaneous Disorders

Chapter 21

Disorders of the Newborn

INTRODUCTION

The care of the newborn infant and the developing relationship between the mother and her infant have been discussed previously. In this section the focus will be on certain disorders of the neonate that are encountered at times in the maternity unit. Fortunately for all concerned, these usually are not seen frequently; yet their appearance, however infrequent, is traumatic for both parents and staff. The principles of supportive care which were delineated in Chapters 15, 16 and 19 are appropriate here; at times modification will be needed, especially when separation of mother and infant is necessary, or when parental response makes the acceptance of the infant difficult. As the various disorders are discussed, the particular aspects, modifications, etc., which are peculiar to the condition will be described. It is important to remember that the parents of babies with disorders have all the usual tasks of adjusting to the coming of a new infant; in addition they must cope with all the restrictions, limitations and complications that the disorder imposes.

PARENTAL AND STAFF REACTIONS TO DEFECTS AND DISORDERS

Working Through a Crisis

Many parents, as we have said, think of labor and delivery as "the end" of something rather than the beginning of a whole new phase in the family cycle. Probably the enormous responsibilities involved in being parents are responsible in part for this psychological adaptation. One can say with certainty, however, that becoming a parent is a turning point in life, and it is particularly so for the parents of a child who has a disorder. They can emerge from this crisis less mentally and emotionally healthy than they were, or they can move on to increased maturity. If they utilize maladaptive coping mechanisms to deal with the crisis, then the former no doubt will occur; if they can be helped to work through positively, then this experience will stand them in good stead for future stressful situations (see Chap. 9).

It is the responsibility of the members of the health team to help them cope with this situation adequately. However, staff members, too, are only human, and at times they are hampered by their own anxieties, feelings and fantasies. Thus, it is especially important for the staff to understand the psychodynamics that are occurring in both the parents and themselves so that they may choose a therapeutic course of action to help the parents.

Avoiding Negative Communication. Whenever a disorder is apparent at birth, especially if it is of any magnitude or of a long-term nature (an anomaly, acute respiratory distress, etc.), the tension in the delivery room may be prolonged and intensified instead of released in the more customary ways. If the mother is conscious, she may sense this heightened tension and become increasingly aware and terrified that all is not well. As was stated in Chapter 19, it is not always possible for the staff to stop their activities and to respond to the mother's questions; not only are their efforts often going into lifesaving measures for the infant, but they are having to cope with their own emotional reactions. For instance, it is not unnatural for the staff (and the parents later) to have, and perhaps to express, death wishes for a severely defective child. They feel frustrated and resentful toward a situation that they can neither control nor in many cases change. It may be an extremely difficult time for the physician, for it may seem to him that he has "failed" somehow, since he cannot heal the patient. The mother, in turn, may sense the attendants' frustration and misinterpret it as hostility or resentment toward her—that she also has "failed." This negative communication only intensifies the trauma that is experienced by all concerned. In addition, the new mother feels sadness, a completely different emotion than the joy she had anticipated; furthermore, it comes at a time when she may be physically and emotionally exhausted (see Chap. 12).

Forming a Relationship of Trust. The total response of the mother will depend on the type and the severity of the disorder and on her past experiences with stress and life in general (see p. 171 and Chap. 9). During this immediate period when the disorder or defect may become apparent, the nurse can be a key person in easing the concern. She should utilize the relationship with the patient that hopefully she has established in the labor room, for it is vitally important that a trust relationship be formed with the patient if she and her husband are to weather this hardship. She should try to communicate her concern and empathy in any way that seems acceptable to the patient. This may be by just staying with the patient and/or holding her hand. Certainly allowing and encouraging the mother to express her feelings, either verbally or by crying, or by letting her be silent, are constructive measures on the part of the nurse. The nurse should never underestimate the importance of her mere presence; she is someone to share the mother's burden. However, she sometimes has

to cope with her own inclinations to flee or to avoid the topic.

Telling the Parents. The parents may not be allowed to see their infant for a time, especially if the child has an obvious abnormality or is in critical condition; therefore, *what* the couple is told about the condition and *how* they are told become critical issues. All too often one hears parents complain bitterly about the "bluntness," "coldness" and "unconcern" that the staff demonstrated. Worse still is the "conspiracy of silence" that tortures the already overwrought pair, in which each professional avoids saying anything, pretending or assuming that the other will handle the matter, or that it is better left alone. It is important to recognize that the so-called "coldness," avoidance, etc., are not really manifestations of the staff's true feelings, but rather are unsuccessful coping mechanisms on their part to allay their feelings of helplessness, anxiety and inadequacy. However, it is part of the nurse's professional responsibility to explore her feelings in these matters and to develop more effective ways of handling them.

Most physicians want to tell the parents of the disorder themselves; on rare occasions the telling may be delegated to the nurse. In any case it is imperative for her to confer with the doctor, so that each can be aware of what is being told to the parents, and thus effective communication is fostered. Moreover, the nurse should maintain communication with the rest of the health team, so that a coordinated effort can be made for comprehensive care.

REALISTIC APPRAISAL AND REASSURANCE. In order to give the parents a realistic appraisal of the situation, many authorities feel that the parents should be informed immediately of the disorder and the prognosis, especially if repair or long-term care is involved. This information, of course, must be explained in terms that the couple can understand, and reinforcement over the days probably will be necessary.

Whatever specifics are told, it is important that two aspects of realistic reassurance be given the mother and father: first, that they and their child are acceptable, and second, that the hospital and personnel are there to render any assistance possible. Particularly in the cases of some defects and deformities, e.g., phocomelia or myelomeningocele, the parents must understand that although their child may not be made whole, he usually may be helped to some degree. This kind of reassurance demonstrates an attitude of understanding and sharing of the parents' feelings of hurt and loss, and at the same time it does not minimize the gravity of the situation.

Acceptance of the Infant by the Staff. It is generally the doctor who determines when the parents, and especially the mother, will see and care for her infant. The parents' first encounter with their infant is another crucial time. Particularly in cases in which there is an obvious anomaly, it is vitally important that the physician or the nurse who is showing the baby demonstrate an attitude of warmth and acceptance of the infant; if revulsion or rejection is manifested, then the parents' own feelings of despair and ostracism will be intensified.

One of the ways that the staff can demonstrate to the parents that their child is valuable and important is to hold him close, cuddle him and call him by name. At this time, if it seems to be indicated, the positive points in the prognosis can be reiterated or reinforced. This may be a difficult time for all concerned, since the staff, too, is trying to cope with their own possible feelings of rejection. Therefore, an attempt should be made to avoid a common type of destructive behavior that tends to be demonstrated unconsciously, that of isolating the patient under the guise of "protecting" the mother. In this kind of destructive behavior the mother may not be allowed to see her infant at all (or very infrequently) until she is "stronger"; no one talks to her of her child's handicap or death, because it will "upset" her, visitors are often restricted, and so on. The baby, in turn, is isolated and often overtreated, i.e., time- and energy-consuming procedures are employed which lead to very little change in the infant's condition. All this only emphasizes the enormity of the problem for the parents and hinders them in attaining a successful resolution of the problem.

Grieving. The staff can expect the parents to show signs of grieving when a substantial defect (or death) occurs. The couple must come to terms with a difficult and perhaps unexpected situation, one in which the prognosis may be poor. Both parents will demonstrate grief, and the father's needs should not be forgotten. He is particularly vulnerable, since it is on him that the early decisions, making arrangements, etc., usually fall, and he often does not have the time or the privacy to express his own sorrow.

SEVERAL PHASES are encountered in the grief reaction,[1] and how intensely the parents experience these will vary according to the nature and the gravity of the disorder.

In the first phase are shock and disbelief; this phase may be manifested by a refusal to accept or to comprehend the fact of the disorder or the loss. The person may appear stunned, immobilized, or may try to carry on ordinary activities; intermittent flashes of anguish and despair occur as reality penetrates. Occasionally, there is an overtly intellectual response to the reality of the situation: the mother or father may try to comfort the other, make any necessary arrangements, etc. This type of response takes place only if the full emotional impact is not allowed to reach the consciousness. The loss, etc., is recognized, but its painful character is muted. This phase may last minutes to days; the longings for a "perfect child" may be recalled, felt intensely and discharged gradually. This process serves to free the parents' feelings so that they may proceed to the next phase. The nurse's presence is beneficial at this time, for it helps the parents to feel that they are not entirely alone.

The second phase, that of developing awareness, involves a *feeling* of loss and disappointment, accompanied at times by affective and physical symptoms, i.e., emptiness in the epigastric or chest regions, sadness, etc. Now the painful feelings are allowed to become conscious. The parents (particularly the mother) may cry, express anger toward a variety of persons and things, talk about the situation, or they may be unable to express any verbal emotions, although they want to. A relationship between the nurse and the parents that is based on helping is most effective at this time; the nurse's approach should be dictated by the parents' reactions. When she is accepting and encourages the expression of feelings (and provides privacy for their expression), she is helping to prepare the way for the next phase. Developing awareness may take a long time— days or months, in fact. The nurse in the hos-

[1] Engel, G. L.: Grief and grieving, Am. J. Nurs. 64:93-98, September, 1964.

pital usually will see its beginning, but very infrequently will she see its termination.

The third and final phase of grieving involves restitution and resolving the experience. During restitution mourning occurs, in which mutual grief and loss are expressed by the parents and sympathetic friends and relatives. At this stage religious beliefs and rituals are helpful, for they help to clarify the ambiguity about suffering, eternity and death. In this, the final phase of grief, resolution of the problem gradually occurs; this phase may take 6 months to a year. Here memories and expectations are intensely experienced by repeated questioning, ruminating and recalling the experience to mind. The wise nurse will listen empathically in this phase, reflect what is being said, and gently probe to help the parents arrive at reality.* As already implied, the nurse in the community health agency will be in the best position to do this, and enlisting her help will entail appropriate referral on the part of the hospital staff.

The Interdisciplinary Team

Many institutions are now employing an interdisciplinary team when the disorder is grave and/or of a long-term nature. In the case of a child who is born with a cleft palate, a pediatrician, plastic surgeon, otologist, orthodontist and psychologist may all be involved in his care. Since the parents easily can become lost in a maze of appointments, it is wise to have one central person, e.g., the private physician or a social worker, to be the mother's liaison with the other members of the team. The nurse can be instrumental in helping to arrange this.

Stillbirth or Neonatal Death

Occasionally, parents and staff will be faced with the unfortunate circumstance of a stillbirth or a neonatal death. All of the responses of both personnel and parents that have just been described may be apparent in these cases. Grief and mourning will be noted particularly,

* The articles in Suggested Reading that deal with grief, stillbirth, deformities, etc., will help the student gain more explicit insight into the process of grief and the specifics of effective communication and intervention that are necessary in these cases.

and it will become the nurse's responsibility to provide an environment in which the mother and father can express their feelings. Nursing care is essentially the same as that just described.

Decisions will be difficult for the parents, and whenever possible, especially in everyday mundane matters concerning hospital routine, the nurse should try to structure the situation so that the mother is not overburdened with choices. It is often easier for the mother to respond to "I thought you would like your bed made now," than to "Would you like to shower now, or should I make your bed?" One other point needs special consideration. The nurse must be careful not to offer the mother unhelpful platitudes, such as, "Please don't feel so bad. You have such lovely children at home." Or "You can always have another baby." Statements of this kind are not only unhelpful but are detrimental to the situation, since they convey to the patient the nurse's great lack of understanding and/or her disinterest in the situation. The parents will trust the nurse to the degree that they perceive her understanding and empathic perception of their problem, and to this same degree will they trust her and permit her to help them arrive at a positive solution of their problem.

Getting Help From Instructors and Supervisors

All of the responses that have been described (both for parents and staff) are related to emotionally charged areas, e.g., disappointment, loss and death. As previously implied, these topics often are not discussed easily, and the nurse may encounter resistance on the patient's part in the form of hostility when she attempts to speak of these subjects. It is one thing to *talk* about letting patients express their feelings; it is quite another to permit them to *do* this. At times the inexperienced nurse may become very uncomfortable if a response of resistance is not anticipated. Since the student must have consistent and supportive help to plan effective care (and to manage her feelings and responses adequately) in these cases, she should turn to her instructors and other supervisory personnel for help in this regard. Faculty and supervisors who make themselves readily available as "supportive listeners" to students and anticipate the need for this role can be key persons in helping all concerned to resolve the trauma associated with a disorder or a loss.[2]

In the foregoing section some general aspects related to parental and staff reactions as well as nursing care have been described. In the following pages the specific disorders and principles of care related to them will be discussed. The student may benefit from review of this section as she proceeds with the specific disorders.

NEONATAL RESPIRATORY DISTRESS

Asphyxia Neonatorum

Normally, the infant cries immediately after delivery—often when the shoulders are being born. If respiration has not begun within 30 seconds or so after birth, the condition usually is referred to as *asphyxia neonatorum*. This complication may show various gradations from brief, transitory apnea (absence of respiration) to fatal respiratory failure. In the milder cases the infant's face and often the entire body are of a livid hue, and the vessels of the umbilical cord are distended with blood; the tone of the muscles is good, so that any attempt to move the extremities or open the mouth will meet with some resistance. This stage of the process is known as *asphyxia livida.* In severe cases the infant's face and body are of a deathlike pallor, the vessels of the cord empty and the muscles relaxed so that the infant is entirely limp. This stage is known as *asphyxia pallida.*

Failure of the infant to breathe at birth usually is due to one of three main causes, or to a combination of them:

1. Anoxia (deprivation of oxygen)
2. Cerebral injury
3. Narcosis

Anoxia. Since the infant in utero is entirely dependent on the placenta for its oxygen supply, any interference with the function of that organ or with that of the umbilical cord will put the infant in grave danger because of

anoxia. If the oxygen supply is entirely cut off for more than a very few minutes, fetal death in utero results; if only partially curtailed, the infant is born in an asphyxiated state and (like all asphyxiated persons) does not breathe.

Intra-uterine asphyxia may be produced in a number of ways. The umbilical cord may prolapse and become pinched between the pelvic brim and the fetal head, with the result that the umbilical vein becomes compressed and unable to carry oxygen to the infant. Premature separation of the placenta often disrupts placental function entirely, so that the baby suffers complete deprivation of oxygen. Extremely severe uterine contractions may so squeeze the placental site as to jeopardize the infant's oxygen supply.

Cerebral Injury. This is a very common cause of apnea at birth, particularly after difficult deliveries. Not only may the associated brain hemorrhage damage the respiratory center itself, but other vital centers may be injured. Cerebral injury at birth may be caused by difficult operative delivery, such as midforceps operations, version and extraction, and breech extraction. Likewise, disproportion between the size of the head and that of the pelvis may bring about such compression of the fetal skull as to damage the brain. Cerebral injury may result also from long, difficult labor when no instruments are used.

Narcosis. The narcosis produced in the fetus by analgesic and anesthetic drugs given to the mother is a frequent cause of sluggish respiration at birth. As a rule, however, this is quite transitory, and statistics indicate that these infants do as well subsequently as infants whose mothers received no such drugs. This explains why nurses with adequate experience should supervise these patients closely.

Prevention of Asphyxia Neonatorum

Preventive treatment is very important but is largely the responsibility of the obstetrician. It begins with the first antepartal visit when he measures the pelvis and makes sure that it is large enough to allow passage of the infant's head without compression. Good diet and hygiene contribute greatly to the health of the infant at birth. During labor, the physician can do much to prevent asphyxia of the infant by care in the use of analgesic and anesthetic

[2] See Quint, J. C., and Strauss, A. L.: Nursing students, assignments and dying, Nurs. Outlook 12: 24-27, January, 1964.

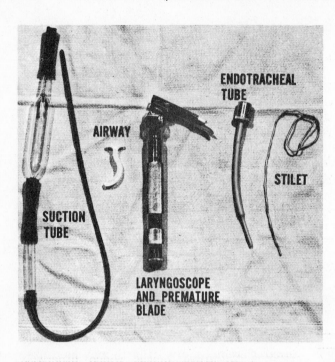

FIG. 21-1. Tray-resuscitation apparatus. (Special Committee on Infant Mortality of the Medical Society of the County of New York: Resuscitation of the Newborn, rev. ed., p. 5, Fig. 4, Philadelphia, Smith Kline & French Laboratories, 1963)

drugs and by avoiding as much as possible the more difficult types of operative delivery: Moreover, by listening regularly to the fetal heart tones, the attendant may detect early signs of impending fetal distress (slow and/or irregular rate), and, with this warning, it may be possible for the physician to deliver the infant before serious trouble develops. The passage of meconium-stained amniotic fluid is another sign of fetal distress but is of no value in breech presentations, since the passage of meconium—ordinarily pure meconium—is the rule in breech cases.

In the past many physicians believed that the administration of vitamin K to the mother late in pregnancy and during labor tended to prevent cerebral hemorrhage in the newborn by improving the clotting power of the fetus' blood. This antihemorrhagic vitamin passes readily through the placenta and raises the prothrombin concentration of the fetal plasma, which ordinarily is low. Recent studies indicate, however, that hyperbilirubinemia is associated with the parenteral administration of a vitamin K analogue antepartally; this is particularly true in the case of premature infants. Therefore, the prophylactic administration of this drug to the mother during labor should be viewed with caution. Current practice is to administer a small dose (1.0 mg.) of water-soluble vitamin K to the infant immediately after birth as a prophylaxis against the coagulation defect related to vitamin K deficiency.

Treatment of Asphyxia Neonatorum

It has been recommended[3] that all members of the delivery room team be trained in methods of resuscitation for mother and baby since both may have difficulty at the same time. Indecisive or ineffective therapy may lose precious moments in which the infant's life can be saved. All equipment necessary for resuscitation (Fig. 21-1) should be checked before each delivery and should include a suction apparatus, a plastic oropharyngeal airway, a laryngoscope equipped with a premature blade (and working batteries) and a Cole plastic endotracheal tube with a stilet. In addition, oxygen should be available.

Generally, the anesthesiologist will assume responsibility for the maintenance of the re-

[3] Manual of Standards in Obstetric-Gynecologic Practice, p. 25, Chicago, The American College of Obstetricians and Gynecologists, 1963; and Special Committee on Infant Mortality of the Medical Society of the County of New York: Resuscitation of the Newborn, rev. ed., p. 5, Philadelphia, Smith Kline & French Laboratories, 1963.

FIG. 21-2. Catheter and glass bulb with a trap, for aspirating mucus in the treatment of asphyxia. (Chicago Lying-in Hospital)

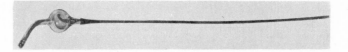

suscitation equipment per se. Since he is usually responsible for the immediate measures of resuscitation, it will fall to the nurse to assist him in any way that she can. Moreover, it is the nurse's function to keep the delivery room prepared for adequate and prompt treatment of asphyxia neonatorum (as well as other emergencies), whether it is expected or not. Therefore, she should have supplies and equipment in readiness. These may include the resuscitator, warm blankets, oxygen and the aforementioned equipment. She should be prepared to position the infant during the procedures, if necessary, and to make and to report accurate observations. Her skill and competence in assisting the physician in caring for the infant and the mother will go far in giving the mother the reassurance and the support that she needs at this time.

In treating an infant which does not breathe at birth, there are 5 main principles to be kept in mind.

1. Gentleness. These infants are often in a state of shock, and rough attempts to resuscitate them—as by vigorous spanking or other overvigorous methods of external stimulation —may do more harm than good. Methods of physical stimulation should be limited to gentle rubbing of the back and, at the most, to light patting of the buttocks. When anoxia is present, oxygen is necessary to overcome it, and the use of measures which act as external irritants will not oxygenate the tissues.

2. Warmth. Heated cribs and other means of maintaining body warmth, such as hot-water bottles and warm blankets, must be in readiness. This is particularly important to remember, because the measures employed to resuscitate infants, unless care be taken, tend to expose their completely naked bodies (accustomed to the temperature in utero) to room temperature; and this may aggravate the state of shock. The body of the infant should be kept covered as much as possible.

3. Posture. Most obstetricians hold the infant up by the feet momentarily after birth in order to expedite drainage of mucus from the trachea, the larynx and the posterior pharynx. The baby is then placed on his back in a slight Trendelenburg position (head turned aside, lower than buttocks), also to favor gravity drainage of mucus.

4. Removal of Mucus. Cleansing the air passages of mucus and fluid is essential, since effective respiration cannot be accomplished through obstructed air passages. The head-down position will promote drainage of mucus and fluid from the respiratory passages, but postural drainage alone is often not adequate for this purpose, and suction of one type or another is frequently necessary. An ordinary catheter is used, size 12 to 14 French; in premature infants a smaller size (8 to 10) is advisable. A glass trap (Fry) is inserted into the catheter to arrest mucus which otherwise might be drawn into the operator's mouth (Fig. 21-2). Milking the trachea upward will help bring mucus and fluid into the posterior pharynx, where it may be aspirated by the catheter. Gentleness is essential, since the mucous membrane of the infant's mouth is delicate. Although the physician occasionally does so, the nurse should not introduce the catheter farther than the posterior pharynx. Mechanical suction devices are provided with most of the modern machines for infant resuscitation and are very convenient (Fig. 12-13).

5. Artificial Respiration. If a newborn infant fails to respond to other resuscitative measures within 1½ minutes after delivery, oxygen must be administered promptly, since diminished muscle tone and lowered heart rate usually result from the progressing asphyxia. The infant should be positioned with his head lower than his torso to facilitate drainage, and with his neck extended as if in a "sniffing posture." Consequently, the infant's natural air passage is straightened (see Fig. 21-3). As oxygen is administered by mask, the infant's chin should be supported by pressing upward with the 4th and the 5th fingers under the angles of the baby's jaw. Because the adult fingers are large in comparison with the smallness of

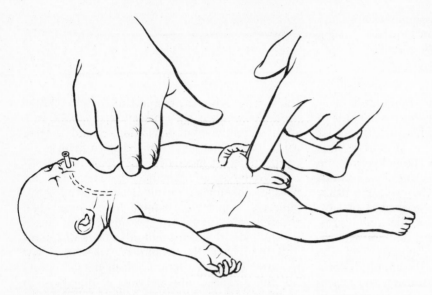

Fig. 21-3. Closed-chest cardiac massage in the newborn infant. *Note:* The infant is placed on a flat surface which is tilted so that his head is on a lower level than his body, facilitating drainage of his airway. In addition, the infant's neck is extended; thus, his natural air passage is straightened.

the infant's jaw, *extreme care* must be taken not to allow the fingers to slip toward the midline under the chin. If this happens, it only contributes to further obstruction of air passages by the infant's tongue. The most effective way to prevent obstruction by the tongue is by insertion of a small oropharyngeal airway into the mouth. Mechanical devices for the controlled administration of oxygen are the most efficient, but resuscitation may be carried out in a number of ways when such equipment is not available.

Probably the oldest method of resuscitation is mouth-to-mouth insufflation, but this is disapproved by some physicians because the method may be dangerous, both from the possibility of rupturing pulmonary alveoli and the risk of infection. Although this procedure is ordinarily performed by the doctor, the nurse may be asked to carry it out if the available physicians are busy attending the mother. The operator stands or sits back of the infant's head. After placing 3 or 4 layers of gauze on the infant's nose and mouth, the operator bends over the infant and puts his opened mouth over the infant's mouth and nose, the gauze intervening. He now exhales gently into the infants respiratory tract. It is advantageous to follow this with light compression of the chest, insufflation and compression being alternated. One does not "blow" into the baby's mouth but simply exhales more or less naturally. As mentioned above, blowing into

the baby's mouth with any degree of force is highly dangerous and may rupture pulmonary alveoli.

A modification of mouth-to-mouth breathing for resuscitation, using instead a mouth-to-airway technic, has been described.[4] This method is accomplished with the use of an S-shaped instrument assembled from 2 standard rubber oropharyngeal airways in such a way as to provide both an oropharyngeal airway for the infant and a mouthpiece for the operator. In the resuscitation of the newborn infant, the operator must "puff" gently into the mouthpiece, a No. 0 airway, using only the air from his oral cavity and not the air from his lungs. It is done in this manner to avoid damage to the infant's lungs. As soon as the chest rises, the operator takes his mouth off the mouthpiece and allows the infant to exhale passively before proceeding with the next "puff" of breath into the airway.

Many hospitals are now using mechanical devices for the resuscitation of the newborn. Such apparatus permits the administration of pure oxygen to the baby's lungs at pressures which are controlled mechanically within safe limits.

Gentle compression of the chest with the *fingers* (external cardiac massage) is usually initiated if the infant's heart has not begun to beat after the administration of oxygen

[4] Safar, P., and McMahon, M.: Mouth-to-airway artificial respiration, J.A.M.A. 166:1459, 1958.

(Fig. 21-3). *Only* a person who fully understands this technic of resuscitation should attempt it, since the procedure *differs* from that used for the adult patient—both in the *manner of applying pressure* and in the *degree of pressure exerted* on the heart (see Suggested Reading at end of chapter).

A RELATIVELY SIMPLE TECHNIC FOR CLOSED-CHEST MASSAGE OF THE NEWBORN has been described as follows:

1. Immediately on delivery the baby is placed in a bassinet with its head on a lower level than its torso in order to facilitate drainage of the airway.

2. The presence or absence of a heartbeat is determined by auscultation.

3. The oropharynx is cleared of meconium so that the vocal chords are visible.

4. Intubation of the trachea is performed under direct vision to ensure access to the pulmonary tree.

5. The trachea and bronchi are rapidly aspirated and cleared of meconium and secretions in order to obtain adequate ventilation.

6. The tracheal tube is held firmly in one hand, and the lungs are expanded by blowing gently down the tube. This is continued intermittently at a rate of 20 per minute.

7. Immediately after filling the lungs, the fingers of the free hand are applied flatly on the midthorax at the level of the sternum, and the latter is compressed firmly in the direction of the vertebral column, and immediately released. This is continued at a rate of approximately 80 to 100 per minute. The degree of pressure exerted on the heart should be enough to obtain a femoral pulse. It is expected that this will suffice to obtain adequate circulation, and yet not inflict trauma on the heart, large vessels, liver, and surrounding tissues. If necessary 0.1 to 0.2 mg. of epinephrine can be injected into the heart.

8. Immediately on the appearance of spontaneous heartbeats, cardiac massage is interrupted, but positive pressure aeration is continued until the baby gasps spontaneously, or under direct external stimulation.

9. Prior to extubation, the trachea, oropharynx, and nasal passages are again aspirated in order to clear any remaining meconium or secretions that may have appeared in the course of treatment.[5]

No drugs have been found to be effective as

[5] Mathews, D. H., *et al.*: Closed-chest massage in the newborn infant, J.A.M.A. 183:964-966, March 16, 1963.

respiratory stimulants for the infant. However, if the infant's respiratory depression is related to maternal narcosis from opiates, then the physician may administer levallorphan (Lorfan, 0.25 mg.) or nalorphine (N-allylnormorphine: Nalline, 0.1 mg. per kilogram of body weight) into the umbilical vein. Respiration may be improved. These drugs should be used only when a specific opiate has been used for the mother, as they otherwise will act as respiratory depressants for the baby (see Suggested Reading).

6. Continued Observation. It is important that close observation be continued after resuscitation methods have ceased. Generally, the baby's condition will improve; occasionally, however, it will worsen, especially if the difficulty is due to mucous obstruction or to drugs administered to the mother. The Apgar method of infant evaluation, as well as the other observations described in Chapter 12, can be utilized in these cases. The continuing observations that should be made when the infant is transferred to the nursery are described in Chapter 15.

Atelectasis

Prior to birth the lungs contain no air and are in a state of collapse. With the first breath, expansion of the lung tissue begins and continues progressively for several days until all parts of the lung are expanded. Feeble respiratory action after birth, incomplete development of the lung, or blockage by mucus or amniotic debris in the small ducts leading to the air sacs may expand the lungs only partially, leaving large areas in a collapsed state. This condition is known as atelectasis. It is particularly common in premature infants. Cyanosis is usually present, because the small areas of expanded lung are inadequate to oxygenate the blood properly. When extensive areas of the lung are involved, there will be irregular, rapid respiration with respiratory grunt, flaring nostrils, intercostal and suprasternal retractions and weakness, in addition to cyanosis.

Atelectasis is treated best by maintaining a clear airway, continuous administration of oxygen, high humidity (to liquefy the secretions so that the infant may cough them up), frequent changes of position, and occasional attempts to stimulate deeper respiration, e.g., short whiffs of carbon dioxide gas. Antibiotics may be utilized, since the inactive portions of the lung are susceptible to infection.

Pneumonia

About 10 per cent of neonatal deaths are due to this complication. In the newborn the condition may be due to bacteria or viruses and is usually of the bronchopneumonic variety rather than the lobar. The birth process itself as well as infection after birth can be etiologic factors. For instance, infection may come from aspiration of infected amniotic fluid or aspiration of secretions from the mother's vagina during delivery, or it may be acquired through the blood stream. Colds are the most common source of infection after birth.

One of the first signs that alerts the nurse is that of rapid respiration (80 per minute or more), accompanied by flaring of the nostrils. The baby is listless, pale or cyanotic and may refuse his feedings; in addition, his temperature may be higher or lower than is usual for him. Oxygen and antibiotics are the treatment of choice. If the pneumonia is due to aspiration of feedings, the first symptom is usually an episode of choking or coughing. The other symptoms soon follow. Careful feeding is a key in prevention. If the infant does choke, he should be placed in a head-down position and the trachea milked to encourage the aspirated fluid to drain from the lungs. After feedings it is wise to place infants on their abdomens or sides to avoid aspiration if regurgitation occurs.

Since many newborn nursery units transfer a baby to a pediatric unit if the infant is born with or develops a serious disorder or infection, separation from her infant may be a problem for the mother. The principles regarding this aspect of nursing care will be essentially the same as those described in Chapter 16.

Idiopathic Respiratory Distress Syndrome (Hyaline Membrane Disease)

Hyaline membrane disease is a syndrome of neonatal respiratory distress in which the alveoli and the alveolar ducts are filled with a sticky exudate, a hyaline material, which prevents aeration. Although it is known that the hyaline material is a protein, the cause of hyaline membrane formation is not definitely known. The condition is observed most frequently in premature infants and infants delivered by cesarean section. A small percentage of infants born at full term are observed to develop this condition, but it is never found in stillborn infants.

The infant may breathe normally at birth and show no signs of respiratory difficulty, but within periods varying from minutes to several hours after birth he develops respiratory distress. This occurs because the hyaline material is deposited and obstructs the flow of air and the exchange of oxygen and carbon dioxide. The cardinal symptoms are cyanosis and dyspnea. If the clinical picture reverses itself promptly, recovery is likely. The infant's color will return to normal, and his respiration will become rhythmic and easy. But if he develops progressive respiratory difficulty and cyanosis and marked sternal retractions increase, death may occur within 48 hours.

It is important that the nurse make meticulous observations and recordings about the respiratory signs and symptoms, especially of infants who are born prematurely or who are delivered by cesarean section. The outcome for the premature is usually poorer and depends a great deal on his birth weight: the smaller he is, the graver is the prognosis. For example, infants who weigh 1,000 Gm. or less generally succumb, since their lungs are not developed enough to make the adjustment to extrauterine life.

Treatment primarily consists of placing the infant in an incubator to facilitate the administration of oxygen and the maintenance of high humidity as soon as the first signs and symptoms are observed. Antibiotics and intravenous feedings also may be employed. Since infants delivered by cesarean section are prone to develop this complication, many physicians prescribe that they be placed in an incubator with oxygen and high humidity immediately on delivery as a prophylactic measure. Moreover, the stomach contents are aspirated, and oropharyngeal suctioning is done to remove mucus and fluid from the nose and the mouth.

INJURIES

Caput Succedaneum

Prolonged pressure on the head during a

FIG. 21-4. Caput succedaneum. (MacDonald House, University Hospitals of Cleveland)

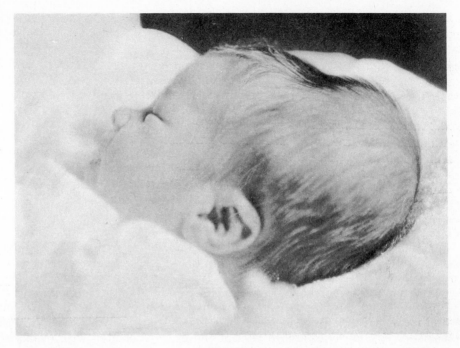

protracted first stage of labor, where the membranes rupture before the cervix is fully dilated, causes an edematous swelling of the soft tissues of the scalp over the area where it is encircled by the cervix (Fig. 21-4). This is called "caput succedaneum," and in its milder forms is very common—so common that it may be regarded as normal.

It is due to an extravasation of serum into the tissues of the scalp at the portion surrounded by the cervix. The term is not confined to vertex cases; the corresponding swelling which forms on any presenting part is also, for the sake of uniformity, known as caput succedaneum. The condition always disappears within a few days without treatment. A prompt and simple explanation should be given to the parents, since this condition, although benign, can be somewhat disfiguring. Once the parents know that the caput will disappear of its own accord, they usually are reassured and will not press for "treatment."

Cephalhematoma

Another swelling of the scalp which resembles caput succedaneum in certain respects is caused by an effusion of blood between the bone and the periosteum (Fig. 21-5). This explains why the swelling appears directly over the bone. It is most common over the parietal bones. It is seldom visible when the infant is born and may not be noticed for several hours or more after delivery, since subperiosteal bleeding occurs slowly. The cephalhematoma increases gradually in size until about the 7th day after labor, when it remains stationary for a time and then begins to disappear. The infant usually recovers without treatment. It may be due to pressure in normal labor, or by forceps; but also it is seen occasionally in breech cases in which no instruments were used or prolonged pressure exerted on the aftercoming head. Such cases, however, are not common. Again, the parents should receive assurance regarding the temporary nature of this condition and its spontaneous disappearance.

Intracranial Hemorrhage
(Cerebral Hemorrhage, Brain Hemorrhage)

In contradistinction to the two conditions just described, intracranial hemorrhage is one of the gravest complications encountered in the newborn. It may occur any place in the cranial vault but is particularly likely to take place as the result of tears in the tentorium cerebelli with bleeding into the cerebellum, the pons and the medulla oblongata. Since these

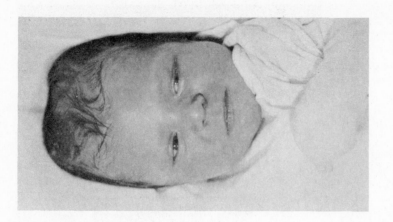

Fig. 21-5. Cephalhematoma. (MacDonald House, University Hospitals of Cleveland)

structures contain many important centers (respiratory center, etc.), hemorrhage in these areas is very often fatal.

Intracranial hemorrhage occurs most often after prolonged labor, especially in primiparae, and is particularly likely to take place in difficult forceps deliveries and in version and extractions. It is also seen more commonly in precipitate deliveries as the result of the rapid propulsion of the infant's head through the birth canal. It is due primarily to excessive or unduly prolonged pressure on the fetal skull. This causes excessive molding of the head and such overriding of the cranial bones that the delicate supporting structures of the brain (tentorium cerebelli, falx cerebri, etc.) are torn, with consequent rupture of blood vessels.

The development of symptoms in cerebral hemorrhage may be sudden or gradual. If the hemorrhage is severe, the infant is usually stillborn; if less marked, apnea neonatorum may result, often with fatal outcome. Many infants who are resuscitated with difficulty at birth succumb later from brain hemorrhage. On the other hand, the infant may appear normal after delivery and develop the first signs of intracranial hemorrhage several hours or several days later.

The nurse should be familiar with the common signs of cerebral hemorrhage, which are described as follows. Any such signs should be reported immediately.

1. Convulsions. These may vary from mild, localized twitchings to severe spasms of the whole body. Twitching of the lower jaw is characteristic, particularly when associated with salivation.

2. Cyanosis. This may be persistent but is more likely to occur in repeated attacks.

3. Abnormal Respiration. Grunting respiration is characteristic; or it may be irregular, of Cheyne-Stokes type, or very rapid and shallow, or very slow. Very slow breathing, usually associated with cyanosis, suggests respiratory paralysis due to pressure on the medulla oblongata and is a grave sign.

4. A Sharp, Shrill, Weak Cry. This is similar to that seen in meningitis.

5. Flaccidity or Spasticity. If the preceding condition is present, it usually portends a fatal outcome. Somnolence also may be present. In other cases there may be generalized spasticity with backward arching of the head and neck and extension of the legs (opisthotonos).

Treatment. Prevention is most important and is largely the responsibility of the physician. It consists in protecting the infant from trauma, particularly in difficult operative delivery. As stated previously, many obstetricians believe that the administration of vitamin K to the mother before delivery decreases the likelihood of cerebral bleeding. This is done less frequently now due to the possibility of hyperbilirubinemia. A small dose of water-soluble vitamin K_1 (1.0 mg.) may be given the infant after birth, however (see p. 354).

Curative treatment can be effective if damage is not too extensive.

Complete rest, with the very minimum amount of handling, is imperative. Infants suspected of having a cerebral hemorrhage should not nurse the breast and should not be weighed or bathed. Since shock often is present, external heat frequently is indicated. Feeding should be carried out in such a manner as to impose on the infant the least possible effort; some of these infants have to be gavaged. Usually the physician will order some form of sedative for convulsions and will prescribe the administration of oxygen for cyanosis. Vitamin C and water-soluble vitamin K may be used to control the hemorrhage, and antibiotics may be given prophylactically. The head of the infant should be kept a few inches above the level of the hips, because this position is believed to lower intracranial pressure. Moreover, the infant should *not* be placed in Trendelenburg position after delivery.

The parents, of course, will need and deserve adequate explanation and reassurance. Since it is difficult to prognosticate in this condition (as well as in several of the other disorders) until the extent and the severity of the injury can be determined, personnel will not want to give the parents false hopes nor yet seem to be unduly pessimistic. The physician and nurse, however, as they report to the parents, can always add an expression like "today" or "at this time" to their explanations, even if the news seems to be unfortunate; e.g., "The baby is responding satisfactorily to the medicines today." "He is progressing at 'this time." This will give the parents a more realistic reassurance and yet subtly alert them to the fluidity of the situation.

Facial Paralysis

Pressure by forceps on the facial nerve may cause temporary paralysis of the muscles of one side of the face so that the mouth is drawn to the other side. This will be particularly noticeable when the infant cries. The condition is usually transitory and disappears in a few days, often in a few hours. Since the infant can look grotesque, the parents will need an explanation concerning the temporary nature of this affliction. If the mother is allowed to feed the baby, the nurse will want to be with her more consistently during the first feedings to help her as necessary. Sucking may be difficult for the infant, and the mother will need to develop patience and skill in the feeding of her baby. If one eye remains open because of the affected muscles, the doctor will prescribe such treatment as is appropriate. Any necessary instruction regarding this continuing care after

discharge should be given the mother before she leaves the hospital. Very often parents are afraid to handle their infants when disorders occur for fear of hurting the child; this may happen even if the condition is short-term and fairly innocuous. Thus, parents should be encouraged to hold and cuddle their infants whenever the condition permits.

Arm Paralysis
(Erb-Duchenne's Paralysis, Brachial Palsy)

This condition results from excessive stretching of the nerve fibers that run from the neck through the shoulder and down toward the arm (brachial plexus). It is a result of forceable pulling of the shoulder away from the head during delivery, usually during a breech extraction. Generally, only the muscles of the upper arm are involved, and the infant holds his arm at the side with the elbow extended and the hand rotated inward. The hand and fingers may not be involved. If the nerves are merely stretched, recovery occurs in several weeks; if they are broken within their sheaths, then healing will not be complete for several months. If healing fails to occur within that time, then surgery is indicated; the outcome for recovery in these cases is guarded. In order to reduce tension on the brachial plexus, the physician usually will place the arm in a splint or cast in an elevated, neutral position. While the arm is healing, the doctor will order gentle manipulation and massage of the muscles to prevent contractures. The mother should be instructed in these procedures so that she may continue the care.

Fractures and Dislocations

Fracture of a long bone or dislocation of an extremity may be the result of a version; or it may occur following a breech delivery in which the arms were extended above the head and are brought down into the vagina. Fractures of the clavicle or of the jaw, or dislocation of either of these bones, may follow forcible efforts to extract the aftercoming head in cases of breech presentation.

Fractures in the newborn baby usually heal rapidly, but it is often difficult to keep the parts in good position during repair. Immobilization of the part often can be achieved by swaddling and positioning the infant on his side. Splints, slings and other apparatus are useful. However, these often make handling the infant difficult and cumbersome; hence parents tend to avoid touching the infant for fear of "hurting" him. Care should be taken by the staff to encourage the parents to give their infant adequate love and attention if these are used. This will mean that the parents will have to be shown how to manipulate the apparatus effectively so that they will not traumatize the injury. Dislocation should be reduced at once, or there will be great danger of permanent deformity in the joint. Follow-up supervision is necessary in order to prevent permanent deformity. Physiotherapy under orthopedic direction is important.

INFECTIONS

Most institutions have an area designated as an isolation nursery where any infant who has or is suspected of having an infection is placed immediately. Once the infant has been transferred to the isolation nursery, he should not be returned to the newborn nursery even though the infection has been treated and/or cured. Strict aseptic technic is used in the care of these babies, and therefore the principles of communicable disease nursing must be understood and carried out by all personnel coming in contact with the infants. Separation of the mother and the infant may be necessary, depending on the type and the severity of the infection. This may require consequent nursing action that has been discussed in Chapter 12.

Ophthalmia Neonatorum (Gonorrheal Conjunctivitis)

This is a serious condition which may result in total blindness, but if suitable treatment is adopted at the very outset of the disease and intelligently carried out, usually the sight can be saved. The entire treatment is, of course, under the direct supervision of the physician.

Fortunately, state laws making the use of silver nitrate prophylaxis compulsory for all infants at birth have reduced the incidence of this infection immeasurably. Before silver nitrate prophylaxis became mandatory, however,

25 to 30 per cent of all children in schools for the blind suffered impaired sight as the result of the infection. This condition is of gonorrheal origin and is characterized by a profuse, purulent discharge in the eyes due to infection, generally from the genital canal at the time of birth. However, the causative organism, *Neisseria gonorrhoeae*, can be transmitted also on the hands of personnel working with infected mothers and by articles, e.g., towels, tissues, etc., that come in contact with the infection. Thus, the importance of proper hygiene for those working with infected persons cannot be stressed enough. Prompt diagnosis and treatment of those suspected of having the disease is also vital, since the mother may reinfect her infant as she handles him.

If the infection occurs at the time of birth, the disease appears within 2 or 3 days; but as the septic discharge may be introduced into the eye at a later period by neglect of the proper care of the infant, the onset may be later. Both eyes are usually affected; and at first they are suffused with a watery discharge and considerable inflammation of the eyelids. Within 24 hours the lids become very much swollen, and a thick, creamy, greenish pus is discharged. Later, unless treatment has been instituted early, the swelling becomes so marked that the eyes cannot be opened, opacities of the cornea occur, the conjunctiva is ulcerated and then perforated, and the eye collapses and finally atrophies.

The preventive treatment consists in the use of 1 per cent silver nitrate, which is instilled into the eyes immediately after birth. However, if infection does occur, penicillin intramuscular injections may be given. If the infection persists, intensive pencillin administration should be carried out. Thanks to this drug, gonorrheal ophthalmia, which used to be one of the most stubborn and grave afflictions and demanded the utmost in elaborate and prolonged nursing and medical care, is now cured within 12 to 24 hours. The swelling and the pus usually disappear in even less time than this.

Ophthalmia neonatorum is a distinctly infectious disease, and there is extreme danger of conveying it to others. This applies not only to other infants' eyes but to the genital tract of other mothers. Even the eyes of the nurse herself may become infected, unless she is most conscientious in her methods. The infant should be isolated, and all articles used should be sterilized.

Staphylococcus of resistant types occasionally cause purulent discharge; all such cases should be under the care of a physician until recovery.

Impetigo

Impetigo is a skin disease of infectious origin and not infrequently occurs in epidemic form in the nursery. For this reason it is often called "impetigo contagiosa." The condition manifests itself by the eruption of small, semiglobular vesicles or pustules. Although these may appear on any part of the body, they are most frequently encountered on moist opposing surfaces, such as the folds of the neck, the axilla and the groin. Thence they may spread rapidly by auto-inoculation to any part of the body. The lesion is small and varies from the size of a pinhead to a diameter of half an inch. It contains yellow pus. The bacterium involved is usually the staphylococcus or the streptococcus.

The treatment is essentially preventive, and cases rarely occur if the nursery technic has been meticulous. The nurse and the physician must wash their hands carefully before handling any infant, and every possible source of skin infection must be eliminated. Constant vigilance is necessary if these cases are to be prevented. Treatment consists of prompt isolation of the infant and local treatment of the lesions. Since these lesions tend to appear on moist or opposing skin surfaces, the infant must be kept clean and dry. Daily baths using hexachlorophene (pHisoHex) may be given. Usually the blebs are broken, and the denuded areas are exposed to dry heat. Gentian violet, alcohol, bacitracin, or neomycin ointment may be applied locally. Systemic antibiotic therapy may be required.

As soon as a lesion develops which resembles impetigo even slightly, strict isolation of the infant is imperative. The physician should be notified at once. If properly treated, the superficial lesions heal quickly and with little scarring. Parenteral antibiotic therapy may be given prophylactically. A high nutritional level must be maintained, and scratching should be controlled. It is important for the nurse to remember that it is the fluid within the bleb which spreads the infection. When impetigo develops in a nursery, it may be stubborn to eradicate, and occasionally it may even become necessary to close the nursery for a few weeks.

Thrush

Thrush is an infection of the mouth caused by the organism *Candida albicans*, the organism which causes monilial vaginitis in the mother (see Chap. 8). The infant may acquire the infection as it passes through the birth canal of a mother so infected. However, the infection may be transferred from infant to infant on the hands of attendants and is favored by lack of cleanliness in feeding, in the care of the mother's nipples, or in the care of the bottles and the nipples. It is most likely to occur in weak, undernourished babies. The condition appears as small white patches (due to the fungus growth) on the tongue and in the mouth. These white plaques may be mistaken at first for small curds of milk. The infant's mouth must be kept clean, but great gentleness is required to avoid further injury to the delicate epithelium, and any attempt to wipe away the plaques will usually cause bleeding.

Some physicians advise painting the spots with an aqueous solution of 1 per cent gentian violet, in which case the spots are touched gently with a sterile, soft cotton swab saturated with the medication. Another method of treatment is with nystatin, an antibiotic specific for infections caused by the monilial organism, *Candida albicans*. Mycostatin, an oral suspension of nystatin (200,000 units per cc.) is dropped into the infant's mouth and thus comes in contact with the affected areas. The usual dosage of Mycostatin is 1 to 4 cc. 3 or 4 times daily, as prescribed by the physician. The nurse will recall that nystatin is poorly absorbed from the gastrointestinal tract and is excreted almost entirely in the feces after oral administration.

Special care must be taken with the bottles and nipples used for infants who have thrush. These bottles and nipples must be kept separated from the others in the nursery until they are soaked in antiseptic solution, washed thoroughly and boiled before they are cared for in the routine way with bottles and nipples of other infants.

Epidemic Diarrhea of the Newborn

During recent years a number of highly fatal epidemics of diarrhea have occurred in nurseries for the newborn throughout the country. Among infants so affected, almost half have died. The mortality rate in premature infants is twice the rate in full-term infants. The onset is sudden, with profuse, watery yellow stools which increase in frequency. Associated with the diarrhea, a precipitous weight loss occurs—often a pound within 24 hours. The appearance of the infant changes rapidly from that of a healthy baby to one of a markedly dehydrated and emaciated infant. In a severe case, death may occur in a day, but more often the baby lingers on in a semi-comatose condition for 4 or 5 days. The spread of the disease is very rapid, and half the infants in a nursery may succumb within a fortnight. Many of the epidemics accordingly are described as "explosive" in character.

The most common offending organisms are strains of a common inhabitant of the intestinal tract, *Escherichia coli*. These pathogenic strains are carried by healthy adults who handle the newborn infant; unfortunately, it is very difficult to diagnose these carriers by the usual means and thus prevent their coming in contact with the newborn.

The symptoms and the mortality rate differ from bacterial types of dysentery or diarrhea. One of the most important predisposing factors is overcrowding in the nurseries. Faulty nursery technic is another—that is, failure to wash the hands before touching a baby, failure to sterilize rubber nipples properly, etc. The guiding principle involved is that everything coming in contact with the baby's mouth and nose should be in a surgically aseptic condition. All obstetric and nursing technics must be planned accordingly. Various health departments have set up rigid regulations along these lines in the hope of preventing epidemics.

Treatment and Prevention. When a case is discovered, immediate and absolute isolation is necessary; therefore, the infant should be transferred from the newborn nursery. A culture of the stools is done to find out the causative organism. This is done so that spe-cific therapy can be instituted as soon as possible.

Neomycin and Colimycin given orally have been found to be most effective against the *E. coli* organisms. These drugs may be given prophylactically to exposed but uninfected infants until their discharge. Penicillin and streptomycin are sometimes administered to prevent or control the secondary infection that might occur in the debilitated infants. Supportive fluid therapy by the intravenous or the subcutaneous route also may be utilized. Oral fluids—water, 5 per cent glucose in water, or Lytren (a commercially prepared electrolyte fluid replacement for oral use)—are given in small amounts. Whole blood is given by transfusion if indicated.

If necessary, the nursery should be closed to new admissions until the epidemic clears up. These nurseries are washed and sometimes even painted before being opened again for new admissions. In the prevention of this disease there seems to be nothing more effective than strict aseptic nursery technic. Hand washing with soap or pHisoHex and water after changing diapers, before feeding the infant and after handling the infant or any of its equipment is a rigid rule that should be stressed.

If an outbreak occurs, there should be a follow-up of all infants discharged in the preceding 2 weeks, and any infants needing treatment should be readmitted to the pediatric service of the hospital. All infants exposed at the time of an outbreak should be given prophylactic therapy. Complete control of this disease, which formerly led to closing of the nursery, can be gained by prompt reporting, rigid technics and immediate treatment.

Syphilis

Even with the rise in the rate of this disease in the general population in recent years, syphilis in the newborn can be prevented when antepartal care is adequate. It has decreased greatly in the 42 states where serologic tests on the blood of all pregnant women are required. This condition shows lesions only if the infant has early prenatal syphilis. They may be present at birth or may appear from a few days up to 4 months of age, predominantly on the face, the buttocks, the palms and the soles. Mucous patches occur in the mouth, and condylomata about the anus. These lesions are highly infectious. The eruption is usually maculopapular and not quite so generalized as in acquired syphilis. Bullae may appear on the palms and the soles, a type of lesion never found in acquired syphilis. The palms and the soles may desquamate as a result of the lesions. Less frequently seen are papular lesions or purely macular or, very rarely, vesicular or somewhat pustular ones. The nails may be deformed, and alopecia may be present. In such cases the blood test for syphilis is usually strongly positive. In addition to the cutaneous manifestations of syphilis, other signs and symptoms may arouse suspicion of the presence of the disease. The infant becomes restless, develops rhinitis (snuffles) and a hoarse voice. The baby does not gain weight as it should. The lymph nodes are enlarged, especially the epitrochlear nodes. The liver and the spleen are enlarged, as are also the ends of the long bones.

In the treatment of syphilis of the newborn, the physicians will rely chiefly on penicillin. The broad-spectrum antibiotics may be used if sensitivity makes the use of penicillin inadvisable. Usually additional therapy is unnecessary; however, most of these infants are kept under surveillance for 1 or 2 years after treatment.

Babies born to mothers who have been treated early in the antepartal period for syphilis are seldom born with the disease.

Staphylococcal Infection

At the present time there is growing concern about the spread of staphylococcal infection in hospitals and its increasing resistance to antibiotic therapy. The newborn nursery is one of the most vulnerable areas because of the infants' low tolerance to infections.

In recent studies of staphylococcal infection of the newborn, the epidemic strain of the organism has been found not only in skin lesions of the infected infants but also in the nasopharynx of a high percentage of apparently well infants. Nurseries at this time must be considered potential epidemic centers. Many factors contribute to the large numbers of infants found to harbor these organisms. *Crowding* of infants in a nursery has always been a serious problem and a contributing factor in

any epidemic disease outbreak. The usually recommended minimum of 24 to 30 square feet of space per infant may actually not be adequate to prevent spread of infection. *Hospital personnel* have been found to be carriers of staphylococcus coagulase-positive organisms. These organisms are highly resistant to most antibiotics in current use, and when they are transmitted to infants, they may result in such manifestations as skin lesions (impetigo; p. 537), pneumonia, septicemia, conjunctivitis, omphalitis, osteomyelitis and other forms of infection from mild infections to those of extremely serious nature. In many studies there appears to be a direct transmission of the offending organisms from hospital personnel to infant, from infant to infant, from infant to mother and to the family at home, and even into the community (see Chap. 20). Hospital sanitation must be critically appraised, since these organisms may be air-borne and can exist in many contaminated or unclean surfaces of the nurseries, wards and other hospital areas. The type of walls, floors and equipment used must be of materials which can be easily and satisfactorily cleaned. Housekeeping personnel, their equipment and methods must be constantly evaluated and supervised. There is no substitute for cleanliness, aseptic technic and isolation of infected patients and staff in controlling the spread of infection.

Manifestations of staphylococcal infection of the newborn frequently appear as pyoderma, stuffy noses, pneumonia and conjunctivitis. Few infants develop serious staphylococcal disease without preceding or accompanying pyoderma. Treatment usually consists of antimicrobial drugs given parenterally.

MALFORMATIONS

In approximately 1 out of 200 cases, an infant is born with some kind of malformation; and about 1 out of every 7 or 8 neonatal and perinatal deaths can be attributed to anomalous development. The incidence of these disorders has not changed greatly over the decades; however, the technics of repair and correction have improved immensely, thus offering a great deal of hope and consolation to the parents and the children who are afflicted with these conditions. Congenital deformities may range from minor abnormalities such as supernumerary digits to grave malformations incompatible with life, such as anencephalia (absence of brain), hydrocephalus (excessive amount of fluid in the cerebral ventricles with tremendous enlargement of head) and various heart abnormalities. In 1963, 20,817 infant deaths (excluding fetal deaths) were attributed to congenital malformations (rate, 11.0%). In the case of hydrocephalus, grave dystocia may occur because of the inability of the huge head to pass the pelvic inlet. Congenital malformations of the heart are a common cause of cyanosis in the newborn. Clubfoot, imperforate anus and meatus, cleft lip and cleft palate are other fairly frequent congenital deformities.

Since these conditions are so numerous and varied, this section will present selected disorders—those more commonly seen that are apparent at birth or soon thereafter and/or those with which the maternity nurse will have to deal. As we indicated on pages 523 to 526, the care of these infants and their parents presents a great challenge to the nurse. She must give competent and, at times, complex nursing care to the babies, and she must help the parents to convert their feelings of disappointment and, often, despair to constructive efforts of habilitation of the infant. In addition, the negative feelings that are aroused in the nurse must be handled. The young student will find that discussing these feelings with her instructor or supervisors will help her to cope with them.

Cleft Lip and Cleft Palate

These deformities, which may occur separately or in combination, result from the failure of the soft and/or bony tissues of the palate and the upper jaw to unite during the 8th to 12th weeks of gestation. The defect may be unilateral or bilateral (Fig. 21-6). Only the lip may be involved, or the disunion may extend into the upper jaw or into the nasal cavity. About 1 in every 1,000 births is so affected; thus, the anomaly is considered to be one of the most common of human birth defects. In some cases heredity seems clearly to be implicated, but in others there is no definite etiologic cause. It occurs in near relations of persons with the defect more often than in the general population.

The plan of treatment and outcome will depend on the severity of the condition. If only the lip is involved, surgery may be performed as early as 12 hours after birth. If the maxilla is involved as well, then surgical repair usually is done within the first few weeks of life. Repair of defects of the palate usually is deferred until about the 2nd year to take advantage of the developmental changes that occur. When surgery is done later, a prosthetic

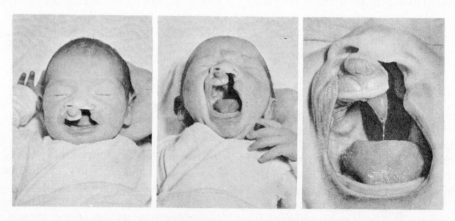

FIG. 21-6. Cleft lip and complete cleft palate. In this case surgical closure of the harelip was performed less than 18 hours following birth, with excellent results. (MacDonald House, University Hospitals of Cleveland)

speech device usually is fitted so that speech development may not be hindered. Cleft palates usually involve other difficulties, frequent respiratory infections, orthodontia and speech problems, etc.; therefore, the care of these children involves the coordinated activities of the pediatrician, plastic surgeon, orthodontist, hospital and public health nurses, speech therapists and, very often, the social worker. Fortunately, modern treatment is so effective that this defect becomes a relatively minor handicap.

Nevertheless, the parents require a great deal of supportive help initially, as mentioned earlier, especially since this disorder is so disfiguring. In our culture a high value is put on physical attractiveness and beauty; and when this condition occurs, particularly if the baby is a girl, it may come as a tremendous shock and burden to the parents. However, repair is generally successful, and it is very helpful if the parents know and understand this. The nurse should emphasize the essential normality of the infant. Babies with this condition may be transferred to the pediatric ward, especially if surgery is to be performed. This will mean separation and loneliness for the mother. If possible, arrangements should be made for the parents to visit the infant whenever possible. (See Chap. 16.)

Feeding is usually one of the most immediate and difficult problems in the daily care of the infant. It can best be accomplished by placing the infant in an upright position and directing the flow of milk against the side of the mouth. This will decrease the possibility of aspiration as well as the amount of air swallowed during feeding. Since sucking strengthens and develops the muscles needed for speech, a nipple should be used for feeding whenever possible. A variety of nipples may be tried, including a regular nipple with enlarged holes, a soft rubber nipple, a cleft palate nipple, or a duck bill nipple. The last two are more expensive and should be used only after the others have been tried. Specific instructions are necessary with their use. If the infant cannot use any of the nipples, then a spoon or a rubber-tipped medicine dropper may be tried. The flow of milk will have to be adjusted to the infant's swallowing and should not be released until the infant attempts to suck. The

feedings should be given at a pace which will neither cause the infant to become unduly tired nor result in aspiration of the liquid. Since these infants tend to swallow a large amount of air, they should be bubbled at frequent intervals, and the mother should be instructed in this technic. The nurse will want to help the mother to attain ease in feeding her baby and should arrange to stay with her during at least several of the sessions. She then can ascertain by demonstration and observation how well the mother is progressing. Gavage feeding usually is unnecessary and should be used only when the other methods fail, since it does not stimulate the sucking and swallowing reflexes and promotes aspiration.

The mother may want to breast-feed her infant, and there is no contraindication as long as the milk can be given the baby in a way that is appropriate. This may mean that the mother will have to pump or express her milk and offer it in a bottle or a medicine dropper. After surgery has been performed, and the infant's sutures have healed, the mother may resume breast-feeding.

Frenum Linguae

The frenum linguae is a vertical fold of mucous membrane under the tongue which is normally short and tight in the newborn infant. If this membrane is *too* short, the activity of the tongue is limited, so-called "tonguetie," and this interferes with sucking and later with the child's speech. This condition should be observed at the time of the initial physical examination or during the inspection bath. The physician will "snip" the margin of the membrane with sterile blunt scissors if necessary.

Hypospadias and Epispadias

In hypospadias the urethra opens on the under surface of the penis proximal to the usual site. Minor degrees of this condition are quite common, and no surgical intervention is necessary. If the opening is at the base of the penis or far back on the shaft, then plastic surgical repair will be necessary. In epispadias the urethral opening is on the dorsal surface of the penis. If the defect is pronounced, then it also will require repair. Surgery usually is deferred in these conditions until childhood or puberty to take advantage of the maturation of the structures. Urination with the penis in the usual elevated position is impossible in these cases when they are severe. Very infrequently the condition occurs in females; in these instances the urethra opens into the vagina.

Spina Bifida

Spina bifida is a rather common malformation and is due to the congenital absence of one or more vertebral arches, usually at the lower part of the spine. When the membranes covering the spinal cord bulge through the opening, the condition is known as meningocele. It forms a soft, fluctuating tumor filled with cerebrospinal fluid. The tumor can be diminished by pressure and enlarges when the baby cries. The extrusion of the cord along with the coverings is known as meningomyelocele. When the tumor is very small and shows no signs of increasing in size, it may merely be protected from injury and infection by carefully applied dressings; but the more severe cases must be treated surgically. Unfortunately, the outlook for surgical repair is discouraging, since hydrocephalus usually occurs, if it is not already present, and fatalities are common. The situation and the prognosis for the infant is discouraging, and the parents will need a good deal of support and instruction about the continuing care of their infant. (See Suggested Reading.) The physician will prescribe regarding the care that is to be carried out at home.

Umbilical Hernia

Umbilical hernia, or rupture at the umbilicus, may appear during the first few weeks of life. The associated protrusion of intestinal contents may be made to disappear entirely on pressure, but it reappears when the pressure is removed, or when the baby cries. This is due to a weakness or an imperfect closure of the umbilical ring and is often associated with nonunion of the recti muscles. The condition usually disappears spontaneously, but should the protrusion of omentum persist, the abdomen may be strapped, using a 2-inch strip of adhesive plaster or a suitable cord bandage. Some mothers may need to be discouraged from placing a coin or a button beneath the umbilical dressing, a practice used many years ago as a "home remedy." This has no value and prohibits adequate approximation of the margins of the hernia.

Obstructions of the Alimentary Tract

Atresia of the Esophagus. This condition, although less common than some which have been mentioned, is quite serious, and immediate steps must be taken to prevent aspiration. The defect, which occurs during embryonic development, results in the esophagus ending in a blind pouch rather than a continuous tube to the stomach. A fistula usually occurs into the trachea near the bifurcation of the esophagus and the trachea. When the baby attempts to swallow liquids or even normal secretions, there is an overflow into the trachea from the blind pouch. This malformation should be suspected whenever the infant demonstrates excessive drooling, coughing, gagging or cyanosis during feeding. The nurse must report these symptoms immediately; unless necessary surgery to correct the defect is prompt, the baby will contract bronchitis or pneumonia from repeated aspiration of milk and secretions. The infant should be placed in the supine position, with his head elevated 30 degrees or more to prevent any gastric secretions from rising into the trachea through the fistula. The baby usually is placed in a heated, humidified incubator after surgery. This atmosphere is needed to liquefy the tenacious mucus that collects. Nasopharyngeal suction is necessary, and the nurse should watch carefully for any cyanosis or labored respiration that indicates the need for this. Blood, plasma, parenteral fluids and antibiotics also are given. The extent of the repair and the condition of the baby determine when oral feeding will be begun.

Pyloric Stenosis. This is a congenital anomaly and usually manifests its symptoms from the first few days to the 2nd or 3rd week by the onset of vomiting which becomes projectile in character and occurs within 30 minutes after every feeding. The infant loses weight, the bowel elimination lessens, highly colored urine becomes scanty, and the symptoms of dehydration appear. Upon examination, gastric peristalsis is found to be present, and the pyloric "acornlike" tumor can be palpated. Usually, thick cereal feedings are prescribed. If no improvement is noted, it is necessary to resort to surgery. Since it is not usually an emergency operation, there is sufficient time for supportive treatment to prepare the infant for surgery by vein and hypoclysis. The preoperative preparation includes intravenous blood and plasma. If the hemoglobin is below 70 per cent, transfusion is indicated. Gastric lavage, from 1 to 2 hours before operation, should be done until returns are clear. Maintaining body heat before and after the operation is essential. Transfusion should be given if indicated. The physician usually orders from 5 to 10 cc. of water to be given within a few hours, then alternated with 10 cc. of milk. As soon as the baby is gaining and consuming from 3 to 4 ounces at each feeding, he is ready for discharge.

Obstruction of the Duodenum and the Small Intestine. These conditions are relatively easy to diagnose. Vomiting occurs with the first feeding, and no meconium is eliminated. The vomitus may or may not be bile-stained, depending on whether the obstruction is high or low in the intestinal tract. If the obstruction is low, usually there is marked distention. A roentgenogram is used to confirm the diagnosis, and immediate surgery is indicated. However, the newborn infant should be allowed at least 12 hours for the respiration and kidney function to become stabilized. The operation is usually accompanied by continuous venous drip and plasma, and blood should be available if needed. Postoperative care includes maintaining body temperature, intravenous fluids until peristalsis is established (about a week), followed by feedings as given in pyloric stenosis. If distention occurs, nasoduodenal suction may be necessary. If the distention is severe, the infant should be in an oxygen tent.

Intussusception. Acute intussusception is the most frequent type of intestinal obstruction and often may be unrecognized. There is usually intermittent abdominal pain, mild or severe, accompanied by blood and mucous intestinal elimination; and the baby may vomit. Upon abdominal examination a mass can be palpated. Immediate surgery is usually indicated. In preparation for surgery a gastric lavage is done, and an indwelling gastric catheter is inserted. Shock, if present, should be treated. Fluids are replaced by the intravenous route. Hypoclysis may be given for 24 hours, followed by water by mouth. Feedings may be started on the 3rd day if retained. Antibiotics may be ordered for the first 3 to 5 days and vitamin C to stimulate healing.

Imperforate Anus. This abnormality consists of atresia of the anus, with the rectum ending in a blind pouch. Careful examination of the infant in the delivery room usually reveals the condition, but it may be discovered by the nurse when attempting to take the first rectal temperature. Surgical treatment is, of course, imperative.

Down's Syndrome

Down's syndrome or mongolism refers to a congenital disorder of genetic origin that is characterized by irreparable brain and body damage. Mental retardation, resulting from malfunction of the cerebral cortex, is usually severe. In addition, other clinical signs involving deformities associated with the disorder, e.g., skull, eyes, etc., may be manifest in variable degrees and frequency. The reader may be more familiar with the term "mongolism" used in reference to this syndrome, but recently this has lost favor, because it bears a connotation which is not only unfortunate but incorrect.

For many years the term "mongolism" has been given to the condition of infants who present a definite clinical picture, the configuration of their faces resembling that of a Mongol or an Oriental. Their eyes are set close together, are slanting, and the palpebral fissures are narrow. The nose is flat. The tongue is large, fissured, and usually is very obvious as it protrudes from the open mouth. The head is small, and posteriorly the occiput appears flat above the broad, pudgy neck. The hands are short and thick, especially the fingers (the little finger is curved), with simian creases apparent on the palmar surfaces. In addition to having defective mentality and the deformities mentioned above, these infants have underdeveloped muscles, loose joints, heart and alimentary tract abnormalities. Although these infants sometimes live past the age of puberty, the majority succumb earlier to some infection.

Incidence and Etiology. The incidence of Down's syndrome has been estimated at 1.5 in 1,000 births. Advanced maternal age has been known to play a very important role in the etiology of this condition, over a third of these children being born to mothers who are 40 years of age or older. Several decades ago it was suggested that this condition might be associated with a chromosomal aberration, but it was not demonstrated until recently that the etiologic factor in Down's syndrome is the result of one of three chromosomal abnormalities (see p. 67).

Types. The most common chromosomal defect of the ovum in Down's syndrome is trisomy of the chromosome 21, resulting in a total chromosomal count of 47 instead of the normal number of 46 (see Chromosomal Aberrations in Chap. 4 and Fig. 4-4). This type, commonly referred to as standard trisomy, usually occurs in infants born to older women and is rarely familial. The incidence of standard trisomy is 1 in 600 births. The second type of abnormality results from a 15/21 translocation; in this type the actual chromosomal count is 46. The translocation type of Down's syndrome usually occurs in infants born to younger parents, is the familial type and is rare. The third type of the disorder, mosaicism, is very rare. A unique factor in mosaicism is that one individual may have cells with different chromosomal counts. Laboratory tests may demonstrate that the affected person's blood cells, for example, have 47 chromosomes, whereas his skin cells may show 46 chromosomes. This is not a familial type of Down's syndrome, and, moreover, the abnormalities may be less.

Help and Emotional Support for the Parents. One can anticipate that the parents will experience an emotional shock on seeing their newborn baby and/or being told that their baby has Down's syndrome. Lay people generally are familiar with the term "mongolian" or "mongolian idiot" and have some idea of the nature of the problem, if not the cause. Their immediate reactions may be manifest in a variety of ways, depending on the individual person, but it is safe to assume that it is difficult for them to accept their baby's condition. Their response is not only related to this infant with obvious abnormalities but also to the implications this has for their future childbearing. Young parents may be afraid to bear more children; on the other hand, the elderly primipara may have more difficulty in accepting her baby's condition because she fears this will be her only child, and he is defective. These examples, of course, are merely illustrative and not meant to imply that the contrast in the response of the young parent and the elderly primipara is in any way stereotyped. Regardless of the situation, these parents require concrete help and emotional support from the professional staff, nurses and physicians, particularly those who are most significant to them in the experience (see pp. 524-525).

Phocomelia

In 1961-62 many thousands of newborns in Germany were afflicted with an extremely pitiful type of malformation characterized either by total absence of the arms and the legs or by such stunting of the extremities that they were mere nubbins. This deformity is known as *phocomelia*. Investigation revealed that practically all the mothers who gave birth to such infants had taken a certain sedative drug, *thalidomide*, during the first part of pregnancy, and that this drug was undoubtedly the cause of the malformations.

Largely as the result of the thalidomide tragedy, the United States Food and Drug Administration, a Federal agency authorized to approve new drugs, tightened greatly the regulations concerning new drug approval. But from the viewpoint of nurses and physicians, the most important lesson to be drawn from this sad experience is that *no pregnant woman should take any drug whatsoever* unless, in the opinion of her physician, it is urgently necessary for her health (see Chaps. 8 and 18). This rule does not apply to the routine administration of vitamins and iron, nor to the use of laxatives when indicated, but it does apply very strongly to most other drugs, particularly those often employed in the treatment of insomnia and nausea.

The child with deformed or missing limbs has special rehabilitation problems that do not occur in the treatment of adults who undergo a loss of a limb (see Suggested Reading). His physical characteristics and contours are different from those of an adult, and they are constantly changing as he grows. This complicates fitting an adequate prosthesis. Furthermore, his psychosocial adjustment demands continued attention, for he does not have the chance to make his adjustment to society as a whole person, and he therefore is likely to have some feelings of inadequacy and devaluation in a culture geared to the nonhandicapped. Fortunately, there are about 15 child amputee clinics throughout this country. They are located in Alabama, California, Connecticut, Florida, Georgia, Illinois, Maryland, Michigan, New York, North Carolina, Oklahoma, Pennsylvania and Washington. These clinics are invaluable in helping parents to learn that their child can be fitted with a functional prosthesis and achieve satisfaction in its use. Even when the deformity is multiple, the child can achieve at least limited function with proper training. Since much of the success of the plan of treatment depends on the parents, it is particularly important that they be informed and reassured of these positive aspects in the situation. It has been demonstrated that the sooner the parents receive this knowledge, the more chance there is of an effective prosthetics program.

German Measles as a Cause of Malformations

The relation of German measles (rubella) in the mother during the first trimester of pregnancy and the occurrence of congenital malformations in her infant has been substantiated. A significant proportion of fetuses will show malformation, principally cataracts, heart disease, deaf-mutism and microcephaly. It should be noted that the disease which produces these harmful effects is German measles, or rubella, and not rubeola, which has no such action. It should also be observed that German measles exerts these effects mainly when it occurs very early, usually before the 12th week of pregnancy; and even then not all infants are affected. Just what proportion of babies are injured cannot be stated in the present stage of our knowledge. Furthermore, there is evidence to indicate that immunity in the pregnant mother from a previous attack may not protect her fetus from the anomalies secondary to an exposure in the first trimester; therefore, even though the mother has had German measles, it is advisable that she avoid exposure during this time. Some authorities recommend that any woman with no history of a previous attack of rubella who is exposed during the first trimester be given 20 cc. of gamma globulin intramuscularly as a protective measure. On the other hand, there is some indirect evidence to indicate that this prophylactic administration of gamma globulin to exposed pregnant women may also lead to masking of clinical symptoms and signs, while permitting the occurrence of viremia (see Suggested Reading). The recent and continuing advances in technology in this area should divulge more definitive information on this problem and its subsequent management.

INBORN ERRORS OF METABOLISM

Numerous metabolic disorders, so-called "inborn errors of metabolism," are now known to originate from mutations in the genes which alter the genetic constitution of an individual to the extent that normal function is disrupted. These biochemical disorders arise because of the disturbance (mutation) in a *molecule of the gene* itself. They *do not* stem from some mishap or alteration during the embryonic development of tissue or organs. The mode of transmission of these "inborn errors" usually is recessive; that is, a child must receive a pair of defective genes (one from his mother and one from his father) to be affected. The mother and the father in these cases would be carriers of the defective genes but would not be affected by the resulting disorder per se. Fortunately, defective genes are found rather infrequently in the general population, and the chance of their joining is even rarer; hence, the diseases they produce are commensurately rare. Some of the more familiar hereditary metabolic disorders and resulting conditions include:

1. Defects in metabolism and transport of amino acids
   A. Phenylketonuria
   B. Maple sugar urine disease
2. Defects in protein metabolism
   A. Agammaglobulinemia
3. Defects in metabolism and transport of carbohydrates
   A. Diabetes mellitus
   B. Gargoylism (Hurler's disease)

C. Galactosemia

D. Arachnodactyly (Marfan's syndrome)

4. Defects in metabolism and transport of lipids

A. Cerebroside lipidosis (Gaucher's disease)

B. Ganglioside lipidosis (Tay-Sach's disease)

C. Sphingomyelin lipidosis (Niemann-Pick disease)

It is important to remember that these inborn errors of metabolism *do not produce symptoms* that are apparent at birth. Therefore, the maternity nurse rarely will see evidence of these disorders. However, one condition does concern us here, since the nursery personnel play an important role in the early detection of the condition. This disorder is phenylketonuria.

Phenylketonuria

This disease, commonly known as PKU, is an inborn error of metabolism of the essential amino acid phenylalanine, characterized by a deficiency in the liver enzyme phenylalanine hydroxylase, which is essential in phenylalanine metabolism. High blood levels of phenylalanine occur, and phenylketone bodies are excreted in the urine. Phenylalanine makes up 5 per cent of the protein factor of all foods. Normally, phenylalanine is converted to tyrosine in the liver and then is further metabolized. The phenylketonuric child is able to digest protein and to absorb the resulting amino acids. However, there is a block in the normal metabolic pathway at this point, and the excess dietary phenylalanine, unable to be converted to tyrosine, builds up in the tissues (blood levels of this enzyme reach as high as 60 mg. per 100 ml., as compared with the normal 1 to 3 mg. per 100 cc.) and spills into the urine in the form of phenylpyruvic acid, excess phenylalanine, phenylacetic acid and orthohydroxyphenylacetic acid. These components, excreted in the urine and the perspiration, give the child a characteristic musty odor.

Without treatment, the condition usually results in mental retardation, although the rest of the clinical picture will vary. Typically, the child with PKU is hyperactive and demonstrates unpredictable erratic behavior. Usually he does not relate well in interpersonal contacts, either within the family or with strangers, and he appears very immature and overly dependent. The three R's, routine, relaxation and repetition (as used with other mentally retarded youngsters), are effective in helping him make a more satisfactory social adjustment. The main foci of management, however, is early detection of the condition and dietary management restricting the phenylalanine intake. If treatment is initiated before 6 months of age, the child probably will fall into the borderline-to-normal range of intelligence (70 to 100 I.Q.).

Diagnosis. This disorder may be diagnosed from both blood and urine tests. The former are more advantageous, since they can be done before the infant leaves the hospital, and they give a low rate of false positive reactions. One of the easiest and most efficient of the blood tests to perform is the Guthrie method. In this test 1 or 2 drops of blood are secured from the infant's heel on the day of discharge and are placed immediately on filter paper. The laboratory then uses a bacterial inhibition assay method on the serum phenylalanine to determine the phenylalanine level. A result of 8 mg. per cent or above is considered to be diagnostic of PKU. The nurse may be asked to collect the specimen for this test and/or to prepare the infants for the doctor. Usually several babies will be tested at one time, therefore, she can facilitate matters by placing the infants in the prone position, which makes the heels easily accessible. The babies then can be covered loosely with a blanket so that they will remain accessible but will not be unduly exposed. After the heel has been wiped with a disinfectant solution, pricked (usually with a disposable blood lancet, and the specimen obtained, the infant should be observed for bleeding from the heel. The test must be repeated in 4 weeks. The test equipment usually is given to the mother at the time of discharge. She should be instructed to take the baby to her physician or baby clinic so that testing may be completed. The other blood tests require 1 to 5 cc. of blood; they are as reliable as the Guthrie method, but many laboratories do not have the facilities required to perform the analysis.

The urine tests utilize ferric chloride as the testing agent; this solution is dropped on a freshly saturated diaper. A green reaction indicates probable phenylketonuria. The urine tests are effective only after the infant is 6 weeks old; they are useful in screening large populations of infants and are most often done in well-baby clinics. Since early diagnosis is imperative, the blood tests are becoming the tests of choice.

Treatment. Restriction of phenylalanine intake is the basis of treatment, and yet enough protein must be available for growth and development; hence the child's diet becomes all-important. Commercial products (e.g., Lofenalac, a special food, which is mixed with water) are available that provide adequate protein for growth with minimal phenylalanine content. The plan of dietary treatment should be reviewed carefully with both parents, and they should have an understanding of how to prepare the formula, use the meal guides and food exchange lists (see Suggested Reading) and prepare menus from them.

Requesting the parents to review their understanding of the problem, diet, etc., often will elicit the areas that need clarification. The parents must be supported until they feel comfortable in discussing the problem; until this happens, they cannot be receptive to further teaching. Since this is a long-term condition and requires consistent counseling and follow-up, the need for a referral to the public health nurse becomes evident.

Care should be taken so that the parents of an affected child are not led to believe that all babies treated will have the usual pattern of growth and development (intellectual development may be slow, for instance). This cannot be guaranteed. *Early detection* and *prompt treatment* prevent mental retardation. The control of this condition demands consistent and disciplined supervision and follow-through on the part of the parents.

HEMOLYTIC DISEASE OF THE NEWBORN

Hemolytic Disease Due to Rh Incompatibility

This condition is a severe hemolytic disease of the newborn due to Rh iso-immunization. It occurs in cases of Rh incompatibility (see Chap. 18). The term "erythroblastosis fetalis" has been applied rather generally to all cases in which there is Rh incompatibility; actually, it is somewhat of a misnomer when used in this way. Erythroblastosis fetalis should be used to designate an illness in the infant which is due to Rh iso-immunization, since this disorder is neither specific nor always present in all instances of Rh incompatibility. The name is derived from *erythros*, red, and *blastos*, a formative cell. It occurs approximately once in every 200 deliveries. The disease may manifest itself in different degrees of severity. About one fifth of the Rh-positive infants born of sensitized Rh-negative mothers may have no clinical manifestations. Others may be mildly or severely affected. If the mother's antibody titer is low, the infant will likely have a mild form of the disease. In mild cases of erythroblastosis fetalis, slight jaundice and anemia may be present at birth or may become evident within a few hours thereafter. These symptoms may be the only clinical manifestations. In more severe cases the jaundice and the anemia are more exaggerated, and the liver and the spleen may be enlarged. Marked anemia with consequent pallor is a characteristic feature due to the destruction of the erythrocytes (see Chap. 18). In making observations the nurse should bear in mind that if the jaundice is pronounced, it may mask the developing pallor. Jaundice and anemia which are present at birth or appear during the first 36 hours are the cardinal clinical symptoms of erythroblastosis. Therefore, the nurse should notify the doctor immediately if any infant is jaundiced on the 1st or the 2nd day of life.

Severe jaundice is a manifestation of hyperbilirubinemia, a condition that occurs when the level of indirect bilirubin (free bilirubin) in the blood reaches 20 mg. per cent. Therefore, the bilirubin level in the blood is increased beyond physiologic limits, since the normal value is usually between 0.2 and 1.4 mg./100 cc. of blood. Even at the peak of physiologic jaundice, often seen in normal newborn infants, the bilirubin level does not exceed 5 to 13 mg./100 cc. of blood. This high serum bilirubin level is caused by the inability of the liver to handle the large amount of bilirubin that is liberated with the destruction of the erythrocytes. So that the indirect bilirubin (free bilirubin) may be excreted after birth properly, it must be converted to direct bilirubin by enzymes in the liver. These enzymes are deficient during the infant's first few days of life. Thus, when hemolysis is excessive (as it is in erythroblastosis), and the bilirubin cannot be converted to the excretable direct variety, the bilirubin accumulates in the blood in such concentration as to cause jaundice and in severe cases to stain the brain cells, causing irreparable damage.

This latter condition is known as *kernicterus*. The infant who has symptoms of kernicterus (jaundice of the nuclear masses of the brain) will take its feedings poorly and show increasing signs of lethargy and loss of normal Moro reflex. It may have convulsions and opisthotonos, often accompanied by a shrill high-pitched cry. Kernicterus due to Rh incompatibility is often fatal, and if the infant survives, it almost always suffers from severe forms of mental retardation and spastic paralysis, and its hearing may be impaired.

Even when kernicterus is not present, the infant with erythroblastosis is usually lethargic, due to the anemia and generalized weakness, and he should have his position changed frequently to prevent atelectasis. Furthermore, special precautions must be exercised to protect these infants from intercurrent infection.

There is some disagreement as to whether or not mothers giving birth to erythroblastotic infants should breast-feed their babies. However, in Nelson's 8th edition of the *Textbook of Pediatrics** it is stated: "Erythroblastosis fetalis is not a contraindication to breast feeding, if the infant's general condition warrants it, since antibodies in the mother's milk are inactivated in the intestinal tract and do not contribute to further hemolysis of the infant's red blood cells."

The most severe manifestation of erythroblastosis affecting the newborn is *hydrops fetalis*. With this condition the infant is tremendously edematous, has marked anemia, jaundice and enlargement of the liver and the spleen. Such infants may be stillborn; otherwise they invariably succumb shortly after birth.

Erythroblastosis fetalis is very likely to repeat itself in subsequent pregnancies, and some unfortunate mothers give birth to a series of such infants. Its cause is immunologic in character and is based on the fact that the

mother in these cases develops in her blood certain antibodies which attack a substance in the baby's red blood corpuscles known as the "Rh factor" (see Fig. 18-17).

The Rh Factor. To understand the phenomenon which causes erythroblastosis fetalis, the nurse must have a knowledge and understanding of the Rh factor. This has already been discussed in some detail in Chapter 18.

Once in every several hundred pregnancies, as the result of an extraordinary combination of chance factors, the Rh substance may be responsible for a chain of events which exerts a harmful effect on the fetus. A number of circumstances must be present before this singular action on the fetus can be exerted. In the first place, the mother must be Rh negative. As indicated in Chapter 18, there is only 1 chance in 7 that any member of the white race belongs to this minority group. In the second place, her husband must be Rh positive; the chances are good—6 out of 7—that he does belong to the positive group, but he may not. In the third place, the fetus must be Rh positive; because the husband is Rh positive, it does not necessarily follow that the baby is positive, because if any large group of Rh-positive men are studied, it will be found that the spermatozoa of about one half are partly Rh negative and will produce an Rh-negative infant. In the fourth place—and this is the crux of the matter—the Rh substance from the Rh-positive fetus must find its way through the placenta and into the blood stream of the mother and build up antibodies therein, as occurs with an Rh-positive blood transfusion. Once these antibodies are developed in the mother, they pass through the placenta into the fetal blood stream, where they cause varying degrees of damage to the infant's red blood cells. Finally, the woman must have had a previous pregnancy or a previous blood transfusion, because, as we have seen, it takes some time for the antibodies to develop.

From the above facts the following rather comforting conclusions can be drawn. Six out of 7 women are Rh positive, and for them there is no possibility whatsoever of complications occurring from this source. Likewise in first pregnancies, even if the expectant mother is Rh negative, the possibility of trouble developing is quite remote unless she has had a previous blood transfusion with Rh-positive

* Page 128.

blood. But if a woman is Rh negative and has had previous pregnancies or previous transfusions, what is her outlook in subsequent pregnancies? So many factors enter into this question that it is impossible to answer it with great precision, but all authorities agree that the vast majority even of this group—from 90 to 95 per cent—go through pregnancy after pregnancy without any suggestion of a complication.

Treatment in Erythroblastosis. When hemolytic disease is suspected, the infant is carefully observed at birth for clinical signs of the disorder. His skin color, the color of the vernix, and the size of his liver and spleen are noted. In addition, a specimen of umbilical cord blood is obtained for the following tests: Coombs' test, Rh determination, blood group, serum bilirubin, reticulocyte, erythrocyte and nucleated red blood cell count, and hemoglobin level. The direct Coombs' test (direct antiglobulin test) is important in accurate diagnosis of hemolytic disease. It reveals the presence of maternal antibodies attached to the red blood cells of an Rh-positive baby (see Chap. 18). The red blood cells of a baby with hemolytic disease may be coated with anti-Rh antibodies, and these antibodies will cause hemolysis of the baby's red blood cells. A positive direct Coombs' test indicates the presence of antibodies on the surface of the infant's blood cells. A negative direct Coombs' test indicates that no antibodies are present on the baby's red blood cells. Depending on the results of the laboratory reports and/or the presence and the severity of the clinical signs, treatment will be instituted.

In live births, that is, except in *hydrops fetalis*, the life of the infant may be saved by exchange transfusion with Rh-negative blood. This provides new red cells and removes the harmful maternal antibodies and products of hemolysis which produce jaundice. Transfusions should be given promptly. The exchange transfusion is accomplished through a polyethylene catheter inserted into the umbilical vein, or other large vein, such as the saphenous. Small amounts of the infant's blood are withdrawn (approximately 10 to 15 cc. at a time) and equal amounts of the Rh-negative donor's blood injected. This procedure is continued until most of the circulating blood of the infant is replaced.

When there is any possibility that exchange transfusion may be required for the infant, the obstetrician invariably will leave the umbilical cord stump longer than usual.

Those infants with hemolytic disease who do not require exchange transfusion should be observed carefully for development of anemia for at least 3 weeks following birth, even when they appear to be doing satisfactorily. The physician will continue to have scheduled determinations of hemoglobin levels done during this period.

The prognosis is favorable for the infant with erythroblastosis fetalis if he survives the first week without developing signs of kernicterus, provided that the severe anemia is given watchful attention and treatment. One may anticipate that hemoglobin and erythrocyte levels will be normal by the time the infant reaches the age of 5 months.

Very recently, a new concept in the management of the Rh problem, i.e., *amniotic fluid evaluation* and *intra-uterine fetal transfusion*, has been introduced to improve the perinatal mortality from erythroblastosis fetalis. It is believed that by the examination of the amniotic fluid of Rh-negative sensitized women, it is possible to predict the presence and the severity of the hemolytic process in the fetus.

The amniotic fluid is obtained by abdominal amniocentesis on pregnant women suspected of bearing infants with erythroblastosis. Then, since there is a relationship of the amniotic fluid bilirubin concentration to the presence of erythroblastosis fetalis in utero, the amniotic fluid can be evaluated by spectrophotometric analysis. Once this has been done, the further management of the pregnancy is determined almost entirely by the results of amniotic fluid analysis, irrespective of the height of the mother's antibody titer levels.

Intra-uterine fetal transfusion is indicated when the fetus is likely to die otherwise before becoming mature enough to survive premature delivery. The fetal transfusion is done on the basis of the mother's past history of having a severely affected infant at birth or a fetal death in utero due to erythroblastosis, in addition to the appearance of an amniotic fluid absorption curve in the spectrometric tracings suggesting a severely affected infant.

The results of this new approach in the management of the Rh problem during prenatal life is encouraging indeed, although it must be remembered that this is still in the investigational stage. The student will benefit from studying the works of Bowes, Freda, Glynn, Liley, Westberg, etc., in the current literature (see Suggested Reading).

ABO Incompatibility

A relatively mild type of hemolytic disease of the newborn is associated with ABO incompatibility. In this disease the father's blood group is A or B and the mother's is Type O. At the time of conception the fertilized ovum receives the genes from both parents, and because the A and B genes are dominant over O, the infant will develop Type A or B blood. During the placental exchange of intra-uterine life, the anti-A or anti-B agglutinins of the mother's blood cross the placental barrier and attack the red blood cells of the infant. Hemolysis of these cells occurs, resulting in severe jaundice and anemia.

This disease occurs in first as well as in subsequent pregnancies, but rarely is it as severe as the hemolytic disease caused by Rh incompatibility. The Coombs' test is invariably negative.

Exchange transfusions are done, as necessary, to keep the serum bilirubin level below 20 mg. per 100 cc. The blood for transfusion should be of appropriate Rh type and Type O, the mother's blood group and not the infant's.

Hyperbilirubinemia of the Newborn

Hyperbilirubinemia, as previously stated, is present beyond physiologic bounds when the total serum bilirubin levels reach 18 to 20 mg. per 100 cc. of blood. This may occur particularly in premature infants as an exaggeration of physiologic jaundice or as a consequence of excessive hemolysis, such as severe hemolytic disease of the newborn. Occasionally, this condition is found in term infants who have no blood group incompatibilities. Therefore some authorities suggest that this term, "hyperbilirubinemia of the newborn," be applied only to those infants whose primary problem is a deficiency or inactivity of bilirubin transference rather than an excessive load of bilirubin for excretion. Certain conditions of the mother, e.g., diabetes, as well as neonatal conditions

arising from the use of certain drugs, bacteremia and prolonged cyanosis, appear to be implicated in causing this condition. Occasionally this disorder appears among breast-fed infants during the 2nd week of life. For some reason the mother manufactures a substance in her milk that inhibits the conjugation of bilirubin. If breast-feeding is discontinued, serum bilirubin levels return to normal within 5 days, and apparently no lasting damage is done to the infant. The significance of hyperbilirubinemia, of course, lies in the high incidence of kernicterus associated with it, which, as previously explained, can be lethal to the baby.

MISCELLANEOUS DISORDERS

Hemorrhage from Cord

Hemorrhage from the cord may be of two types: (1) primary, due to the slipping or loosening of the ligature or umbilical clamp, and (2) secondary, coming from the base of the cord when it separates from the body of the baby. In the first instance, the bleeding is from the end of the cord and not from its base and can be controlled by the proper application of a fresh ligature. The secondary hemorrhage, from the base of the cord, occurs at about the 5th to the 8th day when separation takes place. It is often preceded by a slight jaundice; it is not an actual flow of blood but a persistent oozing which frequently resists treatment. This variety of hemorrhage, which is of rare occurrence, is usually due to one of two causes: (1) the baby may be syphilitic, or (2) the peculiar condition known as hemorrhagic diathesis may be present. In this condition the baby's blood shows no disposition to coagulate, and bleeding from any denuded surface is persistent and often profuse.

The nurse's responsibility in the treatment of secondary hemorrhage from the cord consists in applying a sterile dressing to the bleeding surface. The physician should be notified promptly; and if, by the time he arrives, the use of the dressing has not effectually controlled the oozing, he will doubtless ligate the base of the umbilicus. When this form of bleeding is at all severe and persistent, recovery is doubtful; and even if the umbilical hemorrhage is controlled, bleeding may appear in the nose, the mouth, the stomach, the intestines or the abdominal cavity; or purpuric spots may develop on various parts of the body. The prompt administration of vitamin K has greatly improved the prognosis in these cases.

Retrolental Fibroplasia

Retrolental fibroplasia is an acquired disease, associated with prematurity, in which retinal pathology occurs in those infants receiving continuous oxygen therapy in high concentration. This disease is characterized by proliferation of endothelial cells in the layer of nerve fibers in the periphery of the retina. This leads to the formation of new vessels, and the retina becomes edematous and elevated and finally retinal detachment may follow. Because most of the damage is mechanical, one cannot determine the extent of detachment that will occur. When the condition is detected early, and proper measures are instituted promptly, i.e., reduction in concentration of oxygen administered, the condition in the infant may regress at any stage of the disease, or, on the other hand, partial or complete blindness may result.

Retrolental fibroplasia is no longer considered to be a major problem, because it rarely occurs today. Extensive research, carried on within the past two decades since retrolental fibroplasia was first described, has established the cause and the means of prevention of the disease. It is now a fact that almost all cases of retrolental fibroplasia in the premature infant are the result of intensive oxygen therapy. Today oxygen is administered to an infant in the lowest concentration compatible with life and is discontinued as soon as feasible. The maximum oxygen concentration of the incubator housing the premature infant is kept at less than 40 per cent, with rare exceptions, and this is done only for as long as it is *absolutely* necessary (see Oxygen Therapy, p. 412).

Drug Addiction in the Newborn

Although this condition is still rare, it is seen more frequently with the rise of drug addiction in the general population. Furthermore, it is the nurse who may be the first to discover this condition. The symptoms of the infant are due to withdrawal rather than narcosis; they may appear almost immediately after birth, or they may be delayed for several hours, depending on the time of the mother's last injection of narcotic, the dose, and the interval between the administration of the narcotic and the delivery. The infant may manifest restlessness, tremors, shrill crying, convulsions, or twitchings of the extremities and/or face. The Moro reflex may be incomplete, and the deep tendon reflexes may be increased. Diarrhea, vomiting, anorexia, yawning, sneezing and excessive mucus also may be present. These symptoms parallel somewhat those found in the adult undergoing withdrawal symptoms from narcotics. If the signs of withdrawal are unrecognized, the baby may die; if the infant is treated (hydration, supportive measures, and diminishing doses of sedatives), then recovery and permanent cure are assured since the infant does not have a psychic dependence on narcotics. However, some physicians believe that the infant should be removed from the mother's environment if it carries a threat of readdiction. This possibility will present a problem that will require a multidisciplinary approach, and the nurse can be helpful in beginning the process through appropriate and accurate reporting and recording.

The Infant of the Diabetic Mother

The successful control of diabetes with insulin has led to the survival and fertility of an increasing number of diabetic women (see Chap. 18). The infants of these women and women who have a prediabetic condition exhibit certain characteristics that are distinctive. In addition to having distinctive characteristics, these infants have a higher incidence of intra-uterine deaths after the 36th week of gestation and a higher neonatal mortality rate than the general population. These babies are large, often 10 pounds or over; their increased body weight is due to a combination of obesity and edema. The former is thought to be related to excessive insulin production, and the latter, to excessive intracellular glycogen deposition. Hypoglycemia, hyperbilirubinemia and hypocalcemia also are common. The infants appear to be bloated and tend to be jumpy or trembly after the first 24 hours of life. They are subject to unexplained cyanotic attacks, and the respiratory distress syndrome (see p. 532) is common. The tremulousness appears to be due to the hypoglycemia and hypocalcemia. The increased perinatal mortality is thought to be secondary to such maternal factors as ketosis, hydramnios, preeclampsia and vascular degeneration, which are common accompaniments of the diabetic and prediabetic state.

The management of these infants is all-important. A pediatrician is usually in attendance at the time of delivery, which may be done vaginally, but is more often accomplished by cesarean section (to prevent intra-uterine death, which is common after 36 weeks of gestation). He will institute resuscitation measures in cases of respiratory distress, treat hyperbilirubinemia or infection, if they are present, and examine the infant for congenital anomalies. The infant is usually given an Apgar rating, which gives a more accurate indication of the prognosis than other classifications (see Chap. 12). Aspiration of the infant's gastric contents is done immediately after the airway has been cleared. This procedure is thought to be helpful in reducing the incidence of respiratory distress syndrome through removal of swallowed amniotic fluid, which may be regurgitated and aspirated and contribute to the formation of the syndrome. The child may be transferred to the premature nursery and a low concentration of oxygen given to facilitate respiration. Early feeding (4 to 12 hours after birth) of glucose in water or sodium chloride solution may be instituted to reduce the hypoglycemia. If convulsions occur, especially within the first 6 hours of life, blood will be drawn for sugar determination and a glucose solution started intravenously; intravenous feeding will be continued until the infant is feeding well by mouth.

Nursing Care. The importance of accurate observation and reporting by the nurse regarding these infants cannot be stressed enough. Vital signs must be watched carefully and respiratory function closely observed. Nursing care is similar to that for a premature infant and that for a baby who is being observed for respiratory difficulty. Appropriate explanation and reassurance of the parents also are necessary. They will need counseling regarding future childbearing, since there is no prevention of the problems in these infants as long as diabetes or a prediabetic condition exists. The baby's prognosis is good if he survives the first 48 hours of life; his subsequent progress will be the same as that of an infant of his gestational age.

SUGGESTED READING

Apgar, Virginia: Drugs in pregnancy, Am. J. Nurs. 65:104-105, March 1965, reprinted from J.A.M.A. 190:840-841, 1964.

Atresia of the esophagus, Clin. Sympos. 11:48-53, March-April, 1959.

Benz, G. S.: Pediatric Nursing, ed. 5, St. Louis, Mosby, 1964.

Blake, F. G., and Wright, F. H.: Essentials of Pediatric Nursing, ed. 7, Philadelphia, Lippincott, 1963.

Bowes, W. A., *et al.*: Amniocentesis and intra-uterine fetal transfusion in erythroblastosis, Am. J. Obstet. Gynec. 93, No. 6:822-841, November 15, 1965.

Brody, J. A., *et al.*: Prevention of rubella by gamma globulin during an epidemic in Barrow, Alaska, in 1964, New Eng. J. Med. 272:127-129, January 21, 1965.

Brooks, Milo, *et al.*: The child with deformed or missing limbs—his problems and prosthesis, Am. J. Nurs. 62:88-92, November, 1962.

Bruce, S.: Reactions of nurses and mothers to stillbirths, Nurs. Outlook 10:88-91, February, 1962.

Buchanan-Davidson, D. J.: What can we learn from meconium?, Am. J. Nurs. 63:112-113, July, 1963.

Caplan, Gerald: The mental hygiene role of the nurse in maternal and child care, Nurs. Outlook 2:14-19, January, 1954.

Carson, M. J.: Diabetes mellitus in infants and children, Postgrad. Med. 36:67-75, July, 1964.

Cleft Lip and Cleft Palate, Ross Laboratories, Nursing Education Service, No. 11, Columbus, Ohio, 1962.

Coffelt, R. W.: Unexpected finding from a PKU newborn screening program, Pediatrics 24:889-890, December, 1964.

Committee on Handicapped Child: Statement on treatment of phenylketonuria, Pediatrics 25:501-503, March, 1965.

Cornblath, M., *et al.*: Research and nursing care in the premature nursery, Am. J. Nurs. 62:92-96, July, 1962.

Davens, E.: A view of health services for mothers and children, Children 12:47-54, March-April, 1965.

David, A. J.: The skills of communication, Am. J. Nurs. 63:66-70, January, 1963.

Davidson-Buchanan, D. J.: Erythroblastosis neonatorum, Am. J. Nurs. 64:110-112, April, 1964.

Davis, Louise: PKU testing in older children—follow-up report, Nurs. Outlook 12:55, April, 1964.

Diller, L.: Psychology of disabled children, Am. J. Nurs. 64:131-136, July, 1964.

Duke-Elder, Sir Stewart: Parson's Diseases of the Eye, ed. 14, London, Churchill, 1964.

Eastman, N. J., and Hellman, L. M.: Williams Obstetrics, ed. 13, New York, Appleton, 1966.

Editors: Saving life before birth, Med. World News 6:43-53, January 1, 1965.

Engel, G. L.: Grief and grieving, Am. J. Nurs. 64:93-98, September, 1964.

Falconer, M. W., et al.: The Drug, the Nurse, the Patient, ed. 2, Philadelphia, Saunders, 1962.

Fishbein, M. (ed.): Birth Defects, Philadelphia, Lippincott, 1963.

Fleming, J. W.: Recognizing the newborn addict, Am. J. Nurs. 65:83, January, 1965.

Freda, V. J.: The Rh problem in obstetrics and a new concept of its management using amniocentesis and spectrophotometric scanning of amniotic fluid, Am. J. Obstet. Gynec. 92, No. 3:341-371, June 1, 1965.

Freda, V. J., and Robertson, J. G.: Amniotic fluid analysis in Rh iso-immunization, Am. J. Nurs. 65:64-68, August, 1965.

Gingras, G., et al.: Congenital anomalies of the limbs—medical aspects, Canad. Med. Assoc. J. 91:67-72, July 11, 1964.

Glaser, B. G., and Strauss, A.: The social loss of dying patients, Am. J. Nurs. 64:119-121, June, 1964.

Glynn, E. M.: Nursing support during intrauterine transfusion, Am. J. Nurs. 65:72-73, August, 1965.

Groves, R., and Schlvesser, P. T.: A state program to control phenylketonuria, Am. J. Nurs. 64:74-77, August, 1964.

Guthrie, Robert, and Stewart, W.: Phenylketonuria, Children's Bureau Publication No. 41, Washington, D. C., U. S. Government Printing Office, 1964.

Hagbard, Lars: Pregnancy and Diabetes Mellitus, Springfield, Ill., Thomas, 1961.

Kramm, E. R.: Families of Mongoloid Children, U. S. Children's Bureau, Publication No. 401, Washington, D. C., U. S. Government Printing Office, 1963.

LaDu, B. N.: Inborn errors of metabolism, Am. J. Obstet. Gynec. 90, part 2:1024-1034, December 1, 1964.

Larsen, G. L.: What every nurse should know about congenital syphilis, Nurs. Outlook 13:52-54, March, 1965.

Liley, A. W.: Intrauterine transfusion of foetus in haemolytic disease, Brit. Med. J. 2:1107, November 2, 1963.

Lin-Fu, J. S.: Histidinemia, Washington, D. C., U. S. Children's Bureau, 1964.

Lyon, R. A.: Pediatrics 1960-61, Philadelphia, Davis, 1960.

McCracken, J. S.: Subclinical virology in pregnancy, Nurs. Mirror, p. 247, December 11, 1964.

McDermott, M. M.: The child with cleft lip and palate: the pediatric ward, Am. J. Nurs. 65:122-123, April, 1965.

McDonald, J. C.: Gamma-globulin for the prevention of rubella in pregnancy, Brit. Med. J. No. 5354:416-418, August 17, 1963.

McGowen, Larry: Rubella and pregnancy: a current opinion, Postgrad. Med. 36:88-90, July, 1964.

McKendry, J. B. J.: Jaundice in the newborn infant, Clin. Pediat. 3:209-214, April, 1964.

McLenahan, I. G.: No baby to take home, Am. J. Nurs. 62:70-71, April, 1962.

Maple Syrup Urine Disease, Washington, D. C., U. S. Children's Bureau, 1964.

Marlow, D. R.: Textbook of Pediatric Nursing, ed. 2, Philadelphia, Saunders, 1965.

Mathews, D. H., et al.: Closed chest massage in the newborn infant, J.A.M.A. 183:964-966, March, 16, 1963.

Miller, A. L., and McDonald, E.: Staphylococcal infections—A community problem, Nurs. Outlook 7:584-587, October, 1959.

Nelson, W.: Textbook of Pediatrics, ed. 8, Philadelphia, Saunders, 1964.

Newman, A. J., and Grose, Samuel: Hyperbilirubinemia in breast-fed infants, Pediatrics 32:995-1001, December, 1963.

Newman, D. S., and Sutherland, J. M.: Diagnosing hyaline membrane disease, Am. J. Nurs. 61:72-75, January, 1961.

Odell, G. B.: Hyperbilirubinemia in the neonatal period, Postgrad. Med. 36:280-286, September, 1964.

Owens, C.: Parents' reactions to defective babies, Am. J. Nurs. 64:83-86, November, 1964.

Parmalee, A. H.: The doctor, and the handicapped child, Children 9:189-193, September-October, 1962.

Prinzing, D. M.: Cleft palate habilitation, Nurs. Outlook 7:577-579, October, 1959.

Queenan, J. T.: Intra-uterine transfusion for erythroblastosis fetalis, Am. J. Nurs. 65:68-72, August, 1965.

Queenan, J. T., and Douglas, R. G.: Intrauterine transfusion: a preliminary report, Obstet. Gynec. 25:308-321, March, 1965.

Quint, J. C. and Strauss, A. L.: Nursing students,

assignments and dying, Nurs. Outlook 12:24-27, January, 1964.

Ripley, I. L.: The child with cleft lip and palate: through his years of growth, Am. J. Nurs. 65:124-127, April, 1965.

Root, H. F., and White, Priscilla: Diabetes Mellitus, New York, Landsberger, 1956.

Schild, Sylvia: Parents of children with phenylketonuria, Children 11:92-96, May-June, 1964.

Schwartz, Philip: Birth Injuries of the Newborn, New York, Hafner, 1961.

Stanley, J. L.: Physiology of respiration in newborn infants and in respiratory distress syndrome, Pediatrics 24, No. 6:1069-1101, 1959.

Stephens, J. W., *et al.*: Diabetes and pregnancy, Diabetes 12:213-219, May-June, 1963.

Strassman, S. S.: The respiratory distress syndrome, Ohio Med. J. 60:556-558, June, 1964.

Symposium on congenital defect, Am. J. Obstet. Gynec. 90, No. 7, part 2:983-1250 (entire issue), December 1, 1964.

U. S. Children's Bureau: Galactosemia: A Selected Bibliography, compiled by Donough O'Brien, Washington, D. C., U. S. Government Printing Office, 1963.

U. S. Children's Bureau: The Clinical Team Looks at Phenylketonuria, Washington, D. C., U. S. Government Printing Office, 1964.

Urry, Nellene: Progressive muscular atrophy in an infant, Am. J. Nurs., 63:74-76, November, 1963.

Van Leeuwen, Gerard, and Jackson, R. L.: Infants of diabetic mothers, Clin. Pediat. 4:315-319, June, 1965.

Westberg, J. A., and Margolis, A. J.: Amniotic fluid evaluation and intrauterine transfusions for erythroblastosis fetalis, Am. J. Obstet. Gynec. 92, No. 5:583-591, July 1, 1965.

White, Priscilla: Management of pregnancy in the diabetic patient, Spectrum 6, No. 19:520-521, 1958.

White, P.: The pregnant diabetic, Virginia Med. Monthly 91:102-105, March, 1964.

CONFERENCE MATERIAL

1. In your own hospital setting, evaluate the facilities for and the care of the newborn infants in relation to the prevention of infection.

2. A mother's firstborn infant has a cleft lip and cleft palate. The infant is apparently normal otherwise. The distraught mother can see only "my poor deformed baby girl" and blames herself for this "tragedy," because she did not follow her physician's instructions during pregnancy, particularly in relation to good nutrition. How might the nurse handle the nursing problems in this situation?

3. How do you account for the high infant mortality during the neonatal period?

4. What community agencies in your city render services for handicapped children? What is the procedure for making the referral to such agencies? How can the public health nurse function most effectively in such cases?

5. What legislation in your city or state has contributed to reducing the incidence of congenital syphilis?

6. What methods are used by your hospital, well-baby clinics, and/or other community agencies for the detection of phenylketonuria?

Study Questions

UNIT EIGHT: ABNORMALITIES OF THE FETUS AND THE NEWBORN

Read through the entire question and place your answer on the line to the right.

1. When the newborn infant does not breathe at birth, and modern equipment for infant resuscitation is not available, which of the following procedures are sometimes resorted to?
   A. Hold the infant in the palm of one hand, with head, legs and arms hanging forward, thus compressing the chest wall. Then turn the infant over on its back, in the other hand, in which position the head, legs and arms hang backward, thus expanding the chest.
   B. With one hand grasp the infant by the ankles and hold him suspended head downward, while the other hand is used to "milk the trachea" or gently rub the infant's back.
   C. Mouth-to-mouth insufflation, exhaling through clean dry gauze directly into the infant's mouth at intervals corresponding to those of normal respiration.
   D. Alternately, plunge the infant into tubs of hot and cold water.
   E. Immerse the infant's body in a tub of hot water (110° F.) to prevent chilling and simultaneously dash a little cold water upon the infant's face and chest.

   Select the number corresponding to the correct letters.
   1. A and C
   2. B and C
   3. B and D
   4. C and E

   2

2. The nurse sometimes observes swelling of the newborn infant's scalp which may be due to caput succedaneum or cephalhematoma. Which of the following statements are true concerning cephalhematoma?
   A. It is due to an extravasation of serum into the tissues of the scalp.
   B. It is seldom visible when the infant is born and may not be noticed for several hours or more after delivery.
   C. The infant usually recovers without treatment.
   D. It always disappears within a few days.
   E. It gradually increases in size until about a week after the infant's birth, when it remains stationary for a time and then begins to disappear.

   Select the number corresponding to the correct letters.
   1. A and B
   2. A, C and D
   3. B, C and D
   4. B, C and E

   4

3. What are some of the signs of cerebral hemorrhage which may be observed by the nurse caring for infants in the newborn nursery?
   A. Convulsions
   B. Slow, deep, rhythmic respiration
   C. Twitching of extremities
   D. Flushed face with circumoral pallor
   E. Weak, whining cry

   Select the number corresponding to the correct letter or letters.
   1. A only
   2. A and C
   3. B, C and E
   4. All of them

   2

555

4. A newborn infant develops respiratory distress several hours after birth, and the diagnosis of hyaline membrane disease is made. Which of the following statements have bearing on this condition?
  A. The infant was born prematurely.
  B. The infant is cyanotic and dyspneic.
  C. Progressive respiratory difficulty is evidenced by increased cyanosis and marked sternal retractions.
  D. Treatment primarily consists of the administration of oxygen and maintenance of high humidity.
  E. A protein material is obstructing the flow of air and the exchange of oxygen and carbon dioxide in the lungs.

Select the number corresponding to the correct letters.
  1. A, B and C
  2. B, D and E
  3. C, D and E
  4. All of them

4

5. Which of the following manifestations of staphylococcal infection may appear in the newborn infant?
  A. Impetigo
  B. Milia
  C. Conjunctivitis
  D. Erythema toxicum
  E. Breast engorgement

Select the number corresponding to the correct letters.
  1. A and C
  2. A and D
  3. B, C and E
  4. All of them

1

6. Which of the following conditions are congenital disorders?
  A. Phimosis
  B. Chloasma
  C. Frenum linguae
  D. Retrolental fibroplasia
  E. Seborrhea capitis

Select the number corresponding to the correct letters.
  1. A and C
  2. B, C and D
  3. B, D and E
  4. All of them

1

7. The most effective treatment of erythroblastosis is accomplished by blood transfusion. Which one of the following is the best method to use?
  A. Exchange transfusion with Rh-negative blood
  B. Exchange transfusion with Rh-positive blood
  C. Exchange transfusion with blood plasma
  D. Repeated small transfusions with Rh-negative blood
  E. Repeated small transfusions with Rh-positive blood
  F. Repeated small transfusions with blood plasma

8. Hemolytic disease of the newborn may be produced by the union of parents with which of the following blood types?
  A. Rh-positive mother with Rh-negative father
  B. Rh-negative mother with Rh-negative father
  C. Rh-negative mother with Rh-positive father
  D. Type O mother with Type A father
  E. Type A mother with Type B father

Select the number corresponding to the correct letters.
1. A and C
2. B and D
3. C and D
4. All of them

3

9. Which one of the following infectious diseases, when contracted by the mother during the first trimester of pregnancy, will most often produce congenital anomalies in the infant?
A. Scarlet fever
B. Rubella
C. Diphtheria
D. Rubeola
E. Typhoid fever

B

10. Some disorders which affect the infant in the neonatal period are manifestations of inborn errors of metabolism. Which of the following conditions would this include?
A. Phenylketonuria
B. Icterus neonatorum
C. Galactosemia
D. Down's syndrome
E. Erythroblastosis fetalis

Select the number corresponding to the correct letter or letters.
1. A only
2. A and C
3. B, C and D
4. B, D and E

2

Note: The key to the correct answers to these questions is given on page 598.

Related Information

Home Delivery; Nurse-Midwifery
Obstetrics During Emergency
History of Obstetrics

Chapter 22

Home Delivery; Nurse-Midwifery

Even though at the present time the vast majority of mothers in this country are delivered in hospitals, there is still a small percentage of deliveries attended by physicians and qualified midwives at home, the majority of which take place in rural areas. Therefore, the nurse should know how a home delivery is conducted. In an emergency, too, the nurse may need this knowledge and experience. For the nurse who is interested in obtaining special preparation for this aspect of maternity care, a small number of schools in this country offer nurse-midwifery programs that include education and training for the conduct of home deliveries.

When a home delivery is preferred, such factors as the normalcy of the patient, accessibility of the obstetrician, facilities at home and available care are important considerations.

PREPARATIONS FOR HOME DELIVERY

Preparations for home delivery should be begun early in pregnancy to enable the family to make adequate preparations. Today in many areas the public health nurse visits the patient in her home routinely during the antepartal period and assists the physician in the management and care of the mother. When there is a home delivery service, these nurses may attend the delivery with the physician. The nurse can be most helpful with prepara-

tions for delivery because of her special knowledge.

Many obstetricians give their patients a list of supplies that they will need for delivery at home, but where the matter is left to the parents and the nurse, the following suggestions may be helpful. Even when the mother has been able to avail herself of the opportunity of attending a Mothers' Club or expectant parents' classes and of obtaining suggestions, she may desire to discuss some of them, along with personal problems, with the obstetrician and the nurse.

Supplies for the Mother

The supplies provided by the mother will necessarily vary in the individual situation. The following list contains supplies which will be needed:

Sheets and pillowcases (4)

Bath towels and washcloths (4)

Waterproof material—large enough to protect the mattress (about 1½ yards square). Rubber sheeting, plastic or white table oilcloth are preferable, although heavy brown paper can be used.

Receiving blanket for the infant

Delivery pads (4 to 6). These bed pads are made from 12 thicknesses of newspaper opened to full size (sewed together at the edges) and covered with freshly laundered old or new muslin. The corners of the

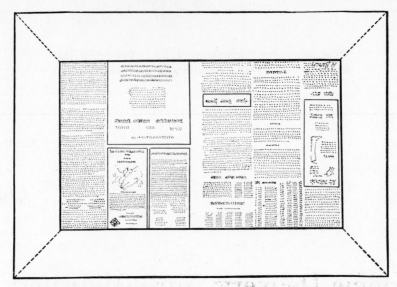

FIG. 22-1. Newspaper pad made of 12 thicknesses of newspaper sewed together at the outer edges and covered with unbleached muslin (viewed from underside). The muslin covers are mitered at the corners so that they may be removed, laundered and used again.

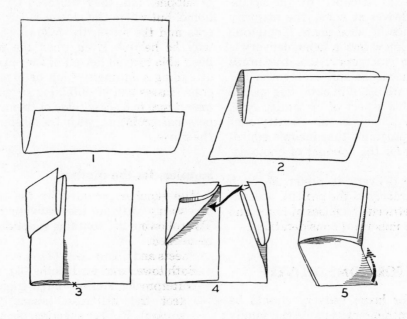

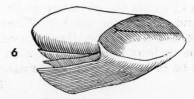

FIG. 22-2. Steps in making a newspaper bag. These are useful receptacles for waste material. They may be made in small and large sizes.

cover may be mitered, so that it can be removed and laundered when necessary and fresh newspaper inserted (Fig. 22-1). Quilted pads or large-size paper diapers may also be purchased for this purpose.

Newspapers. A supply of clean newspapers should be saved for the many uses to which they can be put at this time.

Newspaper bags. The large newspaper bags are especially useful at the time of delivery (Fig. 22-2).

Small enamel wash basins (2 or 3) for solutions and sponges used in cleansing the patient's genitals, to receive the placenta, and a hand basin.

Large pail with cover

Covered kettles or stew pans (2), one for cooled boiled water and one for boiling water

Ladle or dipper

Enema can with tubing and rectal tip

Board for placing under mattress of delivery bed (table leaf or ironing board without legs may be used)

Hot-water bottle and cover

Bedpan

Pair of white stockings (may be inexpensive variety)

Nightgowns or pajama tops (3 or 4)

Brassières (3 or 4) (may be improvised from straight binders, 10 in. wide, or large smooth cotton towels)

Sanitary pads (2 to 3 doz.). If they cannot be purchased, they may be made from freshly laundered, soft, absorbent material, folded and ironed ready for use.

Sanitary belts or T-binders (3 or 4)

Safety pins: 1 doz. small and 1 doz. large

Pitcher or Mason jar with cover

Sterile absorbent cotton (1 lb.) in original package, unopened

Sterile gauze squares 4″ x 4″ (1 doz.)

Mineral oil

Plain white petroleum jelly (tube)

Soap

New nail brush and orangewood stick

Umbilical tape or bobbin tape (narrow cotton) for tying cord (1 yd.)

Scissors

Roll of toilet tissue, unopened

Home Preparations

In preparing for a home delivery, the nurse should explain and demonstrate to the mother how to prepare the articles that are to be used during delivery, viz., sheets to be used for the bed and draping, towels and bed pads of the homemade variety. These articles should be washed with soap and water, dried in the sun if possible, ironed and folded so that the ironed surfaces are folded upon each other. The ironed surface should be used for the field of delivery. These articles should be put away in a pillowcase or wrapped in a piece of ironed paper. The other articles needed at the time of delivery should be laid aside ready for use. Packages of absorbent cotton, gauze squares, sanitary pads and toilet tissue should be put away unopened.

Packages of sterile delivery supplies may be available from a local health agency, or it may be possible to have a package, assembled at home, autoclaved at a local hospital. Although autoclaving is most desirable, it is possible to sterilize dressings, etc., in the oven at home. The simplest method is to place the materials in small muslin bags, or bags of some other heavy white cotton material, and then place these bags in an old pillowcase and pin it shut (double wrapped). This package should be baked on the top shelf in a moderate oven, 325° for 1 hour. If an oven thermometer is not available, place a large white potato (washed and scrubbed) in the oven, and when it is done, the supplies in the pillowcase should be sterilized. The pillowcase should not be opened until the time of delivery, and if it has not been used within a month, it must be resterilized.

The more simple and carefully prepared the preparations are, the more efficient will be the results. The important factor to be achieved in a home delivery is cleanliness. Soap and water, sunshine and a hot iron have proved to be effective. On the whole, only a few articles must be sterile.

Room for Delivery

Deciding on the room in which the patient is to be delivered is one of the "preparations." It should be the room in which the patient will be most comfortable. Many mothers during this period have to assume certain responsibilities for the management of the household, so it means much to be where the household affairs can be directed with the least exertion.

Ideally, it should be a room that is light, airy, quiet, cheerful and comfortable, conveniently near a bathroom. The room furnishings should be simple, so that they are easy to keep clean, as cleanliness is one of the first essentials of good obstetric care. The bed should be so placed that it can be approached from either side, and so that the light is convenient either day or night. Ample light is a necessity.

The nurse may help select the room, but the choice is limited or even fixed by the possibilities of the house. Naturally, the nurse will avoid putting the family to any unnecessary inconvenience, but always her first thought must be in the interest of her patient.

The nurse should make sure that the room has not been occupied recently by a patient suffering from any contagious, infectious or suppurative disease. The instructions set forth in the manual *The Control of Communicable Disease in Man,* American Public Health Association, regulate the isolation, quarantine and disinfection practiced in the care of the patient with communicable disease. In case of such disease, adaptation of procedures to facilities in the home is made as necessary.

In any event, the room should be cleaned thoroughly, and all unnecessary furniture removed, only enough being left to make the room comfortable and cheerful. The obstetrician will need a plain table or a substitute. The nurse will need a table or chair for supplies, unless perhaps the top of the bureau may be used. A card table may be very practical.

Preparation of the Delivery Bed

The mother's bed should be comfortable. The springs should be in good condition, and the mattress firm and level. A single bed is preferable to the wider or double bed, because it is easier for the obstetrician and the nurse to care for the mother. If the bed is low, it may be raised to a more convenient height by using blocks. The bed should be so arranged that after the labor the mother may be made clean and comfortable without too much disturbance. The best way to accomplish this is first to prepare the bed as it is to be used after delivery and then to add the necessary preparations on top for the labor and the delivery.

The mattress should be supported by means of boards placed between it and the springs, so that it will be perfectly firm and level and not sag. Table leaves, a flat ironing board or plain board may be used for this purpose. Such supports should lie crosswise under the mattress at a point directly under the mother's buttocks and should be removed at the conclusion of the delivery. A firm, flat mattress helps to prevent the patient's hips from sinking into the bed.

The mattress should be covered with a piece of waterproof material, if available; if not, heavy brown paper, newspaper or water-repellent paper may be used. Over this covering, a white cotton sheet should be placed and tucked in securely along the edges. The top sheet, the blanket and the spread should be fan-folded to the foot of the bed, where they will be convenient to cover the mother immediately after the delivery. Covered newspaper or moistureproof pads afford excellent protection and are so arranged that they protect the bed at the time of delivery, and a fresh one is left under the mother after delivery.

If these preparations are first demonstrated and their uses explained to the patient and her husband, they may be better able to make adequate preparations and have them ready at the time of labor.

Special Equipment

The physician and the nurse probably will have all the supplies needed for the delivery other than those provided by the mother. As stated previously, sometimes these supplies are provided by a local health agency. The Maryland State Department of Health, Division of Public Health Nursing, provides its staff with a nurse's bag and, since it provides a home delivery service, also makes available a nurse-midwife's delivery bag which contains the following:
1. Newspaper pads
   Safety pins
2. Sterno outfit
3. Box of medicines:
   A. Syntocinon (2 amp.)
   B. Methergine (2 amp.)
   C. Ergotrate tablets (50)
   D. Silver nitrate 1% (2 wax amp.)
   E. Vitamin K_1 (2 amp.)
   F. File

Fig. 22-3. The evolution of a newspaper Kelly pad. When used under a patient, it is lined with a piece of waterproof material and a towel.

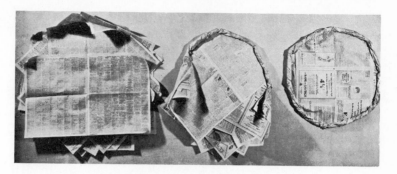

G. Chromic catgut #2 (2 tubes)
4. Sterile gloves:
Size 7 (2 pairs)
Size 7½ (2 pairs)
5. Sterile pack containing:
A. Hand towel (1)
B. Doctor's gown (1)
C. Leggings (2) with towel clips (2)
D. Towels (6)
E. Gauze squares 3" x 3" (12)
F. Cord dressings (2) with cord ties (4)
G. Perineal pads (package)
H. Towels for pelvic examination (package of 5)
6. Case of instruments:
A. 1–2 cc. syringe with No. 25 needles (2)
B. Mayo scissors (1)
C. Metal box with needles
D. Sponge holder (1)
E. Kelly clamps (2)
7. Muslin case with scales, tape measure, bottle of cord tape, 3" x 3" gauze squares (2 pkgs.)
8. Large basins (2)
Liter cup (1)
Bag of cotton (to be placed in cup)
9. Enamel covered container
10. Muslin case containing:
A. Applicators, tongue depressors, razor and box of blades, and finger cots
B. No. 14 catheters (2):
1 for bladder catheterization
1 for suctioning the infant
C. No. 28 rectal tube with glass connecting tip (1)
D. Rubber bulb syringe (1)
11. Muslin case containing enema equipment
12. Muslin case containing:
A. Aprons (2)
B. Caps (2)
C. Masks (4)

13. Brown folder containing:
A. Delivery bag list
B. Labor and delivery procedure
C. Standing orders
D. Procedure for care of premature infants.
E. Birth certificate book
F. Labor and delivery records (12)
G. Infant records (6)
H. Baby's Care (6)
I. Small envelopes (12)
J. Scratch pad and pencil
K. Laundry lists (12)
14. Side pockets of bag:
No. 1. Thermometers
A. Mouth thermometer
B. Rectal thermometer
No. 2. K. Y. jelly
No. 3.
A. Alcohol 70%
B. Green soap
C. Bottle of antiseptic No. 3
D. Mercury cyanide
E. Brush and orangewood stick
F. Paper napkins (12)
G. Paper towels (12)
H. Aromatic spirits of ammonia

If an anesthetic other than Trilene is to be given, the nurse may need to cover the wire mask (Fig. 11-6). A cone may be improvised with a wire sieve, but should not be made from newspaper because of the danger involved (see Chap. 11, Analgesia and Anesthesia in Labor).

DELIVERY IN THE HOME

During the antepartal period the patient and her husband will have prepared the needed supplies and made preparations so that labor should be conducted with comparatively little inconvenience and confusion. They have been

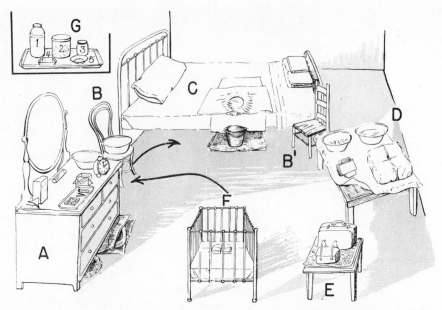

FIG. 22-4. Delivery room in the home, in readiness for the mother in labor.
A. Bureau (newspaper protecting the surface, cloth on top):
1. Flashlight
2. Perineal pads
3. Paper waste bag
4. Clock
5. Basin
6. Enamel tray containing: (a) Thermometer in solution in glass tube, (b) Thumb forceps, (c) Cotton balls in tray
B. Chair at head of bed for enema equipment. *Note.* This chair will be moved down toward the center of the bed later to support the mother's legs for the actual delivery.
B¹ Second chair to be moved toward the center of the bed to support the mother's legs for the delivery.
C. Bed protected with paper pad, Kelly newspaper pad and cloth cover for the delivery. Sheet fanned-folded to foot of bed, extra blanket and sheet. (Bed is made for delivery with the mother lying crosswise.)
D. Table (protected with newspaper covered by cloth):
1. Basin of antiseptic solution
2. Basin with sterile cotton balls in water
3. Sterile gloves and towels
4. Sterile pack (for contents see Special Equipment in this chapter)
E. Small table (protected with newspaper) for nurse's bag and delivery bag (see Special Equipment for contents)
F. Crib containing small bundle of infant's clothes and blankets. *Note.* The crib is moved in place of chair B when that space is available.
G. Improvised toilet tray for the infant:
1. Jars (3) for boiled water, cotton balls and small cotton swabs
2. Soap dish
3. Dish for mineral oil
Note. This tray should be readily available for use when needed for the infant's initial care. Before this time there may be no place for it because the bureau and small table surfaces are occupied by the essentials for the delivery.

FIG. 22-5. The certified nurse-midwife conducting a home delivery. The father at the bedside encourages his wife and simultaneously derives considerable satisfaction from his participation in the birth of their baby. (Catholic Maternity Institute, Santa Fe, N. Mex.)

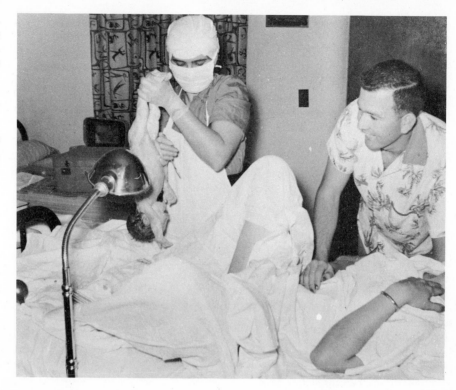

instructed concerning the symptoms of labor and when to call the physician and the nurse. Many physicians wish to be with the mother from the onset of labor; however, this will have been arranged beforehand, and if the nurse's arrival precedes that of the physician, she will make her observations of the mother's condition and proceed accordingly.

A few preparations cannot be made until labor begins, such as boiling the 2 kettles of water (for 20 minutes) in covered vessels and setting 1 aside to cool. It is a good idea also to boil a ladle or dipper in the kettle that is set aside to cool. The bed and the crib should be prepared and the delivery supplies arranged (Fig. 22-4). The nurse should also see that the provisions for lighting the room are ample, and that the room is warm and as comfortable as possible.

The underlying principles for the care of the mother being delivered at home are the same as those for hospital delivery (see Chap. 12), although procedures will necessarily have to be modified because of the home situation. The patient will probably have taken a warm sponge bath, but it may be necessary to assist her with it if this is necessary and time permits. The patient should have special preparation for delivery. These preparations may seem strange to the patient, so the nurse should explain procedures and any developments carefully, so the mother will have less cause to become anxious. According to the physician's specific orders, a low soapsuds enema may be given to empty the lower intestine in order to make more room for the descending head and to prevent fecal discharge during the delivery. The vulva should be shaved and the external genitalia cleansed with aseptic technic. The mother may need to have it explained that the former practice of keeping a perineal pad on while in labor has been largely discarded because of the danger of carrying infection, notably the colon bacillus, to the parturient canal from the anal region.

During the first stage of labor the mother is usually allowed to be up and about until labor becomes very active, or the membranes rupture. The physician may suggest liquids to be given freely and that light nourishment be offered, such as tea and toast or crackers, if delivery is not imminent. As labor progresses, careful explanation will provide comfort and reassurance.

The nursing care of the mother in labor at home is essentially the same as in the hospital. Observations of the mother's temperature, pulse, respirations, blood pressure, intake and output and the progress of labor are made consistently. The fetal heart tones should be checked routinely, and the mother should be watched closely for any complication which might develop. If membranes rupture in the first stage of labor, the danger of prolapse of the cord must be kept in mind. In addition, if the physician is not present, he should be notified immediately, as would be the case if anything unusual developed. If the physician needs to be called for this reason, it should be done without alarming the mother, especially if this is her first labor. From the beginning of true labor, the mother should use a commode or bedpan and should be encouraged to empty her bladder at fairly frequent intervals to avoid bladder distention, as well as to keep her more comfortable.

As soon as it is apparent that the mother is nearing the second stage of labor, she should be put to bed, if she has not been already. The nurse should now have everything in readiness for delivery, if possible. On the arrival of the physician, he will, in all probability, want to make a rectal or a vaginal examination at once to determine the amount of dilatation of the cervix and the progress the mother has made. For the examination the patient should be in lithotomy position, lying on the side of the bed convenient for the physician. The nurse should drape the mother so that she is well protected, but with the perineal region well exposed. Some physicians prefer to make the examination with the patient lying on her back, but across the bed, with the buttocks resting on the edge of the mattress and the patient's feet supported by two chairs. A pillow may be placed under the patient's head for comfort. When a vaginal examination is to be made, the preparation of the perineal area will be according to the wishes of the physician. Although the technic for local preparation of the patient for vaginal examination varies, if the nurse always regards the perineal region as a site for operation and cleanses the immediate area accordingly, she has followed an important principle for safe care.

All instruments required for the delivery are usually provided by the physician and are brought to the home in sterile packages. However, if such equipment as catheters, hypodermic syringes and needles and the various instruments are not sterile, these are boiled in a tightly covered container for 20 minutes. Sterile packages should not be laid open, or sterile equipment laid out, until just before they are to be used for the delivery.

The Delivery. The activities of the nurse in assisting the physician at delivery will vary. Because of the vast differences in home situations, the details in each case are so variable that it would be impossible to describe them here. In general, the conduct of normal labor, as described in Chapter 12, should serve as a guide for the care of the mother and her infant.

Delivery by the Nurse

In certain cases the nurse will find it necessary to manage the entire labor herself, either because of precipitate delivery or through delay in securing the services of a physician.

It is needless to say that labor in such cases progresses rapidly, and that almost before anything else can be done, the contractions are recurring with such frequency and severity that the mother must be put to bed and be given the undivided attention of the nurse. If time permits, much can be done for the comfort of the mother while preparations are made for delivery. Undoubtedly, the calmness of the nurse at the bedside will be transferred to the mother.

It seldom happens that the nurse and her patient are entirely alone; usually the husband, some relative or friend in the home can be called upon to assist and bring the necessary things to the bedside. In an emergency, when there has been no previous preparation, an ordinary pair of scissors and pieces of clean, soft, white cord or tape may be boiled and used for tying and cutting the cord. As there is usually never any special hurry about tying and cutting the umbilical cord, there is time for scissors and tape to be boiled. Time may be saved by using only enough water to cover the instruments, but it must be sufficient to allow for evaporation. Also, anything which will float, such as the tape, should be weighted down with the scissors. The pan may be covered with a second pan, thus sterilizing both.

If the patient is fully dressed, as may be the case in precipitate delivery, the nurse should do what she can to protect the patient's clothing and the bedding and maintain cleanliness to the best of her ability. The procedure is, of course, the same as when the physician is present; but since the nursing care is wholly different, it may help her to have the steps described as they are in the section on Emergency Delivery by the Nurse in Chapter 12, in order to aid her until help arrives.

Nurse-Midwifery

The 12th International Congress of Midwives, held in Rome during the week of October 2, 1960, was attended by representatives from 39 countries, as well as the International Council of Nurses and the World Health Organization. The theme of the Congress, "The Midwife in the World of the Future," was developed through a series of papers on the effect of the changing pattern of civilization on the work of the midwife, the effect of scientific developments on the work of the midwife, and the educational role of the midwife in relation to the individual and the family.

In the inaugural address, Dr. Prawirohardjo presented a comprehensive review of the global situation, contemplating the world of the future and the role of the midwife and reviewing the significant events from the past and the present.[1] Any attempt to summarize the content of this paper would be an injustice; hence, the student is urged to read it in its entirety. However, it seems quite appropriate to quote here certain passages concerning the early history of midwifery:

From the remote past until about three centuries ago midwifery care was practically the sole domain of women-midwives; only in difficult situations with which they could not cope, male doctors were asked to render the necessary assistance. During the era of Greek medicine midwifery progressed, too, but in later centuries much of the knowledge was lost again. During the Middle Ages midwifery care was at a low level.

[1] Prawirohardjo, Sarwono: The midwife in the world of the future, Bull. Am. Coll. Nurse-Midwifery 6, No. 1:4-11, 14-19, March, 1961.

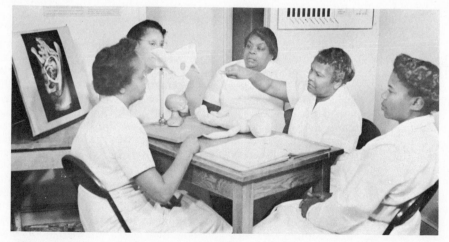

Fig. 22-6. The certified nurse-midwife, a member of the Public Health Nursing staff of Charles County Health Department, LaPlata, Maryland, conducting a class for nonprofessional midwives. (Maryland State Department of Health)

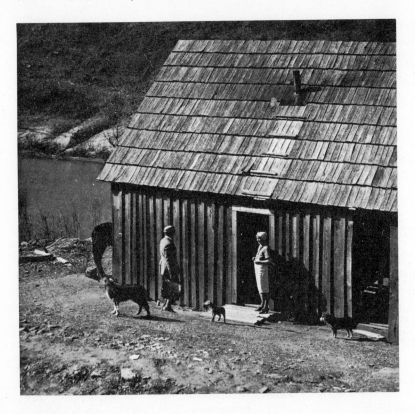

FIG. 22-7. Antepartal visit. Outside the cabin. (Photo by Marvin Breckinridge; Frontier Nursing Service, Wendover, Ky.)

Midwives were generally illiterate and ignorant, and deliveries took place mostly at home, where the conditions were usually unfavorable for safe performance. Abnormalities in pregnancy and labor meant, therefore, great danger to the mother and child.

During the period of the Renaissance two developments were being inaugurated which were destined to have a profound influence on midwifery and its practice. The first was related to efforts to attain a higher standard of professional skill for midwives, while the latter involved the intrusion of male doctors into a so far forbidden domain—that of normal pregnancy and labor.

In 1503 Eucharius Roesslin wrote a book entitled *Der Schwangeren Frauen und Hebammen Rosengarten*. The great significance of this book was that it was the first textbook of midwifery which was accessible for midwives because it was written in a vernacular language. It did meet, indeed, a long-felt need and it was translated into many languages. By means of this book Roesslin became for about a century the teacher of the midwives in Europe. Roesslin's example was later followed by many others. However, something more was needed to give the midwives the necessary competence for a satisfactory performance of their duties. What they most needed was a

better preparation for their work, and this was only possible through systematic training. The beginning of such a training was made in München in 1589 in the Munchener Gebäranstalt, but more famous was the school in the Maternity Department of the Hôtel-Dieu in Paris, opened in 1630. Systematic instruction of midwives is now worldwide in scope, and in practically every country schools of midwifery can be found.

In 1648, for the first time in history, male doctors were permitted to attend normal deliveries in the Hôtel-Dieu in Paris. This revolution, the management of midwifery by men, gradually spread over the whole of Europe and later over the whole world. Objectively viewed, the vesting of midwifery in the hands of men was of great advantage for its development. Without underestimating the work of many eminent midwives, it was mainly due to the achievements of medical men practicing and studying midwifery that obstetrics could raise its status and become a fullfledged discipline of medical learning and practice equal to medicine and surgery.

The increasing knowledge of the physiology and pathology of obstetrics at the end of the 19th century gave rise to that important development of maternity care which we know as "Prenatal Care." Becoming well-known through the efforts

FIG. 22-8. By horse and by jeep. (Louisville Courier-Journal photo — Thomas V. Miller, Jr.; Frontier Nursing Service, Wendover, Ky.)

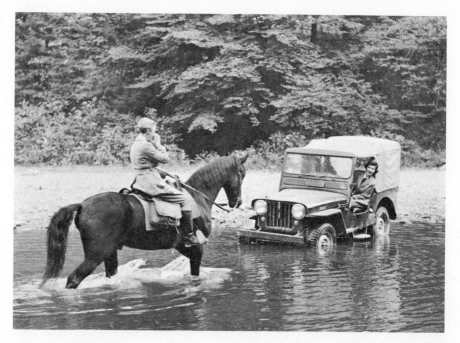

of Professor Budin, who in 1892 in the Charité Hospital in Paris started the famous Consultation des Nourissons, prenatal care is now being practiced everywhere. With its position as a central part of midwifery care, preventive medicine became firmly entrenched in the practice of obstetrics. In stressing the eminent importance of prenatal care, we must not depreciate the role of the other parts of maternity care, such as, for instance, intranatal care. Both prenatal and intranatal care are equally important, and both deserve the greatest attention in any program of maternity care. In this connection it has been rightly stated by Eardly Holland that "antenatal methods could be considered as the strategy and intranatal methods as the tactics of obstetrics, and that no one could be exalted at the expense of the other."

NURSE-MIDWIFERY IN THE UNITED STATES

Organizations

Frontier Nursing Service. The first use of the trained nurse-midwife in this country was made in 1925, when an organization was established in the mountains of eastern Kentucky to handle the maternity problem in the rural and isolated areas of that territory—the now famous Frontier Nursing Service (Figs. 22-7,

8). This organization was founded by the late Mrs. Mary Breckinridge at Wendover, Ky., the headquarters of the public health nurse-midwifery service. Today, FNS is organized with Hayden Hospital, which has a full-time Medical Director (an M.D.), and 5 outpost clinics, each staffed with nurse-midwives. These nurses often travel by horseback from the outposts to serve families in the even more remote areas, but along the highways and roads they travel today by jeep or station wagon (Figs. 22-7, 8). This organization has demonstrated clearly that graduate nurses prepared in midwifery can help to lower mortality rates in a large population in rural and isolated areas.

Frontier Nursing Service gives a wide range of medical care to 10,000 patients annually. In slightly more than the last decade, during which more than 5,000 mothers have been safely delivered by these nurse-midwives, there have been no maternal deaths. In the fall of 1939, the Frontier Nursing Service inaugurated the Frontier Graduate School of Midwifery in Hayden, Ky.

The **Maternity Center Association** was founded in New York in 1918, and in 1932 the Center established its school of nurse-midwifery for graduate nurses. The Lobenstine

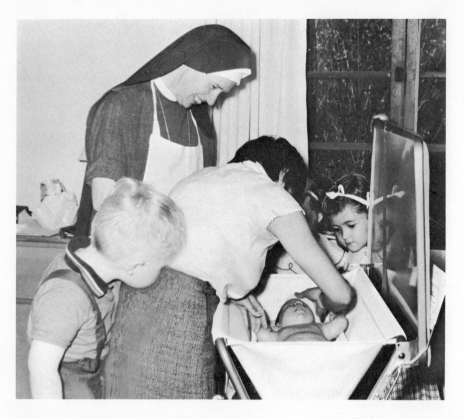

FIG. 22-9. Postpartal care and teaching in the home provided by the certified nurse-midwife. (Catholic Maternity Institute, Sante Fe, New Mexico)

Midwifery Clinic was established to provide a field service for this school. It trained about 12 students a year in a 6-month course which provided obstetric theory and supervised practice by an obstetrician and by graduate nurse-midwives. In 1935, the Maternity Center Association and the Lobenstine Midwifery Clinic applied to the State of New York to consolidate under the name of Maternity Center Association. The progress achieved in this endeavor can best be explained by citing an excerpt from the Center's recent annual report:

WHITHER NURSE-MIDWIFERY?[2]

One of the major projects of the Maternity Center Association since 1932 has been the education of nurse-midwives. These are professional nurses with graduate education in the science and art of obstetrics. The Center's school was the first in the United States.

Working within the framework of organized obstetric services, nurse-midwives provide warm, human, scientific care to mothers in clinics, in

[2] Maternity Center Association: Forty-fifth Annual Report (1918-1963), pp. 6-11, New York, Maternity Center Association, 1964.

labor and delivery rooms, in homes, in parents' classes. They direct maternal and child health programs at different levels of government. They are professors of graduate and undergraduate nursing education. These are superior, dedicated women, a majority of whom have a bachelor's degree, and many their master's degree in Nursing or Public Health. They enter nurse-midwifery because they want to serve well where the need is great.

Wherever nurse-midwives have worked, at large universities and medical centers, in the backwoods of Kentucky or the deserts of the Southwest, the bush country of Africa or the bleak hills of Korea, they have helped to bring confidence and comfort to patients and their families.

In an article in the *American Journal of Nursing*, Miss Mary I. Crawford, who heads the nurse-midwifery program at the Columbia-Presbyterian Medical Center, explained how nurse-midwives can improve maternity care in a large urban hospital. She pointed out that teams consisting of a resident doctor, a nurse-midwife and nurses, working in shifts in prenatal clinics and labor and delivery rooms, could provide greater continuity of care for the mother and more job satisfaction for the professional workers. Nurse-midwives in the United States, she went on to say, are not trying to be poorly prepared doctors but expertly prepared nurses.

Dr. Louis M. Hellman, Professor of Obstetrics and Gynecology at the State University of New York (Downstate Medical Center) and Director of the Department of Obstetrics at Kings County Hospital, recently estimated that by 1975 as many babies will be born in the *hospital ward services* as were born in the whole country in 1950. He foresaw also a rapidly declining number of general practitioners, with only a moderate increase in the number of obstetricians—not nearly enough to provide good care for the on-coming flood of newborn babies.

Who can provide this care? Since the nurse-midwives have been at Kings County Hospital, Dr. Hellman said, the capacity of the hospital has risen from 5,000 to 7,000 deliveries a year, and the perinatal mortality rate is an incredibly low 0.96.

Since 1958, Maternity Center Association's School of Nurse-Midwifery has conducted a joint program with the Downstate Medical Center of State University of New York and Kings County Hospital. In this time it has certified 89 nurse-midwife graduates. Most are Americans planning to practice in this country; some come from other parts of the world. Since the Center's School of Nurse-Midwifery was founded in 1932, 413 graduates have been certified.

The New York City Department of Health provides for the licensing of nurse-midwives, and qualified nurse-midwives, working as such, are employed in two municipal hospitals. The position of nurse-midwife is spelled out on the city's line budget.

If maternity care is to profit fully from what the nurse-midwife can contribute, the existing personnel-structure within the hospital should be restudied and recast. Is the nurse-midwife primarily a nurse working under the director of nurses? Or should she work under the medical director of obstetrics? Dr. Hellman believes she provides "third-party care," that is, between medicine and nursing, and a new pattern for work relationships among the professions must be developed. Unless this is done, most nurse-midwives will continue to work as consultants, educators and administrators rather than in direct patient care.

The American College of Nurse-Midwifery was established in 1955 as an organization of nurse-midwives to study and evaluate the activities of nurse-midwives, to plan and develop educational programs meeting the requirements of the profession, and to perform other related functions. In 1957, the College became a member of the International Confederation of Midwives, a midwifery organization with members from some 31 countries throughout the world.

At the annual meeting of the College in May, 1962, the definitions of the nurse-midwife and nurse-midwifery were accepted by the membership and stated as follows:

The Nurse-Midwife is a Registered Nurse who by virtue of added knowledge and skill gained through an organized program of study and clinical experience recognized by the American College of Nurse-Midwifery, has extended the limits (legal limits in jurisdictions where they obtain) of her practice into the area of management of care of mothers and babies throughout the maternity cycle so long as progress meets criteria accepted as normal.

Nurse-Midwifery is an extension of nursing practice into the area of management of care of mothers and babies throughout the maternity cycle so long as progress meets criteria accepted as normal.

This was a major step in the formulation of a basic policy for the College as a professional organization.

Midwifery Programs

At the present time there are 11 schools of nurse-midwifery in the United States, with several other programs reported to be in the planning stage. All of the schools provide programs of study for registered nurses (graduates from accredited schools of nursing) leading to a Certificate in Nurse-Midwifery. Five of the schools have their programs designed in conjunction with graduate study in nursing, leading to a Master of Science degree beside a Certificate in Nurse-Midwifery.

The American College of Nurse-Midwifery has published the following list of schools in the U.S.A. having programs in nurse-midwifery:[3]

Programs leading to a certificate in nurse-midwifery:

Nurse-Midwifery Program
Maternity Center Association,
48 East 92nd Street, New York, N.Y. 10028
   affiliated with

[3] What Is a Nurse-Midwife?, bulletin of The American College of Nurse-Midwifery, 50 East 92nd Street, New York, N. Y. 10028.

Downstate Medical Center,
State University of New York and
Kings County Hospital

The Johns Hopkins Hospital
Nurse-Midwifery Program
Room 151, Women's Clinic
601 North Broadway
Baltimore 5, Maryland

Catholic Maternity Institute
School of Nurse Midwifery
417 East Palace Avenue
Santa Fe, New Mexico

Graduate School of Nursing
New York Medical College
Nurse-Midwifery Program
Fifth Avenue and 106th Street
New York, N.Y.   10029

Frontier Nursing Service
School of Nurse-Midwifery
Wendover, Leslie County
Kentucky

Puerto Rico Nurse-Midwifery Program
Department of Health
University District Hospital
Caparra Heights
Puerto Rico

Programs leading to a Master's degree and a certificate in nurse-midwifery:

Presbyterian Hospital
Columbia University Graduate Program in
Maternity Nursing
Dept. of Nursing, Faculty of Medicine
Columbia-Presbyterian Medical Center
630 West 168th Street
New York, N.Y.   10032

The Catholic University of America
Washington, D.C.
   affiliated with
Catholic Maternity Institute
Santa Fe, New Mexico

Yale University School of Nursing
Nurse-Midwifery Program
Yale University School of Nursing
New Haven, Connecticut

Graduate School of Nursing
New York Medical College
Nurse-Midwifery Program
Fifth Avenue and 106th Street
New York, N.Y.   10029

Nurse-Midwifery Program*
University of Utah Medical Center
50 North Medical Drive
Salt Lake City, Utah

SUGGESTED READING

Home Delivery

Bookmiller, Mae, and Bowen, George: Textbook of Obstetrics and Obstetric Nursing, ed. 4, Philadelphia, Saunders, 1963.

Davis, M. E., and Rubin, Reva: DeLee's Obstetrics for Nurses, ed. 17, Philadelphia, Saunders, 1962.

Frontier Nursing Service, Wendover, Ky.: Thirty Years Onward (1925-1955), 1955.

Maryland State Department of Health, 301 West Preston St., Baltimore, Md.: Division of Public Health Nursing, Manual of Nursing and Special Procedures, 1955.

Maryland State Department of Health, Bureau of Preventive Medicine: Midwifery in the Counties of Maryland, The Maryland Law, Senate Bill No. 115, Enacted 1924, and Regulations of the State Board of Health Governing the Licensing of Midwives, Adopted February 1, 1957.

Newman, Margaret: The "mountain granny" bows out, Nurs. Outlook 6:680, 1958.

U. S. Children's Bureau: Prenatal Care, Publication No. 4, Washington, D. C., U. S. Government Printing Office, 1962.

Ziegel, Erna, and Van Blarcom, C. C.: Obstetrical Nursing, ed. 5, New York, Macmillan, 1964.

Nurse-Midwifery

Anniversary issue (10th), Bull. Am. Coll. Nurse-Midwifery 10, No. 1, Spring, 1965.

Clem, Alfred, and Haedenbrook, Harry: Edge of dark land, Abbottempo 2:15-21, February, 1964.

Corbin, Hazel, and Hellman, L. M.: The nurse-midwife in American obstetrics, Bull. Maternal Infant Health 7, No. 2:13-18, 1960.

Crawford, Mary: Potential of the urban nurse-midwife, Am. J. Nurs. 63:129-131, September, 1963.

Education issue, Bull. Am. Coll. Nurse-Midwifery 10, No. 2, Summer, 1965.

Frontier Nursing Service: Thirty Years Onward (1925-1955), Wendover, Ky., Frontier Nursing Service, 1955.

*New program-evaluation pending.

Gentile, Louis: A resident looks at the nurse-midwifery program, Bull. Am. Coll. Nurse-Midwifery 7, No. 3:68-72, Fall, 1962.

Hellman, Louis, and O'Brien, Francis: Nurse-midwifery, an experiment in maternity care, Obstet. Gynec. 24, No. 3:343-349, September, 1964.

Hershey, Nathan: Putting the legal aspects of nurse-midwifery in perspective, Bull. Am. Coll. Nurse-Midwifery 8, No. 3:65-75, 1963.

Prawirohardjo, Sarwono: The midwife in the world of the future, Bull. Am. Coll. Nurse-Midwifery 6, No. 1:4-11, 14-19, March, 1961.

Runnerstrom, Lillian: The contributions of nurse-midwifery to maternity care, Bull. Am. Coll. Nurse-Midwifery 5:44-45, June, 1960.

Sevcovic, Lorraine: The nurse-midwife—a clinical specialist, Bull. Am. Coll. Nurse-Midwifery 8, No. 4:93-102, Winter, 1963.

Twenty Years of Nurse Midwifery, New York, Maternity Center Association, 1955.

Whither nurse-midwifery?, Maternity Center Association: Forty-fifth Annual Report (1918-1963), pp. 6-11, New York, Maternity Center Association, 1964.

Whitridge, J. J.: Nurse-midwife fills a gap in obstetric care, Bull. Am. Coll. Nurse-Midwifery 5:28-35, June, 1960.

Wiedenbach, Ernestine: Nurse-midwifery—purpose, practice and opportunity, Nurs. Outlook 8:256-259, May, 1960.

Woodville, Lucille: Descriptive Data, Nurse Midwives—U.S.A., New York, American College of Nurse-Midwifery, 1963.

Chapter 23

Obstetrics During Emergency

When any large-scale emergency arises, it is usually sudden and calls for immediate action, whether it is caused by hurricane, flood, fire or war. In the event of such catastrophe, babies are likely to be born rapidly, and many women may abort. When organized rescue work is hampered, it may fall to those who are in the immediate area to manage as best they can. The nurses in the area should be able to assist with measures for the safety and the welfare of maternity patients and their newborn infants.

All nurses who have completed the basic course in maternity nursing are familiar with antepartal care, the conduct of labor and the immediate care of the newborn infant, but their preparation has been carried out, for the most part, in an organized environment (such as a hospital) where supplies, equipment and medical direction are available. It requires considerable imagination on the part of a nurse to conceive of an emergency situation in which she might be required to work. Communities may be isolated and temporarily left to their own resources if telephone and radio communications are wrecked; roads may be impassable if they are inundated by water and blocked by débris, and an area may be without safe water, means of power and light and medical supplies.

DISASTER INSURANCE FOR MOTHERS AND BABIES*

Sara E. Fetter, John Whitridge, Jr., and Col. John Welch

Insuring the lives and health of pregnant women and newborn infants during national or extensive local disasters requires planning for this purpose predicated on the belief that plans and preparations *prior* to disasters are essential and imperative.

With the advent of the H-bomb and the rapid advance in the development of ballistics and intercontinental missiles, the earlier concept of planning for the care of pregnant

* Reprinted from The Bulletin of Maternal Welfare 4:9, 1957.

women and newborn infants, based on the Hiroshima experience, has changed in some ways, because the degree and the extent of man-made hazard have increased. Protection from radioactive fallout must be provided; evacuation from expected target areas will be 20 to 50 miles distant, instead of the 8 to 10 miles originally considered necessary, and, in all probability, the care of women in labor must be provided en route. Large-scale plans are under way for evacuees to be cared for in reception areas—including pregnant women and newborn infants. As the national defenses are strengthened and increased, there is logical expectation that there may be prior warning of an attack and time to put into effect large-scale evacuation of priority groups, such as pregnant women, to predesignated reception areas. However, evacuation is cumbersome, time-consuming and requires several hours' advance warning. Provision must also be made for protection in shelters, pits, etc., to care for those who cannot be evacuated.

Although early planning for the protection of the civilian population recognized the need for pacts of mutual assistance mostly with state coordination, disaster planning now includes nationwide and continental participation. The concept is still valid that official state and community agencies, in cooperation with civil defense planners, medical and welfare, assume the major responsibility, not only for planning prior to disasters, but for the administration and operation of emergency services for expectant mothers and infants through local and regional health units.

In planning for the safeguarding of mothers and newborn infants prior to a disaster, certain assumptions can be made and specific factors considered:

Pregnant women will be subject to all of the risks and injuries to which men and nonpregnant women will be exposed. Their general care should be in accordance with provisions made for the population at large. However, their obstetric care does require additional planning and facilities, for it should be separate from hospital and emergency facilities for casualties. Two lives are at stake, lives of particular import to the future of the country. The need for care of the pregnant woman is predictable, since sooner or later she must inevitably be delivered, and in the process will need medical attention to a greater or lesser extent. In the vast majority of instances, probably in 90 per cent of all cases, the birth process, whether it results in a viable infant or abortion, will be essentially uncomplicated. The most formidable complications to be encountered with any frequency will be hemorrhage, obstructed or prolonged labor, infection, mild and severe toxemias of pregnancy with convulsions and miscellaneous medical and surgical conditions accompanying pregnancy.

It is estimated that at any given time approximately 2 per cent of the total population will consist of women in various stages of pregnancy. In applying this prevalence rate to a given geographic area, allowance must be made for the character of the area, since the rate will, of course, be affected by the presence of large industrial plants and offices employing large numbers of males.

On the basis of the Hiroshima experience with the A-bomb, it can be anticipated that approximately one quarter of all surviving pregnant women on the periphery of the atomic explosion will abort or deliver shortly thereafter. Furthermore, approximately 10 per cent of pregnant women within range of the effects of a nuclear explosion will have abortions or premature deliveries.

It is possible, therefore, that in the affected blast area there may be as many as 500 to 700 deliveries or abortions per 100,000 population shortly after an explosion. In areas more remote from the explosion the number of deliveries or abortions will more nearly approximate that occurring during normal times.

If the foregoing concepts are accepted and remain valid in disaster planning, what then should be the planning for minimal essential care for mothers and newborn infants in disaster situations? To the extent that it is possible, the facilities which are normally available for pregnant women during the antepartal, delivery and postpartal periods should be available.

Preparation for the care of mothers and babies during a disaster requires that thought be given and plans made for the training of families for their own protection and survival and for the training of a large percentage of the population to carry out minimal essentials of care to save the lives of other people.

It can be assumed that in any major disaster, physicians, nurses and other specially trained professional personnel will be almost completely absorbed in the task of caring for casualties; normal women in labor at such times will have to rely largely on nonprofessional personnel for their needs. Just who will these nonprofessional people be? They will have to be other women who have received instruction in the procedures described. In other words, each community must contain a corps of lay women who understand the basic concepts contained in this brief review and have been given at least minimal training in providing this type of care. Preparation for civil defense is a family affair. Every citizen and every family needs to have the information necessary to protect himself, his family and his community well in advance of a disaster or an enemy attack. Those responsible for planning and implementing disaster plans have the unique responsibility for making this information available to individuals in communities in a way which they can understand and accept.

The only hope we have for the saving of lives of mothers and newborn infants depends on the family's ability to carry out the plans made with and for them.

Every expectant mother needs to know her physician's expectation of the kind of delivery she will have, so that if she needs any special facilities, she will be able to go where these are available. She needs to understand the care she and her baby will need during delivery and immediately afterward.

There are differences of opinion about how much information pregnant women should have about their own condition and the conduct and the outcome of the delivery. It is assumed that in the event of large-scale disasters, women will have to carry much of the responsibility for their own safety. Therefore, adequate information about what to do, where to go and what constitutes essential equipment will be comforting to them rather than alarming.

Essential equipment is quite minimal and is available to almost every woman in her own home. A package should be made up and kept accessible with other emergency supplies. Contents include a clean sheet, towels, washcloth and soap; blankets, clothing, a nipple and a bottle for the baby; a pair of blunt scissors; 2 pieces of clean linen tape, 6 inches long and ¼ inch wide, wrapped separately from the other articles, and a package of powdered milk for the mother.

Those who are giving care to pregnant women need to understand that the pregnant woman's normal dependent needs may be greatly enhanced by separation from and concern for her husband and family and by increased fear for herself and her baby. Understanding in meeting this exaggerated need for mothering and providing a warm accepting environment will increase the confidence of the pregnant woman in her ability to have her baby and will comfort her and relieve some of her fear and apprehension. Every effort should be made to have someone with the patient throughout labor. The emotional support which patients in labor (who have had some preparation) derive from each other should be utilized.

Essentials of care during the first stage of labor include the maintenance of physical and emotional reserves, the interpretation of the progress of labor to the patient and the family, the provision of rest and fluids, the maintenance of asepsis and preparation for the second stage of labor, including frequent emptying of the bladder.

There should be constant review of progress and observation of signs of complications. As the patient approaches the completion of the first stage of labor, she will need special care and encouragement and should not be left alone. If care is delegated, it should be assigned to a nursing auxiliary or to a relative or a friend who is kindly, understanding and responsible.

During the second stage of labor, constant observation, encouragement and interpretation are all-important. A clean delivery area should be maintained, and there should be continual observation of the patient's general condition for signs of exhaustion and other complications. The maternal pulse rate and the quality should be observed.

A progress report to the supervising physician should be made by the person giving the care. In the absence of the physician during the delivery, the nurse, the nurse-midwife or the attendant who is helping the patient can teach her that when the baby's head is in sight to take a deep breath at the beginning of each contraction, to hold her breath and exert downward pressure, while the infant's head is controlled. As soon as the contraction is over, the patient should be encouraged to relax completely and wait for the next contraction.

Supportive care is especially important. The back can be rubbed for low back pain and the legs stretched for muscle cramps. The explanation of the progress of labor often provides the encouragement which the patient needs to complete the second stage of labor with minimal emotional stress.

When the head crowns, the perineum should be supported and protected with a clean towel if a sterile towel is not available. Gentle pressure is applied against the head as it emerges to prevent too rapid delivery of the head, which is supported as it is born. Immediate removal of the membranes from around the baby's head is important. If the umbilical cord is around the neck, it is slipped over the head whenever it can be done easily. The mucus should be wiped from the baby's mouth and nose. Occasionally, spontaneous rotation of the head to one side or the other will not take place within a reasonable period of time. Under such circumstances, gentle rotation of the head in the direction toward which it tends to go more easily will suffice to bring one shoulder anteriorly behind the symphysis.

To deliver the anterior shoulder of the baby, the head is grasped with both hands, and gentle but steady pressure toward the floor is applied until the anterior shoulder slips under the symphysis pubis, and the upper portion of the arm can be seen. Then the direction of traction is reversed upward in order to deliver the posterior shoulder over the perineum. The above maneuvers should be carried out slowly and carefully; there is no pressing need to hurry.

The baby's body is supported as it is born and is wrapped in a warm sterile towel or clean cloth and placed on the mother's abdomen with the head lower so that the mucus will drain out. Pulling on the cord should be avoided. The mother will want to know about the baby and see it as soon as it is born. If the baby does not cry immediately, or if there is mucus, the nose and the mouth should be cleared and postural drainage instituted. Gentle rubbing of the back helps to stimulate the baby's breathing. When the cord stops pulsating, it is tied in two places and cut between the two ties. After the cord is cut, the baby is warmly wrapped and placed in the mother's arms.

During the delivery of the baby and the beginning of the third stage of labor there should be constant observation of the mother's general condition and of signs indicating the separation of the placenta. If the attendant assisting with the delivery places her hand on the mother's fundus, she can report the changes to the person conducting the delivery. When the uterus rises upward in the abdomen and becomes globular and firm, and the umbilical cord extends 3 or 4 inches out of the vagina and there is a gush of blood, the patient can be asked to bear down with the next contraction. This pressure is usually sufficient to expel the placenta, which is received in a clean receptacle. In order to express the placenta, it may be necessary occasionally to apply gentle pressure on the fundus of the uterus when it is well contracted. The direction of pressure should be toward the vaginal outlet. Following the expulsion of the placenta, if the uterus tends to become soft, and bleeding occurs, the uterus should be massaged vigorously with the fingertips to promote uterine contraction, and the baby put to the breast.

The placenta and membranes should be examined to determine whether there are any missing portions.

If the uterus remains small and firm, nothing should be done other than to keep the hand on the fundus for 1 hour following the delivery of the baby. The patient should be made comfortable, given nourishment, encouraged to void and allowed to rest.

As soon as the mother can be left, the baby should be identified, according to the method established by the particular health department, and carefully examined for injuries and congenital malformations.

Essentials of nursing care for the baby include gentle handling, observation of breathing, color, appearance, activity, skin and body temperature, stools, weight (if possible), and umbilical cord for bleeding and healing; provision should be made for warmth, proper food and protection from infection.

Mother and newborn baby should be considered an inseparable unit. If a mother cannot take care of her baby, full-time mothering care must be provided to enhance the baby's chances of survival and promote his well-being. Irregularities in breathing, mucus in air passages, weak sucking reflex, skin irritation and unstable temperature-regulating mechanism point to the importance of constant observation and an environment adapted to meet the needs of the individual infant.

The infant should be put to breast 24 hours after birth and at 4-hour intervals for periods of 5 minutes until the milk supply is established. Once the supply of milk is sufficient to satisfy the infant, feedings should be given as often as necessary to meet his need. Artificial feedings may be necessary until the mother's milk supply is adequate or in instances in which the mother is unable to nurse the infant.

The newborn is particularly susceptible to infection. Anyone with any evidence of infection, such as rash, diarrhea or upper respiratory infection, should not give infant care.

When the infant is found to be premature and in need of special care, or to have congenital malformations, the emergency facilities which have been developed for such conditions should be utilized.

When the mother and infant are to be discharged from the place where care has been given during labor and delivery, it is essential for arrangements to be made with the family and others for the mother to be relieved of responsibilities except the care of her baby and herself. The mother, the family and the attendant should know where and whom to call if she or the baby have any conditions or symptoms needing medical care.

To increase the number of people with some training in the care of pregnant women and newborn infants, the existing educational programs need to be expanded. These include mother and baby care classes, such as those given by the Red Cross and other health agencies, parent education groups, home nursing classes, first-aid training, classes for baby sitters and junior and senior high school students and the midwifery training programs. Planning for training and the achievement of the training of persons who carry this responsibility in a disaster are not easy.

During a disaster, it is assumed that it will be the responsibility of nurses, certified nurse-midwives and licensed nonprofessional midwives to carry on an intensive program of on-the-job training of whoever is available to help and to supervise the care of mothers and babies.

SUGGESTED READING

Green, J. M.: Emergency care of the obstetric patient, Nurs. Outlook 6:694, 1958.

Hogan, Aileen: Bomb-born babies, Pub. Health Nurs. 43:383, 1951.

————: If disaster strikes—are we ready?, Briefs 21:8, 1957.

Maryland State Department of Health, Division Public Health Nursing: Suggested Content for the Training Program in Civil Defense Nursing, Parts III and IV, Maryland State Department of Health, January, 1952.

New York State Department of Health, Bureau of Maternal and Child Health: Assisting at the Birth of a Baby If No Doctor Is Available, New York State Department of Health, 1954.

Rayner, J. F.: How do nurses behave in disaster?, Nurs. Outlook 6:572, 1958.

Work Conference on Disaster Nursing: Text of addresses, Norfolk, Va., November 12-16, 1956.

Obstetrics Among Primitive Peoples • Egyptian Obstetrics • Oriental Obstetrics • Grecian Obstetrics • Byzantine, Mohammedan, Jewish and Medieval Periods • The Renaissance Period • The Seventeenth Century • The Eighteenth Century • The Nineteenth and the Twentieth Centuries • Background and Development of Antepartal Care in the United States

Chapter 24

History of Obstetrics*

In the course of one chapter it is impossible to give a detailed history of obstetrics. This account does not purport to be a complete survey of the progress of obstetrics through the ages but merely a skeletal outline on which the interested may place significant facts by additional reading. Sufficient references will be given to enable the student to obtain more complete information.

For greater simplicity and more ready understanding, the ages of obstetrics have been divided arbitrarily as set forth at the beginning of this chapter.

OBSTETRICS AMONG PRIMITIVE PEOPLES

We know little about obstetrics among the primitive races, but from careful study of the customs of the aboriginal American Indians and the African Negroes we are able to learn some of the customs which were part of the obstetric practice of the ancients. Childbirth in primitive times was a relatively simple process. The mother retired to a place apart from the tribe and there gave birth to her child without great difficulty. It is known that intertribal marriages were relatively rare; therefore, there was not the conglomeration of mingled races which exists today. A realization of this fact alone makes possible an under-

*By Douglas E. Cannell, M.B., B.Sc. (Med.), F.R.C.S. (C), Toronto, Canada.

standing of the relative simplicity of childbirth under these circumstances. The fetal head and body were accommodated satisfactorily within the anatomic range of the maternal pelvis. The lack of mixed marriages prevented the resultant disproportion between passenger and pelvic passages. It became customary for women who had attended other women in labor to be asked to assist or accompany more of them, and they became the primitive counterpart of our latter-day midwife. The only real danger a primitive mother faced was that of abnormal presentation, which usually terminated fatally for both mother and child. Toxemias and other complications are largely the products of more advanced civilization and were rarely if ever met among primitive peoples.

EGYPTIAN OBSTETRICS

In Egypt a highly organized state of society existed, and with it there arose a more complicated, if not more advanced, type of obstetrics. The priesthood in Egypt was interested in all the activities of society, and obstetrics was not neglected. They had a supervisory interest in it and took an active part in the care of abnormal or operative cases. They are known to have had obstetric forceps, to have performed cesarean sections on dead mothers, and podalic version was a part of their art.

ORIENTAL OBSTETRICS

Hindu medicine was probably the first authentic system of medicine to be given to the world. Among the earliest Hindus of whom there is written record was Susrata, one of the most prolific of Hindu writers. The exact date of his existence is still a matter of dispute, but he is variously stated to have worked and written between 600 B.C. and A.D. 500, more probably about the latter date. His knowledge of menstruation and gestation was quite modern. He knew and described intelligently the management of normal and abnormal labor. He described the use of forceps and cesarean section upon dead mothers to remove living children, and gave excellent prenatal and post-partal advice. He advised cleanliness on the part of the obstetrician; cutting the beard, the hair and the nails closely; the wearing of clean gowns; and thorough disinfection of the operating rooms prior to operation or delivery. His surgical antiseptic technic seems remarkable to modern students.

Chinese obstetrics was largely of a legendary nature until the publication of a Chinese household manual of obstetrics, *Ta Sheng P'Ien*, which, according to the author's own statement, "is correct and needs no change or addition of prescription." There were monographs on obstetrics prior to this, but none so complete. Many of his statements are unfounded; in fact, the knowledge is scanty or incorrect, but the author had the saving grace of objecting to unnecessary interference and counseled patience in the treatment of labor. He had a poor opinion of midwives in general, stating that "the majority of them are fools." The reviews of Chinese obstetrics and obstetric drugs by Maxwell are excellent and give a detailed account of an interesting phase of obstetrics, which for lack of space we are forced to dispense with in this account.

GRECIAN OBSTETRICS

Prior to Hippocrates, the Asclepiads, or followers of Aesculapius, the Father of Medicine, had a slight and largely supervisory interest in obstetrics. Abortions were not illegal. There is little definite knowledge concerning this period, but it seems probable that obstetric treatment was of a primitive nature.

The Hippocratic Period. During this age normal obstetric cases were handled by midwives under the supervision of the physicians. Abnormal labor was entirely in the hands of the medical profession. To Hippocrates is accredited the Hippocratic oath, which is still a part of the exercises for all students graduating from medical school. Treatises upon obstretrics attributed to Hippocrates are the oldest records available of the Western World's obstetric methods.

Greco-Roman Obstetrics. This period was one of progress, which was due largely to the work of Celsus, Aëtius and Soranus (second century). The last reintroduced podalic version and is responsible for the first authentic records of its use in the delivery of living children. He gave an excellent technical description of the procedure and the indications for its use.

BYZANTINE, MOHAMMEDAN, JEWISH AND MEDIEVAL PERIODS

These may be said to have been characterized by a complete absence of progress, and as a corollary, a retrogression and loss of previously known practice resulted. This was due in large part to the general failure of science in the medieval period, but the interference of the Roman Church in secular matters, particularly those of a scientific nature, must be held responsible for a large share of it. The paucity of operative treatment in difficult labor may be judged from the recommendations contained in the only textbook of the day on obstetrics and gynecology, which read as follows: "Place the patient in a sheet held at the corners by four strong men, with her head somewhat elevated. Have them shake the sheet vigorously by pulling on the opposite corners, and with God's aid she will give birth." However, hospitals and nursing services were organized in this age.

Although the ancient Jews gave very little assistance to the woman during labor and delivery, they were interested in the hygiene of pregnancy and cleanliness at the time of childbirth. Hygiene and sanitation were apparently a part of their religion. At the time of difficult deliveries, the women "were comforted until they died." The stool or obstetric chair was used at this time and continued to be used until about the 19th century A.D. Reference is made to this chair in the Bible, in the first chapter of Exodus, "when you do the office of the midwife to the Hebrew women, and see them upon the stools. . . ."

THE RENAISSANCE PERIOD

The Renaissance was characterized by advances in medicine and obstetrics commensurate with those in other fields. During this time appeared the first English text on obstetrics, the *Byrthe of Mankynde*, published by Raynalde. Both it and its German counterpart by Roesslin are copies of Soranus, and with their publication podalic version was reintroduced to obstetric practice. Many famous men were responsible for the progress in obstetrics—among them Leonardo da Vinci (who made the first accurate sketches of the fetus in utero) and Vesalius (who accurately described the pelvis for the first time).

To Ambrose Paré, the dean of French surgeons and obstetricians, must go the chief credit for making podalic version a useful and practicable procedure. Due to his skill, he preferred its use to cesarean section in difficult labor. By his careful studies of its indications and technic, he made possible the removal of obstetrics from the hands of the midwives, where it had rested since the fall of the Roman Empire, and its establishment as an independent branch of medicine. Regulations were enacted for the practice of midwives, and schools were established during this period for their training. Paré's work on version and his discouragement of cesarean section were opportune.

Sections had been practiced since antiquity upon dead mothers, but the first authentic section performed upon a living mother is credited to Trautman, of Wittenberg, in 1610. This was done upon a woman with a large ventral hernia which contained the uterus. Prior to this, Nufer, a sow gelder, is reputed to have performed the operation on his wife, after obstetricians and midwives had failed to deliver her. It has been stated that Jane Seymour was delivered by a section done by Frère, a noted surgeon of the time, at the request of Henry VIII. That she died a few days after the birth of Edward VI adds credence to the story, but no absolute confirmation is available. Due to the frightful mortality from hemorrhage, sepsis, etc., it did not become popular in spite of the advocacy of the Church. Through the following centuries it was done occasionally, but not until the advent of uterine sutures and aseptic technic did it become a practical procedure.

The origin of its name has been ascribed to Julius Caesar, but, as his mother lived many years after his birth, this seems improbable—considering the high mortality of all abdominal operations before the time of Lister. A more accurate explanation is that Numa Pompilius, one of the earlier Roman kings, passed a law making it compulsory to perform the operation upon all mothers who died while pregnant in order that the mother and the child might be buried separately. This was known as the "Lex Regis" and with the advent of the Caesars as the "Lex Caesaris"—and subsequently "cesarean section." The name has been attributed to *cedere*, the Latin verb meaning to cut, but the former explanation seems to be more reasonable.

THE SEVENTEENTH CENTURY

This century was notable for many famous obstetricians. Mauriceau, of Paris, was the first to correct the view that the pelvic bones separated in normal labor. He was also the first man to refer to epidemic puerperal fever. His description of an obstetrician, or rather of the qualities an obstetrician should possess, is both interesting and amusing. He stated:

He must be healthful, strong and robust; because this is the most laborious of all the Operations of Chirurgery; for it will make one sometimes sweat, so he shall not have a dry Thread, tho' it were the coldest Day in Winter. . . . He ought to be well shaped, at least to outward appearance, but above all, to have small hands for the easier Introduction of them into the Womb when necessary; yet strong, with the Fingers long, especially the Fore-finger, the better to reach and touch the inner orifice. He must have no Rings on his Fingers, and his Nails well pared, when he goeth about the Work, for fear of hurting the

Womb. He ought to have a pleasant Countenance, and to be as neat in his Clothes as in his person, that the poor women who have need of him be not affrighted at him. Some are of the opinion, that a Practitioner of this Art ought on the contrary to be slovenly, at least very careless, wearing a great Beard, to prevent the Occasion of the Husband's Jealousy that sends for him. Truly some believe this Policy augments their Practice but 'tis fit they should be disabused; for such a Posture and Dress resembles more a Butcher than a Chirurgeon, whom the woman apprehends already too much, that he needs not such a Disguise. Above all he must be sober, no Tipler, that he may at all times have his Wits about him. . . ."

Van Deventer, of Holland, has been called the Father of Modern Obstetrics and is credited with the first accurate description of the pelvis, its deformities and their effect on parturition. He also shares with Ould, of Dublin, the first description of the mechanism of labor. As time passed, customs changed, and the term "accoucheur" replaced the objectionable "midman" and "man-midwife." Obstetric forceps were invented, probably about 1580, by Peter Chamberlen but were kept as a family secret until 1813 in an effort of the Chamberlens to monopolize the field. In 1699, Hugh Chamberlen sold one half of the instrument to Amsterdam but added fraud to infamy by selling the vector or worthless half. Prior to that, in 1670, he had demanded the equivalent of $7,500 for the secret and, in an attempt to show their worth, had killed a woman and baby before Mauriceau, who craftily chose for the demonstration a woman with a distorted pelvis, upon whom he previously had planned to do a cesarean section. After some hours of fruitless effort, Chamberlen failed in his attempts at delivery, with the resultant double fatality. When the Chamberlen forceps were finally revealed to the profession in 1813, their need had been met by other men, and the Chamberlens were thus justly punished for the discredit they had brought upon their calling.

THE EIGHTEENTH CENTURY

The eighteenth century was marked by a succession of famous men such as Palfyne, the Hunters, Smellie, White and others. The first named is credited with the invention of obstetric forceps, as he presented a copy in 1770 to the Academy of Medicine of Paris.

Smellie taught obstetrics with a manikin and made improvements on the obstetric forceps in use at that time, adding a steel lock and curved blades. He also laid down the first principles for their use and differentiated by measurement between contracted and normal pelves.

William Hunter, though a pupil of Smellie, was opposed to the use of forceps, and frequently exhibited his rusted blades as evidence of their uselessness. In conjunction with his brother he laid the foundation of modern knowledge of placental anatomy.

Charles White published an obstetric thesis advocating the scrubbing of the hands and general cleanliness on the part of the accoucheur; he was the pioneer in aseptic midwifery. John Harvie, 90 years before Crede, advocated external manual expression of the placenta, and it is known that a similar procedure was in use in Dublin at that time. One of the most active and famous English obstetricians of the time, John Clarke, had his fame commemorated in this epitaph:

Beneath this stone, shut up in the dark
Lies a learned man-midwife y'clep'd Dr. Clarke.
On earth while he lived by attending men's wives,
He increased population some thousands of lives;
Thus a gain to the nation was gain to himself,
An enlarged population, enlargement of pelf.
So he toiled late and early, from morning to night,
The squalling of children his greatest delight;
Then worn out with labours, he died skin and bone
And his ladies he left all to Mansfield and Stone.

There were many famous obstetricians on the Continent in this period, chief among them being Baudelocque, who invented the pelvimeter and named and described positions and presentations. In America, prejudices against men in midwifery were carried over from Europe; as late as 1857 a demonstration before the graduating class at Buffalo roused such a storm of criticism that the American Medical

Association had to intervene. Their judgment was that any physician who could not conduct labor by touch alone should not undertake midwifery.

This 18th century produced such men as Moultrie, Lloyd and Shippen. The last was a pupil of Smellie and Hunter; in 1762, he opened a school for midwifery in Philadelphia, and, since he provided convenient lodgings for the accommodation of poor women during confinement, he may be said to have established the first lying-in hospital in America. With Morgan, he founded the School of Medicine of the University of Pennsylvania, becoming its first Professor of Anatomy, Surgery and Midwifery.

THE NINETEENTH AND THE TWENTIETH CENTURIES

The increased knowledge, interest and ability which physicians brought to obstetrics were largely offset by the increased mortality due to puerperal fever. During the 17th, the 18th and the 19th centuries it became a pestilence, at times wiping out whole communities of puerperal women. The mortality rates varied in the best European clinics at Paris and Vienna from 10 to 20 per cent. The origin and the spread of the disease were little understood or studied. Obstetricians wasted futile hours on a study of minor alterations in instruments or technic and ignored the vast loss of life from puerperal fever. Oliver Wendell Holmes, of Harvard, first presented his views on the contagiousness of puerperal fever in 1843, and in 1855 he reiterated them in a monograph on *Puerperal Fever as a Private Pestilence*. This was, and still remains, a medical classic on the subject. His statements aroused great controversy in America, and he received a great deal of abuse and criticism from Meigs and Hodge, two of the foremost American obstetricians of the day. One of them stated that it was ridiculous to conceive of any gentleman carrying contamination on his hands from patient to patient.

The following is Holmes' summary of his observations on the prevention of puerperal sepsis. Written in 1843, before the discovery of any human pathologic organism, and before

the adoption of disinfection in surgical procedures, it is a truly remarkable summary.[1]

1. A physician holding himself in readiness to attend cases of midwifery, should never take any active part in the postmortem examination of cases of puerperal fever.

2. If a physician is present at such autopsies, he should use thorough ablution, change every article of dress, and allow twenty-four hours or more to elapse before attending to any case of midwifery. It may be well to extend the same caution to cases of simple peritonitis.

3. Similar precautions should be taken after the autopsy or surgical treatment of cases of erysipelas, if the physician is obliged to unite such offices with his obstetrical duties, which is in the highest degree inexpedient.

4. On the occurrence of a single case of puerperal fever in his practice, the physician is bound to consider the next female he attends in labor, unless some weeks, at least, have elapsed, as in danger of being infected by him, and it is his duty to take every precaution to diminish her risk of disease and death.

5. If within a short period two cases of puerperal fever happen close to each other, in the practice of the same physician, the disease not existing or prevailing in the neighborhood, he would do wisely to relinquish his obstetrical practice for at least one month, and endeavor to free himself by every available means from any noxious influence he may carry about with him.

6. The occurrence of three or more closely connected cases, in the practice of one individual, no others existing in the neighborhood, and no other sufficient causes being alleged for the coincidence, is prima facie evidence that he is the vehicle of contagion.

7. It is the duty of the physician to take every precaution that the disease shall not be introduced by nurses or other assistants, by making proper inquiries concerning them, and giving timely warning of every suspected source of danger.

8. Whatever indulgence may be granted to those who have heretofore been the ignorant causes of so much misery, the time has come when the existence of a *private pestilence* in the sphere of a single physician should be looked upon not as a misfortune but as a crime; and in the knowledge of such occurrences, the duties of the practitioner to his profession should give way to his paramount obligations to society.

While Holmes first conceived the correct idea of the nature of the disease, it is to Ignaz

[1] From Abraham Levinson, *Pioneers of Pediatrics*.

Philipp Semmelweiss that the glory must go of finally proving without question the nature of its source and transmission. He was an assistant in the Viennese clinic for women, and while his associates fussed with unimportant details of technic, he was studying and mourning the tremendous death rate among puerperal women in the clinic. He observed that the death rate in Clinic I, where women were delivered by medical students or physicians, was always higher than that of Clinic II, where midwives officiated or received instruction. After fruitless study and manifold changes in technic in order to follow more closely that of Clinic II, the cause of the disease was brought home to him in a desperate and startling fashion. His friend, Kalletschka, an assistant in pathology, died after performing an autopsy upon a victim of puerperal fever, during which Kalletschka had sustained a slight cut on his finger.

At postmortem the findings were identical with those of puerperal sepsis, and Semmelweiss concluded that the disease was transmitted from the dead, by contact from the physicians and the students, who often went directly from the postmortem room to deliveries. Accordingly, he immediately instituted and enforced a ruling which made it obligatory that all physicians and students wash their hands in a solution of chloride of lime after attending autopsies and before examining or delivering mothers. In 7 months he had reduced the mortality in Clinic I from 12 to 3 per cent, and in the subsequent year had a mortality lower than Clinic II, a hitherto unheard-of feat. Subsequently, he observed that puerperal sepsis could be transmitted from patient to patient by contact of contaminated material, or attendants, as well as from the postmortem room, and in 1861 he published his immortal work on *The Cause, Concept and Prophylaxis of Puerperal Fever*.

Medicine provides pitiful figures in profusion, but none, it seems, met such a cruel reception and ultimate fate as Semmelweiss. His colleagues (for the most part, but with a few notable and loyal exceptions) distorted and criticized his teachings. Had they stopped there, it might have been bad enough, but they carried their distaste for his views to the stage of persecution. He was forced to leave Vienna and go to Budapest, where a similar attitude —if possible a more malignant one—awaited him. A disappointed man, he died in 1865 from a brain abscess which may have originated in an infection similar to that of his friend Kalletschka. To the tragedy of his life, his death added satire. His work, however, has lived on; Pasteur and Lister added to it; and with a more modern and tolerant age his worth has been recognized.

The organisms causing puerperal fever probably were seen by several early workers beginning with Mayrhofer, who, in 1863, described "cylindrical vibrios" or "strings of pearls" in the lochia of puerperal sepsis. In 1864, 310 deaths occurred in the 1,350 confinement cases in the Maternité hospital in Paris, and that "Vestibule of Death" had to be closed in 1865.

Pasteur, in 1879, saw "cocci in chain" in cases of puerperal sepsis and contributed definitely to our knowledge of the causal streptococci, demonstrating to doctors the "presence of the invisible foe" in a drop of blood obtained by a "simple pin-prick on the finger tip of the unhappy woman doomed to die the next day" and recommending methods of aseptic technic for their control.

The 19th and the 20th centuries were largely notable for their utilization of drugs to alleviate the pains of childbirth. The use of ether as an anesthetic was first discovered in America, but it was first utilized for childbirth by Simpson in Great Britain. He brought back the lost art of version by making it a safer procedure and eventually substituted chloroform for ether. As with almost every advance in medicine, it was opposed bitterly. The opposition was loudest and most vehement from the clergy, but, in 1853, Queen Victoria accepted it for delivery and by her action silenced most of the criticism. Nitrous oxide had been used in 1880 and has continued to be popular ever since that time.

Obstetric analgesia and anesthesia have made great strides during the 20th century (see Chap. 11, Analgesia and Anesthesia in Labor).

The present century will be remembered largely for the development of antepartal clinics and the more concentrated care of the expectant mothers that came with them. The application of advances in general medicine, metabolism and public health to obstetrics has led to a marked decrease in mortality and morbidity from cardiac, pulmonic, metabolic, venereal and associated medical conditions complicating pregnancy. The consideration of adequate vitamin, mineral and caloric contents in connection with the diet of pregnant and puerperal women not only has decreased the morbidity but also has enhanced the health of all mothers and children who receive adequate obstetric care.

Many other contributions have been made and are being added constantly to the science of obstetrics, not the least of which is more intensive training and study in this specialty demanded by the public as well as the medical profession. The advent of routine external expression of the placenta, silver nitrate prophylaxis in the eyes of the newborn, purified ergot and pituitary preparations in hemor-rhage control and prevention are but a few of the methods and medications which have marked the early 20th century.

The morphologic and anthropologic studies of Naegele, Roberts, Williams, Goodwin, Caldwell, Moloy and others have done much to improve our understanding of the various types of pelves and some of their importance in labor. Roentgenologic pelvimetry and cephalometry have greatly advanced our knowledge of the probable course of labor and delivery; Thoms, Caldwell and Moloy, Hanson, Jarcho and countless others have contributed to our advances in this field (see Chap. 2).

In a necessarily brief and incomplete fashion, an endeavor has been made to touch upon some of the more interesting phases of the history of obstetrics—a delightful and fascinating subject.

Background and Development of Antepartal Care in the United States

As we know it today, antepartal care developed into its present status through devious avenues of investigation and many bypaths of interrelated activity and work. Individuals, both from the profession and the laity, as well as private and municipal organizations, contributed time, money and interest until, at last, Government action was obtained.

The background of our present maternity situation is of interest both as a history and a story. Antepartal care in the United States had its beginnings in the days of slavery. The intelligent slaveowners paid special attention to the diet and the care of pregnant slaves. Healthy slaves were more valuable, were worth more money and produced stronger offspring. From this beginning the chronologic efforts which led to our present-day antepartal care follow.

1866. A story was written which concerned cruelty to a child. Some thoughtful person referred the case to *The Society for the Prevention of Cruelty to Animals.* Henry Bergh, a former diplomat to Russia, was the founder and director of this association and was influ-ential in having the judgment pronounced on the ground that a child was a human animal. This incident stimulated interest in the general treatment of children.

1873. *The New York Diet Kitchen Association*, the oldest public health organization in America, was opened at the request of doctors from "de Milt Dispensary" on the lower East Side of New York City. It was first organized as a soup kitchen, and milk, gruel, beef tea and cooked rice were taken to the sick in their homes, with the idea of restoring health. In 1892, they began to make formulas for sick babies and still later dispensed free milk or sold it at 3 cents a quart. Maria L. Daniels was the first nurse director and contributed much for many years to public health progress. In 1926, this group was organized as *The Children's Health Service of New York.* The organization grew with the times, changing its program from curing the sick to preventive work—keeping well babies well. Although the organization devoted its major effort to work with babies and preschool children, it also included antepartal care in its program.

1876. The beginning of child-welfare legislation in the United States was the Act passed by the New York State Legislature, granting to *The Society for the Prevention of Cruelty to Children* a charter that gave it wide power with regard to the protection of child life. The inception of this legislation was based on the incident of the "child as a human animal" (1866).

1893. The first *Infant Milk Station* in the United States was established in New York City by Nathan Strauss. Through his persistence, milk was finally made "safe" through pasteurization; and many such stations were set up.

1900. *The United States Census Bureau* was made a permanent organization. Up to this time, *vital statistics* were considered to be of so little importance in the United States that, as soon as the population was tabulated and classified, the bureau was disbanded, to be re-established and reorganized every 10 years.

1906. *The United States Census Bureau* published mortality statistics which drew attention to the appalling loss of life among babies and children. Up to this time, very little thought had been given to maternity and infant protection.

1907. Due to the growing interest, Mr. George H. F. Schrader was stimulated to give money to *The Association for Improving Conditions of the Poor* (now the *Community Service Society*) for the salaries of two nurses to do antepartal work. This was the first consistent effort to prevent deaths of babies by caring for the mothers *before* the babies were born. Two reasons were given as to why antepartal care would be of value: (1) nurses in convalescent homes for postpartal mothers thought that if patients had better care during pregnancy, the health of mothers would be improved; (2) social workers going into the homes felt that they were not adequately prepared to advise pregnant mothers.

1907. *The New York Milk Committee* was organized. Its object was the reduction of infant mortality through the improvement of the city's milk supply. It established milk depots which proved beyond question their great value in the reduction of infant mortality by dispensing clean pasteurized milk and by educating mothers.

1908. In this year the *Division of Child Hy-giene* was established in New York City, the first in the United States, and it was important enough to be recognized nationally. Josephine Baker, M.D., was appointed chief. This was a pioneer achievement, and the methods that were evolved had no precedent.

1909 to 1914. At approximately this time, Mrs. William Lowell Putnam, of Boston, promoted a demonstration of organized antepartal care. It was called *The Prenatal Care Committee* of the Women's Municipal League. The members of this committee worked in cooperation with the Boston Lying-In Hospital through Robert L. DeNormandie, M.D., of Harvard Medical School, Dr. Ruggles, of the then Homeopathic Hospital, and the Instructive District Nurses Association. The committee functioned long enough to establish the fact that good obstetric care was not possible without antepartal care.

1909. In this year *The American Association for the Study and Prevention of Infant Mortality* was organized and held its first meeting in New Haven, Connecticut. This committee was composed of both professional and lay members and devoted itself entirely to problems connected with child life, particularly to studying and trying to correct the high mortality rate. At this time there were no records of births or deaths, and the causes of deaths were unknown. The education of physicians and nurses was shamefully unsatisfactory; there was no public health in the schools, and practically no activity on the part of municipal, state or the Federal Government to prevent infant mortality. The first president of this association was J. H. Mason Knox, M.D., and Gertrude B. Kipp was the first secretary. The committee consisted of the Honorable Herbert Hoover, Livingston Ferrand, M.D., L. Emmet Holt, M.D., Richard Bolt, M.D., and Philip Van Ingen, M.D. The work of this organization was of profound significance. In 1918, its expanding activities caused it to change its name to *The American Child Hygiene Association*, and in 1923 the name was changed to the *American Child Health Association*. In 1935, after having contributed to every angle of this pioneer work, the association was disbanded.

1909. *The First White House Conference*, on "The Dependent Child," was called by President Theodore Roosevelt. These investigations resulted in the establishment of the U. S. Children's Bureau in 1912. According to some authorities, this conference was called through the influence of a public health nurse.

1910. *The Census Bureau* published another report, this time on the mortality of infants under 1 year of age and at "special ages." As a result of this report maternity hospitals made an effort to improve the care given to infants.

1911. In New York City *the first strictly municipal baby-health stations* were organized under the jurisdiction of the Department of Health, and the full cost of the work was borne by the municipality. Soon the dispensing of milk was of minor importance, and emphasis was placed on prevention—keeping well babies well. They are now called *Child-Health Stations*.

1911. *The New York Milk Committee* (1907) made an investigation at the baby-health stations and found that 40 per cent of all infant deaths (112 per 1,000) occurred within the 1st month of life before the mothers registered their babies at the health stations. This indicated the necessity for care *before* birth. The committee then decided to carry on an experiment in antepartal work. (See 1917.) They were convinced that much could be hoped for as a result of organized antepartal care.

1912. *The Babies' Welfare Association* (formerly *The Association of Infant Milk Stations* [1893]) represents the first comprehensive and successful attempt to coordinate the various child-welfare agencies in any community. All of the organizations of this type agreed to coordinate their activities by preventing duplication and overlapping without interfering with the organizations. In 1922, the name was changed to the *Children's Welfare Federation* of New York City. It continued to act as a clearing house and, among its other activities, managed the *Mother's Milk Bureau*.

1912. The *U. S. Children's Bureau* was established. It began in the Department of Commerce and Labor; in 1913 it was made a part of the Department of Labor and, in 1946, was transferred to the Federal Security Agency. This was created by Congress through a Federal Act (Government sanction). This bureau was to set up special machinery to study and protect the child and to study all matters pertaining to the welfare of children and child life among all classes of our people, to assemble and accumulate factual information and to disseminate this information throughout the country. Miss Julia Lathrop was chosen as chief. Much of the success of this bureau is credited to Miss Lathrop's vision. Fortunately, her successor, Miss Grace Abbott, continued the work with equal zeal.

1915. *The Birth Registration Area* was established as a Federal Act. The information is compiled in a uniform manner, giving the birth and the death statistics on which are based our information on mortality rates. The New England States, New York, Pennsylvania, Michigan, Minnesota and the District of Columbia were the first states to comply. At the present time all 50 states and the District of Columbia require registration of every birth. (See p. 11 and Tables 1 and 2.)

1915. Dr. Haven Emerson, Health Commissioner of New York City, appointed a special committee (Ralph W. Lobenstine, M.D., Clifton Edgar, M.D., and Philip Van Ingen, M.D.), in cooperation with the New York Milk Committee, to make an analysis of the facilities for maternity care in the city. The result of the survey showed that there was little antepartal work and no uniformity, and that only a very small number of pregnant mothers were receiving care. It showed also that hospitals took care of 30 per cent of the deliveries, midwives delivered 30 per cent, general practitioners delivered 30 per cent, and private doctors, who might be classified as obstetricians, delivered 10 per cent. Previous to this time little or nothing had been done to regulate or control the midwives.

1916. *The National Society for the Prevention of Blindness* was created after much pioneer work and investigation, locally and throughout the states, by Carolyn Van Blarcom, R.N. She was chosen to be the executive secretary. Through these investigations it was learned that by far the greatest cause of blindness was ophthalmia neonatorum. These findings led to the passing of a law compelling all physicians and midwives to use prophylaxis in newborn babies' eyes. Also, as a direct result of Miss Van Blarcom's surveys, a school for lay midwives was started, Belleview School for Midwives (no longer in existence). Miss Van Blarcom took out a midwife's license and was the first nurse in the

United States so to register. The first obstetrical nursing textbook to be written by a nurse is to Miss Van Blarcom's credit. Her later contribution to the better care of mothers and babies was to secure for Johns Hopkins Hospital the E. Bayard Halsted Fund for medical research.

1917. The Women's City Club of New York City and the New York Milk Committee opened three antepartal centers. The one sponsored by the Women's City Club was organized as the *Maternity Service Association* and, with Frances Perkins as the first executive secretary and Miss Mabel Choate as president, provided stimulating leadership. Dr. Ralph W. Lobenstine, a famous obstetrician, gave much time, labor, authority and direction as chairman of the medical board. In 1918, this organization was incorporated as the *Maternity Center Association* and carried out the first extensive piece of organized antepartal work in the United States. Miss Anne Stevens was director. Miss Annie W. Goodrich's wise counsel, as a member of the nursing committee, gave impetus to the organization's accomplishments. Louis I. Dublin, Ph.D., associated with this movement from the beginning, made an analysis of the first 4,000 records collected by the association. This revealed the startling fact that, through antepartal care, 50 per cent of the lives of mothers might be saved and 60 per cent of the lives of babies. Antepartal training and experience were extended to nurses throughout the world. This piece of intensive antepartal work fired increased interest in the care of mothers and babies. In 1929, the Maternity Center Association opened a school for the training of nurse midwives.

1919. *The Second White House Conference* was called by President Woodrow Wilson as a result of the activities of the U. S. Children's Bureau. It was organized in five sections. Each section was interested in a different phase of maternity and child care.

1919. *The American Committee on Maternal Welfare* was founded. The object of the committee was:

To awaken and stimulate the interest of members of the medical profession in cooperating with public and private agencies for the protection of the health of mothers and their offspring before and during pregnancy and labor and after confinement to the end that the conditions which

menace and interfere with the health or life of the mother or infant may be improved or prevented, disease and disorder corrected, health promoted and life saved; to teach the principles and practices of general and personal hygiene and health to parents and to improve and generalize the standards and methods of training physicians, nurses and others dealing with the problems of maternity.

The Committee was incorporated as a nonprofit organization in 1934 for the purpose of studying the maternal mortality rate in the United States and the management of obstetric problems generally. For more recent progress, see 1957 and 1964.

This organization publishes the magazine *The Bulletin of Maternal and Child Health*. It also promoted the American Congress of Obstetrics and Gynecology, which was held every 3 years. Seven such Congresses have been held, in 1939, 1942, 1947, 1950 (the first International Congress to be held in the United States), 1952, 1954 and 1957.

1921. *The Sheppard-Towner Bill* was passed by Congress, an Act for the Promotion of the Welfare and Hygiene of Maternity and Infancy, to be administered by the Children's Bureau. This bill was introduced in the 65th Congress by Congresswoman Jeanette Rankin of New Jersey. It was reported out of committee favorably but failed to pass. A second bill was introduced in the 66th Congress. It passed in the Senate but, through delays, was not considered by the House. In the first session of the 67th Congress the bill was again introduced by Senator Sheppard and Congressman Towner and, after much agitation, finally passed—an epoch in child-welfare legislation. An appropriation of $1,240,000 per year was granted for 5 years. The Cooper Bill, passed in 1927, extended it for 2 more years. This law was accepted by all of the states except 3. This legislation gave a tremendous impetus to the education not only of laity but also of physicians. Because of this legislation there was created at once, in the states which did not already have them, departments which now are quite uniformly labeled Divisions or Bureaus of Maternity and Child Health. In 1935, the Social Security Act was passed, following the plan of the Sheppard-Towner Bill. This Act appropriated $3,800,000. In 1939, the Social Security Act was amended, increasing the appropriation to $5,820,000. The amount has been increased gradually, and by 1952 (82nd Congress), $30,000,000 was appropriated for Maternal and Child Health, Crippled Children and other Child Health Services.

1923. *The National Committee for Maternal Health* was formed with Robert L. Dickinson, M.D., as secretary and later as president. This was a clearing house and a center of information on certain medical aspects of human fertility. The object was to gather and analyze material, to stimulate research, to issue reports to the medical profession and to persuade it to take a leading part in the scientific investigations of these problems in preventive medicine. No other group existed for this purpose. It was dissolved in 1950.

1923. *The Margaret Sanger Research Bureau* came into being, an affiliation of the Planned Parenthood Federation of America, Inc., for research in the field of infertility, contraception and marriage counseling.

1923. Mary Breckinridge began her investigations in Kentucky, which led to the organization of the *Frontier Nursing Service*. With this concentrated effort of all phases of maternity and infant care, the striking results proved the value of prenatal care. Through her vision, determination and unfaltering energy, Mary Breckinridge has made this organization one of worldwide renown. In 1936, the Frontier Nursing Service opened a school for the training of nurse midwives.

1925. *The Joint Committee on Maternal Welfare* was formed. This consisted of the American Gynecological Society, the American Association of Obstetrics and Gynecology and Abdominal Surgeons and the American Child Health Association (1909). Later the section of Obstetrics, Gynecology and Abdominal Surgeons of the American Medical Association was represented. The Committee issued a pamphlet entitled *An Outline of Delivery Care*. This stimulated the Children's Bureau to publish a concise pamphlet, *Standards of Prenatal Care* (1925), an outline for the use of physicians, which did much to standardize routine procedures.

1930. *The Third White House Conference* was called by President Herbert Hoover. Mr. Hoover's interest in child welfare was very evident. The conference was very comprehensive and far-reaching and was devoted to all aspects of maternity and child care. The Children's Charter was adopted and became a Federal Act. The 45,000,000 children were analyzed in chart form to show the paramount importance of care during pregnancy and the early years.

1938. *The Conference on Better Care for Mothers and Babies* was called by the Children's Bureau. This was the first time that representatives from the states, private and public organizations, both lay and professional people, met to pool ideas.

1939. The *Maternity Consultation Service* in New York City was organized to further prenatal education and care.

1940. The *Fourth White House Conference on Children in a Democracy* was called by President Franklin D. Roosevelt. It considered the aims of our American civilization for the children in whose hands its future lies; how children can best be helped to grow into the kind of citizens who will know best how to preserve and protect our democracy. By 1940, the 48 states, the District of Columbia, Puerto Rico, Alaska and Hawaii (then Territories) were cooperating with the Children's Bureau in its administration of child-welfare services.

1940. *The Cleveland Health Museum* was opened to the public—the first health museum in the Western Hemisphere. It is significant in the maternity field because, in its workshops, it is reproducing the *Dickinson-Belskie models*, acquired in 1945. Dr. Bruno Gebhard, Director, says that, in his belief, the use of this sculptural series in professional and lay education will advance knowledge on this all-important subject more quickly and more accurately than any other visual means thus far available.

1943. *The Emergency Maternity and Infancy Care Program* was launched to care for the wives and the babies of enlisted men in the armed forces. From $17,000,000 to $45,000,000 per year was appropriated. This Act also furthered interest in prenatal and child care.

1946. The *World Health Organization*—an agency of the United Nations—became a reality. At the first meeting in Paris, 64 nations signed the constitution. The membership now (1965) totals 117 countries. The object of the organization is "the attainment of the highest possible level of health of all the peoples." So far, much has been accomplished toward that end.

1950. *The Fifth White House Conference*, with emphasis on children and youth, was called by President Harry S. Truman.

1950. *The Fred Lyman Adair Foundation* of the American Committee on Maternal Welfare was established. Its purpose is to collect funds from charitable sources to underwrite research and educational projects in this field.

1955. The *American College of Nurse-Midwifery* was established as an organization of nurse-midwives to study and evaluate the activities of nurse-midwives, to plan and develop educational programs meeting the requirements of the profession and to perform other related functions. In 1957, the College became a member of the International Confederation of Midwives, a midwifery organization with members from some 30 countries throughout the world.

1957. The *American Association for Maternal and Infant Health* (formerly the American Committee on Maternal Welfare) was activated at the Seventh American Congress held in July. Prompted by the spectacular improvements and advances in maternity care which have taken place since its founding, the Board of Directors of the Committee voted unanimously to change the name, the role and the character of the organization. The new American Association for Maternal and Infant Health provides close integration of the various disciplines which participate in providing modern maternity care, and will serve as a forum for their mutual problems related to maternal and infant health.

1960. The *Sixth White House Conference*, concerned with the nation's children and youth, was called by President Dwight D. Eisenhower. The theme of this "Golden Anniversary" Conference was "Opportunities for Children and Youth to Realize Their Full Potential for Creative Life in Freedom and Dignity."

1963. *The Maternal and Child Health and Mental Retardation Planning Amendments of 1963* was enacted. This law will make it possible for the Children's Bureau to carry out some of the major recommendations of the President's Panel.

1964. *The American Association for Mater-*

nal and Child Health (formerly the American Association for Maternal and Infant Health), as a multidisciplinary organization, is one of the most potentially valuable groups interested in matters concerning infant, child and maternal health. The Board of Directors of the Association altered the official title of the organization, not to imply any change in its proposed program but to present a more accurate definition of the organization in terms of its aims and objectives.

Although there is yet much to be done, encouraging advances have been made over the years. During this seemingly disconnected sequence of activities, from cruelty to a child, care of the sick, keeping the well babies well, mortality studies and then to antepartal care, the aim for well mothers and healthy babies has finally been reached.

Today, in contrast with the past, the general public, including mothers and fathers, through education and publicity realizes the need for antepartal care. Physicians encourage early antepartal supervision in order to keep the mother well and to prevent complications during the maternity cycle.

The credit for the advancement of antepartal care and child care in the United States cannot be assigned to any individual or any one organization. Our present improved conditions are the results of extended public health education, organized efforts through private and public agencies (national, state and local), the intelligent interest and cooperation of public-spirited citizens who gave time and real sums of money, public officials, physicians, nurses, social workers, teachers, dentists and many others who made possible the putting into action of these ideas.

SUGGESTED READING

Bookmiller, Mae, and Bowen, George: Textbook of Obstetrics and Obstetric Nursing, ed. 4, Philadelphia, Saunders, 1963.

Corbin, Hazel: Maternity care today and tomorrow, Am. J. Nurs. 53:201, 1953.

Findley, Palmer: Priests of Lucina, Boston, Little, 1939.

Graham, Harvey: Eternal Eve, Garden City, Doubleday, 1951.

Heaton, C. E.: Obstetrics and gynecology in America, N. Carolina Med. J. 8:35, 1947.

Heaton, Claude: Fifty years of progress in obstetrics and gynecology, New York J. Med. 51: 83, 1951.

Hingson, R. L., and Hellman, L. M.: Anesthesia for Obstetrics, Philadelphia, Lippincott, 1956.

Kirkwood, S. B.: Twenty years of maternity care, Children 2:133, 1955.

Lesser, A. J.: Mental retardation and the maternal and child health amendments of 1963, Pediatrics 33:3, 1964.

Mack, H. C.: Back to Sacajawea, Am. J. Obstet. Gynec. 69:933, 1955.

Speert, Harold: Obstetric and Gynecologic Milestones, New York, Macmillan, 1958.

Ziegel, Erna, and Van Blarcom, C. C.: Obstetric Nursing, ed. 5, New York, Macmillan, 1964.

Appendix

Answer Key for Study Questions
Glossary
Conversion Table for Weights of Newborn
Aid for Visualization of Cervical Dilatation

Answer Key for Study Questions

UNIT ONE

1: 3
2: A
3: B
4: A. External conjugate
   B. Diagonal conjugate
   C. Intercristal
   D. Conjugata vera
   E. Intertuberous diameter
5: A. D
   B. D
   C. C
6: C
7: A. 4
   B. 3
   C. 1
   D. 2
8: C
9: B
10: A. 2
    B. 2
    C. 3
11: B
12: C
13: C
14: D
15: 2
16: A
17: A. L.O.T.
    B. L.O.A.
    C. R.O.P.
    D. L.S.P.
    E. R.M.A.
    F. R.A.D.P.

UNIT TWO

1: 2
2: A. 3
   B. 3
3: B
4: B
5: F
6: C
7: C
8: A. 2
   B. 3
9: A. 1
   B. 3
   C. 3
10: A. 3
    B. 1

11: B
12: D
13: A
14: D
15: 1
16: 2
17: D

UNIT THREE

1: A. Full dilatation
   B. Effacement
   C. Amnesic
   D. Uterine atony
   E. Episiotomy
   F. Lightening
2: Situation No. 1: 3
   Situation No. 2: 2
   Situation No. 3: 2
3: A. 2
   B. 3
   C. 2
4: 1
5: 3
6: C
7: B
8: 4
9: 2
10: 1
11: 3
12: A. 3
    B. 2
13: A. 3
    B. 1
    C. 4
    D. 4

UNIT FOUR

1: 3
2: 2
3: 1: G
   2: D
   3: B
   4: C
   5: G
   6: G
   7: D
   8: G
4: 4
5: 2
6: 1
7: 3
8: 1

UNIT FIVE

1: 1
2: 2
3: D
4: E
5: B
6: C
7: C
8: D
9: 2
10: 3
11: 3
12: 2
13: 1
14: 1
15: 2

UNIT SIX

1: 3
2: 2
3: 2
4: 1
5: 3
6: 1

UNIT SEVEN

1: 1
2: 1
3: 3

4: 4
5: 1
6: 2
7: 3
8: 1
9: 2
10: 4
11: 3
12: 3
13: 2
14: 2
15: 3
16: A. Mastitis
    B. Endometritis
    C. Pelvic cellulitis or parametritis
    D. Subinvolution
    E. Engorgement

UNIT EIGHT

1: 2
2: 4
3: 2
4: 4
5: 1
6: 1
7: A
8: 3
9: B
10: 2

Glossary

Note: The pronunciations as indicated in the following paragraph in this Glossary follow Webster's Second International Dictionary.

āle, châotic, câre, ădd, ăccount, ärm, ȧsk, sofȧ; ēve, hēre, ĕvent, ĕnd, silĕnt, makēr; īce, ĭll, charĭty; ōld, ôbey, ôrb, ŏdd, sôft, cŏnnect; fōōd, fŏŏt; out; oil, cūbe, ūnite, ûrn, ŭp, circŭs, menü; chair; go; sing; then, thin; natūre; verdūre; k = ch in German ich or ach; bon; yet zh = z in azure

abdominal (ăb-dŏm′ĭ-năl). Belonging to or relating to the abdomen.

a. delivery, delivery of the child by abdominal section. See *cesarean section.*

a. gestation, ectopic pregnancy occurring in the cavity of the abdomen.

a. pregnancy. See *gestation* above.

ablatio placentae. See *abruptio placentae.*

abortion. The termination of pregnancy at any time before the fetus has attained a stage of viability, i.e., before it is capable of extra-uterine existence.

abruptio placentae (ăb-rŭp′shĭ-ō plȧ-sen′-tē). Premature separation of normally implanted placenta.

acromion (ȧ-krō′mĭ-ŏn). An outward extension of the spine of the scapula, used to explain presentation of the fetus.

adnexa (ăd-nĕk′sȧ). Appendages.

a., uterine (ū′tēr-ĭn), the fallopian tubes and ovaries.

afibrinogenemia (ȧ-fī″brin-ō-jen-ē′mē-ȧ). Lack of fibrinogen in the blood.

after-birth (ȧf′tēr-bûrth″). The structures cast off after the expulsion of the fetus, including the membranes and the placenta with the attached umbilical cord; the secundines.

after-pains (ȧf′tēr-pāns″). Those pains, more or less severe, after expulsion of the after-birth, which result from the contractile efforts of the uterus to return to its normal condition.

agalactia (ăg′ȧ-lăk′shĭ-ȧ). Absence or failure of the secretion of milk.

allantois (ȧ-lăn′tō-ĭs). A tubular diverticulum of the posterior part of the yolk sac of the embryo; it passes into the body stalk through which it is accompanied by the allantoic (umbilical) blood vessels, thus taking part in the formation of the umbilical cord; and later, fusing with the chorion, it helps to form the placenta.

amenorrhea (ā-měn″ō-rē′ȧ). Absence or suppression of the menstrual discharge.

amnesia (ăm-nē′zhĭ-ȧ). Loss of memory.

amnion (ăm′nĭ-ŏn). The most internal of the fetal membranes, containing the waters which surround the fetus in utero.

amniotic (ăm″nĭ-ŏt′ĭk). Pertaining to the amnion.

a. sac, the "bag of membranes" containing the fetus before delivery.

analgesia (ăn″ăl-jē′zĭ-ă). Drug which relieves pain, used during labor.

androgen (ăn′drȯ-jěn). Any substance which possesses masculinizing activities, such as the testis hormone.

android (ăn′droid). The term adopted for the male type of pelvis.

anencephalia (ăn-ěn″sė̇-fā′lĭ-ȧ). Form of monstrosity with absence of a brain.

anovular (ăn-ōv′ū-lēr). Not accompanied with the discharge of an ovum; said of cyclic uterine bleeding.

anoxia (an-ox′e-ah). Oxygen deficiency; any condition of absence of tissue oxidation.

antenatal (ăn-tē-nā′tȧl). Occurring or formed before birth.

antepartal (ăn″tė-pär′tal). Before labor and delivery or childbirth; prenatal.

areola (ȧ-rē′ȯ-lȧ). The ring of pigment surrounding the nipple.

secondary a., a circle of faint color sometimes seen just outside the original areola about the 5th month of pregnancy.

articulation (är-tĭk″ū-lā′shŭn). The fastening together of the various bones of the skeleton in their natural situation; a joint. The articulations of the bones of the body are divided into two principal groups—*synarthroses*, immovable articulations, and *diarthroses*, movable articulations.

Aschheim-Zondek test (ăsh″hīm-tsŏn′děk). A test for the diagnosis of pregnancy. Repeated injections of small quantities of urine voided during the first weeks of pregnancy produce in infantile mice, within 100 hours, (1) minute intrafollicular ovarian hemorrhage and (2) the development of lutein cells.

asphyxia (ăs-fĭk′sĭ-à). Suspended animation; anoxia and carbon dioxide retention resulting from failure of respiration.

    a. neonatorum (nē″ô-nà-tō′rŭm), "asphyxia of the newborn," deficient respiration in newborn babies.

attitude (ăt′ĭ-tūd). A posture or position of the body. In obstetrics, the relation of the fetal members to each other in the uterus; the position of the fetus in the uterus.

axis (ăk′sĭs). 1. A line about which any revolving body turns. 2. **Pelvic a.,** the curved line which passes through the centers of all the anteroposterior diameters of the pelvis.

bag of waters. The membranes which enclose the liquor amnii of the fetus.

ballottement (bă-lŏt′měnt). Literally means tossing. A term used in an examination when the fetus can be pushed about in the pregnant uterus.

Bandl's ring (Băn′dls). A groove on the uterus at the upper level of the fully developed lower uterine segment; visible on the abdomen after hard labor as a transverse or slightly slanting depression between the umbilicus and the pubis. Shows overstretching of lower uterine segment. Resembles a full bladder.

Bartholin's glands (Bär′tô-lĭn). Glands situated one on each side of the vaginal canal opening into the groove between the hymen and the labia minora.

bicornate uterus (bī-kôr′năt). Having two horns which, in the embryo, failed to attain complete fusion.

bimanual (bī-măn′ŭ-ăl). Performed with or relating to both hands.

    b. palpation, examination of the pelvic organs of a woman by placing one hand on the abdomen and the fingers of the other in the vagina.

blastoderm (blăs′tô-dûrm). Delicate germinal membrane of the ovum.

    b. vesicle, hollow space within the morula formed by the rearrangement of cells, and by proliferation.

Braxton Hicks sign. Painless uterine contractions occurring periodically throughout pregnancy, thereby enlarging the uterus to accommodate the growing fetus.

    B.H. version, one of the types of operation designed to turn the baby from an undesirable position to a desirable one.

breech (brēch). Nates or buttocks.

    b. delivery, labor and delivery marked by breech presentations.

bregma (brĕg′mà). The point on the surface of the skull at the junction of the coronal and sagittal sutures.

brim (brĭm). The edge of the superior strait or inlet of the pelvis.

caked breast. See *engorgement.*

caput (kā′pŭt). 1. The head, consisting of the cranium, or skull, and the face. 2. Any prominent object, such as the head.

    c. succedaneum (sŭk″sē-dā′nē-ŭm), a dropsical swelling which sometimes appears on the presenting head of the fetus during labor.

catamenia (kăt-à-mē′nĭ-à). See *menses.*

caudal (kô′dăl). The term applied to analgesia or anesthesia resulting from the introduction of the suitable analgesic or anesthetic solution into the caudal canal (nonclosure of the laminae of the last sacral vertebra).

caul (kôl). A portion of the amniotic sac which occasionally envelops the child's head at birth.

cephalhematoma (sĕf″ăl-hē″mà-tō′-mà). A tumor or swelling between the bone and the periosteum caused by an effusion of blood.

cephalic (sē-făl′ĭk). Belonging to the head.

    c. presentation, presentation of any part of the fetal head in labor.

cervix (sûr′vĭks). Necklike part; the lower and narrow end of the uterus, between the os and the body of the organ.

cesarean section (sē-zâ′rē-ăn). Delivery of the fetus by an incision through the abdominal wall and the wall of the uterus.

Chadwick's sign (tshăd′wĭks). The violet color on the mucous membrane of the vagina just below the urethral orifice, seen after the 4th week of pregnancy.

change of life. See *climacteric.*

chloasma (klô-ăz′mă). Pl. *chloasmata.* A cutaneous affection exhibiting spots and patches of a yellowish-brown color. The term chloasma is a vague one and is applied to various kinds of pigmentary discoloration of the skin.

c. gravidarum, c. uterinum, chloasma occurring during pregnancy.

chorioepithelioma (kō′rĭ-ō-ĕp-ĭ-thē-lĭ-ō′-mȧ). Chorionic carcinoma; a tumor formed by malignant proliferation of the epithelium of the chorionic villi.

chorion (kō′rĭ-ŏn). The outermost membrane of the growing zygote, or fertilized ovum, which serves as a protective and nutritive covering.

chromosome (kro′mo-sōm). One of several small, dark-staining and more or less rod-shaped bodies which appear in the nucleus of the cell at the time of cell division and particularly in mitosis.

circumcision (sûr″kŭm-sĭzh′ŭn). The removal of all or part of the prepuce, or foreskin of the penis.

cleft palate (klĕft păl′ĭt). Congenital fissure of the palate and the roof of the mouth.

climacteric (klī-măk-tĕr′ĭk). A particular epoch of the ordinary term of life at which the body undergoes a considerable change; especially, the menopause or "change of life."

clitoris (klī′tȯ-rĭs). A small, elongated, erectile body, situated at the anterior part of the vulva. An organ of the female homologous with the penis of the male.

coitus (kō′ĭt-ŭs). Sexual intercourse; copulation.

colostrum (kȯ-lŏs′trŭm). A substance in the first milk after delivery, giving to it a yellowish color.

c. corpuscles, large, granular cells found in colostrum.

colporrhaphy (kŏl-pōr′ȧ-fē). 1. The operation of suturing the vagina. 2. The operation of denuding and suturing the vaginal wall for the purpose of narrowing the vagina.

colpotomy (kŏl-pŏt′o-mē). Any surgical cutting operation upon the vagina.

conception (kŏn-sĕp′shŭn). The impregnation of the female ovum by the spermatozoon of the male, whence results a new being.

condyloma (con-dil-o′mah). Pl. *condylomata.* A wartlike excrescence near the anus or the vulva; the flat, moist papule of secondary syphilis.

confinement (kŏn-fīn′mĕnt). Term applied to childbirth and the lying-in period.

congenital (kŏn-jĕn′ĭ-tĕl). Born with a person; existing from or from before birth, as, for example, congenital disease, a disease originating in the fetus before birth.

conjugate (kŏn′jŏŏ-gȧt). The anteroposterior diameter of the pelvic inlet.

contraception (kŏn″trȧ-sĕp′shŭn). The prevention of conception or impregnation.

coronal (kŏr′ȯ-năl). Belonging to, or relating to, the crown of the head.

c. suture, the suture formed by the union of the frontal bone with the two parietal bones.

corpus luteum (kôr′pŭs lū′tĕ-ŭm). The yellow mass found in the graafian follicle after the ovum has been expelled.

cotyledon (kŏt″ĭ-lē′dŭn). Any one of the subdivisions of the uterine surface of the placenta.

cul-de-sac (kōōl′dē-săk′) of Douglas. A pouch between the anterior wall of the rectum and the uterus.

cyesis (sī-ē′sĭs). Pregnancy.

decrement (dĕk′rē-mĕnt). Decrease; also the stage of decline.

delivery (dē-lĭv′ēr-ĭ). [French, *délivrer,* to free, to deliver.] 1. The expulsion of a child by the mother, or its extraction by the obstetric practitioner. 2. The removal of a part from the body; as *delivery* of the placenta.

dizygotic (dī″zī-gŏt′ĭk). Pertaining to or proceeding from two zygotes (ova).

Döderlein's bacillus (ded′er-līnz). The large gram-positive bacterium occurring in the normal vaginal secretion.

Douglas' cul-de-sac (kōōl′dē-săk′). A sac or recess formed by a fold of the peritoneum dipping down between the rectum and the uterus. Also called *pouch of Douglas* and *recto-uterine pouch.*

ductus (dŭk′tŭs). A duct.

d. arteriosus (är-tē″rĭ-ō′sŭs), "arterial duct," a blood vessel peculiar to the fetus, communicating directly between the pulmonary artery and the aorta.

d. venosus (vē-nō′sŭs), "venous duct," a blood vessel peculiar to the fetus, establishing a direct communication between the umbilical vein and the inferior vena cava.

Duncan (dŭng′kăn) mechanism. The position of the placenta, with the maternal surface outermost; to be born edgewise.

dystocia (dĭs-tō′shĭ-ȧ). Difficult, slow or painful birth or delivery. It is distinguished as *maternal* or *fetal* according as the difficulty is due to some deformity on the part of the mother or on the part of the child.

d., placental, difficulty in delivering the placenta.

eclampsia (ĕk-lămp′sĭ-ȧ). Acute "toxemia of pregnancy" characterized by convulsions and coma which may occur during pregnancy, labor or the puerperium.

ectoderm (ĕk′tō-dûrm). The outer layer of cells of the primitive embryo.

ectopic (ĕk-tŏp′ĭk). Out of place.

    e. gestation, gestation in which the fetus is out of its normal place in the cavity of the uterus. It includes gestations in the interstitial portion of the tube, in a rudimentary horn of the uterus (cornual pregnancy) and cervical pregnancy as well as tubal, abdominal and ovarian pregnancies. See also *extra-uterine pregnancy.*

    e. pregnancy, same as *ectopic gestation.*

effacement (ĕ-fās′mĕnt). Obliteration. In obstetrics, refers to thinning and shortening of the cervix.

ejaculation (ē-jăk″ū-lă′shŭn). A sudden act of expulsion, as of semen.

embryo (ĕm′brĭ-ō). The product of conception in utero from the 3rd through the 5th week of gestation; after that length of time it is called the fetus.

empathy (ĕm′pȧ-thĭ). The projection of one's own consciousness into that of another. Empathy may be distinguished from sympathy in that the former state includes relative freedom from emotional involvement.

endocervical (ĕn′dō-sûr′vĭ-kăl). Pertaining to the interior of the cervix of the uterus.

endometrium (ĕn″dō-mē′trĭ-ŭm). The mucous membrane which lines the uterus.

engagement (ĕn-gāj′mĕnt). In obstetrics, applies to the entrance of the presenting part into the superior pelvic strait and the beginning of the descent through the pelvic canal.

engorgement (ĕn-gôrj′mĕnt). Hyperemia; local congestion; excessive fullness of any organ or passage. In obstetrics, refers to an exaggeration of normal venous and lymph stasis of the breasts which occurs in relation to lactation.

entoderm (ĕn′tō-dûrm). The innermost layer of cells of the primitive embryo.

enzygotic (ĕn-zī-gŏt′ĭk). Developed from the same fertilized ovum.

episiotomy (ĕp″ĭs-ĭ-ot′ō-mĭ). Surgical incision of the vulvar orifice for obstetric purposes.

Erb's paralysis. Partial paralysis of the brachial plexus, affecting various muscles of the arm and the chest wall.

ergot (ûr′gŏt). A drug having the remarkable property of exciting powerfully the contractile force of the uterus, and chiefly used for this purpose, but its long-continued use is highly dangerous. Usually given in the fluid extract.

erythroblastosis fetalis (ĕ-rĭth″rō-blăs-tō′sĭs). A severe hemolytic disease of the newborn usually due to Rh incompatibility.

estrogen (ĕs′trō-jĕn). A hormone secreted by the ovary and the placenta.

extraperitoneal (ĕks″trȧ-pĕr-ĭ-tō-nē′ăl). Situated or occurring outside the peritoneal cavity.

extra-uterine (ĕks″trȧ-ū′tĕr-ĭn). Outside of the uterus.

    e. pregnancy, pregnancy in which the fetus is contained in some organ outside of the uterus, i.e., tubal, abdominal and ovarian pregnancies.

fallopian (fȧ-lō′pĭ-ăn). [Relating to G. *Fallopius,* a celebrated Italian anatomist of the 16th century.]

    f. tubes, the oviducts—two canals extending from the sides of the fundus uteri.

fecundation (fē″kŭn-dā′shŭn). The act of impregnating or the state of being impregnated; the fertilization of the ovum by means of the male seminal element.

fertility (fĕr-tĭl′ĭ-tĭ). The ability to produce offspring; power of reproduction.

fertilization (fûr-tĭ-lĭ-zā′shŭn). The fusion of the spermatozoon with the ovum; it marks the beginning of pregnancy.

fetus (fē′tŭs). The baby in utero from the end of the 5th week of gestation until birth.

fimbria (fĭm′brĭ-ȧ). A fringe; especially the fringelike end of the fallopian tube.

fontanel (fŏn″tȧ-nĕl′). The diamond-shaped space between the frontal and two parietal bones in very young infants. This is called the *anterior f.* and is the familiar "soft spot" just above a baby's forehead. A small, triangular one (*posterior f.*) is between the occipital and parietal bones.

foramen (fō-rā′mĕn). A hole, opening, aperture or orifice—especially one through a bone.

    f. ovale (ō-vā′lē), an opening situated in the partition which separates the right and left auricles of the heart in the fetus.

foreskin (fōr′skĭn). The prepuce—the fold of skin covering the glans penis.

fornix (fôr′nĭks). Pl. **fornices** (fôr′nĭ-sēz). An arch; any vaulted surface.

    f. of the vagina, the angle of reflection of the vaginal mucous membrane onto the cervix uteri.

fourchet (foor-shĕt'). [French, "fork."] The posterior angle or commissure of the labia majora.

frenum (frē'nŭm). Lingual fold of integument or of mucous membrane that checks, curbs or limits the movements of the tongue (ankyloglossia). Congenital shortening.

Friedman's test (frēd'măn). A modification of the Aschheim-Zondek test for pregnancy; the urine of early pregnancy is injected in 4-cc. doses intravenously twice daily for 2 days into an unmated mature rabbit. If, at the end of this time, the ovaries of the rabbit contain fresh corpora lutea or hemorrhagic corpora, the test is positive.

F.S.H., FSH. Abbreviation for follicle-stimulating hormone.

fundus (fŭn'dŭs). The upper rounded portion of the uterus between the points of insertion of the fallopian tubes.

funic souffle (fū'nĭc soo'f'l). A soft, blowing sound, synchronous with the fetal heart sounds and supposed to be produced in the umbilical cord.

funis (fū'nĭs). A cord—especially the umbilical cord.

galactagogue (ga-lăk'ta-gŏg). 1. Causing the flow of milk. 2. Any drug which causes the flow of milk to increase.

galactorrhea (gă-lak-tō-re'ă). Excessive flow of milk.

gamete (găm'ēt). A sexual cell; a mature germ cell, as an unfertilized egg or a mature sperm cell.

gastrula (găs'troo-la). The early embryonic stage which follows the blastula.

gene (jēn). An hereditary germinal factor in the chromosome which carries on an hereditary transmissible character.

genitalia (jĕn-ĭtăl'ĭ-a). The reproductive organs.

gestation (jĕs-tā-shŭn). The condition of pregnancy; pregnancy; gravidity.

gonad (gŏn'ăd). A gamete-producing gland; an ovary or testis.

gonadotropin (gŏn"ăd-ô-trō'pĭn). A substance having an affinity for or a stimulating effect on the gonads.

Goodell's sign (good'elz). Softening of the cervix, a presumptive sign of pregnancy.

graafian follicles or **vesicles** (gräf'ĭ-ăn). Small spherical bodies in the ovaries, each containing an ovum.

gravida (grăv'ĭd-ä). A pregnant woman.

habitus (hăb'ĭt-ŭs). Attitude, disposition or tendency; to act in a certain way; position acquired by frequent repetition.

Hegar's sign (hā'gärz). Softening of the lower uterine segment; a sign of pregnancy.

homologous (hô-môl'ô-gŭs). Corresponding in structure or origin; derived from the same source.

hormone (hôr'mōn). A chemical substance produced in an organ, which, being carried to an associated organ by the blood stream, excites in the latter organ a functional activity.

hydatidiform (hi"dah-tid'ĭ-form) **mole.** Cystic proliferation of chorionic villi, resembling a bunch of grapes.

hydramnios (hī-drăm'nĭ-ŏs). An excessive amount of amniotic fluid.

hymen (hī'mĕn). A membranous fold which partially or wholly occludes the external orifice of the vagina, especially in the virgin.

hypofibrinogenemia (hī"pô-fī-brĭn"ô-jen-ē'-mē-ă). Deficiency of fibrinogen in the blood.

hypogalactia (hī"pô-gă-lăk'she-ă). Deficiency in the secretion of milk.

hypoxia (hī-pŏks'ĭ-a). Insufficient oxygen to support normal metabolic requirements.

iliopectineal line (ĭl"ĭ-ô-pĕk-tĭn'ē-ăl). The linea terminalis.

impregnation (ĭm"prĕg-nā'shŭn). See *fertilization*.

increment (ĭn'krĕ-mĕnt). That by which anything is increased.

inertia (in-ûr'shĭ-a). Inactivity; inability to move spontaneously. Sluggishness of uterine contractions during labor.

infant (ĭn'fănt). A baby; a child under 2 years of age.

infertility (ĭn-fûr-tĭl'ĭ-tĭ). The condition of being unfruitful or barren; sterility.

inlet (ĭn'lĕt). The upper limit of the pelvic cavity (brim).

introitis (ĭn-trō'ĭ-tŭs). A term applied to the opening of the vagina.

in utero. Inside the uterus.

inversion (ĭn-vûr'shŭn). A turning upside down, inside out, or end for end.

    i. of the uterus, the state of the womb being turned inside out, caused by violently drawing away the placenta before it is detached by the natural process of labor.

involution (ĭn"vô-lū'shŭn). 1. A rolling or pushing inward. 2. A retrograde process of change which is the reverse of evolution: particularly applied to the return of the uterus to its normal size and condition after parturition.

ischium (ĭs'kĭ-ŭm). The posterior and inferior bone of the pelvis, distinct and separate in the fetus or the infant, or the corresponding part of the innominate bone in the adult.

jelly (jĕl'ĭ). A soft substance which is coherent, tremulous and more or less transparent.

    j. of Wharton, the soft, pulpy, connective tissue that constitutes the matrix of the umbilical cord.

labia (lā'bĭ-à). The nominative plural of *labium.* Lips or liplike structures.

    l. majora (mà-jō'rà), the folds of skin containing fat and covered with hair which form each side of the vulva.

    l. minora (mĭ-nō'rà), the nymphae, or folds of delicate skin inside of the labia majora.

labor (lā'bēr). Parturition; the series of processes by which the products of conception are expelled from the mother's body.

lactation (lăk-tā'shŭn). The act or period of giving milk; the secretion of milk; the time or period of secreting milk.

lambdoid (lăm'doid). Having the shape of the Greek letter λ (lambda).

    l. suture, the suture between the occipital and two parietal bones.

lanugo (là-nū'gō). The fine hair on the body of the fetus. The fine, downy hair found on nearly all parts of the body except the palms of the hands and the soles of the feet.

leukorrhea (lū''kŏ-rē'à). A whitish discharge from the female genital organs.

L.H. Abbreviation for luteinizing hormone.

lightening (līt'n-ĭng). The sensation of decreased abdominal distention produced by the descent of the uterus into the pelvic cavity, which occurs from 2 to 3 weeks before the onset of labor.

linea (lĭn'ē-à). Pl. *lineae* (lĭn'ē-ē). A line or thread.

    l. alba (ăl'bà), the central tendinous line extending from the pubic bone to the ensiform cartilage.

    l. nigra (nī'grä). A dark line appearing on the abdomen and extending from the pubis toward the umbilicus—considered one of the signs of pregnancy.

    l. terminalis. The oblique ridge on the inner surface of the ilium, continued on the pubis, which separates the true from the false pelvis. Formerly called the iliopectineal line.

lingua (lĭng'gwà). Tongue.

    l. frenum, tonguetie.

liquor (lĭk'ēr). A liquid.

    l. amnii (lĭ'kwôr ăm'nĭ-ī), the fluid contained within the amnion in which the fetus floats.

lochia (lō'kĭ-à). The discharge from the genital canal during several days subsequent to delivery.

mask (màsk) of pregnancy. See *chloasma.*

maturation (măt''û-rā'shŭn). In biology, a process of cell division during which the number of chromosomes in the germ cells is reduced to one half the number characteristic of the species.

meatus (mē-ā'tŭs). A passage; an opening leading to a canal, duct or cavity.

    m. urinarius (ū''-rĭ-nā'rĭ-ŭs), the external orifice of the urethra.

mechanism (mĕk'à-niz'm). The manner of combinations which subserve a common function. In obstetrics refers to labor and delivery.

meconium (mē-kō'nĭ-ŭm). The dark-green or black substance found in the large intestine of the fetus or newly born infant.

menarche (mē-när'kē). The establishment or the beginning of the menstrual function.

menopause (mĕn'ô-pôz). The period at which menstruation ceases; the "change of life."

menorrhagia (mĕn''ô-rā'jĭ-à). An abnormally profuse menstrual flow.

menses (mĕn'sēz). [Pl. of Latin *mensis,* month.] The periodic monthly discharge of blood from the uterus; the catamenia.

menstruation (mĕn''strŏŏ-ā'shŭn). The cyclic, physiologic uterine bleeding which normally recurs at approximately 4-week intervals, in the absence of pregnancy, during the reproductive period.

mentum (mĕn'tŭm). The chin.

mesoderm (mĕs'ô-dûrm). The middle layer of cells derived from the primitive embryo.

metrorrhagia (mē-trŏ-rā'jĭ-à). Abnormal uterine bleeding.

migration (mī-grā'shŭn). In obstetrics refers to the passage of the ovum from the ovary to the uterus.

milia (mĭl'ē-ă). Plural of *milium.*

milium (mĭl'ē-ŭm). A small white nodule of the

skin, usually caused by clogged sebaceous glands or hair follicles.

milk-leg. See *phlegmasia alba dolens.*

miscarriage (mĭs-kăr'ĭj). Abortion.

molding (mōld'ĭng). The shaping of the baby's head so as to adjust itself to the size and shape of the birth canal.

monozygotic (mŏn″ȯ-zī-gȯ'tĭk). Pertaining to or derived from one zygote.

    m. twins (mŏn″ȯ-zī-gȯ'tĭk). Pertaining to or derived from one zygote.

mons veneris (mŏnz vĕn'ĕ-rĭs). The eminence in the upper and anterior part of the pubes of women.

Montgomery's tubercles (mŭnt-gŭm'ĕr-ĭz). Small, nodular follicles or glands on the areolae around the nipples.

multigravida (mŭl″tĭ-grăv'ĭ-dȧ). A woman who has been pregnant several times, or many times.

multipara (mŭl-tĭp'ȧ-rȧ). A woman who has borne several, or many, children.

navel (nāv'ĕl). The umbilicus.

neonatal (nē″ȯ-nā'tăl). Pertaining to the newborn, usually considered the first 4 weeks of life.

nevus (nē'vŭs). A natural mark or blemish; a mole, a circumscribed deposit of pigmentary matter in the skin present at birth (birthmark).

nidation (nĭ-dā'shŭn). The implantation of the fertilized ovum in the endometrium of the pregnant uterus.

nullipara (nŭ-lĭp'ȧ-rȧ). A woman who has not borne children.

occipitobregmatic (ŏk-sĭp″ĭt-ȯ-brĕg-măt'-ĭk). Pertaining to the occiput (the back part of the head) and the bregma (junction of the coronal and sagittal sutures).

oligohydramnios (ŏl″ĭ-gȯ-hī-drăm'nĭ-ŏs). Deficiency of amniotic fluid.

omphalic (ŏm-făl'ĭk). Pertaining to the umbilicus.

oocyesis (ō'ȯ-sī-ē'sĭs). Ovarian pregnancy.

ophthalmia neonatorum (ŏf-thăl'mĭ-ȧ). Acute purulent conjunctivitis of the newborn usually due to gonorrheal infection.

os (ŏs). Pl. *ora* (ō'rȧ). Mouth.

    o. externum (*external os*), the external opening of the canal of the cervix.

    o. internum (*internal os*), internal opening of canal of cervix.

    o. uteri, "mouth of the uterus."

ova. Plural of ovum.

ovary (ō'vȧ-rĭ). The sexual gland of the female in which the ova are developed. There are two ovaries, one at each side of the pelvis.

ovulation (ō-vŭ-lā'shŭn). The growth and discharge of an unimpregnated ovum, usually coincident with the menstrual period.

ovum (ō'vŭm). The female reproductive cell. The human ovum is a round cell about 1/120 of an inch in diameter, developed in the ovary.

oxytocic (ŏk″sĭ-tō'sĭk). 1. Accelerating parturition. 2. A medicine which accelerates parturition.

oxytocin (ŏk-sĭ-tō-sĭn). One of the two hormones secreted by the posterior pituitary.

palsy (pôl'zĭ). A synonym for paralysis, used in connection with certain special forms.

    Bell's p., peripheral facial paralysis due to lesion of the facial nerve, resulting characteristic distortion of the face.

    Erb's p., the upper-arm type of brachial birth palsy.

para (pär'ä). The term used to refer to past pregnancies which have produced an infant which has been viable, whether or not the infant is dead or alive at birth.

parametrium (păr-ȧ-mē'trĭ-ŭm). The fibrous subserous coat of the supravaginal portion of the uterus, extending laterally between the layers of the broad ligaments.

parity (păr'ĭ-tĭ). The condition of a woman with respect to her having borne children.

parovarian (păr-ȯ-vâr'ĭ-ăn). Pertaining to the residual structure in the broad ligament between the ovary and the fallopian tube.

parturient (pär-tŭ'rĭ-ĕnt). Bringing forth; pertaining to child-bearing. A woman in childbirth.

parturition (pär″tŭ-rĭsh'ŭn). The act or process of giving birth to a child.

patulous (păt'ŭ-lŭs). Spreading somewhat widely apart; open.

pelvimeter (pĕl-vĭm'ē-tēr). An instrument for measuring the diameters and capacity of the pelvis.

pelvimetry (pĕl-vĭm'ē-trĭ). The measurement of the dimensions and capacity of the pelvis.

penis (pē'nĭs). The male organ of copulation.

perineorrhaphy (pĕr″ĭ-nē-ŏr'ȧ-fĭ). Suture of the perineum; the operation for the repair of lacerations of the perineum.

perineotomy (pĕr'ĭ-nē-ŏt'ō-mĭ). A surgical incision through the perineum.

perineum (pĕr″ĭ-nē'ŭm). The area between the vagina and the rectum.

peritoneum (pĕr″ĭ-tô-nē′ŭm). A strong serous membrane investing the inner surface of the abdominal walls and the viscera of the abdomen.

phimosis (fī-mō′sĭs). Tightness of the foreskin.

phlegmasia alba dolens (flĕg-mā′zhĭ-à ăl′bà dō′lĕnz). Phlebitis of the femoral vein, occasionally following delivery.

Pitocin (pĭ-tŏ′sĭn). A proprietary solution of oxytocin.

placenta (plà-sĕn′tà). The circular flat, vascular structure in the impregnated uterus forming the principal medium of communication between the mother and the fetus.

　ablatio p. See *abruptio placentae.*

　abruptio p., premature separation of the normally implanted placenta.

　previa p., a placenta which is implanted in the lower uterine segment so that it adjoins or covers the internal os of the cervix.

polygalactia (pŏl″ē-gà-lăk′shē-à). Excessive secretion of milk.

polyhydramnios (pŏl″ĭ-hī-drăm′nĭ-ŏs). Hydramnios.

position (pô-zĭsh′ŭn). The situation of the fetus in the pelvis; determined by the relation of some arbitrarily chosen portion of the fetus to the right or the left side of the mother's pelvis.

postnatal (pōst-nā′tăl). Occurring after birth.

postpartal (pōst-pär′tal). After delivery or childbirth.

preeclampsia (prē-ĕk-lămp′sĭ-à). A disorder encountered during pregnancy or early in the puerperium, characterized by hypertension, edema and albuminuria.

pregnancy (prĕg′năn-sĭ). [Latin, *praeg′nans,* literally "previous to bringing forth."] The state of being with young or with child. The normal duration of pregnancy in the human female is 280 days, or 10 lunar months, or 9 calendar months.

premature infant. An infant which weighs 2,500 Gm. or less at birth.

prepuce (prē′pūs). The fold of skin which covers the glans penis in the male.

　p. of the clitoris, the fold of mucous membrane which covers the glans clitoris.

presentation (prĕ″zĕn-tā′shŭn). Term used to designate that part of the fetus nearest the internal os; or that part which is felt by the physician's examining finger when introduced into the cervix.

primigravida (prī″mĭ-grăv′ĭ-dà). Pl. *primigravidae* (prī″mĭ-grăv′ĭ-dē). A woman who is pregnant for the first time.

primipara (prī-mĭp′à-rà). Pl. *primiparae* (prī-mĭp′à-rē). A woman who has given birth to her first child.

primordial (prī-môr′dĭ-ăl). Original or primitive; of the simplest and most undeveloped character.

prodromal (prŏ-drŏ′măl). Premonitory; indicating the approach of a disease.

progesterone (prō-jĕs′tĕr-ōn). The pure hormone contained in the corpora lutea whose function is to prepare the endometrium for the reception and development of the fertilized ovum.

prolactin (prŏ-lăk′tĭn). A proteohormone from the anterior pituitary which stimulates lactation in the mammary glands.

prolan (prŏ′lăn). Zondek's term for the gonadotropic principle of human-pregnancy urine, responsible for the biologic pregnancy tests.

promontory (prŏm′ŭn-tō″rĭ). A small projection; a prominence.

　p. of the sacrum, the superior or projecting portion of the sacrum when in situ in the pelvis, at the junction of the sacrum and the last lumbar vertebra.

pseudocyesis (sū″dō-sī-ē′sĭs). An apparent condition of pregnancy; the woman really believes she is pregnant when, as a matter of fact, she is not.

puberty (pū′bĕr-tĭ). The age at which the generative organs become functionally active.

pubic (pū′bĭk). Belonging to the pubis.

pubiotomy (pū′bī-ŏt′ô-mĭ). The operation of cutting through the pubic bone lateral to the median line.

pubis (pū′bĭs). The os pubis or pubic bone forming the front of the pelvis.

pudendal (pū-dĕn′dăl). Relating to the pudenda.

pudendum (pū-dĕn′dŭm). [Latin, *pude′re,* to have shame or modesty.] The external genital parts of either sex, but especially of the female.

puerperium (pū″ĕr-pē′rĭ-ŭm). The period elapsing between the termination of labor and the return of the uterus to its normal condition, about 6 weeks.

quickening (kwĭk′ĕn-ĭng). The mother's first perception of the movements of the fetus.

rabbit test. See *Friedman's test.*

Rh. Abbreviation for *Rhesus,* a type of monkey. This term is used for a property of human blood cells, because of its relationship to a similar property in the blood cells of *Rhesus* monkeys.

Rh factor. A term applied to an inherited antigen in the human blood.

Ritgen maneuver (rĭt′gĕn). Delivery of the infant's head by lifting the head upward and forward through the vulva, between contractions, by pressing with the tips of the fingers upon the perineum behind the anus.

Schultze's mechanism (shōŏlt′sĕz). The expulsion of the placenta with the fetal surfaces presenting.

secundine (sĕk′ŭn-dīn). The afterbirth; the placenta and membranes expelled after the birth of a child.

segmentation (sĕg″mĕn-tā′shŭn). The process of division by which the fertilized ovum multiplies before differentiation into layers occurs.

semen (sē′mĕn). 1. A seed. 2. The fluid secreted by the male reproductive organs.

show (shō). 1. Popularly, the blood-tinged mucus discharged from the vagina before or during labor.

Skene's gland. Two glands just within the meatus of the female urethra; regarded as homologues of the prostate gland in the male.

smegma. A thick cheesy secretion found under the prepuce and in the region of the clitoris and the labia minora.

souffle (sōōf′f'l). A soft, blowing, auscultatory sound.

    funic s., a hissing souffle synchronous with the fetal heart sounds and supposed to be produced in the umbilical cord.

    placental s., a souffle supposed to be produced by the blood current in the placenta.

spermatozoon (spûr″mȧ-tŏ-zō′ŏn). Pl. *spermatozoa* (spûr″mȧ-tŏ-zō′ȧ). The motile microscopic sexual element of the male, resembling in shape an elongated tadpole. The male reproductive cell.

stillborn (stĭl′bôrn″). Born without life; born dead.

stria (strī′ȧ). Pl. *striae* (strī′ē). A Latin word signifying a "groove," "furrow" or "crease."

    striae gravidarum (grăv-ĭ-där′ŭm), shining, reddish lines upon the abdomen, thighs and breasts during pregnancy.

subinvolution (sŭb′ĭn-vŏ-lū′shŭn). Failure of a part to return to its normal size and condition after enlargement from functional activity, as subinvolution of the uterus which exists when normal involution of the puerperal uterus is retarded.

succedaneum (sŭk′sē-dā′nē-ŭm). See *caput.*

superfecundation (sū′pēr-fē-kŭn-dā′shŭn). The fertilization at about the same time of two different ova by sperm from different males.

superfetation (sū′pēr-fē-tā′shŭn). The fecundation of a woman already pregnant.

symphysis (sĭm′fĭ-sĭs). The union of bones by means of an intervening substance; a variety of synarthrosis.

    s. pubis (pū′bĭs), "symphysis of the pubis," the pubic articulation or union of the pubic bones which are connected with each other by interarticular cartilage.

synchondrosis (sĭng″kŏn-drō′sĭs). A union of bones by means of a fibrous or elastic cartilage.

testicle (tĕs′tĭ-k'l). One of the two glands contained in the male scrotum.

thrush. An infection caused by the fungus *Candida albicans*, characterized by whitish plaques in the mouth.

tonguetie. See *lingua frenum.*

toxemia (tŏks-ē′mĭ-ȧ). The toxemias of pregnancy are disorders encountered during gestation, or early in the puerperium, which are characterized by one or more of the following signs: hypertension, edema, albuminuria, and in severe cases, convulsions and coma.

trichomonas (trĭk-ŏm′ŏ-nȧs). A genus of parasitic flagellate protozoa.

    t. vaginalis, a species sometimes found in the vagina.

trophectoderm (trŏf-ĕk′tŏ-dûrm). The outer layer of cells of the early blastodermic vesicle; it develops the trophoderm—the feeding layer.

umbilical (ŭm-bĭl′ĭ-kȧl). Pertaining to the umbilicus.

    u. arteries, the arteries which accompany and form part of the umbilical cord.

    u. cord [Latin, *funis umbilicalis*], the cord connecting the placenta with the umbilicus of the fetus, and at the close of gestation principally made up of the two umbilical arteries and the umbilical vein, encased in a mass of gelatinous tissue called "Wharton's jelly."

    u. hernia, hernia at or near the umbilicus.

    u. vein, forms a part of the umbilical cord.

uterus (ū'tẽr-ŭs). The hollow muscular organ in the female designed for the lodgement and nourishment of the fetus during its development until birth.

vagina (vȧ-jī'nȧ). [Latin, a sheath.] The canal in the female, extending from the vulva to the cervix of the uterus.

vernix caseosa (vûr'nĭks kā"sê-ō'sȧ). "Cheesy varnish." The layer of fatty matter which covers the skin of the fetus.

version (vûr'shŭn). The act of turning; specifically, a turning of the fetus in the uterus so as to change the presenting part and bring it into more favorable position for delivery.

vertex (vûr'tĕks). The summit or top of anything. In anatomy, the top or crown of the head.
    v. presentation, presentation of the vertex of the fetus in labor.

vestibule (vĕs'tĭ-būl). A triangular space between the labia minora; the urinary meatus and the vagina open into it.

viable (vī'ȧ-b'l). A term in medical jurisprudence signifying "able or likely to live"; applied to the condition of the child at birth.

villus (vĭl'ŭs). A small vascular process or protrusion growing on a mucous surface, such as the chorionic villi seen in tufts on the chorion of the early embryo.

vulva (vŭl'vȧ). The external genitals of the female.

Wharton's jelly (hwôr'tŭnz). [Thomas *Wharton,* English anatomist, died 1673.] The jellylike mucous tissue composing the bulk of the umbilical cord.

witches' milk (wĭch'ĕz). A milky fluid secreted from the breast of the newly born.

womb (wōōm). See *uterus.*

zona pellucida (zō'nȧ pĕll-ū'sĭd-ä). A transparent belt; translucent or shining through.

zygote (zī'gōt). A cell resulting from the fusion of two gametes.

CONVERSION TABLE FOR WEIGHTS OF NEWBORN

(Gram equivalents for pounds and ounces)

For example, to find weight in pounds and ounces of baby weighing 3315 grams, glance down columns to figure nearest 3315 = 3317. Refer to number at top of column for pounds and number to far left for ounces = 7 pounds, 5 ounces.

Pounds→ Ounces↓	3	4	5	6	7	8	9	10
0	1361	1814	2268	2722	3175	3629	4082	4536
1	1389	1843	2296	2750	3203	3657	4111	4564
2	1417	1871	2325	2778	3232	3685	4139	4593
3	1446	1899	2353	2807	3260	3714	4167	4621
4	1474	1928	2381	2835	3289	3742	4196	4649
5	1503	1956	2410	2863	3317	3770	4224	4678
6	1531	1984	2438	2892	3345	3799	4252	4706
7	1559	2013	2466	2920	3374	3827	4281	4734
8	1588	2041	2495	2948	3402	3856	4309	4763
9	1616	2070	2523	2977	3430	3884	4338	4791
10	1644	2098	2551	3005	3459	3912	4366	4819
11	1673	2126	2580	3033	3487	3941	4394	4848
12	1701	2155	2608	3062	3515	3969	4423	4876
13	1729	2183	2637	3090	3544	3997	4451	4904
14	1758	2211	2665	3118	3572	4026	4479	4933
15	1786	2240	2693	3147	3600	4054	4508	4961

Or, to convert grams into pounds and *decimals* of a pound, multiply weight in grams by .0022. Thus, 3317 × .0022 = 7.2974, i.e., 7.3 pounds, or 7 pounds, 5 ounces.

To convert pounds and ounces into grams, multiply the pounds by 453.6 and the ounces by 28.4 and add the two products. Thus, to convert 7 pounds, 5 ounces, 7 × 453.6 = 3175; 5 × 28.4 = 142; 3175 + 142 = 3317 grams.

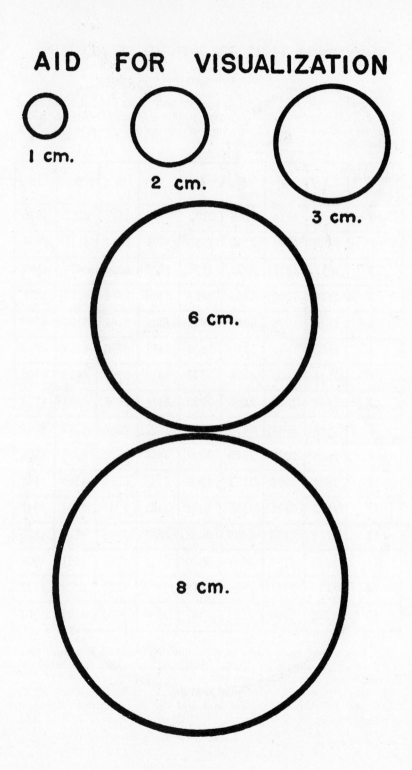

OF CERVICAL DILATATION

4 cm.

5 cm.

10 cm.
COMPLETE (OR FULL)
DILATATION

Index

Abbott, Grace, 589
Abdomen, changes, as probable
   sign of pregnancy, 123-124
  examination, in labor, 249
  muscles, control, antepartal,
   178-179
  "stitch" sensation, antepartal
   period, treatment, 178
  support, maternity girdle,
   159
   in puerperium, 321-322
  wall, changes, in pregnancy,
   111, 114-116
    contour, 111, 112
    muscles, diastasis, 116
    stria gravidarum, 114-
    115, 117-118
    in puerperium, 299
Abortion, 456-460
  causes, 458-459
  clinical picture, 457-458
  complete, 455, 457
  criminal, 457
   major considerations, 17
   potential infection, 460
  deaths, maternal, United
   States (1963), 444
  definitions, 456
  habitual, 457
  incomplete, 455, 457
  induced, 456
  inevitable, 455, 456
  missed, 457
  rate, 17
  responsibility of nurse, 460
  spontaneous, 456
  stages, 455

Abortion—(Cont.)
  terminology, 456-457
  therapeutic, 457
  threatened, 455, 456
  treatment, 458-460
   instruments, 458-460
Abruptio placentae, 465-466
Abscess, breast, puerperal, epidemic, 511-513
   symptoms, 512
    treatment and care,
    512-513
Accouchement. *See* Labor
Acetazolamide (Diamox) therapy, preeclampsia, 448
Acini cells, 50
Activity, antepartal period,
  176-177
Adams, Martha, quoted, 394-
  395
Adrenal glands, cortex, changes
  in pregnancy, 119
Aëtius, 582
After-pains, in puerperium,
  300-301
Agammaglobulinemia, 545
Age, as factor in incidence,
  eclampsia, 450
Albuminuria, in eclampsia, 450
  in preeclampsia, 446, 447
  test in antepartal care, 134
Alimentary tract, obstructions,
  in newborn infant, 542-543
N-allylnormorphine (Nalor-
  phine) therapy, asphyxia
  neonatorum, 531
Ambulance for premature infant, 411

Ambulation, early, in puer-
  perium, 314
Amenorrhea, 59, 68
American Academy of Pedi-
  atrics, 374
American Association for Ma-
  ternal and Child Health, 592
American Association for Ma-
  ternal and Infant Health,
  592
American Association of Ob-
  stetrics and Gynecology and
  Abdominal Surgeons, 591
American Association for the
  Study and Prevention of Infant Mortality, organization,
  588
American Child Health Association, 588, 591
American Child Hygiene Association, 588
American College of Nurse-
  Midwifery, 573, 592
  programs, 573-574
American Committee on Ma-
  ternal Welfare, 590, 592
American Congress of Obstetrics and Gynecology, 590
American Gynecological Society, 591
American Home Economics Association, information on nutrition, 151
American Hospital Association,
  recommendations, identification of newborn infant, 282-
  283

613

American Medical Association, endorsement of family planning, 341

information on nutrition, 151

American Public Health Association, *The Control of Communicable Disease in Man*, 564

endorsement of family planning, 341

information on nutrition, 151

American Red Cross, classes in preparation for parenthood, 171

Ammonium chloride therapy, preeclampsia, 448

Amnesia, narcotic, in obstetrics, 228-229

barbiturates, 229

meperidine hydrochloride (Demerol), 226, 229

paraldehyde, 229

scopolamine, 226, 228-229

Amnion, 77, 78

Amniotic fluid, embolism, as complication of labor, 497

evaluation, in erythroblastosis fetalis, 549

Amobarbital sodium (Amytal Sodium), as analgesic agent in obstetrics, 229

therapy, eclampsia, 452

hyperemesis gravidarum, 471

Amputees, child, clinic for, 545

Amytal Sodium (amobarbital sodium), as analgesic agent in obstetrics, 229

therapy, eclampsia, 452

hyperemesis gravidarum, 471

Analgesia, in labor, first (dilating) stage, 259-260

obstetric, 226, 228-230

amnesia, narcotic, 228-229

barbiturates, 229

meperidine hydrochloride (Demerol), 226, 229

paraldehyde, 229

scopolamine, 226, 228-229

inhalation, 229-230

paracervical block, 230

"twilight sleep," 228

Anatomy, related to reproductive system. *See individual anatomic parts*

Anesthesia, forceps delivery, 428

in labor, normal, second (expulsion) stage, 266

obstetric, 226, 230-239

inhalation, 233-238

gas anesthetics, 237-238

cyclopropane, 226, 229, 238, 239

nitrous oxide, 226, 229, 237

volatile anesthetics, 233-237

chloroform, 226, 229, 233, 236-237

ether, 226, 233-236

trichlorethylene (Trilene), 233, 237

intravenous, 238-239

thiopental sodium (Pentothal Sodium), 226, 238-239

regional, 230-233

continuous caudal, 231-233

possible complications, 232-233

local infiltration, 230-231

pudendal block, 231

spinal, 233

hyperbaric, low-dosage (saddle block), 233

saddle block, 233

Aneuploidy, 68

Anomalies, congenital. *See* Congenital malformations

Anoxia, asphyxia neonatorum from, 527

Antepartal care, 131-189

discomforts, 163-170

backache, 165-166

constipation, 165

cramps, 168, 169

diarrhea, 165

dyspnea, 166

edema, 166, 169, 170

flatulence, 165

heartburn, 164-165

hemorrhoids, 169

nausea, 163-164

urination, frequency, 163

vaginal discharge, 170

Antepartal care, discomforts—(*Cont.*)

varicose veins, 166-169

symptoms, 166

treatment, 166-169

vomiting, 163-164

hygiene (general), 153-163

bowel habits, 160-161

breast care, 157-158

clothing, 159-160

dental care, 160, 161

diversion, 156

douches, 161-162

employment, 154-156

standards recommended by Children's Bureau, 155-156

exercise, 154

marital relations, 162-163

rest, relaxation and sleep, 153-154

skin care, 157

smoking, 163

traveling, 156-157

medical, 132-137

danger signals to be reported to physician, 137

examination, general, 134

laboratory tests, 134-135

obstetric, 134

history of patient, 133-134

instructions to patients, 137

return visits, 136

weight, 132, 135-136

nursing, 137-145

community settings, 142-143

comprehensive antepartal care, 143

home visits, 142-143

public health nurse serving in an agency, 142

medical social workers, 143, 145

office and clinic settings, 138-142

examination, physical, 136, 139-141

cervix, 140-141

pelvis, 140-141

family relationships, 141-142

problem of limited time, 138

Antepartal care, nursing, office and clinic settings—(*Cont.*)
  teaching the patient, 138-139
    group approach, 139
    referrals, 139
    visual aids, 139
  nutrition in pregnancy, 144-153
    bread and cereals, 149
    fluids, 149
    information, 151
    minerals, 150-151
    planning diet, balance, 146-151
      counseling and planning sessions, 144, 146
      religious, racial and ethnic background of patient and family, 146
      psychological aspects, 146-147
    dairy foods, 148
    general factors, 145-146
    meats, 148-149
    salt, restriction, 145-146
    vegetables and fruits, 149
    vitamins, 150
    weight control, 151-153
  pioneer efforts, 13-14
  plans for after-care of mother and baby, 188-189
  return to employment, 188-189
  preparation(s), for baby, 185-188
    layette, 184-186
    nursery equipment, 186-188
    for parenthood, 170-174
    classes, 171
    conventional type of program, 171-172
    natural childbirth, 172-174
    psychoprophylactic childbirth, 174
    psychophysical, for childbearing, 174-185
      avoidance of stress, 175-183
      activity, 176-177
      relaxation, general, 175-176

Antepartal care, preparation, psychophysical, for childbearing—(*Cont.*)
      neuromuscular control, 178-183
        muscles of trunk and pelvic floor, 178-180
        relaxation, of rest of body during uterine contraction, 180-181
        selective, 180
      respiration, 180-183
      accelerated breathing, application to labor, 182-183
      panting, 183
      for second stage of delivery, 182, 183
      shallow breathing, 181-183
      slow breathing, application to labor, 181-182
      transition breathing, 182, 183
    postpartum restoration, 183-185
    relief of common minor discomforts, 177-178
  prevention, of calamities, 131-132
  of maternal mortality, 13
  in United States, background and development, 587-592
Antibiotics, therapy, infection, puerperal, 507
Antisepsis, in labor, normal, second (expulsion) stage, 265
Anuria, in eclampsia, 450
Anus, anatomy, 50
  imperforate, 543
  muscles, 50
  patulous and everted, in labor, second stage, 218, 219
Anxiety, allaying by nurse in postpartal hemorrhage, 495
Aorta, 45
Apgar Scoring System of condition of newborn infant, 279-280
Apresoline Hydrochloride (hydralazine hydrochloride) therapy, eclampsia, 452

Aquamephyton (phytonadione solution), for hypothrombinemia prophylaxis, 282
Arachnodactyly, 546
Areola, 46, 51
Arm, paralysis, in newborn, 535
Artery(ies), fallopian tubes, 44, 45
  hemorrhoidal, median, 50
  hypogastric, 45
  iliac, 45
  intercostal, 50
  mammary, internal, 50
  ovaries, 43, 45, 47
  pudic, internal, 50
  renal, 45
  spermatic, internal, 51
  testes, 51
  uterine, 45, 47, 50
  vagina, 50
  vesical, inferior, 50
Aschheim-Zondek test of pregnancy, 118, 125-126
Asepsis in labor, normal, second (expulsion) stage, 265
Asphyxia neonatorum, 527-531
  causes, 527
  prevention, 527-528
  treatment, 528-531
    artificial respiration, 529-531
    closed-chest massage, 530-531
    equipment, 528
    gentleness, 529
    observation, continued, 531
    posture, 529
    removal of mucus, 529
    warmth, 529
Association for Improving the Conditions of the Poor, New York City, 13, 588
Association of Infant Milk Stations, 589
Atelectasis, 531-532
Atresia, of esophagus, in newborn infant, 542
Aureomycin (chlortetracycline) therapy, brucellosis, 476
Auscultation, in diagnosis of fetal position, 100-101

Babies' Welfare Association, 589
Baby, preparations for birth, 185-188
  layette, 184-186

Baby, preparations for birth—
  (*Cont.*)
    nursery equipment, 186-188
  See also Newborn infant
Baby-health stations, munici-
  pal, first organized, 589
Bacillus, colon, as causitive
  agent, puerperal infection,
  503
  Welch, as causitive agent,
    puerperal infection, 503
Bacitracin therapy, impetigo,
  in newborn infant, 537
Backache, antepartal, 165-166
  treatment, 177-178
Baker, Josephine, 588
Ballottement as indication of
  pregnancy, 125
Bandage, Ace, for varicosities
  or edema of legs, 167
  elastic, for varicose veins in
    leg, 167-168
Baptism of infant, postpartal,
  283-284
Barbiturates, as analgesic agents
  in obstetrics, 229
  therapy, eclampsia, 452
    uterine dysfunction, hyper-
      tonic, 484
Bartholin's glands, 40, 41
Barr, M. L., 72
Bassinet infant Kreiselman resuscitator, 263, 265
Bath(s) and bathing, of newborn infant, 374-375, 380-
  381
    basic principles, 380-381,
      384
    concern of mother about,
      394
    demonstration by nurse,
      337, 381
  in puerperium, 314-315
Baudelocque, invention of pelvimeter, 584
Beck, A. C., 430
Bed for delivery in home, preparation, 564
Behavior and physiologic re-
  sponses of newborn infant,
  373-374
Bergh, Henry, founder of Society for the Prevention of
  Cruelty to Animals, 587
Bibring, Grete, 401
Binder, for breast support, in
  mastitis, 511
  in puerperium, 317-318

Birth(s), certificate, 10, 11
  injuries, death from, 16
  live, percentage distribution
    color, U. S. (1963), 14, 15
    United States (1930-63),
      10-12
  rate, definition, 9
  registration, as legal respon-
    sibility, 11
  time, exact, recording, 268
Birth Registration Area, established as Federal Act, 589
Bladder, anatomy, 50
  complications, in puerperium,
    513-514
  distention, in labor, first (di-
    lating) stage, 258-259
  dystocia, in labor, first (di-
    lating) stage, 258
Blakely, P. L., quoted, 284
Blood, cells, white, count in
  newborn infant, 354
  changes in pregnancy, nor-
    mal, 116-117
  in puerperium, 300
  coagulation, in newborn in-
    fant, 354
  groups, 466-467
  pressure, measurement, in
    antepartal care, 133,
    134
    in hemorrhage, postpar-
      tal, 495-496
    in labor, first (dilating)
      stage, 258
    newborn infant, 354
  Rh factor, 467-469
    considerations in preg-
      nancy, 468-469
    development of antibodies
      against, 467
    differences in mates, 468,
      469
    effect, 469
    iso-immunization, 468, 469
    transfusions, 467-468
  tests, syphilis, 478
  transfusion, intra-uterine fe-
    tal, in erythroblastosis fe-
    talis, 549
    as therapy, peritonitis, 507
  types, incompatibility, ABO,
    550
  volume, total, of newborn in-
    fant, 353
"Blues," postpartal, 310-311
Body of newborn infant, appearance, 361

Bolt, Richard, 588
Bones, cranium (skull), 92-93
  innominate, 21-23
  pelvis, 21
Boyd, J. D., 68
Brain, hemorrhage, of newborn,
  533-535
  injury, asphyxia neonatorum
    from, 527
Brassière for breast support, in
  mastitis, 511
  maternity, 159
  in puerperium, 317-318
Braxton Hicks, contractions, as
  probable sign of preg-
  nancy, 125
  as prelude to labor, 242-243
  version, 429
Bread in diet, antepartal care,
  149
Breast(s), care, antepartal, 157-
  158
  changes, in pregnancy, nor-
    mal, 116
    as presumptive sign of
      pregnancy, 122
  disorders, in puerperium, 509-
    513
    abscess, epidemic, 511-
      513
        symptoms, 512
        treatment and care,
          512-513
    drying up, 299, 318, 509
    engorgement, 299, 509
    mastitis, 510-511
    nipples, abnormalities,
      510
    secretion abnormalities,
      509-510
  engorgement, in newborn in-
    fant, 364, 365
  in puerperium, 299, 509
  exercises, in breast-feeding
    period, 335
  feeding. *See* Feeding of new-
    born infant, breast
  milk, variation in quality and
    quantity, 299-300
  nursing care, in puerperium,
    317-319
    cleansing, 317
    drying up milk, 318, 509
    support, 317-318
  in puerperium, anatomic
    changes, 299-300
  shield, 326, 327

Breasts—(*Cont.*)
support, maternity brassière, 159
See also Glands, mammary
Breckinridge, Mary, 571, 591
Bruce, S. J., quoted, 5
Brucellosis (undulant fever, Malta fever), with pregnancy, 475-476
"Bubbling" of infant during feeding, 358, 392
Bulletin of Maternal and Child Health, 590
Buttocks, nursing care, continuing, 380-382
Byrthe of Mankyinde, first English text on obstetrics, 583

Calcium in diet in antepartal period, 144, 150
Caldwell, W. E., 28-30
Calories, requirements of newborn infant, 355
Candida albicans as etiologic agent, moniliasis, in pregnancy, 170
thrush, in newborn infant, 537
Cannell, Douglas E., 581
Cap of nurse, adjusting and wearing, correct and incorrect methods, 264, 265
Caplan, Gerald, 402, 415
Caput succedaneum, 532-533
Carter, P. J., 89
Catheterization, bladder, in forceps delivery, 428
in labor, first (dilating) stage, 259
second (expulsion) stage, 266-267
in puerperium, 316
Cells, acini, 50
Celsus, 582
Cephalhematoma, 533
Cereals in diet, antepartal care, 149
Cervix, changes, in pregnancy, normal, 112-114
"mucous plug," 113-115
"show," 113
as probable sign of pregnancy, 125
dilatation, aid for visualization, 610-611
in labor, first stage, 214, 217, 218

Cervix—(*Cont.*)
examination, in antepartal care, 140, 141
lacerations, as cause of postpartal hemorrhage, 494
normal, nonpregnant, 115
os, incompetent, 460-461
in primigravida, 216
in puerperium, anatomic changes, 298
Cesarean section. *See* Operative obstetrics, cesarean section
Chadwick, sign of, 114
Chamberlen, Hugh, 584
Chamberlen, Peter, invention of obstetric forceps, 584
Channing, Walter, 226
Cheeks, of newborn infant, 361
sucking pads, 358
Child Health Stations, 589
Childbirth, mental hygiene. *See* Mental hygiene of pregnancy and childbirth
natural, preparation of parents, 172-174
preparation, psychophysical. *See* Antepartal care, preparation, psychophysical, for childbearing
psychoprophylactic, 174
Children's Bureau, Standards for Maternity Care and Employment of Mothers in Industry, 155-156
Children's Charter, adoption, 591
Children's Health Service of New York, 587
Children's Welfare Federation, New York City, 589
Chloasma ("mask of pregnancy"), 117
Chloral hydrate therapy, eclampsia, 452
Chloroform as agent in inhalation anesthesia in obstetrics, 226, 229, 233, 236-237
administration, 236-237
analgesia á la reine, 230, 236
possible dangers, 237
Chloroprocaine hydrochloride (Nesacaine) as agent in continuous anesthesia in obstetrics, 232
Chlorothiazide (Diuril) therapy, preeclampsia, 448
Chlorotrianisene (Tace), 58

Chlortetracycline (Aureomycin) therapy, brucellosis, 476
Choate, Mabel, 590
Chorion, 77, 78
frondosum (leafy), 78
laeve (bald), 78
villi, 74, 75, 78
Chorioncarcinoma as complication of hydatidiform mole, 463
Chorionic gonadotropin hormone, 118
Chromatin, sex, 72, 73
Chromosomes, 64-68
aberrations, 67-68
determination of sex, 69, 72, 73
form and size, 65
karyotypes, 65, 66
malformations, 67
number, 64-65, 69
variation in preparation for reproduction, 67
"polar bodies," 65
possible combinations, 67
X, 64, 69, 72-73
Y, 64, 69, 72-73
Circulation, change at birth, 88, 89
fetal, 87, 88
newborn infant, changes. *See* Newborn infant, physiology, changes, circulatory
path after birth, 88, 90
peripheral, of newborn infant, 353
placental, 87
Circumcision, postoperative nursing care, 376-377
inspection for bleeding, 364
preparation, 362, 364
technic, 362-364
Clamp(s), umbilical, 268, 269, 272
Cleft lip, 540
Cleveland Health Museum, 591
Clitoris, 39-41
Clothing, antepartal period, 159-160
Coccyx, 21-24
Coitus. *See* Intercourse, sexual
Colimycin therapy, epidemic diarrhea of newborn, 538
Color, as basis of classification of births in U. S., 9
of newborn infant, Apgar Scoring System, 279, 280
observation, 374

Colostrum, 116
  appearance, 324
  in puerperium, 299
Coma in eclampsia, 450
Committee on Infant Social Service of the Women's Municipal League, Boston, 13, 15
Common cold, with pregnancy, 475
Community Service Society, 588
Community services for antepartal care, 142-143
  public health nurse, 142
  home visits, 142-143
Conference on Better Care for Mothers and Babies, 591
Confinement. *See* Labor
Congenital malformations, death from, 16
Constipation, antepartal, 161, 165
Contractions, Braxton Hicks, as prelude to labor, 242-243
Convulsions, in eclampsia, 450-451, 452-454
  in hemorrhage, intracranial, in newborn, 534
Cooke, W. R., 455
Coombs test, erythroblastosis fetalis, 549
Cooper Bill, passage, 590
Corbin, Hazel, 174
Cord, umbilical. *See* Umbilical cord
Corner, G. W., Sr., 73
Corpus, albicans, 55
  luteum, changes in ovulation and menstruation, 55
    secretion of progesterone, 55, 56
Cramps, muscular, in legs, antepartal, 168
Cranium (skull), bones, 92-93
Crying by newborn infant, 379
  concern of mother about, 394
  initiation after delivery, 277-278
Crawford, Mary I., 572
Cul-de-sac of Douglas, 42, 44, 45
Curette, sharp, of Sims, 458
Cyanosis in hemorrhage, intracranial, in newborn, 534
Cyclopropane as agent in inhalation anesthesia in obstetrics, 226, 229, 238, 239

Cystocele from lacerations of perineum, 497

Dairy foods in diet, antepartal care, 148
Daniels, Maria L., 587
Death(s), classification, by WHO Manual of International Classification of Diseases, injuries and Causes of Death, 9
  maternal, from abortion, United States (1963), 444
    disorders associated with pregnancy, United States (1963), 444
    from ectopic pregnancy, 462
    from puerperal infection, 503
  neonatal, from disorders, United States (1963), 444
    from prematurity, causes, 407
    reactions of parents and staff, 526
  rate, fetal ("stillbirth") definition, 9
    neonatal, definition, 9
  See also Mortality
Decidua, 75, 77
  basalis (serotina), 75, 77, 78
  capsularis (reflexa), 75, 77, 78
  vera, 75, 77, 78
Dehydration in hyperemesis gravidarum, 471
Deladumone therapy in puerperium, drying up breasts, 318
Delalutin (progesterone), 58
Delestrogen (estrogen), 58
Delirium in hyperemesis gravidarum, 472
Delivery in home, 561-569
  preparations, 561-565
    bed, 564
    room, 563-564, 566
    special equipment, 564-565
    supplies for mother, 561-563
Demerol Hydrochloride (meperidine hydrochloride), as analgesic agent in obstetrics, 226, 229

Demerol Hydrochloride— (*Cont.*)
  therapy, incompetent cervical os, 460-461
DeNormandie, Robert L., 588
Deutsch, Helene, 402
  quoted, 192
Diabetes mellitus, mother, infant of, 551-552
  with pregnancy, 474
Diamox (acetazolamide) therapy, preeclampsia, 448
Diaphragm, urogenital, 41-42
Diarrhea, antepartal, 165
  epidemic, of newborn, 538
Dickinson-Belskie models, 212-214, 217, 219, 223, 591
Dicumarol therapy, embolism, pulmonary, 514
  thrombophlebitis, 506
Diet, balanced, in antepartal care. *See* Antepartal care, nutrition, diet, balance
  iron-rich, for anemia, 473
  in lactation, 313
  low sodium, in preeclampsia, 447, 448
  mother, in breast-feeding period, 333-334
  in pregnancy, planning, general factors, 145-146
    salt restriction, 145-146
Diethylstilbestrol, 58
  therapy, in puerperium, drying up breasts, 318
Digestion, changes in pregnancy, normal, 117
  of newborn infant, changes, 358-359
  in puerperium, 301
Dilator, Goodell-Ellinger, modified, 458
  Hegar, 459
"Disaster Insurance for Mothers and Babies," by Fetter, Whitridge and Welch, 576-580
Dislocations in newborn, 535-536
Diuresis, promotion of, in eclampsia, 453
Diuretics, therapy, preeclampsia, 448
Diuril (chlorothiazide) therapy, preeclampsia, 448
Division of Child Hygiene, New York City, first in United States, 588

Douches, vaginal, in antepartal period, 161-162
vinegar, therapy, leukorrhea, 170
Douglas, cul-de-sac. *See* Cul-de-sac of Douglas
Down's syndrome (mongolism), 67, 543-544
Draping, in labor, normal, second (expulsion) stage, 266, 267
Drug, addiction, in newborn, 551
excretion in milk of mother, possible harmful effects to infant, 334
Dublin, Louis I., 590
Duct, ejaculatory, 52
Ductus, deferens, 51
venosus, 88, 89
Duncan, mechanism of extrusion of placenta, 221, 224
Duodenum, obstruction, in newborn infant, 542
Dyk, R. B., 194
Dysfunction, uterine, types, hypotonic, treatment, 484-487
Dysmenorrhea, 59
Dyspnea, antepartal, 166
Dystocia, from bladder distention in labor, first (dilating) stage, 258
mechanical, 482-493
abnormal fetal positions, 485-491
breech presentations, 485-490
classification, complete, 489
footling, 485, 489
frank, 485, 489
delivery, 486-490
footling breech, 486-489
persistent occiput posterior, 487-489
transverse arrest, 488
shoulder, face and brow presentations, 490-491
disproportion, contracted pelvis, 491, 492
hydrocephalus, 493
oversize baby, 492-493
uterine dysfunction, 483-487
causes, 483
complications, 483
definition, 483

Dystocia, mechanical, uterine dysfunction—(*Cont.*)
types, hypertonic, 483-484
intrapartal infection, 484
treatment, 484
hypotonic, 484-487
explanations to parents, 484-485

Ears, and hearing, of newborn infant, 361
Eastman, N. J., 86, 119
Eclampsia, 445, 450-454
clinical picture, 450-451
coma, 450
stages, contraction, 450
convulsion, 450
invasion, 450
incidence, 450-451
prognosis, 451
treatment, 451-453
conservative, 451-452
nurse's responsibilities, 453-454
prevention, 451
promotion of diuresis, 453
protection, from extraneous stimuli, 453
from self-injury, 452-453
sedation, 452
Ectoderm, 74, 76, 77
Edema, in eclampsia, 450
lower extremities, antepartal period, 166, 169, 170
in preeclampsia, 446
Edgar, Clifton, 589
Edwards, W. B., 233
Eisenhower, Dwight D., 592
Elimination, intestinal, antepartal, habits, 160-161
newborn infant, nursing care, continuing, 383-384
in puerperium, 301, 316
urinary, newborn infant, nursing care, continuing, 384
in puerperium, 315-316
catheterization, 316
Embolism, amniotic fluid, as complication of labor, 497
pulmonary, in puerperium, 514
Embryo(s), growth, in early weeks of pregnancy, 79
twin, 73
Emergency Maternity and Infancy Care Program, 591

Emerson, Haven, 589
Employment, in antepartal period, 154-156
standards recommended by Children's Bureau, 155-156
return after birth of baby, 188-189
Endometritis, 505
Endometrium, 46
Enema, administration, at onset of labor, 248
Entoderm, 74, 76, 77
Epididymis, 51
Episiotomy, anesthesia, local infiltration, 230
and repair of lacerations, 286-288, 425
Epispadias, 541-542
Erb-Duchenne's paralysis in newborn, 535
Ergonovine therapy, endometritis, 505
hemorrhage, postpartal, 496
to increase uterine contractions and minimize bleeding, 273-276
Erysipelas with pregnancy, 476
Erythema toxicum, 362, 364
Erythroblastosis fetalis, 468-469, 548
Rh factor, 548-549
treatment, 549-550
Erythrocytes, count, newborn infant, 354
Escherichia coli as causative agent, epidemic diarrhea of newborn, 538
Esidrix (hydrochlorothiazide) therapy, preeclampsia, 448
Esophagus, atresia, in newborn infant, 542
Estrogen (Theelin, Delestrogen, Premarin), 58
therapy, menopausal disorders, 63
Ether as agent in inhalation anesthesia in obstetrics, 226, 233-236
administration, 234-236
stages of anesthesia, 236
Examination(s), in labor, 249-251
abdominal, 249
general, 249
rectal, 249-250
vaginal, 250-251

Examination(s)—(*Cont.*)
  medical, general, in pregnancy, 134
  obstetric, in antepartal care, 134
  physical, in antepartal care, 136, 139-141
    cervix, 140
    pelvis, 140-141
  in puerperium, 302
Exercise(s), in antepartal period, 154
  pelvic rocking, antepartal period, 176
  for posture, antepartal period, 176
Eyelids, edema, in preeclampsia, 446
Eyes, of newborn infant, nursing care, continuing, 375
  and visual perception, of newborn infant, 360-361

Face, and brow, presentation, as complication of labor, 490-491
  paralysis, in newborn, 535
Facies in preeclampsia, 446
Fallopian tubes, 42-45, 48
  arteries, 44, 45
  ligaments, in puerperium, anatomic changes, 299
  ligation, 455
  nerves, 44
  transport of ovum through, 68-71
  veins, 44, 45
Family(ies), expansion in America, 5-8
  living quarters, small, 6-7
  mobility of population, 6-7
  planning, 341-343
    methods, conventional, 342-343
      newer, 342
    need for, population explosion, 341
  relationships, in antepartal care, 141-142
  relatives, assistance in management of household during hospitalization of mother, 8
  size, average, 6
Fatigue as presumptive sign of pregnancy, 123

Fear of pregnancy and childbirth. *See* Mental hygiene of pregnancy and childbirth, attitude of mother, fear
Feces, expulsion, in labor, second (expulsion) stage, 267
  transfer of matter to vagina, as causative agent in puerperal infection, 504
Federal Bureau of Narcotics, 229
Feeding of newborn infant, 385-394
  ability of baby to handle food, 385-386
    stomach and intestines, 385-386
    sucking and swallowing reflexes, 385
  artificial, 383, 386-392
    assisting mother, 392-394
      environmental climate, 393
      expanding contacts with baby, 393
      insight into her goals and problems, 393-394
    bubbling, 392
    cow's, composition, 387
    nutrition, hunger, 391-392
      requirements, 387-389
        formula, aseptic method, 389-391
          bottles and nipples, 389, 390
          computation, 388-389
          directions for making, 389
          terminal sterilization, 390, 391
        nutrients, 387-388
    regurgitation, 392
  breast, 322-335
    advantages, 322
    attitudes of doctor and nurse, 322
    bubbling, 327-328
    complemental feedings, 329
    engorgement, 323-324
    expression of milk, 329-333
      electric-pump, 332-333
      hand-pump, 333
      manual, 330-332
    hygiene of mother, 333-334
    initiation, 324-328
      colostrum, 324
      orientation of infant, 326

Feeding of newborn infant, breast, initiation—(*Cont.*)
      sucking behavior of infant, 326-327
      support and supervision by nurse, 328
    length of nursing time, 327, 329
    making the decision, 322
    mechanisms in lactation, 322-323
      milk-ejection reflex, 323
      secretion of milk, 323
    nipples, care, 328-329
    position of mother and baby, 325-326
    schedule, 329
    weaning, 334-335
    See also Lactation
  concern of mother about, 394
  milk, human, composition, 386, 387
  nutrition, progress in scientific developments, 386
  premature, 413-414
  self-regulation, 396
  twins, 501
Ferrand, Livingston, 588
Ferrous sulfate therapy, anemia, 473
Fertility, rate, definition, 9
Fetter, Sara E., 576
Fetus, abnormal positions complicating labor, 485-491
  breech presentations, 485-490
    classification, complete, 489
    footling, 485, 489
    frank, 485, 489
    delivery, 486-490
      footling breech, 486-489
    persistent occiput posterior, 487-489
    transverse arrest, 488
  shoulder, face and brow presentations, 490-491
  amnion, 77, 78
  chorion, 77, 78
  circulation, 87, 88
    at birth, 88, 89
    path after birth, 88, 90
  decidua, 75, 77
  derivation of various parts of body by progressive differentiation and divergent specialization, 76

Fetus—(*Cont.*)
determination of sex, 69, 72, 73
development, month by month, 81-85
periods, 90
fertilization and changes following fertilization, 73-75
germ layers, 77
growth, in early weeks of pregnancy, 79
habitus, 92
head, 92-93
diameters, anteroposterior, 97
transverse, 96
implantation of ovum, 75
maternal impressions, 91
maturation of ovum and sperm cells, 64-69
chromosomes, 64-68
spermatozoa, 69
transport of ovum through fallopian tube, 68-71
movements, felt by examiner, as positive sign of pregnancy, 129
nutrition, 86-88
outline, by palpation of abdomen, as probable sign of pregnancy, 124
physiology, 86-90
placenta, 78, 80-81
transmission, 86-88
pregnancy, calculation of expected date of confinement, 86
duration, 85-86
size and position in pelvis at various months, 81-83, 112-114
Fever, in eclampsia, 450
childbed. *See* Infection, puerperal
in hyperemesis gravidarum, 472
Malta (brucellosis), with pregnancy, 475-476
puerperal. *See* Infection, puerperal
scarlet, with pregnancy, 476
transitory, of newborn, 355-356
typhoid, with pregnancy, 475
undulant (brucellosis), with pregnancy, 475-476
Fibroplasia, retrolental, in newborn infant, 551

Flatulence, antepartal, 165
Floraquin therapy, trichomoniasis, 170
Fluids, administration, in hyperemesis gravidarum, 471
in diet, antepartal care, 149
intake, in labor, first (dilating) stage, 258
requirements, of newborn infant, 355-356
Fontanels, 92-93
Food, intake, in labor, first (dilating) stage, 258
Food and Nutrition Board, National Research Council, information on nutrition, 151
recommended dietary allowances, in lactation, 313
during pregnancy and lactation, 144, 145
minerals, 144, 150
vitamins, 144, 150
Foramen, ovale, 88, 89
Forceps, bullet, 458
obstetric, delivery, indications, 425, 426
technic, 427-428
types of operations, 427
invention, 584
types, 425-426
placental, 458
Foreskin, adherent, nursing care, continuing, 376
Formula in artificial feeding of newborn infant, computation, 388-389
directions for making, 389
requirements, aseptic methods, 389-390
bottles and nipples, 389, 390
nutrients, 387-388
terminal sterilization, 390, 391
Fornix(ces), 47
Fourchet, 39, 40
Fractures in newborn, 535-536
Frank-Berman test of pregnancy, 126
Fred Lyman Adair Foundation of American Committee on Maternal Welfare, 592
Frenulum (frenum) of clitoris, 39, 40
Frenum linguae, 541
Frère, 583

Friedman, E. A., 215, 216
Friedman, M. H., 126
Friedman test of pregnancy, 118, 126
Frog test, male, of pregnancy, 126
Frontier Graduate School of Midwifery, Hayden, Ky., 571
Frontier Nursing Service, 570, 571
organization, 591
Fruits in diet, antepartal care, 149
Funis. *See* Umbilical cord

Galactorrhea, 510
Galactosemia, 546
Gametogenesis, 65
Gantrisin therapy, puerperal infection, 507
Gargoylism, 545
Garters, antepartal period, 159-160
Gastrointestinal system, of newborn, changes, 358-359
Gaucher's disease, 546
Gebhard, Bruno, 591
Genes, 67
Gentian violet therapy, impetigo, in newborn infant, 537
German measles (rubella), as cause of malformations in newborn infant, 545
with pregnancy, 475
Gilbert, M. S., 69
Girdle, maternity, 159
Gland(s), Bartholin's, 40, 41
bulbo-urethral, 52
Cowper's, 52
mammary, 46, 50-51
structure, external, 46, 51
internal, 46, 50-51
mammary. *See also* Breasts
prostate, 49, 52
Skene's, 40, 41, 50
gonorrhea, 50
Glucose, administration, in hyperemesis gravidarum, 471
Gonorrhea, in pregnancy, 479
Skene's glands, involvement, 50
Goodell, sign of, as indication of pregnancy, 125
Goodell-Ellinger dilator, modified, 458
Goodrich, Annie W., 590
Goodrich, F. W., Jr., 172

Graafian follicle, 54-55, 57
Greisheimer, E. M., 65, 74, 75
Group teaching and counseling, in antepartal care, 139

Hall, E. J., quoted, 5
Ham, A. W., 72
  quoted, 67
Hamilton, W. J., 68
Harelip, 540
Harrison Act, 229
Harvie, John, 584
Hayden, C. T., 30
Head of infant, birth of, 267-269
  emergency (precipitate) delivery by nurse, 284-285
  fetal. *See* Fetus, head
  newborn, appearance, 360
Health, maternal, and child, concept, 5
    nursing, interpretations, 5
    programs, development in State Departments of Health, 15
  services, costs, increased, as problem in maternity care, 17
Heart, beat, rate, of newborn infant, Apgar Scoring System, 279
  changes in pregnancy, normal, 117
  fetal, sound, as sign of pregnancy, 127
  tones, of fetus, in labor, first (dilating) stage, 256-257
Heartburn, antepartal, 164-165
Hegar, dilator, 459
  sign of, as indication of pregnancy, 124
Hellman, Louis M., 119, 573
Hematoma(s), vulvar, as complication of puerperium, 508-509
Hemoglobin, concentration, in newborn infant, 354
  test, in antepartal care, 134
Hemolytic disease of newborn, 547-550
  due to Rh incompatibility, 547-550
    erythroblastosis fetalis, 548
    hydrops fetalis as manifestation, 548
    jaundice as sign, 547-548
    kernicterus as sign, 548
  treatment, 549-550

Hemorrhage, cerebral, of newborn, 533-535
  in childbirth, death from, 13
  complications, 455-456
    abortion. *See* Abortion
    abruptio placentae, 465-466
    ectopic pregnancy. *See* Pregnancy, ectopic
    hydatidiform mole, 463
    incompetent cervical os, 460-461
    placenta previa, 463-465
    supine hypotensive syndrome, 466
  concealed, in abruptio placentae, 465
  diagnosis, mistaken, 466
  external, in abruptio placentae, 465
  intracranial, in newborn, 533-535
    in newborn, signs, 534
    treatment, 534-535
  maternal mortality from, 13
  in placenta previa, 464
  postpartal, clinical picture, 494
    as complication of labor, 493-497
      causes, 493-494
      definition, 493
      incidence, 493
      predisposing factors, 494
    late, 496
    treatment, 494-496
  puerperal. *See* Hemorrhage, postpartal
  in retina, in hyperemesis gravidarum, 472
  from umbilical cord, 550-551
Hemorrhagic disease, neonatal, preventive measure, 282
Hemorrhoids, antepartal period, 169
Hendricks, C. H., 87
Heparin therapy, thrombophlebitis, 506
Heredity, as causative factor, twin pregnancy, 500
Hernia, umbilical, in newborn infant, 542
Hesseltine umbilical clamp, 269, 272, 352
Hexachlorophene (pHisoHex) therapy, impetigo, in newborn infant, 537
Hingson, R. A., 233

Hippocrates, 582
History of obstetrics, 581-592
  Byzantine period, 582-583
  Egyptian period, 581
  Grecian period, 582
  Jewish period, 582-583
  medieval period, 582-583
  Mohammedan period, 582-583
  oriental, Chinese, 582
    Hindu, 582
  primitive peoples, 581
  Renaissance period, 583
  17th century, 583-584
  18th century, 584-585
  19th century, 585-587
  20th century, 587
History of patient, in antepartal care, 133-134
Hogben test of pregnancy, 126
Holmes, Oliver Wendell, "Puerperal Fever as a Private Pestilence," quoted, 585
Holt, L. Emmet, 588
Home, antepartal care, visits of public health nurse, 142-143
  supervision of family health by public health nurse, during antepartal care, 143
Hoover, Herbert, 588, 591
Hormone(s), chorionic gonadotropin, 118
  control of menstruation, 56-58
  estrogen, 58
  follicle-stimulating (FSH), 57, 58
  lactogenic (mammogenic), 119
  suppression in puerperium, 318
  luteinizing (LH), 57, 58
  luteotrophin (LTH), 58, 119
  mammogenic (lactogenic), 119
  oxytocin, 58
  progesterone, 58
  prolactin, 58, 119
Hospital, admission, procedures, knowledge of, before onset of labor, 243
    at onset of labor, 246
Hospitalization, for childbirth, trend toward, 14, 15
Hunger, newborn infant, 391-392
Hunter, William, 584

Hurler's disease, 545

Husband, accompaniment of wife on visits to obstetrician, 6

participation in care and emotional support of wife, in labor, 252

presence with wife during labor, 6

Hyaline membrane disease of newborn, 532

Hydatidiform mole, 462, 463

Hydralazine hydrochloride (Apresoline Hydrochloride) therapy, eclampsia, 452

Hydrocephalus, as complication of labor, 493

Hydrochlorothiazide (Esidrix) therapy, preeclampsia, 448

Hydrops fetalis, in hemolytic disease of newborn, due to Rh incompatibility, 548

Hygiene, general, in antepartal period. *See* Antepartal care, hygiene (general)

Hymen, 39, 41

Hyperbilirubinemia, of newborn, 550

Hyperemesis gravidarum ("morning sickness"), 163-164, 469-472

cause, 470

clinical picture, 470-471

neurotic factor, 470

treatment and nursing care, 471-472

Hypertension, essential. *See* Hypertensive vascular disease, chronic

in preeclampsia, 446, 447

vascular disease, chronic, 445, 454-455

Hypofibrinogenemia, 457, 466

Hypospadias, 541-542

Hypotension, material, as possible complication in continuous caudal anesthesia, 232-233

Hypothrombinemia prophylaxis, newborn infant, 282

Hypoxia, fetal, as disadvantage in intravenous anesthesia, thiopental sodium as agent, 239

Hysterectomy, 431

Icterus neonatorum, 361-362

Identification, infant, newborn, 282-283

Ilium, 21-23

Impetigo, contagiosa, 537

in newborn infant, 537

Incubator, air-conditioned, 412-413

Armstrong Universal, 409

homemade, 412

Isolette, 408

portable, 410

Infant, care, postpartal, immediate, 277-284

appraisal, 279-280

Apgar Scoring System, 279-280

baptism, 283-284

clearing upper respiratory passage, 277, 278

eyes, 280-282

silver nitrate instillation, 280-282

hypoprothrombinemia prophylaxis, 282

identification methods, 282-283

initiation of crying, 277-278

observation by nurse at frequent intervals, 283

placement in heated crib or resuscitator, 278

suctioning, 278, 279

umbilical cord, 280, 282

full-term, 456

immature, 456

Infant Milk Station, New York, first in United States, 588

Infection(s), in newborn infant, 536-539

conjunctivitis, gonorrheal, 536-537

ophthalmia neonatorum, 536-537

in placenta previa, 464, 465

prevention, in newborn infant, 365-366, 371-372

puerperal, 503-508

causative factors, 503-504

death in childbearing from, 13, 503

prevention, 13, 504-505

summary of observations by Oliver Wendell Holmes, 585

signs and symptoms, 507

treatment, 507-508

Infection(s), puerperal— (*Cont.*)

types, 505-507

endometritis, 505

lesions of perineum, vulva and vagina, 505

pelvic cellulitis or parametritis, 507

peritonitis, 506-507

thrombophlebitis, 505-506

staphylococcal, in newborn, 539

Infertility, 62

Influenza with pregnancy, 475

Injection, intramuscular, of newborn infant, 378

Instructive Nursing Association, initiation of antepartal care, 13

Instruments, table, delivery room, preparation, 262, 265

Intercourse, sexual, in antepartal period, 162

coitus interruptus, 343

in pregnancy, late, puerperal infection from, 504

International Confederation of Midwives, 573

Intestine(s), newborn infant, ability to handle food, 385-386

changes, 358

small, obstruction, in newborn infant, 543

Intussusception in newborn infant, 543

Iodine, in diet, antepartal period, 150-151

protein-bound (PBI), increase in pregnancy, 119

Iron in diet, antepartal period, 144, 150

Ischium, 21-23

Jackson, Edith, quoted, 372

Jaundice, in hemolytic disease of newborn, due to Rh incompatibility, 547-548

in hyperemesis gravidarum, 472

physiologic, in newborn infant, 354

Joint Committee on Maternal Welfare, 507, 591

Kahn test for syphilis, 478

Kane umbilical clamp, 269, 272

Kelly umbilical clamp, 268, 271

Kernicterus, in hemolytic disease of newborn, due to Rh incompatibility, 548
Kidneys, function, of newborn infant, changes, 359
urine, secretion, in puerperium, 301
Kielland obstetric forceps, 426
Kipp, Gertrude B., 588
Klein, H. R., 194
Kline test, for syphilis, 478
Klinefelter's syndrome, 68
Knox, J. H. Mason, 588
Kreiselman infant resuscitator, 432

Labium (labia), majora, 39, 40
in puerperium, anatomic changes, 299
minora, 39, 40
in puerperium, anatomic changes, 299
Labor, attitude of mother toward, 197-198
calculation of expected date, 86
complications, 482-501
accidental, 497-498
inversion of uterus, 498
lacerations of perineum, 497-498
prolapse of umbilical cord, 497, 498
amniotic fluid embolism, 496
dystocia, mechanical. *See* Dystocia, mechanical
hemorrhagic, 493-497
postpartal, 493-496
causes, 493-494
clinical picture, 494
definition, 493
incidence, 493
late, 496
predisposing factors, 494
treatment, 494-496
rupture of uterus, 496-497
multiple pregnancy, 499-501
definition, 211
false, 211, 213
vs. true, differential factors, 243
induction, artificial rupture of membranes, 436
medicinal, 434-436

Labor, induction, medicinal— (*Cont.*)
oxytocin, 435-436
mechanism, first description, by Ould, of Dublin, 584
normal, conduct of, 241-288
care of infant, immediate. *See* Infant, care, postpartal, immediate
emergency (precipitate) delivery by nurse, 284-286
body delivery, 285
head delivery, 284-285
immediate care of infant, 285
placenta delivery, 286
precautions concerning cord, 285
rupture of membranes, 285
umbilical cord, care, 285-286
episiotomy and repair, 286-288
first (dilating) stage, 244-245, 251-261
analgesia, 259-260
bladder, 258-259
blood pressure, 258
contractions, uterine, 253-256
anticipation of pain, 254
interval and duration, 254-255
"unprepared" mother, 256
fluid and food intake, 258
heart tones of fetus, 256-257
progression of active phase, 253
pulse, 257-258
respiration, 257-258
show, 256
signs of second stage, 260-261
support, emotional and physical, 251-253
by husband, 252
temperature, 257-258
lacerations of birth canal, 285, 286
second (expulsion) stage, 245, 261-269

Labor, normal, conduct of, second (expulsion) stage—(*Cont.*)
"bearing down," 261-262
delivery, 264-269
anesthesia, 266
asepsis and antisepsis, 265
catheterization, 266-267
cord, clamping, 268-269, 271
cutting, 268, 271
tying, 268, 272
draping, 266, 267
head, 267-269
matter, escape from rectum, 267
positioning of patient, 266
Ritgen's maneuver, 267, 269
room, preparation, 262-265
instrument table, 262, 265
shoulder and body, 268, 270
transfer of mother to, 265-266
muscular cramps in legs, 265
recording exact time of birth, 268
signs, 260-261
transfer to delivery room, attendance by same nurse, 262-264
third (placental) stage, 245, 269-277
delivery of placenta. *See* Placenta, delivery
immediate postpartal care, 276-277
See also Labor, stages
continuing care, 247-249
enema, 248
preparation of vulva and perineum, 248-249
prior to examination by physician, 248
establishment of nurse-patient relationship, 246-247
awareness of physical and behavioral signs, 246

Labor, normal, establishment of nurse-patient relationship —(*Cont.*)
  encouragement, 246
  first impressions, 247
  orientation, 247
  rapport, 246-247
  examination, abdominal, 249
  general, 249
  rectal, 249-250
  vaginal, 250-251
  nursing care, dimensions, 241-242
  onset, 243, 244
  participation, of mother, guidelines, 244-245
  prelude, 242, 244
    preparations for hospitalization and absence from family, 243
  onset, 214-215
  "appearance of show," 113
  phenomena of, 211-224
  premature, definition, 456
  signs, premonitory, 211, 213-214
    "lightening," 211
    "show," 213-214
  rupture of membranes, 214
  stages, 216-224
    first, 214, 216-218, 222
      dilatation of cervix, 214, 217, 218
      effacement, 214, 218
    second (expulsion), 217-222
      anus, patulous and everted, 218, 219
      appearance of head, 219
      birth of "caul," 218
      "crowning," 219
      positional changes of head in passing through birth canal, descent, 220
      extension, 220, 221, 223
      flexion, 220-221
      restitution, 221-223
      rotation, external, 221-223
      internal, 220, 221
      rupture of membranes, 218
      straining of "bearing down," 218

Labor, stages, second (expulsion)—(*Cont.*)
    uterine contractions and intra-abdominal pressure, 215-216, 219-220
    third, 217, 222, 224
      placenta, expulsion, 221, 222, 224
        Duncan's mechanism, 221, 224
        Schultze's mechanism, 221, 224
      separation, 222, 224
    See also Labor, normal, conduct, first, second and third stages
  time factor, graphic appraisal, 215, 216
  true, vs. false, differential factors, 243
Lacerations, in delivery repair, 425
Lactation, diet, 313
  mechanisms, 322-323
    milk-ejection reflex, 323
    secretion of milk, 323
  postponement of conception, 343
Lactogenic (mammogenic) hormone, 119
Laryngospasm, maternal, as disadvantage in intravenous anesthesia, thiopental sodium as agent, 239
Lathrop, Julia, 589
Latsko, W., 431
Laxative(s), antepartal period, 161
Legs, cramps, antepartal period, 168, 169
Leopold maneuvers in diagnosis of fetal position, 99-100
Lesser, A. J., quoted, 17, 18
Leukorrhea in pregnancy, 170
Levallorphan (Lorfan) therapy, asphyxia neonatorum, 531
Levin tube in hyperemesis gravidarum, 471, 472
Lex Caesarius (Lex Regis), 583
Lidocaine (Xylocaine), as agent in continuous anesthesia in obstetrics, 232
Ligament(s), broad, 44, 46, 47
  cardinal, 44, 47
  mesovarian, 42
  ovarian, 42
  rectovaginal, 44

Ligament(s)—(*Cont.*)
  round, 42, 44-47
  sacrosciatic, 27
  suspensory, 42
  uterosacral, 42, 44, 46, 47
  uterus, 44, 46-47
    ovaries and fallopian tubes, in puerperium, anatomic changes, 299
"Lightening," 111, 114, 211, 242
Linea nigra, 117
Lip(s), cleft, 540-541
  of newborn infant, 361
Lipidosis, cerebroside, 546
  ganglioside, 546
  sphingomyelin, 546
Lithopedion formation, 457
Liver, function, of newborn, changes, 359
Lobenstein Midwifery Clinic, New York, 572
Lobenstine, Ralph W., 589, 590
Lochia, alba, rubra and serosa, in puerperium, 298
Lorfan (levallorphan) therapy, asphyxia neonatorum, 531
Luminal Sodium (phenobarbital sodium) therapy, eclampsia, 452
Lung(s), cancer, cigarette smoking as possible cause, 163
  complications, in puerperium, embolism, 514
Luteotrophin (LTH, prolactin, lactogenic or mammogenic hormone), 58, 119
  activity in puerperium, 299
Lymphatics, uterus, 47
  vagina, 50

Macintyre, M. N., 66, 80
Magnesium, citrate of, therapy, preeclampsia, 448
  sulfate therapy, eclampsia, 452
  preeclampsia, 448
Malaria with pregnancy, 476
Malformations, congenital. *See* Congenital malformations newborn. *See* Newborn, disorders, malformations
Malta fever (brucellosis), with pregnancy, 475-476
Mammogenic (lactogenic) hormone, 119
Marfan's syndrome, 546

Margaret Sanger Research Bureau, 591
Marital relations. *See* Intercourse, sexual
Marriage(s), age (average), bride, 6
    groom, 6
    rate, definition, 9
Maryland State Department of Health, Division of Public Health Nursing, equipment for nurse-midwife's delivery bag, 564-565
Massage, closed chest, for asphyxia neonatorum, 530-531
Massé Nipple Cream, application after nursing period, 328
Mastitis, 510-511
Maternal and Child Health and Mental Retardation Planning Amendments of 1963, enactment, 592
Maternity Center Association, New York, 571-573
    annual report, "Whither Nurse-Midwifery?" 572-573
    classes in preparation for parenthood, 171
    psychophysical preparation for childbearing, 174-175
Maternity Consultation Service, New York City, 591
Maternity nursing, current problems, 17-18
    definition, 4
    scope, 4-5
Maternity Service Association, organization, 590
Maturity, sexual, 53-55
    menstruation. *See* Menstruation
    ovulation, 53-55, 57
    puberty, 53
Mauriceau, of Paris, quoted, 583-584
Mayrhofer, 586
Mazzini test for syphilis, 478
Measles, German (rubella), as cause of malformations in newborn infant, 545
    with pregnancy, 475
Meats in diet, antepartal care, 148-149
Medical care, in pregnancy. *See* Antepartal care, medical
Meiosis, 67

Menarche, 58-59
Menopause (climacteric), 59, 62-63
    disorders, estrogen therapy, 63
Menstruation, 53-59
    clinical aspects, 58-59
    control by hormones, 56-58
        phases, menstrual, 57
            proliferative, 56, 57
            secretory, 56-57
        role of pituitary gland, anterior lobe, 57-58
            posterior lobe, 58
    corpus luteum changes, 55, 57
    cycle, 55-59
    disturbances, 59
    graafian follicle, 54-55, 57
    by newborn infant, 364
    normal, 59
    onset (menarche), 58-59
        average age, 58-59
    in puerperium, 301-302
    relation to pregnancy, 55-56
    suppression, as presumptive sign of pregnancy, 121-122
    temperature, basal, use of graphs, 61-62
        directions, 61
        plotting, 61
        variations, 59-60
        oral, 61-62
Mental hygiene of pregnancy and childbirth, 191-203
    attitude of mother, fear, for child, 193-194
        effect of, 196-197
        for herself, 192-193
        toward labor, 197-198
        toward newborn, 198-200
            open hostility and neglect, 199
            overprotection, 199-200
            perfectionism, 199
        toward her pregnancy, 192-197
            fear, 192-194
            rejection, 194-196
                effect of, 196-197
        contribution of nurse, 201-203
            guidance, 201-203
            listening, 201
            understanding, 201
    psychoses, 200
Meperidine hydrochloride (Demerol), as analgesic

Meperidine hydrochloride (Demerol)—(*Cont.*)
    agent in obstetrics, 226, 229
    therapy, incompetent cervical os, 460-461
Mesoderm, 74, 76, 77
Metabolism, basal, changes in newborn infant, 355-356
    errors, inborn, 545-547
Methergine, administration, to increase uterine contractions and minimize bleeding, 276
Metycaine as agent in anesthesia, caudal, in obstetrics, 232
    regional, local infiltration, 230
Micrococcus gonorrhoeae as causative agent of gonorrhea, 479
Micturition, frequency, as presumptive sign of pregnancy, 122
Midwifery, early history, 569-571
Midwives, International Confederation of, 573
    12th International Congress, Rome (1960), 569
Milia, 364
Milk, breast, variation in quality and quantity, 299-300
    cow's, composition, 387
    human, composition, 386, 397
    "witch's," 87
Milk-fever in puerperium, 300
Miscarriage, 456
Mitosis, 67
Moloy, H. C., 28-30
Mongolism (Down's syndrome), in newborn infant, 67, 543-544
Moniliasis, antepartal period, 170
Monoploidy, 68
Monosomy, 68
Mons veneris, 39, 40
Moore, K. L., 72
Morbidity, puerperal, definition, 507
"Morning sickness." *See* Hyperemesis gravidarum
Moro or startle reflex of newborn infant, 355-357, 360
Morphine, as analgesic agent in obstetrics, 228

Morphine—(*Cont.*)
  therapy, eclampsia, 451, 452
    embolism, pulmonary, 514
    preeclampsia, severe, 448
Mortality, infant, 15-17
    by age, United States
      (1963), 14
    causes, United States
      (1963), 16
    by color, 15
    definition, by WHO, 15
    perinatal, 15
    rate, definition, 9
    subgroups, by gestation
      age in weeks, 15-16
  maternal, 12-13, 15
    causes, 12-13
    by color, 12
    prevention, antepartal
      care, 13
      change in attitude of
        doctors, nurses and
        parents, 13
    rate, 12
      definition, 9
    reduction, factors, 13
  perinatal, definition, 9
  See also Death
Morton, D. G., 30
Morula, 72, 74
Mosaicism, 68
Mossman, H. W., 68
Mother, understanding of newborn infant, assessment, 373,
  375
Mother's Milk Bureau, 589
Mouth, gag, improvised, for
    prevention of tongue in-
    jury in eclampsia, 453
  of newborn infant, 361
Movements of newborn infant,
  360
Mucus, plug, in cervix in pregnancy, 113-115
Muscle(s), anus, 50
  bulbocavernosus, 41, 42
  coccygeus, 41
  control, antepartal. *See* An-
    tepartal care, psychophysi-
    cal preparation for child-
    bearing, neuromuscular
    control
  gluteus, 41
  iliococcygeus, 41, 42
  legs, cramps, antepartal pe-
    riod, 168, 169
    in labor, second (expul-
      sion) stage, 264

Muscle(s)—(*Cont.*)
  levator ani, 41, 42
  perineum, 41-42
  pubococcygeus, 41
  puborectalis, 42
  recti abdominis, diastasis, in
      pregnancy, 116
    in puerperium, 299
  sphincter ani, external, 41, 42
  tone, of newborn infant, Ap-
    gar Scoring System, 279,
    280
  transverse, superficial, of per-
    ineum, 41, 42
  uterus, changes in preg-
    nancy, 109-110
Mycostatin therapy, thrush, in
  newborn infant, 537

Nalline therapy, asphyxia neonatorum, 531
Nalorphine (N-allylnormorphine) therapy, asphyxia neonatorum, 531
Narcosis, asphyxia neonatorum
    from, 527
  fetal, as disadvantage in in-
    travenous anesthesia, thio-
    pental sodium as agent,
    238-239
Natality, 9, 11
  fluctuations, 9
  live births and population,
    United States (1930-63),
    10-12
  marriages, annual number,
    as factor, 11
  size and age composition of
    female population of child-
    bearing age as factor, 9, 11
  twins, frequency, 9
National Committee for Maternal Health, 591
National Society for the Prevention of Blindness, 589
Nausea, antepartal, 163-164
  in hyperemesis gravidarum,
    469-472
  in peritonitis, 507
  as presumptive sign of preg-
    nancy, 122
Neisseria gonorrhoeae as causi-
    tive agent, conjunctivitis,
    gonorrheal, 536-537
  gonorrhea, 479
Nelson, W. E., 387

Nembutal (pentobarbital so-
    dium), as analgesic agent, in
    obstetrics, 229
Neonatal, definition, 9
Neomycin, ointment, therapy,
    impetigo, in newborn in-
    fant, 537
  therapy, epidemic diarrhea
    of newborn, 538
Nerve(s), control, antepartal.
    See Antepartal care, psy-
    chophysical preparation for
    childbearing, neuromuscu-
    lar control
  fallopian tubes, 44
  ovaries, 43
  pudendal, block, in regional
    anesthesia, local infiltra-
    tion, 231
  testes, 51
  uterus, 47
Nervous system, changes in
    pregnancy, normal, 118
  of newborn infant, changes,
    reflexes. *See* Newborn in-
    fant, physiology, changes,
    neurologic, reflexes
Nesacaine (chloroprocaine hy-
    drochloride), as agent in
    continuous anesthesia in ob-
    stetrics, 232
New York City Department of
    Health, 573
New York Diet Kitchen Asso-
    ciation, 587
New York Milk Committee,
    588, 589
Newborn infant, attitude of
    mother toward, 198-200
  open hostility and neglect,
    199
  overprotection, 199-200
  perfectionism, 199
  characteristics, 359-364
    appearance, general, 359-
      361
      body and skin, 361
      ears and hearing, 361
      eyes and visual per-
        ception, 360-361
      head, 360
      lips, mouth and
        cheeks, 361
      position and move-
        ments, 360
    deviations from normal,
      breast engorgement,
      364, 365

Newborn infant, characteristics, deviations from normal—(*Cont.*)
    erythema toxicum, 362, 364
    icterus neonatorum, 361-362
    menstruation, 364
    milia, 364
    phimosis, 364
  disorders, 523-552
    drug addiction, 551
    fibroplasia, retrolental, 551
    infections, 536-539
      conjunctivitis, gonorrheal, 536-537
      diarrhea, epidemic, 538
      impetigo, 537
      ophthalmia neonatorum, 536-537
      staphylococcal, 539
      syphilis, 538-539
      thrush, 537-538
    injuries, 532-536
      caput succedaneum, 532-533
      cephalhematoma, 533
      fractures and dislocations, 535-536
      hemorrhage, intracranial (brain, cerebral), 533-535
      paralysis, arm (Erb-Duchenne's, brachial), 535
      facial, 535
    hemolytic disease, 547-550
      ABO incompatibility, 550
      hyperbilirubinemia, 550
      from Rh incompatibility, 547-550
      Rh factor, 548-549
      treatment in erythroblastosis, 549-550
    hemorrhage, from umbilical cord, 550-551
    infant of diabetic mother, 551-552
    malformations, 539-545
      cleft lip and palate, 540-541
      Down's syndrome, 543-544

Newborn infant, disorders, malformations—(*Cont.*)
    epispadias, 541-542
    from German measles, 545
    harelip, 541
    hernia, umbilical, 542
    hypospadias, 541-542
    incidence, 539-540
    frenum linguae, 541
    obstructions of alimentary tract, 542-543
      atresia of esophagus, 542
      duodenum and small intestine, 543
      imperforate anus, 543
      intussusception, 543
      stenosis, pyloric, 542-543
    phocomelia, 544-545
    spina bifida, 542
  of metabolism, 545-547
    phenylketonuria, 546-547
  reactions of parents and staff, 523-527
    getting help from instructors and supervisors, 525-527
    interdisciplinary team, 526
    stillbirth or neonatal death, 526
    working through a crisis, 523-526
      acceptance of infant by staff, 525
      avoiding negative communication, 523-524
      forming a relationship of trust, 524
      grieving, 525-526
      telling the parents, 524-525
  respiratory distress, 527-532
    asphyxia neonatorum. *See* Asphyxia neonatorum
    atelectasis, 531-532
    hyaline membrane disease, 532
    idiopathic syndrome, 532

Newborn infant, disorders, respiratory distress—(*Cont.*)
    pneumonia, 532
  environment, 365-372
    prevention of infection, 365-366, 371-372
    types of care, 366-372
      central nursery system, 366-367, 369-370
      crib and general supplies, 367, 369-370
      observation nursery, 368, 370
      rooming-in, 368-372
  nursing care, 373-384
    continuing, 374-384
      assessment of mother's understanding, 373, 375
      after circumcision, 376-377
      cleansing, 374-375, 380-381
      crying, 379
        "hypertonic" babies, 379
      elimination, intestinal, 383-384
        urinary, 384
      eyes, 375
      foreskin, adherent, 376
      girl babies, 377-378
      pulse and temperature, 379
      skin, 379-382
        bathing, 380-381
          basic principles, 380-381, 384
          demonstration and practice, 381
        buttocks, 380-382
        umbilical cord tie, 381
      sleeping, 382-383
      umbilical cord, 375-376
      weight, 378-379
    feeding. *See* Feeding of newborn infant
    initial, 373
    observations, 373-374
      behavior and physiologic responses, 373-374
      respiration and color, 374
      skin, 374
      temperature, 374
      umbilical cord, condition, 374

Newborn infant—(*Cont.*)
  physiology, 351-359
    changes, circulatory, 353-354
      blood, coagulation, 354
        pressure, 354
        volume, total, 353
        white cells, count, 354
      erythrocyte count and hemoglobin concention, 354
      jaundice, physiologic, 354
      peripheral, 353
      pulse rate, 353-354
    gastrointestinal, 358-359
    hepatic function, 359
    kidney function and urinary secretion, 359
    metabolism, basal, 355-356
      requirements, caloric, 355
        fluid, 355-356
    neurologic, 356-358
      reflexes, 356-358
        blinking, 358
        cough, sneeze and yawn, 358
        gag, 357
        grasp, 357-358
        Moro or startle, 355-357, 360
        rooting, 357
        stepping or dancing, 358
        sucking, 356, 357, 385
        swallowing, 357, 385
        tonic neck, 356, 357, 360
    respiratory, 352-353
      first and second periods of reactivity, 353
      initiation of respiration, 352-353
      normal respiration, 353
    temperature regulation, 354-355
  and primigravida. *See* Primigravida and her newborn
Niemann-Pick disease, 546

Nipple(s), 46, 51
  abnormalities, in puerperium, 510
  care, 328-329
    antepartal, 158
    cleanliness, 328
    depressed, 510
    after nursing period, 328
    fissures and erosion, nursing care, 328-329
    flat, 510
    galactorrhea, 510
    inverted, 510
    shield, protection of fissured or eroded nipples in breast-feeding, 326, 328
    types, 157, 158
Nitrous oxide as agent in inhalation anesthesia in obstetrics, 226, 229, 237-238, 586
Nufer, 583
Numa Pompilius, 583
Nurse-midwife, conduct of home delivery, 565, 567-569
  delivery bag, contents, 564-565
Nurse-midwifery, 569-574
  in United States, 571-574
    organizations, 571-573
      American College of Nurse-Midwifery, 573
      Frontier Graduate School of Midwifery, Hayden, Ky., 571
      Frontier Nursing Service, 570, 571
      Lobenstine Midwifery Clinic, New York, 572
      Maternity Center Association, New York, 571-573
    programs, 573-574
Nursery, for care of newborn infant, central system, 366-367, 369-370
  crib and general supplies, 367, 369-370
  observation type, 368, 370
  "receiving," on labor and delivery division, 373
  rooming-in plan, 368-372
  home, equipment, 186-188
  for premature infant, 411
Nurses, shortage, as problem in maternity care, 18

Nutrients, requirements, in artificial feeding of newborn infant, 387-388
Nutrition, of fetus, 86-88
  mother, in breast-feeding period, 333
  newborn infant, progress in scientific developments, 386
  in pregnancy. *See* Antepartal care, nutrition
  in puerperium, 307, 313

Obstetrics, definition and etymology, 3-4
  in emergency, 576-580
Oliguria in eclampsia, 450
Oocyte(s), 65
Oogenesis, stages, 65
Oogonium, 65
Operative obstetrics, 425-436
  cesarean section, 429-434
    first authentic operation performed on living mothers, 583
    hypertonic uterine dysfunction, intrapartal infection, 484
    hypotonic uterine dysfunction, 484
    indications, 429
    nursing care, 432-434
      oxytocics therapy, 432-434
      retention catheter, 434
      sedative drugs, 434
    origin of term, 583
    preparation, 431-432
    types, 429-431
      classic, 430, 431
      extraperitoneal, 431
      hysterectomy, 431
      low cervical, 430-433
  destructive operations, 434
  episiotomy and repair of lacerations, 425, 428
  forceps delivery, 425-428
    anesthesia, 428
    high forceps, 427
    indications, 426-427
    low (outlet) forceps, 427
    midforceps, 427
    types of instruments, 425-426
    vacuum extractor, 428
  induction of labor, 434-436
    artificial rupture of membranes, 436

Operative obstetrics, induction of labor—(*Cont.*)
  medicinal, 434-436
    oxytocin, 435-436
  version, 428-429
    Braxton Hicks, 429
    external, 428-429
    internal, 429
Opium derivatives, as analgesic agents in obstetrics, 228
Ould, of Dublin, first description of mechanism of labor, 584
Ovary(ies), 42-44, 48
  arteries, 43, 45
  graafian follicle, 54-55, 57
  ligaments, in puerperium, anatomic changes, 299
  nerves, 43
  veins, 43, 45
Ovulation, 53-55, 57
Ovum, development, stages, early, 74
  fertilization, 73-75
  fertilized, cleavage, 72
  growth, in early weeks of pregnancy, 79
  implantation, stages, 75
  maturation, 64
  size, 65, 68
  transport through fallopian tube, 68-71
Oxygen therapy, embolism, pulmonary, 514
  peritonitis, 507
  premature infant, 412
Oxytocin (Pitocin, Syntocinon), 58, 119
  administration, to increase uterine contractions and minimize bleeding, 275
  therapy, cesarean section, 432-434
    for facilitation of milk flow in puerperium, 323
    hemorrhage, postpartal, 496
    induction of labor and to minimize bleeding, 273-276, 435-436
    intrapartal infection, in hypertonic uterine dysfunction, 484

Pain(s), after delivery, 300-301
  relief, general principles, 226-228

Pain(s), relief, general principles—(*Cont.*)
    attention, constant and meticulous, 227-228
    environment, 227
    explanations by nurse about the therapy, 227
    psychological preparation of patient, 226-227
    recovery, 228
    removal of dentures and foreign objects from mouth, 228
    safety of mother and child, 227
  types, analgesia, obstetric. *See* Analgesia, obstetric
    anesthesia, obstetric. *See* Anesthesia, obstetric
Palate, cleft, 540-541
Palsy, brachial, in newborn, 535
Papanicolaou test, in antepartal care, 134-135
Paraldehyde, as analgesic agent in obstetrics, 229
  therapy, eclampsia, 452
    preeclampsia, severe, 448
Paralysis, arm, in newborn, 535
  Erb-Duchenne's, in newborn, 535
  facial, in newborn, 535
Parathyroid glands, changes in pregnancy, 119
Paré, Ambroise, 583
Parenthood, preparation, 170-174
  classes, 171
  conventional type of program, 171-172
  for natural childbirth, 172-174
Parents, expectant, classes, 6
  tour of maternity hospital, 7
  reactions to disorders of newborn. *See* Newborn, disorders, reactions of parents and staff
Pasteur, Louis, 586
PBI (protein-bound iodine), increase in pregnancy, 119
Pelvimeter, invention by Baudelocque, 584
  Williams, 37

Pelvimetry, as basis of preventive care, 39
  x-ray, 38-39
Pelvis, anatomy, 21-39
  android, 29
  anthropoid, 29
  articulations, 22
  bones, 21
  canal, 24-25
  cavity, 24-25, 28
  contracted, as complication of labor, 491, 492
  divisions, 22-23
  examination, in antepartal care, 140-141
  false, 22-23, 25
  floor, muscles, control, antepartal, 178-180
  gynecoid, 29
  inlet, 23, 26, 38
  maturity, ages, 28
  measurements, 31-38
    anteroposterior, 23, 24, 26, 27
    conjugate, Baudelocque's (external), 33, 34
      diagonal, 23, 33-35
      external (Baudelocque's), 33, 34
      obstetric, 35, 36
      true, 35, 36
    intercristal, 26, 32
    interspinous, 26, 32, 33
    intertrochanteric, 32-33
    ischial tuberosities, 27, 36-37
    oblique, 26, 33-34
    transverse, 23, 24, 26
    external, 32-34
    internal, 34-37
  outlet, 23-24, 27
  platypelloid, 29
  in puerperium, anatomic changes, 298-299
  rocking exercises, antepartal period, 176
  size and position of fetus by months, 112-114
  structure, 21
  surfaces, 22
  true, 23, 25
  types, 28-30
  variations, 25, 28
Penicillin therapy, epidemic diarrhea of newborn, 538
  erysipelas, 476
  gonorrhea, 479
  infection, puerperal, 507

Penicillin therapy—(*Cont.*)
mastitis, 511
syphilis, 478
Penis, 49, 51
Pentobarbital sodium (Nembutal), as analgesic agent in obstetrics, 229
Pentothal Sodium (thiopental sodium), as agent in intravenous anesthesia, 226, 238-239
Perineum, 39, 41-42
lacerations, as accidental complication of labor, 497-498
as cause of postpartal hemorrhage, 494
in delivery, repair, 425
nursing care in puerperium, 319-321
discomfort, relief measures, 320, 321
teaching self-care, 320-321
preparation, at onset of labor, 248-249
wounds, as portals of entry for puerperal infection, 504, 505
Peritonitis, 506-507
Perkins, Frances, 590
Perspiration, excessive, in puerperium, 301
Phenobarbital sodium (Luminal Sodium) therapy, eclampsia, 452
preeclampsia, 448
Phenylketonuria, 546-547
Phimosis, 364, 376
pHisoHex (hexachlorophene) therapy, impetigo, in newborn infant, 537
Phocomelia, 544
Phosphorus in diet, antepartal period, 150
Physicians, shortage, as problem in maternity care, 18
Phytonadione solution (Aquamephyton), for hypoprothrombinemia prophylaxis, 282
Pitocin. *See* Oxytocin
Pituitary gland, anterior lobe, hormonal influences in pregnancy, 119
posterior lobe, hormonal influences in pregnancy, 119
Pituitrin, administration, to increase uterine contractions and minimize bleeding, 275

Placenta, 78, 80-81
abruptio placentae, 465-466
changes, endocrine, in pregnancy, 118-119
circulation, 87
delivery, 269-270, 273-276
agents to increase uterine contractions and minimize bleeding, 273-276
"bearing down," 273, 274
emergency (precipitate) delivery by nurse, 286
"expression," 273, 274
inspection, 273, 275
separation, signs suggesting, 270, 273
expulsion, in labor, third stage, 221, 222, 224
low implantation, 463, 464
previa, 463-465
partial, 463, 464
total, 463, 464
treatment, 464-465
types, 463, 464
retained fragments, as cause of postpartal hemorrhage, 494
separation, in labor, third stage, 222, 224
transmission, 86-88
Planned Parenthood Federation of America, Inc., 591
Plexus, venous, uterovaginal, 47
Pneumonia, of newborn, 532
with pregnancy, 475
Polak, J. O., 503
Poliomyelitis with pregnancy, 477
Polocyte(s), 65
Polygalactia, 510
Polyploidy, 68
Pontocaine as agent, in continuous caudal anesthesia in obstetrics, 232
in low-dosage hyperbaric spinal (saddle block) anesthesia, 233
Population, shifts, as problem in maternity care, 17
United States (1930-63), 10
increases, determining factors, 11
predicted, 11
Porro operation, 431
Position(s), lithotomy, in labor, normal, second (expulsion) stage, 266

Position(s)—(*Cont.*)
of newborn infant, 360
presenting part of baby. *See* Presentations and positions
Sims, modified, in anesthesia, continuous caudal, 231, 232
for varicosities of vulva and rectum, 168
Potter, H. W., 194
Prawirohardjo, Sarwono, 569
Preeclampsia, 445-450
mild, 445
nursing care, 449-450
postpartum, 449
severe, 445
signs and symptoms, 446-447
treatment, 447-450
ambulatory patient, 447
delivery, 449
diet, 448
drugs, 448-449
hospital patient, 447-448
prophylaxis, 447
Pregnancy, calculation of expected date of confinement, 86
coincidental diseases, 472-479
anemia, 473
cardiac complications, 474-475
diabetes mellitus, 474
infection, 475-479
brucellosis (undulant fever, Malta fever), 475-476
common cold, 475
erysipelas, 476
influenza, 475
malaria, 476
measles (rubeola), 475
German (rubella), 475
pneumonia, 475
poliomyelitis, 477
scarlet fever, 476
smallpox, 476
tuberculosis, 476-477
typhoid fever, 475
venereal diseases, 477-479
gonorrhea, 479
syphilis, 477-479
physiologic disturbances, general, 473-475
ptyalism, 475
urinary tract infection, 474-475

Pregnancy—(*Cont.*)
   complications, 443-479
      toxemias. *See* Toxemias of
         pregnancy
   definitions, 115
   duration, 85-86
   early weeks, growth of ovum,
      embryo and fetus, 79
   ectopic, 461-462
      abdominal, 461
      causes, 461-462
      definition, 461
      incidence, 461
      interstitial, 461
      maternal death from, 462
      nursing care, 462
      recurrence, 462
      tubal, 461
      types, 461
   mental hygiene. *See* Mental
      hygiene of pregnancy and
      childbirth
   multiple, as complication of
      labor, 499-501
      delivery, 501
         nursing care, 501
      discomforts and hazards,
         500-501
      incidence, 500
      problems, feeding, 501
         psychological and eco-
            nomic, 501
   normal, 109-119
      changes, endocrine, 118-
         119
         adrenal glands, 119
         parathyroid   glands,
            119
         placenta, 118-119
         pituitary body, ante-
            rior and posterior
            lobes, 119
         thyroid gland, 119
      local, 109-116
         abdominal wall, 111,
            114-116
         contour, 111, 112
         diastasis, 116
         stria   gravidarum,
            114-115, 117-118
         breasts, 116
         uterus. *See* Uterus,
            changes in preg-
            nancy
         metabolic, 116
         physiologic, 109

Pregnancy, normal, local—
   (*Cont.*)
      in systems, cardiovascu-
         lar, blood, 116-117
         heart, 117
         digestive, 117
         nervous, 118
         respiratory, 117
         skin, 117-118
         urinary, 118
   posture, correct, in standing,
      110
   psychoses, 200
   rejection by mother, 194-196
      effect of, 196-197
   signs and symptoms, 121-129
      classification, 121
      positive, 121, 127-129
         heart sounds, fetal, 127-
            128
         movements of fetus felt
            by examiner, 129
         roentgenogram, 128, 129
         souffle, funic and uterine,
            128
      presumptive, 121-123
         breast changes, 122
         fatigue, 123
         menstrual   suppression,
            121-122
         micturition, frequent, 122
         nausea and vomiting, 122
         "quickening," 122-123
         skin changes, 123
         vaginal changes, 123
      probable, 121, 123-127
         abdominal changes, 123-
            124
         Braxton Hicks contrac-
            tions, 125
         cervical changes, 125
         fetal outline, 124
         tests, 125-127
            Aschheim-Zondek,
               125-126
            Frank-Berman, 126
            Friedman, 126
            frog, male, 126
            Hogben, 126
            immunologic, 126-127
            toad, male, 126
         uterus changes, 124-125
Premarin (estrogen), 58
Premature infant, description
   at birth, 407-408
   growth and development, 417
   nursing care, 406-417

Premature infant, nursing care
   —(*Cont.*)
      continuing, 411-413
         feeding, 413-414
         incubator,   homemade,
            412
            modern   air-condi-
               tioned, 412-413
         oxygen therapy, 412
         rest, 413
         skin care, 413
         special nursery in hospi-
            tal, 411-412
         transportation to and
            from hospital, 410, 411
      immediate, 409-411
         incubator or heated bed,
            408-410
         resuscitation, 410
         umbilical cord, clamped
            or tied, 409-410
      parental reactions, 414-417
         guilt feelings, 415
         supportive care required,
            415-417
Prematurity, causes, 407
   death from, causes, 407
   definition, 406, 456
   incidence, 406
   prevention, 406
Prenatal   Care   Committee,
   Women's Municipal League,
   Boston, 588
Prepuce of clitoris, 39, 40
Presentations and positions, 92-
   101
   breech, 93, 96, 129
      frank, 93
      full, 93-94
   diagnosis, 97-101
      auscultation, 100-101
      inspection, 97-98
      palpation, 98-100
         Leopold maneuvers, 99-
            100
      roentgenograms, 101
      vaginal examination, 100
   face, 93, 96
   head (cephalic), 93
   shoulder, 94, 96-97
   vertex, 93, 94, 96, 129, 212
Preventive   care,   importance,
   131-132
Primigravida and her newborn,
   394-403
   clinical study, a nurse and a
      new mother, 395-403
      clinical experience, 395

Primigravida and her newborn, clinical study—(*Cont.*)
  comments and conclusions, 401-402
  components of crisis situation, 402-403
  first 7 days, 395-398
  after first 52 hours at home, 398-401
  concern about baby, 394-395
    bathing, 394
    crying, 394
    feeding, 394
    relation of teaching to, 395
Procaine as agent for regional anesthesia, local infiltration, 230
Progesterone (Delalutin, Proluton), 58
  secretion by corpus luteum, 55, 56
Progestins, oral, in family planning, 342
Prolactin, 58, 119
Prolapse, umbilical cord, as accidental complication of labor, 498
Proluton (progesterone), 58
Pruritus in antepartal period, 170
Psychological considerations, in puerperium. *See* Puerperium, nursing care, changes and reactions, physiologic and psychological
Psychotherapy, hyperemesis gravidarum, 471
Ptyalism with pregnancy, 475
Puberty, 53
Pubis, 21-23
  arch, 27
    in males and females, contrasted, 24, 29-31
Pulse rate, measurement, in hemorrhage, postpartal, 495-496
  in labor, first (dilating) stage, 257-258
  newborn infant, 353-354
    nursing care, continuing, 379
  in puerperium, 300, 312-313
  steady rise, in hyperemesis gravidarum, 472
Putnam, Mrs. William Lowell, 588

Puerperium, complications, 503-514
  bladder, 513-514
  breast disorders, 509
    abscess, epidemic, 511-513
    drying up, 509
    engorgement, 509
    mastitis, 510-511
    nipples, 510
    in secretion, 509-510
  hematomas, vulvar, 508-509
  infection. *See* Infection, puerperal
  pulmonary embolism, 514
  subinvolution of uterus, 508
  examinations, postpartal, 302
  nursing care, 304-343
    breast-feeding. *See* Feeding of newborn infant, breast
    changes and reactions, 304-316
      physiologic and psychological, 305-312
      phases of restorative period, taking-hold, 308-310
        "taking-in," 306-308
          psychological adjustment, 307-308
          sleep and food, 306-307
        postpartal blues, 310-311
      immediate, 312
    parental guidance and instruction, 335-343
      discharge instructions, 340-341
      exercises, postpartal, 339-340
      family-planning, 341-343
        methods, conventional, 342-343
          newer, 342
        need for, population explosion, 341
      group classes, 337-338
        setup for baby bath demonstration, 337
      individual teaching, 338-339
    physical, 312-316
      ambulation, early, 314
      bathing, 314-315

Puerperium, nursing care, physical—(*Cont.*)
      elimination, intestinal, 316
        urinary, 315-316
      nutrition, 313
      pulse, 312-313
      rest and sleep, 313-314
      special aspects, 316-322
        abdomen, support, 321-322
        breasts, 317-319
          cleansing, 317
          drying up milk, 318
          engorgement, relief measures, 318-319
          support, 317-318
        perineum, 319-321
          discomfort, relief measures, 321
          teaching self-care, 320-321
      temperature, body, 312-313
  physiology, 297-302
    anatomic changes, 297-300
      abdomen, wall, 299
      breasts, 299-300
      cervix, 298
      pelvis, 298-299
      uterus, 297-298
      lochia, 298
    clinical aspects, 300-302
      after-pains, 300-301
      blood, 300
      digestion, 301
      elimination, intestinal, 301
      kidneys, 301
      menstruation, 301-302
      pulse, 300
      skin, 301
      temperature, 300
      weight loss, 301

Quadruplets, incidence of birth, 500
Queen Victoria, acceptance of use of chloroform in delivery, 586
"Quickening" as presumptive sign of pregnancy, 84, 112, 122-123
Quintuplets, incidence of birth, 500

Race, as basis of classification of births in U. S., 9

Rankin, Jeannette, 590

Read, Grantly Dick, 140, 172, 174

Recreation, in antepartal period, 156

Rectocele, from lacerations of perineum, 497

Rectum, examination, in labor, 249-250

varicose veins, Sims's position, 168

Reflex(es), of newborn infant, irritability, Apgar Scoring System, 279, 280

Regurgitation by newborn infant, 358, 392

Relaxation, in antepartal period, 153-154, 175-176

during uterine contraction, 180-181

selective, antepartal, 180

Reproduction, organs, female, 39-48, 50

external, 39-42

internal, 42-48, 50

male, 49, 51-52

external, 49, 51

internal, 49, 51-52

See also individual names

physiology, 53-63

infertility. *See* Infertility

menopause. *See* Menopause (climacteric)

sexual maturity, 53-55

menstruation. *See* Menstruation

ovulation, 53-55, 57

puberty, 53

Respiration, artificial, for asphyxia neonatorum, 529-531

changes in pregnancy, normal, 117

control in labor, 180-183

accelerated breathing, 182-183

panting, 183

second stage, 182, 183

shallow breathing, 181-183

slow deep breathing, 181-182

transition breathing, 182, 183

distress, neonatal, 527-532

asphyxia neonatorum. *See* Asphyxia neonatorum

atelectasis, 531-532

Respiration, distress, neonatal —(*Cont.*)

hyaline membrane disease, 532

idiopathic syndrome, 532

pneumonia, 532

effort, of newborn infant, Apgar Scoring System, 279-280

measurement in labor, first (dilating) stage, 257-258

newborn infant, changes, 352-353

first and second periods of reactivity, 353

initiation, 352-353

normal, 353

observation, 374

Respiratory tract, upper, infant, after delivery, clearance of mucus and amniotic fluid, 277, 278

Rest, in antepartal period, 153-154

in breast-feeding period, 333

for premature infant, 413

in puerperium, 313-314

Restoration, postpartum, 183-185

Resuscitation, premature infant, 410

Retina, hemorrhages, in hyperemesis gravidarum, 472

Retractor, Schroeder vaginal, 458

Rh factor, test, in antepartal care, 134

Rheumatic heart disease, with pregnancy, 473

Ritgen, maneuver of, in labor, second (expulsion) stage, 267, 269

Robinson, Alice M., quoted, 341

Roentgenogram(s), as positive sign of pregnancy, 129

Roesslin, Eucharius, *Der Schwangeren Frauen und Hebammen Rosengarten*, 570

Rooming-in plan, 368-372

Roosevelt, Franklin D., 591

Roosevelt, Theodore, 5, 588

Rubella (German measles), with pregnancy, 475

Rubeola (measles), with pregnancy, 475

Rubin, Reva, 402

Ruggles, Dr., 588

Sacrum, canal, placement of needle in continuous caudal anesthesia, 231, 232

Salt, in diet, restriction, in pregnancy, 145-146

Sacrum, 21-24

promontory, as obstetric landmark, 21, 23, 24, 26

Scarlet fever with pregnancy, 476

Scheinfeld, Amran, 469

Schrader, G. H. F., 13, 588

Schroeder vaginal retractor, 458

Schultze, mechanism of extrusion of placenta, 221, 224

Scopolamine as analgesic agent in obstetrics, 226, 228-229

Scrotum, 49, 51

Secobarbital sodium (Seconal Sodium) as analgesic agent in obstetrics, 229

Seconal Sodium (secobarbital sodium) as analgesic agent in obstetrics, 229

Seminal vesicles, 49, 52

Semmelweiss, Ignaz Philipp, proof of nature and source of puerperal infection, 585-586

Sepsis, puerperal. *See* Infection, puerperal

Septicemia, puerperal. *See* Infection, puerperal

Sex, chromatin, 72, 73

determination, 69, 72, 73

Seymour, Jane, 583

Sheppard-Towner Bill, passage, 590-591

Shippen, William, establishment of first lying-in hospital in America, 585

Shirodkar technic, modified, prevention of relaxation and dilatation of cervix, 460

Shock, from hemorrhage, postpartal, 496

in placenta previa, 464

Shoes, antepartal period, 160

Shoulder, of infant, birth of, 268, 270

presentation, as complication of labor, 490-491

"Show" at onset of labor, 113, 213-214, 256

Sign, Braxton Hicks, as indication of pregnancy, 125

of Chadwick, 114

of Goodell, as indication of pregnancy, 125

Sign—(*Cont.*)
  of Hegar, as indication of pregnancy, 124
Silver nitrate, instillation in eyes of newborn infant, 280-282
Silverman, W. A., quoted, 411-412
Simpson, J. Y., 226, 236
  first use of ether and chloroform for childbirth, 586
Simpson obstetric forceps, 426
Sims, curette, sharp, 458
  position of, for varicosities of vulva and rectum, 168
  speculum, 458
Skene, glands of. *See* Glands, of Skene
Skin, care, antepartal, 157
  premature infant, 413
  changes, in pregnancy, normal, 117-118
    as presumptive sign of pregnancy, 123
  of newborn infant, appearance, 361
    nursing care, continuing, 379-382
      bathing, 380-381
        basic principles, 380-381, 384
        demonstration and practice, 381
        buttocks, 380-382
        umbilical cord, tie, 381
      observation, 374
  perspiration, excessive, in puerperium, 301
Sleep, in antepartal period, 153-154
  newborn infant, nursing care, continuing, 382-383
  in puerperium, 306, 313-314
Smallpox, with pregnancy, 476
Smegma, newborn infant, female, 377
  male, 376
Smellie, improvements on obstetric forceps, 584
Smith, Clement, 385
Smoking, antepartal period, 163
Social Security Act, passage, 590
Society for the Prevention of Cruelty to Animals, founded by Henry Bergh, 587
Society for the Prevention of Cruelty to Children, 588

Social Service workers, medical, aid in antepartal care, 143, 145
  function, 143
  shortage, as problem in maternity care, 18
Soranus, 582
Souffle, funic and uterine, as positive sign of pregnancy, 128
Sound, uterine, 458
Sparteine sulfate (Tocosamine) therapy, to increase uterine contractions and minimize bleeding, 275-276
  uterine dysfunction, 497
Speculum, Sims, 458
Spermatids, 65
Spermatocytes, primary and secondary, 65
Spermatogenesis, 65
Spermatozoon(a), 69
  fertilization, 73-75
"Spiders," vascular, in pregnancy, 117
Spina bifida, 542
Spirochaeta pallida as causitive organism of syphilis, 477
Sponge holder, 458
Staphylococcus aureus as causitive agent, abscess, breast, puerperal, epidemic, 511, 512
  mastitis, 510
Staphylococcus as causitive agent, puerperal infection, 503
Starvation in hyperemesis gravidarum, 471
Statistics (vital), 8-9
Stenosis, pyloric, in newborn infant, 542
Stethoscope, Leff, with interchangeable bells, 127
Stevens, Anne, 590
Stillbirth, reactions of parents and staff, 526
Stocking, support, for varicose veins in leg, 167-168
Stomach, newborn infant, capacity for milk, 385-386
  changes, 358
Stone, Abraham, 62
Stools of newborn infant, 359, 383-384
Strauss, Nathan, 588

Streptococcus as causative agent, puerperal infection, 503
Streptomycin, epidemic diarrhea of newborn, 538
Streptomycin-sulfadiazine therapy, brucellosis, 476
Stress, avoidance, antepartal period. *See* Antepartal care, psychophysical preparation for childbearing
Stria gravidarum, 114-115, 117-118
Stroganoff regimen in treatment of eclampsia, 451
Sugar, in urine, test, in antepartal care, 134
Sulfadiazine therapy, infection, puerperal, 507
Sulfonamides, therapy, infection, puerperal, 507
  urinary tract infection, with pregnancy, 474
Superstitions relating to childbearing, 91
Supine hypotensive syndrome, 466
Sussman, M. B., quoted, 8
Sutures of cranium, 92, 93
Symphysis pubis, 21-23, 26, 27
Syntocinon. *See* Oxytocin
Syphilis, causitive organism, 477
  diagnosis, blood tests, 478
  in pregnancy, clinical symptoms, 477
  in newborn, 538-539
  with pregnancy, 477-479
    previous history, 477-478
    tests, to determine condition of infant, 478
    treatment, 478-479
  types, 477
  Wassermann test, in antepartal care, 134

Tace (chlorotrianisene), 58
Taeuber, Irene, 341
Tarnier axis-traction obstetric forceps, 425, 426
Tay-Sach's disease, 546
Teeth, care, antepartal, 160, 161
Temperature of body, basal, use of graphs, 61-62
  directions, 61
  plotting, 61
  variations, 59-60

Temperature of body—(*Cont.*)
measurement, in labor, first (dilating) stage, 257-258
newborn infant, nursing care, continuing, 377, 379
observation, 374
oral, 61-62
in puerperium, 300, 312-313
regulating mechanism, changes in newborn infant, 354-355
Test(s), albumin in urine, in antepartal care, 134
Aschheim-Zondek, of pregnancy, 118, 125-126
blood, for syphilis, 134, 478
Coombs, erythroblastosis fetalis, 549
erythroblastosis fetalis, 549
Frank-Berman, of pregnancy, 126
Friedman, of pregnancy, 118, 126
frog, male, of pregnancy, 126
hemoglobin, in antepartal care, 134
Hogben, of pregnancy, 126
immunologic, of pregnancy, 126-127
Kahn, for syphilis, 478
Kline, for syphilis, 478
laboratory, in antepartal care, 134-135
Mazzini, for syphilis, 478
Papanicolaou, in antepartal care, 134-135
of pregnancy, 118, 125-127
Rh factor and blood type, in antepartal care, 134
sugar, in urine, in antepartal care, 134
toad, male, of pregnancy, 126
urinalysis, in antepartal care, 134, 135
Wassermann, for syphilis, 134, 478
Testis(es), 49, 51
Tetany in pregnancy, 119
Thalidomide, phocomelia from, 544
Theelin (estrogen), 58
Thiamine chloride therapy, hyperemesis gravidarum, 471
Thiopental sodium (Pentothal Sodium) as agent in intravenous anesthesia, 226, 238-239

Thrombophlebitis, 505-506
femoral, 506
pelvic, 506
Thoms, Herbert, 38, 172, 174
Thrush, antepartal period, 170
in newborn infant, 537-538
Thyroid gland, changes in pregnancy, normal, 119
Toad test, of pregnancy, 126
Tocosamine (sparteine sulfate) therapy, to increase uterine contractions and minimize bleeding, 275-276
uterine dysfunction, 497
"Tonguetie," 541
Toxemias of pregnancy, 444-455
classification, 445
deaths from, United States (1963), 444
definition, 444
eclampsia. *See* Eclampsia
incidence, 444
maternal death from, 13
preeclampsia. *See* Preeclampsia
prevention, 13
Transfusion, fetal, intra-uterine, 549-550
Trautman, of Wittenberg, first authentic section performed on living mother, 583
Travail. *See* Labor
Traveling in antepartal period, 156-157
Treponema pallidum as causitive organism of syphilis, 477
Trichlorethylene (Trilene) as agent in inhalation anesthesia in obstetrics, 233, 237
Trichomonas vaginalis as etiologic agent, leukorrhea, in pregnancy, 170
Trilene (trichlorethylene) as agent in inhalation anesthesia in obstetrics, 233, 237
Triplets, incidence of birth, 500
Triploidy, 68
Trisomy, 67, 68
Tuberculosis with pregnancy, 476-477
Tubes, fallopian. *See* Fallopian tube(s)
Tube, Levin, in hyperemesis gravidarum, 471, 472
Tucker McLane obstetric forceps, 425, 426
Turner's syndrome, 68

"Twilight sleep," 228
Twins, "double-ovum" and "single-ovum," 500
heredity as causitive role in pregnancy, 500
identical and nonidentical, 500
incidence of birth, 500
problems, in feeding, 501
psychological and economic, 501
Typhoid fever with pregnancy, 475

Umbilical cord, 80-81
care, immediate postpartal, 285-286
clamping, 268-269, 271, 352
cutting, 268, 271
hemorrhage from, 550-551
nursing care, continuing, 375-376
observation of condition, 374
precautions, emergency (precipitate) delivery by nurse, 285
premature infant, clamped or tied, 409-410
prolapse, as accidental complication of labor, 498
tying, 268, 272, 381
Undulant fever (brucellosis), with pregnancy, 475-476
United States, Census Bureau, 588, 589
Children's Bureau, 5, 589
Department of Health, Education, and Welfare, National Statistics Division, Public Health Service, registration of births, 11
Public Health Service, Communicable Disease Center, 476, 477
National Center for Health Statistics, Vital Statistics Division, definitions, 9
Ureter(s), 50
Urethra, 50
female, 39-41
male, 49, 52
Urinalysis, in antepartal care, 134, 135
catheterized specimens, in urinary tract infection, with pregnancy, 474

Urinary system, changes in pregnancy, 118
Urinary tract, infection, with pregnancy, 474-475
Urination, frequency, antepartal, 163
Urine, excretion, by newborn, changes 359
retention, in puerperium, 513
secretion, in puerperium, 301
Uterus, anatomy, 42-48
arteries, 45, 47
atony, as cause of postpartal hemorrhage, 493-494
cavity, 45
cervix. *See* Cervix
changes, in pregnancy, 109-114
size increase, 109-110
weight increase, 111-112
as probable sign of pregnancy, 124-125
compression, bimanual, as therapy, in hemorrhage, postpartal, 495, 496
contractions in labor, 215-216, 219-220
first (dilating) stage, 253-256
frequency, duration and intensity, 254-255
dysfunction, mechanical dystocia from. *See* Dystocia, mechanical, uterine dysfunction
implantation of ovum, 75
inversion, as accidental complication of labor, 498
ligaments, 44, 46-47
in puerperium, anatomic changes, 299
lymphatics, 47
massage, as therapy, for hemorrhage, postpartal, 494-495
measurements, 44, 45
nerves, 47
palpation, after delivery, 275, 277, 311, 312
in pregnancy, 3rd to 9th months, 110-111
prolapse, from lacerations of perineum, 497
in puerperium, anatomic changes, involution, 297-298
lochia, 298

Uterus—(*Cont.*)
rupture, hemorrhage, postpartal, 496-497
subinvolution, as complication of puerperium, 508
weight, 44

Vacuum extractor instead of forceps delivery, 428
Vagina, 47, 48, 50
arteries, 50
changes, as presumptive sign of pregnancy, 123
discharge, antepartal period, 170
examination, in diagnosis of fetal position, 100
in labor, 250-251
functions, 47, 50
Vagina, lacerations in delivery, as cause of postpartal hemorrhage, 494
repair, 425
lymphatics, 50
varicosities, 169
veins, 50
wounds, as portals of entry for puerperal infection, 504, 505
Van Blarcom, Carolyn, 589-590
Van Deventer, Father of Modern Obstetrics, 584
Van Ingen, Philip, 588, 589
Vegetables in diet, antepartal care, 149
Vein(s), fallopian tubes, 44, 45
hypogastric, 45, 47, 50
iliac, common, 45
internal, 45, 47
mammary, 50
ovaries, 43, 45
renal, 45
vagina, 50
varicose, antepartal period, 166-169
support stocking or elastic bandages, 167-168
symptoms, 166
treatment, 166-169
prevention, 169
Vena cava, inferior, 45
Venereal diseases, incidence, 477
with pregnancy, gonorrhea, 479
syphilis, 477-479

Veratrone therapy, eclampsia, 452
Version, 428-429
Braxton Hicks, 429
external, 428-429
internal, 429
Vestibule, 39-41
Villi, chorionic, 74, 75, 78
Visiting Nurse Associations, classes in preparation for parenthood, 171
Visual aids, teaching patient, in antepartal care, 139
Vitamin(s), A, and D Ointment, application to nipples after nursing period, 328
therapy, antepartal period, 150
B complex, therapy, antepartal period, 150
C, therapy, antepartal period, 150
D, therapy, antepartal period, 150
K, therapy, hemorrhage, intracranial, in newborn, 535
Vomiting, antepartal, 163-164
in hyperemesis gravidarum, 469-472
by newborn infant, 358-359
in peritonitis, 507
pernicious, in hyperemesis gravidarum, 470
as presumptive sign of pregnancy, 122
Vulva, 39-41
cleansing, in labor, normal, second (expulsion) stage, 266
hematomas, as complication of puerperium, 508-509
preparation at onset of labor, 248-249
varicosities, treatment, 168
wounds as portals of entry for puerperal infection, 504, 505

Wassermann test, for syphilis, 134, 478
Waters, E. G., 431
Weight, control, in antepartal care, 151-153
in pregnancy, 132, 135-136
gain, in pregnancy, 116
sudden, in preeclampsia, 446, 447

Weight—(*Cont.*)
  loss, in hyperemesis gravidarum, 471
  loss, in puerperium, 301
  of newborn, conversion table, pounds and ounces to grams, 609
  nursing care, continuing, 378-379
  oversize baby, as complication of labor, 492-493
Welch, John, 576
Wharton's jelly, 81
White, Charles, 584
Whitridge, John, Jr., 576
White House Conference, 1st, Theodore Roosevelt, 588-589
  2nd, Woodrow Wilson, 590
  3rd, Herbert Hoover, 591
  4th, Franklin D. Roosevelt, 591

White House Conference—(*Cont.*)
  5th, Harry S Truman, 592
  6th, Dwight D. Eisenhower, 592
Williams, J. F., 90
Wilson, Woodrow, 590
"Witch's milk," 87
Wolff, I. S., 416
World Health Organization (WHO), United Nations, Expert Committee on Maternal and Child Health, quoted, 417
  Expert Committee on Maternity Care, definition of maternity care, 4
  Manual of International Classification of Diseases, Injuries and Causes of Death, definitions, 9

World Health Organization, (WHO), United Nations—(*Cont.*)
  definition of fetal death, 15
  new definitions, 456
  organization, 591-592
Wounds, vulvar, vaginal and perineal, as portals of entry for puerperal infection, 504

Xylocaine (lidocaine), as agent in continuous anesthesia in obstetrics, 232

Yellen clamp in technic of circumcision, 363

Zeigler umbilical clamp, 269, 272
Zuspan, F. P., 87